Handbook of Experimental Pharmacology

Volume 182

Jürgen Schüttler • Helmut Schwilden
Editors

Modern Anesthetics

Contributors

J. Ahonen, G. Akk, B. Antkowiak, M. Arras, V. Billard, P. Bischoff, T.W. Bouillon, J.G. Bovill, D. Brian, F. Camu, A. De Wolf, B. Drexler, J. Fechner, B.M. Graf, C. Grashoff, J.F.A. Hendrickx, T.K. Henthorn, R. Jurd, E. Kochs, K. Kück, G. Kullik, S. Lambert, J. Manigel, M. Maze, S. Mennerick, J.-U. Meyer, C. Nau, K.T. Olkkola, M. Perouansky, U. Rudolph, R.D. Sanders, W. Schlack, G. Schneider, J. Schüttler, H. Schwilden, F. Servin, S.L. Shafer, B. Sinner, D.R. Stanski, J.H. Steinbach, B.W. Urban, C. Vanlersberghe, N.C. Weber, N. Wruck, A. Zeller

Springer

Prof. Dr. h.c. Jürgen Schüttler
Klinik für Anästhesiologie
Friedrich-Alexander-Universität
Erlangen-Nürnberg
Krankenhausstr. 12
D-91054 Erlangen
Germany
Juergen.Schuettler@kfa.imed.uni-erlangen.de

Prof. Dr. Dr. Helmut Schwilden
Klinik für Anästhesiologie
Friedrich-Alexander-Universität
Erlangen-Nürnberg
Krankenhausstr. 12
D-91054 Erlangen
Germany
Schwilden@kfa.imed.uni-erlangen.de

ISBN 978-3-540-72813-9 ISBN 978-3-540-74806-9 (eBook)

Handbook of Experimental Pharmacology ISSN 0171-2004

Library of Congress Control Number: 2007936361

Cover Design: WMXDesign GmbH, Heidelberg

Printed on acid-free paper

9 8 7 6 5 4 3 2 1

springer.com

Preface

Some important constraints of anesthesia must be taken into consideration when the pharmacological properties of modern anesthetics are discussed. The most important of these could be that the target effect be achieved preferably within seconds, at most within a few minutes. Similarly, offset of drug action should be achieved within minutes rather hours. The target effects, such as unconsciousness, are potentially life-threatening, as are the side effects of modern anesthetics, such as respiratory and cardiovascular depression. Finally, the patient's purposeful responses are not available to guide drug dosage, because, either the patient is unconscious, or more problematically, the patient is aware but unable to communicate pain because of neuromuscular blockade.

These constraints were already recognised 35 years ago, when in 1972 Volume XXX entitled "Modern Inhalation Anesthetics" appeared in this Handbook Series. The present volume is meant as a follow up and extension of that volume. At the beginning of the 1970's anesthesia was commonly delivered by inhalation, with only very few exceptions. The clinical understanding of that time considered anesthesia as a unique state achieved by any of the inhalation anesthetics, independent of their specific molecular structure. "The very mechanism of anesthetic action at the biophase" was discussed within the theoretical framework of the "unitary theory of narcosis". This theoretical understanding was based on the Meyer-Overton correlation and the apparent additivity of MAC when several inhalational anesthetics were given simultaneously, MAC being the measure of anesthetic potency and anesthetic depth developed in the mid-1960's. Since the 1980's this understanding has changed completely. Today "general anesthesia" is commonly considered a collection of neurophysiologically very different states, achieved by a multitude of very different drugs (delivered not only by inhalation) acting on a plethora of subcellular structures. Unconsciousness and absence of pain are always included in this collection of different states.

Three main factors contributed to this changed understanding:

1) the increasing use of intravenous anesthesia, facilitated by the development of new intravenous anesthetics, not only for the induction but also for the maintenance of anesthesia
2) the discovery of non-additive types of anesthetic interactions,

3) the development of molecular techniques (biological, pharmacological and physiological) to study the interaction of anesthetic drug molecules with receptive cell structures.

For these reasons, when the outline of this Handbook was discussed at a brainstorming meeting in Erlangen in February 2005, it became clear that it should be entitled "Modern Anesthetics" and contain in addition to a section on "Inhalation Anesthetics" one on "Intravenous Anesthetics", preceded by another on "Molecular Mechanisms of Anesthetic Action". Emphasis was put on the term "molecular" to draw attention to the discovery in the past decades of a great many findings on the interaction of anesthetic compounds with subcellular entities. On the other hand, this emphasis was to underline the lack of our understanding concerning the summation of all the different interactions from the molecular level through the progressive stages of integration within the CNS, which needs to be studied in the future. While these considerations may be considered mainstream of current research in experimental anesthetic pharmacology, it was strongly felt that the particularities of anesthetic drug therapy discussed above require not only specific drugs, but also very particular modes of their delivery and administration. It is not only the properties of the compounds but the combination of compounds plus drug delivery system which turns the compounds into a clinically effective and safe drug. It was therefore thought necessary to integrate a fourth section on "Pharmacokinetics-Pharmacodynamics based Administration of Anesthetics". This final section illustrates a strategy, still at an experimental stage, in which the integration of drug, medical technology and computational medicine leads to optimized anesthetic therapeutic systems.

We wish to thank all colleagues and authors for their endurance and willingness to contribute all their efforts and a considerable amount of time, to share freely their outstanding expertise and knowledge for this Handbook. Special thanks go to those who took responsibilities for each of the four sections: to Bernd Urban for "Molecular Mechanisms of Anesthetic Action", to Jim Bovill for "Modern Inhalation Anesthetics", to Frederic Camu for "Modern Intravenous Anesthetics", and to Don Stanski for "Phamacokinetics-Pharmacodynamics based Administration of Anesthetics".

Erlangen, Germany

Jürgen Schüttler
Helmut Schwilden

Contents

Contributors

J. Ahonen
Helsinki University Central Hospital, Department of Anesthesia and Intensive Care Medicine, Women's Hospital, P.O. Box 140 (Haartmaninkatu 2), FIN-00029 Hus, Finland, jouni.ahonen@hus.fi

G. Akk
Department of Anesthesiology, Washington University School of Medicine, 660 South Euclid Avenue, Saint Louis, MO 63110, USA

B. Antkowiak
Section of Experimental Anesthesiology, University of Tübingen, Tübingen, Baden-Württemberg, Germany

M. Arras
Institute of Laboratory Animal Sciences, University of Zurich, Zurich, Switzerland

V. Billard
Institut Gustave Roussy, 39, rue Camille Desmoulins, 94805 Villejuif Cedex, France, billard@igr.fr

P. Bischoff
Klinik und Poliklinik für Anästhesiologie, Universitätsklinikum Hamburg-Eppendorf, Gebäude O50, Martinistraße 52, 20246 Hamburg, Germany, bischoff@uke.uni-hamburg.de

T.W. Bouillon
Novartis Pharma AG, PH346, Modeling & Simulation, CHBS, WSJ-027.4.048, Lichtstraße 35, CH-4056 Basel, Switzerland, thomas.bouillon@novartis.com

J.G. Bovill
Department of Anaesthesiology, Leiden University Medical Centre, P.O. Box 9600, NL-2300 RC Leiden, The Netherlands, j.g.bovill@lumc.nl

D. Brian
Academic Anaesthetics, Imperial College, Chelsea & Westminster Hospital, 369 Fulham Road, London SW10 9NH, UK

F. Camu
Department of Anesthesiology, V.U.B. Medical Center, University of Brussels, Laarbeeklaan 101, B-1090 Brussels, Belgium, frederic@fcamu.telenet.be

A. De Wolf
Department of Anesthesiology, Feinberg School of Medicine, Northwestern University, 251 E. Huron St, F5-704, Chicago, IL 60611, USA, a-dewolf@northwestern.edu

B. Drexler
Section of Experimental Anesthesiology, University of Tübingen, Tübingen, Baden-Württemberg, Germany

J. Fechner
Klinik für Anästhesiologie, Universität Erlangen-Nürnberg, Krankenhausstr. 12, 91054 Erlangen, Germany, joerg.fechner@kfa.imed.uni-erlangen.de

B.M. Graf
Zentrum Anästhesiologie, Abt. Anästhesiologie I, Universitätsklinikum Göttingen, Robert-Koch-Str. 40, 37075 Göttingen, Germany, bgraf@zari.de

C. Grashoff
Section of Experimental Anesthesiology, University of Tübingen, Tübingen, Baden-Württemberg, Germany

J.F.A. Hendrickx
Department of Anesthesiology and Intensive Care, OLV Hospital, Moorselbaan 164, 9300 Aalst, Belgium, jcnwahendrickx@yahoo.com

T.K. Henthorn
Department of Anesthesiology, University of Colorado HSC, 4200 E. 9th Avenue, Denver, CO 80262, USA, Thomas.Henthorn@uchsc.edu

R. Jurd
Institute of Pharmacology and Toxicology, University of Zurich, Zurich, Switzerland

E. Kochs
Klinik für Anästhesiologie, Klinikum Rechts der Isar, Technische Universität München, Ismaninger Str. 22, 81675 München, Germany, E.F.Kochs@lrz.tu-muenchen.de

K. Kück
Drägerwerk Aktiengesellschaft, Moislinger Allee 53-55, 23542 Lübeck, Germany

G. Kullik
Drägerwerk Aktiengesellschaft, Moislinger Allee 53-55, 23542 Lübeck, Germany

S. Lambert
Institute of Pharmacology and Toxicology, University of Zurich, Zurich, Switzerland

J. Manigel
Drägerwerk Aktiengesellschaft, Moislinger Allee 53-55, 23542 Lübeck, Germany

M. Maze
Head of Department of Anaesthetics, Imperial College London, Chelsea and Westminster Hospital, 369, Fulham Road, London SW10 9NH, UK, m.maze@imperial.ac.uk

S. Mennerick
Departments of Psychiatry and Anatomy & Neurobiology and the Neurosciences Program, Washington University School of Medicine, 660 South Euclid Avenue, Saint Louis, MO 63110, USA

J.-U. Meyer
Drägerwerk Aktiengesellschaft, Moislinger Allee 53-55, 23542 Lübeck, Germany, joerg-uwe.meyer@draeger.com

C. Nau
Klinik für Anästhesiologie, Universität Erlangen-Nürnberg, Krankenhausstr. 12, 91054 Erlangen, Germany, carla.nau@kfa.imed.uni-erlangen.de

K.T. Olkkola
Department of Anaesthesiology, Intensive Care, Emergency Care and Pain Medicine, Turku University Hospital, PO Box 52 (Kiinamyllynkatu 4-8), FI-20521 Turku, Finland, klaus.olkkola@utu.fi

M. Perouansky
Department of Anesthesiology, Room 43, Bardeen Labs, 1300 University Ave., Madison, WI 53792-3272, USA, mperouansky@wisc.edu

U. Rudolph
Laboratory of Genetic Neuropharmacology, McLean Hospital, Department of Psychiatry, Harvard Medical School, Belmont, MA 02478, USA, urudolph@mclean.harvard.edu

R.D. Sanders
Academic Anaesthetics, Imperial College, Chelsea & Westminster Hospital, 369 Fulham Road, London SW10 9NH, UK

W. Schlack
Department of Anaesthesiology, University of Amsterdam (AMC), Meibergdreef 9, NL-1100 DD Amsterdam, The Netherlands, W.S.Schlack@amc.uva.nl

G. Schneider
Klinik für Anästhesiologie, Klinikum Rechts der Isar, Technische Universität München, Ismaninger Str. 22, 81675 München, Germany

J. Schüttler
Klinik für Anästhesiologie, Universität Erlangen-Nürnberg, Krankenhausstr. 12, 91054 Erlangen, Germany, Juergen.Schuettler@kfa.imed.uni-erlangen.de

H. Schwilden
Klinik für Anästhesiologie, Universität Erlangen-Nürnberg, Krankenhausstr. 12, 91054 Erlangen, Germany, Schwilden@kfa.imed.uni-erlangen.de

F.S. Servin
Service d'Anesthésie-Réanimation chirurgicale, Hôpital Bichat, 46, rue Henri-Huchard, 75877 Paris Cedex 18, France, fservin@magic.fr, frederique.servin@bch.ap-hop-paris.fr

S.L. Shafer
Department of Anesthesiology, Stanford University School of Medicine, 300 Pasteur Dr., Stanford, CA 94305A, USA, steven.shafer@stanford.edu

B. Sinner
Zentrum für Anaesthesie, Rettungs- und Intensivmedizin, Georg August Universität Göttingen, Robert-Koch-Str. 40, 37075 Göttingen, Germany

D.R. Stanski
3903 Albemerle N.W., Washington, DC 20016, USA, drstanski@prodigy.net

J.H. Steinbach
Department of Anesthesiology, Washington University School of Medicine, 660 South Euclid Ave, Saint Louis, MO 63110, USA, jhs@morpheus.wustl.edu

B.W. Urban
Klinik für Anästhesiologie, Universität Bonn, Sigmund-Freud-Str. 25, 53127 Bonn, Germany, bwurban@uni-bonn.de

C. Vanlersberghe
Department of Anesthesiology, V.U.B. Medical Center, University of Brussels, Laarbeeklaan 101, B-1090 Brussels, Belgium, anesvec@uz.brussel.be

N.C. Weber
Department of Anaesthesiology, University of Amsterdam (AMC), Meibergdreef 15, M0-128, NL-Amsterdam 1105 AZ, The Netherlands, NinaC.Hauck@amc.uva.nl

N. Wruck
Drägerwerk Aktiengesellschaft, Moislinger Allee 53-55, 23542 Lübeck, Germany

A. Zeller
Institute of Pharmacology and Toxicology, University of Zurich, Zurich, Switzerland

Part I
Molecular Mechanisms of Anesthetic Action

Section Editor: B.W. Urban

The Site of Anesthetic Action

B.W. Urban

Abstract The mechanisms of general anesthesia constitute one of the great unsolved problems of classical neuropharmacology. Since the discovery of general anesthesia, hundreds of substances have been tested and found to possess anesthetic activity. Anesthetics differ tremendously in their chemical, physical, and pharmacological properties, greatly varying in size, in chemically active groups, and in the combinations of interactions and chemical reactions that they can undergo. The

B.W. Urban
Klinik für Anästhesiologie und Operative Intensivmedizin, Universitätsklinikum Bonn, Sigmund-Freud-Straße 25, 53127 Bonn, Germany
bwurban@uni-bonn.de

J. Schüttler and H. Schwilden (eds.) *Modern Anesthetics.*
Handbook of Experimental Pharmacology 182.

large spectrum of targets makes it obvious that dealing with anesthetics pharmacologically is different from dealing with most other drugs used in pharmacology. Anesthetic potency often correlates with the lipophilicity of anesthetic compounds, i.e., their preference for dissolving in lipophilic phases. This suggests as a main characteristic of anesthetic interactions that they are weak and that for many of them there is overall an approximate balance of nonspecific hydrophobic interactions and weak specific polar interactions. These include various electrostatic (ions, permanent and induced dipoles, quadrupoles), hydrogen bonding, and hydrophobic interactions. There are many molecular targets of anesthetic action within the central nervous system, but there are many more still to be discovered. Molecular interaction sites postulated from functional studies include protein binding sites, protein cavities, lipid/protein interfaces, and protein/protein interfaces.

1 Introduction

The mechanisms of general anesthesia remain one of the great unsolved problems of classical neuropharmacology (Miller 1985). Definitions, concepts, and hypotheses concerning general anesthesia have been discussed at length elsewhere (Urban and Bleckwenn 2002; Urban 2002; Campagna et al. 2003; Sonner et al. 2003; Rudolph and Antkowiak 2004; Franks 2006; Evers and Crowder 2005; Koblin 2005). Since there is no agreement on the mechanisms of general anesthesia, sites for interactions of general anesthetics will be discussed without attempting to decide whether or not they are relevant for general anesthesia.

The first section will review which drugs produce general anesthesia both clinically and experimentally, and which targets they affect. The next section will describe the molecular interactions that anesthetics are capable of undergoing with their targets. The final section will discuss molecular sites of anesthetic actions that have been investigated in detail.

2 Anesthetics and Their Targets

Since the discovery of general anesthesia hundreds of substances have been tested and found to possess anesthetic activity (Urban et al. 2006). Only very few of these have ever been introduced into clinical practice. The ability of an anesthetic drug to produce experimental general anesthesia is a necessary but not a sufficient condition for its use in humans. It is their side effects that rule out most general anesthetics for clinical use.

2.1 General Anesthetics in Clinical Use

Only a few anesthetics are listed by Goodman and Gilman's *The Pharmacological Basis of Therapeutics* (Hardman et al. 2001) as being used in clinical practice today. They comprise the halogenated ethers sevoflurane, desflurane, isoflurane and enflurane, the halogenated alkane halothane, nitrous oxide, a few barbiturates, a few benzodiazepines, etomidate (imidazole derivative), propofol (phenol derivative), ketamine (phencyclidine derivative), and the opioid analgesics (Fig. 1). While the use of halothane, enflurane, and nitrous oxide is clearly declining, the noble gas xenon is about to be introduced into clinical practice. Barbiturates serve mainly as agents for induction of anesthesia. Opioids are predominantly used as analgesics. Although their use as general anesthetics is controversial (Hug 1990), as an adjuvant they help to reduce the amount of other anesthetic agents needed.

Most of these compounds, however, be they modern halogenated inhalation anesthetics or intravenous anesthetics, cannot be used by themselves as universally as diethyl-ether once was. For example, the intravenous anesthetic ketamine is not

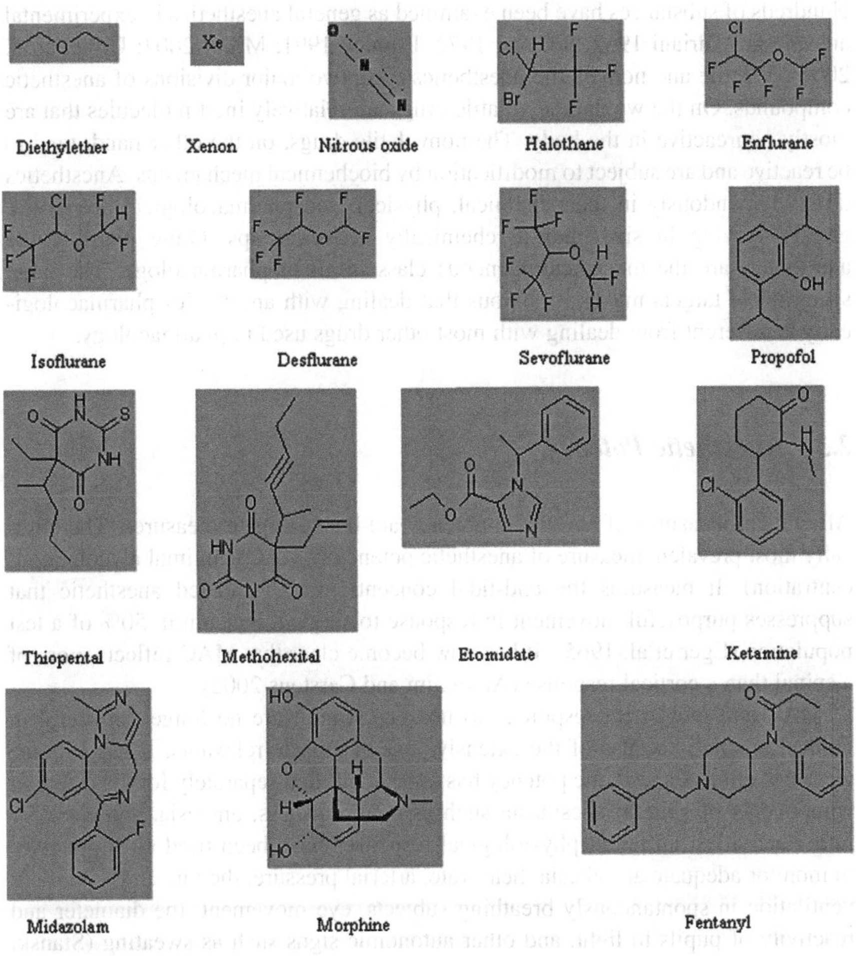

Fig. 1 Anesthetics and anesthesia adjuvants widely used in clinical practice, except for diethyl ether, which is shown for historical reasons

given by itself, but is commonly co-administered with benzodiazepines to counteract the possible undesirable psychological reactions which occur during awakening from ketamine anesthesia (Reves et al. 2000). Almost all halogenated ethers such as isoflurane or desflurane lack sufficient analgesic potency and may even possess hyperalgesic properties (Antognini and Carstens 2002). Intravenous anesthetics such as barbiturates or propofol also lack analgesic potency. Modern general anesthetic techniques in clinical use typically involve the co-administration of a hypnotic drug, an analgesic drug, and possibly a muscle relaxant, allowing the reduction of hypnotic drug concentrations and thereby reducing side effects.

2.2 General Anesthetics in Experimental Use

Hundreds of substances have been examined as general anesthetics in experimental anesthesia (Adriani 1962; Seeman 1972; Lipnick 1991; Miller 2004; Urban et al. 2006). Volatile and nonvolatile anesthetics form two major divisions of anesthetic compounds. On the whole, the volatile drugs are relatively inert molecules that are mostly nonreactive in the body. The nonvolatile drugs, on the other hand, tend to be reactive and are subject to modification by biochemical mechanisms. Anesthetics differ tremendously in their chemical, physical, and pharmacological properties, greatly varying in size, and in chemically active groups. Quite possibly the anesthetics are the most heterogeneous class in all of pharmacology. The large spectrum of targets makes it obvious that dealing with anesthetics pharmacologically is different from dealing with most other drugs used in pharmacology.

2.3 Anesthetic Potency

All clinical measures of anesthetic potency are but surrogate measures. The clinically most prevalent measure of anesthetic potency is MAC (minimal alveolar concentration). It measures the end-tidal concentration of inhaled anesthetic that suppresses purposeful movement in response to surgical incision in 50% of a test population (Eger et al. 1965). It has now become clear that MAC reflects more of a spinal than a cortical response (Antognini and Carstens 2002).

MAC and movement responses to noxious stimuli are no longer as useful in clinical practice because of the extensive use of muscle relaxants. It has become clear that clinical anesthetic potency has to be quantified separately for the different components of general anesthesia such as consciousness, amnesia, analgesia, or reflex activities. Different physiological responses have been tried as alternatives to monitor adequate anesthesia: heart rate, arterial pressure, the rate and volume of ventilation in spontaneously breathing subjects, eye movement, the diameter and reactivity of pupils to light, and other autonomic signs such as sweating (Stanski and Shafer 2004). Using a combination of some of these parameters, Evans (1987) developed the PRST score (pressure, heart rate, sweating, tear production) that, however, is not widely used. Spontaneous electroencephalograms (EEG) and evoked potentials (EG) are electrical brain activities that have been employed to quantify the hypnotic component (Stanski and Shafer 2004).

Stanski criticized the fact that clinical measures with poor or unpredictable utility when evaluated scientifically (blood pressure or pulse) have become the mainstay of clinical assessments of depth of anesthesia in routine clinical practice (Stanski and Shafer 2004). It still remains true today that no numerical measure of clinical potency and no monitor, but rather many years of experience, will tell an anesthesiologist whether or not a patient is adequately anesthetized. The only "hard numbers" available at present are either MAC values and their equivalent Cp_{50} values for intravenous agents (Glass et al. 2004) or empirical doses and concentrations recommended by textbooks and typically given in the operating rooms.

The importance of carefully defining functional endpoints when assessing anesthetic potency of in vivo or in vitro experiments has been discussed elsewhere (Urban et al. 2006); there is also a need to establish complete concentration-response curves for each functional endpoint.

2.4 Identifying Molecular Targets

As the publications from the most recent Seventh International Conference on Molecular and Basic Mechanisms of Anaesthesia and previous conferences (Fink 1975; Fink 1980; Roth and Miller 1986; Rubin et al. 1991; Richards and Winlow 1998; Urban and Barann 2002; Mashimo et al. 2005) have shown, there are a great many molecular targets of anesthetic actions within the central nervous system. While in the past much attention has focused on ion channels, other proteins have been found to be sensitive to anesthetics as well (Urban et al. 2006). Currently under investigation and definitely of interest are, for example, metabotropic receptors, which modulate synaptic transmission and partly bind the same ligands as ligand-gated ion channel receptors. Other proteins affected by anesthetics are protein pumps, G proteins, protein kinases, and phosphatases, as well as adrenergic receptors, prostanoid receptors, motility proteins, SNARE (soluble *N*-ethylmaleimide-sensitive factor attachment protein receptor) proteins, or fatty acid amide hydrolase (FAAH) (Urban et al. 2006).

Still, relatively speaking, the anesthetic sensitivities of only a few proteins have been investigated, when compared with the estimated number of at least 12,000 different membrane proteins, of which ion channels are only a small fraction. The known list of molecular anesthetic targets (Urban et al. 2006) is steadily increasing as ongoing research on other molecular targets is constantly revealing new targets.

There is a great deal of discussion and dissent on which molecular targets and which molecular mechanisms are relevant for general anesthesia (Urban and Bleckwenn 2002; Urban 2002; Campagna et al. 2003; Sonner et al. 2003; Rudolph and Antkowiak 2004; Franks 2006; Evers and Crowder 2005; Koblin 2005). This is perhaps not surprising since many levels of integration within the central nervous system have to be passed before an anesthetic action at the molecular level is sensed at the systemic level. As long as the detailed architecture of these pathways and networks remains mostly obscure, a final judgment on the relevance of molecular anesthetic targets should be postponed.

Several points can be made by surveying the existing information on anesthetic actions on the molecular targets: (1) Even at clinical concentrations, anesthetics act on many different molecular targets. (2) Wherever investigated in detail, it has been found that any single anesthetic suppresses proteins by more than one action, i.e., anesthetics affect not just one but several different aspects of any particular molecular target. (3) No two anesthetics appear to act alike on the same target; they all have their individual spectra of effects. (4) Anesthetics differ not only quantitatively in the relative strengths of their various effects but also qualitatively, in that both suppression as well as potentiation may occur.

3 Physical and Chemical Nature of Anesthetic Interactions

Two fundamentally different approaches have been used in order to characterize interactions between anesthetics and their targets: thermodynamic descriptions and molecular descriptions. Thermodynamic descriptions consider averages over many individual interactions, while molecular descriptions attempt to measure directly individual interactions between anesthetic molecules and their molecular targets. The thermodynamic approach has been largely replaced by molecular approaches as increasingly refined molecular methods have become available to investigate interactions between anesthetics and their targets.

3.1 Thermodynamic Approaches

3.1.1 Solution Theories

Although anesthetically active substances may vary greatly in size and in other physical and physiochemical properties—not to mention their pharmacological behavior—they do have something in common. More than 100 years ago Meyer and Overton independently discovered that anesthetic potency correlated with the preference of anesthetics to dissolve in lipophilic rather than in polar phases (Urban et al. 2006). They found a linear relationship between the logarithm of anesthetic potency and the logarithm of the oil/water partition coefficients, with unity slope, now called the Meyer-Overton correlation (Urban et al. 2006).

The Meyer-Overton correlation was found long before the concept of cell membranes existed, and the researchers therefore concluded that anesthesia was brought about by anesthetics dissolving the lipophilic moieties of a cell. A thermodynamic description of solutions and interactions of solutes with solvents was used in order to describe anesthetic action. These descriptions of anesthetic interactions could be easily transferred to membranes once their concept had been established. Anesthetic potencies were described in terms of chemical potentials partitioning between different solvents and various solubility parameters (Butler 1950; Ferguson 1939; Kaufman 1977; Mullins 1954; Hildebrand and Scott 1964). These descriptions did not concentrate so much on how these interactions brought about anesthesia. Instead, they sought to identify parameters that would predict at what concentration any given substance would produce anesthesia.

3.1.2 Meyer-Overton Rule

To date, no other rule based on physiochemical or structural parameters has been as useful as the Meyer-Overton rule in predicting anesthetic potency. The knowledge of the partition coefficient of a substance is in most cases sufficient to predict its anesthetic potency quite accurately, provided the substance is chemically not too complex (Urban et al. 2006).

When anesthetic potency data collected from various in vivo and in vitro systems were plotted against the same consistent set of octanol/water partition coefficients, comparison of the resulting different lipophilicity plots led to the following observations (Urban et al. 2006). First, different classes of anesthetics give rise to different correlations that are shifted with respect to each other. Second, intravenous anesthetics are, on the whole, considerably more potent than inhalation anesthetics. Third, different proteins may differ in their sensitivities to anesthetics, depending on the group of anesthetics involved.

The macroscopic Meyer-Overton rule does not provide any direct microscopic insight. However, the existence of so many Meyer-Overton correlations appears to imply that the hydrophobic component of the anesthetic interaction is roughly equal to weak polar components and therefore is not being masked by them (Urban et al. 2006). Consistent with anesthetic interactions being weak is the observation that IC_{50} values in the millimolar and micromolar range are characteristic in general anesthesia, and that large quantities of anesthetic drugs (in the order of grams or at least milligrams) have to be administered during inhalation anesthesia and intravenous anesthesia (barbiturate, propofol, ketamine, etomidate).

3.1.3 Multiple Linear Regression Analyses of Various Physical Properties

Without examining hydrophobic and weak polar interactions directly on the molecular level, attempts have been made to identify their contributions by using multiple linear regression analysis on thermodynamic parameters. Equations similar to the following have been used to quantify the relative contributions of various physical properties of an anesthetic (i.e., its ability to donate or accept a hydrogen bond, its dipolarity and polarizability, and its size) to the magnitude of partition coefficients or concentrations of anesthetic endpoints (Abraham et al. 1991; Davies et al. 1974):

$$\log(P) = c + s\cdot\pi + d\cdot\delta + a\cdot\alpha + b\cdot\beta + v\cdot V$$

where P is the partition coefficient between two solvents or the potency of an anesthetic. The solute parameters in this equation represent the following interactions: π, the solute dipolarity/polarizability; δ, a polarizability correction term; α, the solute (hydrogen-bond donor) acidity; β, the solute (hydrogen-bond acceptor) basicity; and V, the solute volume. Solute volume is so closely correlated with lipophilicity (or hydrophobicity) that the coefficient (v) of V can be considered to be a measure of the lipophilicity of the condensed phase being investigated. The constants c, s, d, a, b, and v are determined, for a large set of anesthetics, using the method of multiple linear regression analysis. The results obtained (Abraham et al. 1991; Davies et al. 1974) suggest that all the factors contained in the equation, i.e., hydrophobicity, dipolarity, polarizability, and hydrogen-bonding, contribute to the overall interaction.

3.2 *Weak Forces Stabilizing Structures of Biological Macromolecules*

Biological macromolecules, the complex functional units of biochemical systems, are held together by several reversible and noncovalent interactions and associations. These play a pivotal role in the folding of proteins, the recognition of substrates, and the interactions between receptors and ligands. The weak forces responsible for the right structure and functioning of biological macromolecules consist of electrostatic interactions, van der Waals forces, hydrogen bonds, and hydrophobic interactions (ChemgaPedia 2006).

The process of the breaking and remaking of hydrogen bonds enables functional proteins to change from one conformation to another. For example, neurotransmitter substances, themselves capable of forming hydrogen bonds and interacting through van der Waals forces and hydrophobic forces, lead to conformational changes by breaking hydrogen bonds in proteins (Celie et al. 2004; Reeves et al. 2003). Not only neurotransmitter molecules but many anesthetic molecules are capable of interacting by such weak forces also, and they have therefore the potential of disrupting functions of biologically important macromolecules such as proteins.

As already suggested in the previous section when multiple linear regression analyses of thermodynamic parameters were discussed, different weak forces may combine and superimpose in anesthetic actions. For example, the functional effects of the binding of ligands such as the neurotransmitter acetylcholine or serotonin are thought to depend on the simultaneous interactions involving several hydrogen bonds, cation–π interactions, dispersion forces, and hydrophobic forces (Celie et al.

2004; Reeves et al. 2003; Thompson et al. 2005). The effect of a combination may well be more than just the sum of the different interaction energies and lead to synergistic effects. Therefore, even small contributions may become very important in a combination of different contributing forces. Depending on the proteins and neuronal networks involved for any particular effect of anesthesia, different combinations of these weak forces may become relevant.

3.3 Ion–Ion Interactions

Ion–ion interactions involve the strongest of the Coulombic electrostatic forces (ChemgaPedia 2006). Typical energies for ion–ion interactions at a distance of 0.5 nm are 250 kJ/mol (ChemgaPedia 2006). Many intravenous anesthetics can be ionized and are present, at neutral pH, both in their neutral and their charged forms. Clinical compounds that are partly ionized at neutral pH include, for example, the barbiturates, ketamine, etomidate, and the benzodiazepines. There are examples demonstrating distinct actions of charged intravenous anesthetics and their neutral counterparts (Kendig 1981; Frazier et al. 1975). While direct evidence for ion–ion interactions is yet lacking for general anesthetics, electrostatic repulsion between the charged form of lidocaine and a Na^+ ion in the selectivity filter has been suggested to occur in voltage-dependent sodium channels (Tikhonov et al. 2006).

3.4 Ion–Dipole Interactions

The strength of ion–dipole interactions is weaker than that of ion–ion interactions, and it decreases rapidly with distance (ChemgaPedia 2006). The typical energies for ion–dipole interactions at a distance of 0.5 nm are 15 kJ/mol (ChemgaPedia 2006). In biochemical processes this type of interaction plays an important role, e.g., during hydration, complex formation, and cation–π interactions. For the squid axon, it has been suggested that alcohols and anesthetics adsorb at the membrane interface, thereby changing its electric field and the membrane potential through their dipole moments (Haydon and Urban 1983). These changes are then postulated to impact on the gating mechanisms that involve the translocation of net charges (Hille 2001). In gramicidin A pores, it has been proposed that their electrical conductance, i.e., ion flow through them, is affected by dipole potentials generated by *n*-alkanols adsorbed at the membrane interface (Pope et al. 1982).

3.4.1 Hydration

When ions dissolve in water, the dipolar water molecules will be attracted to them and associate with them depending on their partial charges (ChemgaPedia 2006). The water molecules form several layers (hydration shells), the first layer depending primarily on ion–dipole interactions, and further layers being held together by hydrogen bonds. The number of coordinating water molecules depends on the size of the ion and its charge. The hydration shells of ions effectively increase the ionic radius, thereby influencing their diffusion through pores and ion channels (Hille 2001). The selectivity filters of ion channel proteins contain such ions that are in contact with water (Hille 2001). In addition, most biological macromolecules carry negative charges and are surrounded by their own hydration shells that help in stabilizing their conformations. The water molecules in these hydration shells are much more ordered and structured than they are in bulk water. Anesthetics can through the process of clathrate formation interfere with the structure of water in these hydration shells, as was first observed by Pauling (1961) and Miller et al. (1961) independently.

3.4.2 Cation–π Interactions

Cation–π interactions are strong electrostatic interactions that occur between a π-electron cloud and an atom that carries a full or partial positive charge (ChemgaPedia 2006). Cations involved are mainly metal ions or partially positively charged side chains that interact with the aromatic side chains of phenylalanine, tyrosine, or tryptophane (Fig. 2). Thus these positive charges can interact with the surfaces of nonpolar, aromatic structures. As a first approximation, these interactions arise from electrostatic attraction between the positive charge of the cation and the quadrupole moment of the aromatic system. Studies to estimate the strength of such interactions suggest that it may contribute as much as several kilocalories per mole of energy to stabilize the binding of ligand to protein (Beene et al. 2002). Because binding affinity is related logarithmically to binding energy, cation–π interactions may enhance binding affinity by several orders of magnitude (Raines 2005).

Cation–π interactions have been recognized as an important noncovalent force in biochemical macromolecules, particularly in proteins. They have been identified in the function of acetylcholine receptor channels and 5-HT_3 receptor channels (Beene et al. 2002), generally as a component in ligand-receptor interactions and in

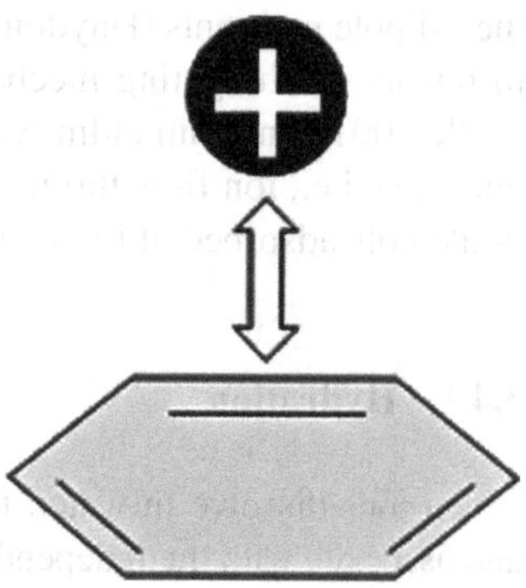

Fig. 2 Cation–π interaction: strong electrostatic interactions between a π-electron cloud of an aromatic ring and an atom that carries a full or partial positive charge

the stabilization of α-helices, in the binding reaction between proteins and DNA, and for the permeation of metal ions through ion channels. Thus by virtue of their π-electron clouds, aromatic anesthetics may engage in attractive electrostatic interactions with cationic atomic charges on protein targets. For example, volatile aromatic drugs inhibit *N*-methyl-d-aspartate (NMDA) receptor-mediated currents with potencies that are highly correlated with their abilities to engage in cation–π interactions (Raines 2005).

3.5 *Van der Waals Interactions (Dipole–Dipole)*

Often the term "van der Waals interaction" is loosely used as a synonym for weak intermolecular forces (ChemgaPedia 2006). In the narrower sense it describes intermolecular forces with attractive interaction energies that decrease with the sixth power of distance, because they arise from dipole–dipole interactions (ChemgaPedia 2006). These interactions occur between all kinds of atoms and molecules, even when those are nonpolar. Van de Waals forces can be attractive and repulsive, attraction dominating for larger distances between the interacting parts. Typical energies for dipole–dipole interactions at a distance of 0.5 nm are 0.3–2 kJ/mol (ChemgaPedia 2006). Thus van der Waals forces are quite weak, but they are additive. Their strengths grow with increasing sizes and polarizabilities of the molecules involved. When contact becomes too close, there will be strong repulsion caused by positively charged nuclei as well as by fully occupied orbitals (Pauli exclusion principle). The attractive and repulsive forces of van der Waals interactions are described mathematically by the Lennard-Jones potential.

Van der Waals interactions become particularly important in biological systems when two molecules consisting of many atoms approach each other. The interaction between ligand and receptor is primarily of electrostatic origin. Electrostatic forces govern the approach and the alignment of the ligand toward the protein. The probability that a sizable number of atoms of a ligand have by chance just the right distance to the atoms of the binding regions is very low. Thus the high selectivity and stereospecificity of ligand and protein interactions arises quite substantially from van der Waals interactions (ChemgaPedia 2006). Three components of van der Waals interactions are distinguished and described in the following: permanent dipole–permanent dipole, permanent dipole–induced dipole, and fluctuating dipole–induced dipole.

3.5.1 Permanent Dipole–Permanent Dipole

Of the three kinds of dipole interactions those between permanent dipoles (Fig. 3) are the strongest (ChemgaPedia 2006). There are many anesthetics that possess a permanent dipole moment, including the halogenated ethers and alkanes, while cyclopropane and xenon have none. The dipole moment of sevoflurane (3.3 debye) is quite similar in magnitude to that of a peptide bond (3.7 debye). Therefore, apart

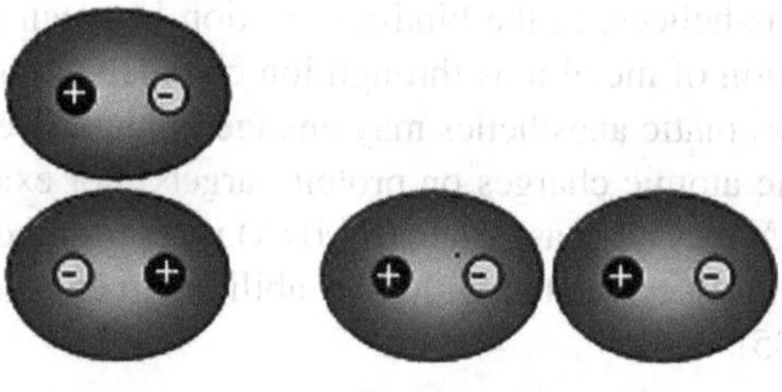

Fig. 3 Permanent dipole–permanent dipole interaction: dipoles can associate either head to tail or in an antiparallel orientation

from interactions with side chains of amino acids, anesthetics carrying permanent dipole moments may interact with proteins in several ways at many positions. Binding of anesthetics to human serum albumin has been suggested to involve permanent dipole interactions (Eckenhoff 1998).

3.5.2 Permanent Dipole–Induced Dipole (Induction Effect)

Dipole interactions may be observed between a dipole and a nonpolar molecule if the latter is polarizable (ChemgaPedia 2006). Polarizability arises if the electron cloud of an atom is distorted in the presence of a strong dipole moment (Fig. 4). For example, as noble gases are polarizable, a permanent dipole will be able to induce a dipole in them, giving rise to electrostatic Debye forces between the permanent and the induced dipole. Thus even the inert gas and anesthetic xenon are capable of interacting with proteins.

Polarizability increases with atomic size, and thus should become more prominent in those inhalation anesthetics that contain larger halogens such as chlorine or bromine. Eckenhoff and Johansson (1997) have observed that, for a given structure, both anesthetic potency and degree of metabolism are progressively increased as heavier halogens are substituted (Harris et al. 1992; Targ et al. 1989), suggesting that this type of van der Waals force may be important in producing anesthetic binding interactions in some relevant target.

3.5.3 Fluctuating Dipole–Induced Dipole (Dispersion or London Forces)

Dispersion forces, also called London forces, arise from spontaneous fluctuations of electron densities within atoms and molecules (ChemgaPedia 2006). The constant motion of the electrons in the molecule causes rapidly fluctuating dipoles even in the most symmetrical molecule such as monatomic molecules and noble gases. These fluctuations give rise to the formation of temporary electric dipoles that, in turn, will induce further dipoles in adjacent molecules (Fig. 5). Dispersion forces may act between completely apolar molecules. They are the weakest of all dipole–dipole interactions.

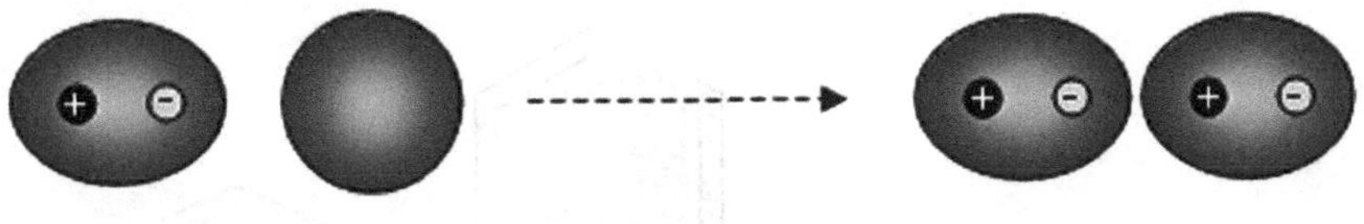

Fig. 4 Permanent dipole–induced dipole interaction: a strong permanent dipole can induce a temporary dipole in a polarizable nonpolar molecule

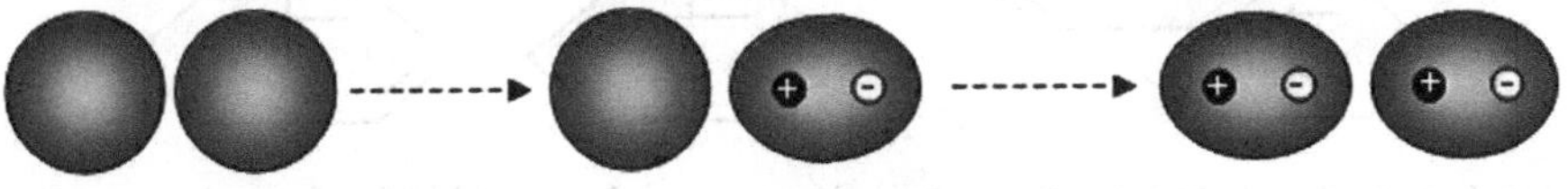

Fig. 5 Fluctuating dipole–induced dipole interaction: spontaneous fluctuations of electron densities within a symmetrical, apolar molecule create dipoles that, in turn, can induce dipoles in another polarizable, nonpolar molecule

The ease with which the electrons of a molecule, atom or ion are displaced by a neighboring charge is called polarizability. Anesthetic molecules are polarizable, even noble gases such as helium or the clinical anesthetic xenon. Thus, contrary to what their names suggest, they are not completely inert. The more electrons there are, and the larger the distance over which they can move, the bigger the possible temporary dipoles and therefore the bigger the dispersion forces. This is why bigger molecules can interact more strongly and why the boiling points of the noble gases increase from helium (–269°C) to xenon (–108°C).

A special case of London forces are π–π interactions between aromatic rings (ChemgaPedia 2006). They are stronger than ordinary London forces because the charges are more mobile in conjugated π-systems. These aromatic interactions occur either as π-stacking or as face-to-face interactions (Fig. 6). π–π interactions are particularly responsible for shaping the tertiary structure of proteins with aromatic side chains. Propofol, etomidate, ketamine, benzodiazepines (such as midazolam), droperidol, morphine, and its fentanyl derivatives are but some examples of intravenous anesthetic compounds containing aromatic rings.

3.6 Hydrogen Bonding

Interactions of the form *D*-H···|*A* between a proton donor *D*-H and a proton acceptor |*A* are called hydrogen bonds (ChemgaPedia 2006). *D* and *A* are generally strongly electronegative atoms such as F, O, and N. The most common hydrogen bonds are formed between oxygen and nitrogen atoms, which can act both as proton acceptors and as proton donors due to their free electron pairs (Fig. 7). In many hydrogen bonds the distance between the atoms *A* and *D* is shorter than the sum of the van der Waals radii. Hydrogen bonds are directional and strongest when all three atoms involved in the bond are on a straight line. The interaction energy of

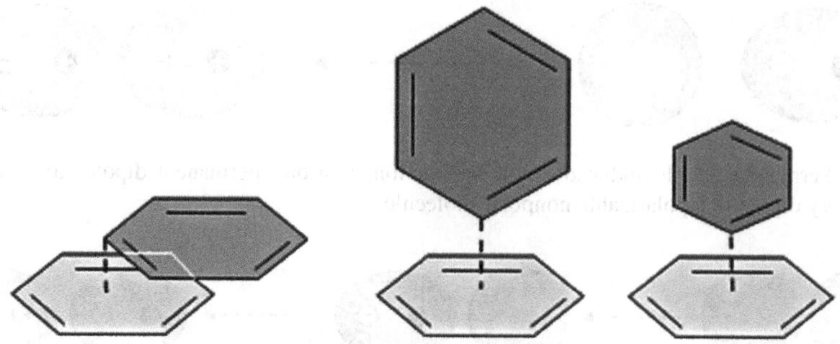

Fig. 6 π–π interactions between aromatic rings: a special case of London forces but stronger, these occur either as π-stacking or as face-to-face interactions

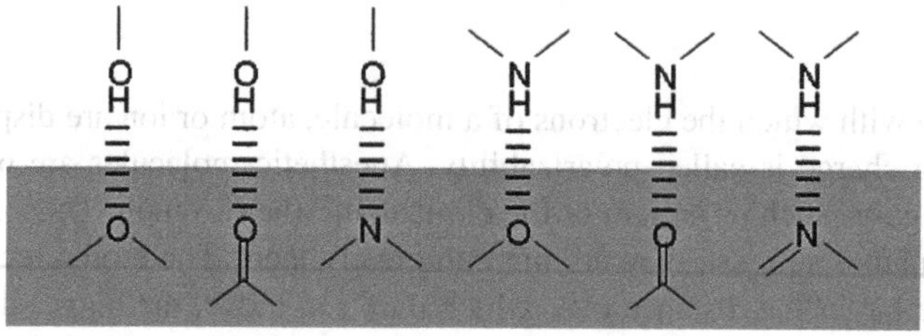

Fig. 7 Hydrogen bonds: the most common hydrogen bonds are formed between oxygen and nitrogen atoms, which can act either as proton acceptors (*shaded area*) or as proton donors (*not shaded area*) due to their free electron pairs

hydrogen bonds consists both of electrostatic contributions (dipole–dipole and dipole–ion interactions) and covalent contributions (three-center four-electron bonds). Energies for hydrogen bonds *D*-H···*A* range between 1 and 50 kJ/mol, energies between 10 and 50 kJ/mol are typical. In low barrier hydrogen bonds (F-H···F, O-H···O^-) the hydrogen atom is evenly spaced between the donor and the acceptor. This bridge is symmetrical with an angle of 180°, F-H···F being the strongest of all hydrogen bonds. All other hydrogen bonds are high-barrier bonds. Of these, O-H···O, O-H···N, N-H···O are the strongest. N-H···N form weaker hydrogen bonds, and the weakest are between O-H and π-electrons.

Infrared spectroscopists have known for more than half a century that aromatic rings (*Ar* in the following) can serve as acceptors for weak hydrogen bonds, with typical interaction energies of 4–8 kJ/mol (Sandorfy 2004). Indeed, amino acids like tryptophan, tyrosine, and phenylalanine possess aromatic rings. The existence of N-H···*Ar*, or OH···*Ar* hydrogen bonds in proteins was successfully demonstrated (Sandorfy 2004). These H-bonds are thought to play a pivotal role in determining the conformations and motions of proteins (Sandorfy 2004). They could be targets for a number of intravenous anesthetics that also possess aromatic rings. For example, the effect of aromatic amino acid side-chain structure on halothane binding to four-helix bundles has been studied in detail (Johansson and Manderson 2002).

Hydrogen bonds are formed between single molecules (intermolecular) or within a molecule (intramolecular); they are the most important inter- and intramolecular interactions of all of biochemistry. Protein function depends on transitions between different conformations, which involve the breaking of old and remaking of new hydrogen bonds. Any substance such as anesthetics that can compete for hydrogen bonds would be disruptive to protein function. Polar interactions and the breakage of hydrogen bonds appear to be important factors for halogenated hydrocarbons containing an acidic hydrogen (Abraham et al. 1971; Davies et al. 1976; Urban and Haydon 1987), including the clinical anesthetics isoflurane, enflurane, sevoflurane, desflurane, halothane, and the obsolete clinical anesthetic chloroform. Hydrogen bonds may even be broken by substances that by themselves do not form hydrogen bonds as has been suggested for the interaction of *n*-alkanes with gramicidin A (Hendry et al. 1978; Elliott et al. 1983).

3.7 Hydrophobic Interactions

Hydrophobic interactions are weak interactions resulting from the tendency of hydrophobic molecules or hydrophobic portions of macromolecules to avoid contact with water (ChemgaPedia 2006; Tanford 1980; Tanford 1997). Hydrophobic forces are responsible for generating lipid bilayers that form the backbone of biological membranes. In aqueous solutions, water molecules close to hydrophobic interfaces are arranged such that their hydrogen bonds point away from the hydrophobic areas. This reduces the mobility of water molecules, leading to a breakdown of the free cluster structure of water. Because water molecules adjacent to a hydrophobic interface are highly ordered, they exist in a thermodynamically unstable state, favoring self-aggregation and minimization of the hydrophobic interfaces (Fig. 8). Thus hydrophobic interactions do not result from the van der Waals attraction of hydrophobic moieties but rather from the exclusion of water molecules from areas between hydrophobic interfaces (Fig. 8), resulting in a gain of entropy within the system. In contrast to hydrogen bonds, hydrophobic interactions are not directional.

The hydrophobic effect contributes significantly to the binding energies of ligands, for example, in 5-HT_3 receptors (Thompson et al. 2005) or nicotinic acetylcholine receptors (Schapira et al. 2002). Hydrophobic interactions are also important for the stabilization of peptide conformations by aliphatic and aromatic side chains (Lins and Brasseur 1995; Kauzmann 1959; Tanford 1997). In processes such as the hydrophobic collapse it plays an important role in protein folding. The contribution is proportional to the surface of the hydrophobic moieties involved. The observation that the Meyer-Overton rule holds in so many interactions between proteins and anesthetics (Urban et al. 2006) underscores the importance of hydrophobic effects in anesthetic action.

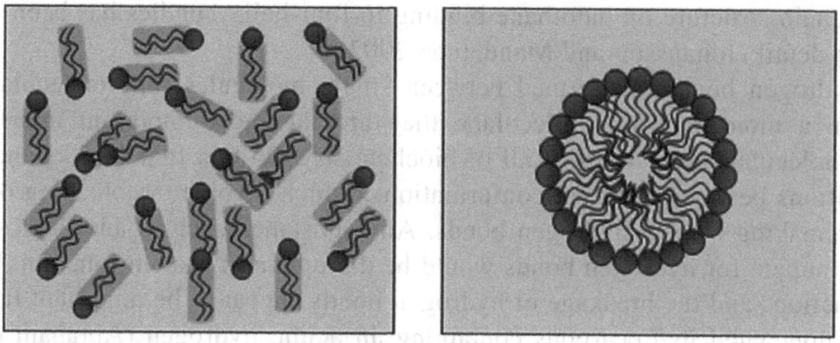

Fig. 8 Hydrophobic interactions: water molecules adjacent to a hydrophobic interface (*shaded areas*) are highly ordered, thus in a thermodynamically unstable state. Self-aggregation minimizes the hydrophobic interfaces

4 Molecular Sites of Anesthetic Action

4.1 Introduction

Following the previous sections' review of anesthetic targets and the various interactions that anesthetics can undergo, we shall finally consider molecular sites of anesthetic action that have been identified. This subject has been reviewed extensively, so only a selection of references is given here (Evers and Crowder 2005; Franks 2006; Koblin 2005; Urban et al. 1997; Sonner et al. 1950; Rudolph and Antkowiak 2004; Richards 1980; Miller 1985; Little 1996; Campagna et al. 1954; Urban 2002; Urban and Bleckwenn 2002; Overton 1901; Seeman 1972). Unfortunately, in the end, most investigations still represent black box approaches, despite the fact that the molecular configuration of the investigated anesthetics and related drugs can be varied systematically and although the molecular structure of the target sites can be altered methodically through site-directed mutagenesis. However, the spatial and temporal resolution needed for visualizing directly anesthetic action on molecular structures at the atomic scale is mostly beyond anything that is technically feasible today; the resolution of the static ion channel structure is currently limited to about 0.2 nm (Valiyaveetil et al. 2006; Unwin 2005). Therefore, for any one particular interaction it is in most cases impossible to be certain of which and how many molecular structures a drug is contacting, which conformational changes are triggered, and whether amino acid substitutions have altered the secondary and tertiary structures of proteins even before drugs interact with them.

The simpler the molecular constitution of an anesthetic-related drug, the more likely it is that it interacts not only with several molecular sites within a biological macromolecule but also with a whole range of different biological macromolecules. Thus the functional endpoint determined in experiments will only in very rare circumstances result from just a single molecular interaction but rather from an integration over time and space of several and dynamic molecular actions. Even seemingly small molecular changes in either drug constitution or target site structure may thus not be attributable to a change in just a single molecular force or site. Unless time-resolved visualization in the 0.1-nm range and below can be achieved for interactions between drugs and their molecular targets, their identification will remain indirect, depending on the observation of function instead.

4.2 *Lipid Bilayers*

Lipid bilayers consisting of a bimolecular leaflet of lipids are the backbone of biological membranes. In the early 1960s it became possible to form artificial lipid bilayers. Their physicochemical properties were systematically characterized (Tosteson 1969; Haydon and Hladky 1972) and it was discovered that anesthetics have many actions on lipid bilayers (Koblin 2005; Miller 1985; Seeman 1972). Purely hydrophobic anesthetics were found to be located preferentially in the lipid membrane hydrocarbon core, while amphipathic molecules tended to be localized predominantly in the membrane interface (North and Cafiso 1997; Tang et al. 1997; Pohorille et al. 1996). Purely hydrophobic anesthetics increase membrane thickness and raise their surface tension (Haydon et al. 1977). Lateral pressure profiles in membranes are also changed (Cantor 1997). The insertion of anesthetic molecules into lipid membranes causes them to become more fluid and disordered (Firestone et al. 1994). The increase in lipid fluidity resulting from the absorption of inhaled agents can vary considerably (Ueda et al. 1986) and depends on the lipid system examined, the position within the membrane, and the method of fluidity measurement (Baber et al. 1995; North and Cafiso 1997; Tsuchiya 2001; Vanderkooi et al. 1977). Phase transition temperatures of bilayer membranes may decrease (Galla and Trudell 1980; Tsuchiya 2001; Vanderkooi et al. 1977). Lateral phase separation may result (Trudell 1977). Anesthetics may also change membrane electrical properties such as membrane dielectric constant (Enders 1990) or surface dipole potentials (Reyes and Latorre 1979). Inhaled agents have been reported to increase the ion permeability of liposomes in a concentration-related manner (Andoh et al. 1997; Barchfeld and Deamer 1985; Miller et al. 1972).

4.3 *Protein Binding Sites*

While there are many studies showing effects of anesthetics on protein function, in general they often fail to prove that anesthetics first bind to the proteins involved before they bring about the observed effects (Eckenhoff and Johansson 1997). Even in reconstituted lipid bilayer systems, for example, consisting only of highly purified sodium channels and no more than two different kinds of lipid molecules (Wartenberg et al. 1994), it is difficult to prove that the observed functional effects of anesthetics are only due to anesthetic binding to the protein. Indeed, it could be shown that lipid bilayer composition modulated some functional anesthetic effects on purified sodium channels (Rehberg et al. 1995). Thus caution is advised when making inferences about binding based on functional studies.

Nuclear magnetic resonance (NMR) spectroscopy and photoaffinity labeling have been used as more direct approaches to study anesthetic binding to proteins (Evers and Crowder 2005). ^{19}F-NMR spectroscopic studies showed that isoflurane binds to approximately three saturable binding sites on bovine serum albumin, a fatty acid-binding protein (Dubois and Evers 1992). These results were confirmed by Eckenhoff and colleagues when they used ^{14}C-labeled halothane to photoaffinity label anesthetic binding sites on bovine serum albumin (Eckenhoff and Shuman 1993). They were able to identify the specific amino acids that were photoaffinity labeled by [^{14}C]halothane.

This binding was eliminated by co-incubation with oleic acid, consistent with the assumption that isoflurane binds to the fatty acid-binding sites on albumin. Other clinical anesthetics, such as halothane and sevoflurane, competed with isoflurane for binding to bovine serum albumin (Dubois et al. 1993). These studies provide suggestive evidence that at least certain anesthetics can compete for binding to the same site on a protein.

Currently, NMR and photoaffinity labeling techniques can only be applied to purified proteins available in relatively large quantities. The muscle-type nicotinic acetylcholine receptor is one of the few membrane proteins that has been purified in large quantities. It could be shown that halothane binds to this protein, but the pattern of photoaffinity labeling is complex, indicative of multiple binding sites (Eckenhoff 1996). Binding to specific sites on the nicotinic acetylcholine receptor could also be shown with a new and different technique involving 3-diazirinyloctanol. Most recently, Miller and colleagues have developed a general anesthetic that is an analog of octanol and functions as a photoaffinity label (Husain et al. 1999).

Other approaches to identify the location and structure of anesthetic binding sites have involved site-directed mutagenesis of candidate anesthetic targets in combination with molecular modeling. Using this strategy the location and structure of the alcohol binding site on γ-aminobutyric acid $(GABA)_A$ and glycine receptors has been predicted (Wick et al. 1998). An additional approach involves the use of model proteins such as gramicidin A (Hendry et al. 1978; Tang and Xu 2002; Pope et al. 1982) or four α-helix bundles with a hydrophobic core that can bind volatile anesthetics (Johansson et al. 1998).

4.4 Hydrophobic Pockets (Cavities) in Proteins

Considerable attention has been focused on preformed cavities within proteins as binding sites for inhaled anesthetics. Hydrophobic cavities within proteins are apparently quite common in proteins (Eckenhoff 2001). When proteins fold into complex structures, packing defects known as "cavities" are generated. These cavities are thought to introduce the necessary instabilities that facilitate conformational changes accompanying protein function (Eckenhoff 2001). The size of some of these cavities permits the occupation by anesthetic molecules. A recent screen of the Protein Data Bank for potential targets of halothane identified 394,766 total cavities, of which 58,681 cavities satisfied the fit criteria for halothane (Byrem et al. 2006). Experimental data support the hypothesis that small molecules can bind in cavities formed between α-helices in proteins (Trudell and Bertaccini 2002).

X-ray diffraction crystallography has been used to reveal details of the three-dimensional structure of anesthetic sites that NMR and photoaffinity techniques cannot provide (Evers and Crowder 2005). Because X-ray diffraction requires crystallized membrane proteins, it has so far only been used for a small number of proteins. One of the first studies of this type was performed with myoglobin. It was shown that the anesthetic molecules xenon and cyclopropane were able to bind in the hydrophobic core of a protein and that the size of the hydrophobic binding pocket could account for a cutoff in the size of anesthetic molecules that can bind in that cavity (Schoenborn et al. 1965; Schoenborn 1967).

Another example of a hydrophobic pocket has been demonstrated with X-ray diffraction for halothane binding deep within the enzyme adenylate kinase (Sachsenheimer et al. 1977). The halothane binding site was identified as the binding site for the adenine moiety of adenosine monophosphate, a substrate for adenylate kinase. Another example of anesthetics binding to endogenous ligand binding sites is provided by firefly luciferase, where two molecules of the anesthetic bromoform bind in the luciferin pocket, one of them competitively with luciferin and the other one noncompetitively (Franks et al. 1998). Human serum albumin has also been successfully crystallized and the X-ray crystallographic data show binding of propofol as well as of halothane to preformed pockets that had been shown previously to bind fatty acids (Bhattacharya et al. 2000).

The binding energies of anesthetics to these sites of action appear to be small, so that these molecules bind presumably adventitiously to preexisting cavities or sites. Consequently, the binding event is not thought to cause an "induced fit" in a protein site or even provide substantial reorganization of an internal cavity (Harris et al. 2002). Anesthetic binding to these cavities affects protein stability depending on their native sizes: proteins having intermediate pre-existing cavities are destabilized, presumably resulting from preferential binding of the anesthetic to less stable intermediates with enlarged cavities. Proteins containing larger cavities are stabilized by the anesthetic, indicative of binding to the native state (Miller 2002; Eckenhoff 2002).

The volume of the cavity or binding pocket constitutes a constraint on the anesthetic molecules that may bind. This volume may depend on the conformation of the protein. This has been shown for glycine receptor channels, possessing binding pockets with volumes that are different in the resting (smaller) and in the activated (larger) state (Harris et al. 2002). The volume of the cavity and proposed anesthetic binding site in $GABA_A$ receptor channels is estimated to range between 0.25 and 0.37 nm^3, quite likely constituting a common site of action for the anesthetics isoflurane, halothane, and chloroform (Jenkins et al. 2001). Modulation of human

5-HT_{3A}-mediated currents by volatile anesthetics exhibits a dependence on molecular volume similar to *n*-alcohols, suggesting that both classes of agents may enhance 5-HT_{3A} receptor function via the same mechanism (Stevens et al. 2005). The data suggest an apparent size of 0.120 nm^3 for the cavity (Stevens et al. 2005), which modulates anesthetic and *n*-alcohol enhancement of agonist action on the 5-HT_{3A} receptor.

These and other studies have demonstrated that possible sites of anesthetic action exist within the transmembrane subunits of the superfamily of ligand-gated ion channels. The exact molecular arrangement of this transmembrane region remains at intermediate resolution with current experimental techniques (Eckenhoff 2001). In order to produce a more exact model of this region, homology modeling methods combined with experimental data have been used. This approach produced a final structure possessing a cavity within the core of a four-helix bundle. Converging on and lining this cavity are residues known to be involved in modulating anesthetic potency. Thus cavities formed within the core of transmembrane four-helix bundles may be important binding sites for volatile anesthetics in the ligand-gated ion channels (Bertaccini et al. 2005).

4.5 Hydrophilic Crevices in Proteins

Water-filled crevices in proteins, apart from hydrophobic cavities, have also been implicated as molecular sites of anesthetic action. Akabas et al. (2002) suggest that crevices and cavities form in the membrane-spanning domains during $GABA_A$ receptor gating. Since a vacuum is energetically unfavorable, water moves in, thereby facilitating conformational change. These water-filled crevices extend from the extracellular surface into the interior of the $GABA_A$ receptor protein. Anesthetics, by preferentially filling these crevices/cavities, could stabilize receptor conformations other than the resting state, altering the probability of channel opening (Akabas et al. 2002). While this site is still quite hypothetical at present, it considers the possibility that anesthetics may enter proteins by transfer to an annular ring formed by the four-component interface of the ligand-binding and transmembrane domains of the protein, the phospholipid bilayer, and the interfacial water layer. This route that anesthetics may take constitutes an alternative to diffusion down the water-filled lumen of the ion channel or dissolution in the phospholipid bilayer followed by transfer through the lipid–protein interface of the ion channel (Trudell and Bertaccini 2002).

4.6 Lipid/Protein Interfaces

Integral membrane proteins are essential for mediating numerous physiological functions. In order to function successfully, membrane proteins must perform properly within, and at the same time interact with, the lipid membrane in which they undergo conformational changes while carrying out their complex functions. There is much evidence for a strong effect of the properties of lipid bilayers on the function of membrane proteins (Trudell and Bertaccini 2002; Rebecchi and Pentyala 2002).

Reconstitution studies have provided the best evidence that the lipid environment may significantly affect the properties of integral membrane proteins. In reconstitution studies it is actually possible to reinsert proteins, which have been removed from their native membranes, into artificial lipid bilayer membranes of defined lipid composition. A number of diverse reconstituted proteins have been found to have altered functions, depending on the composition of the surrounding lipids (Zakim 1986). Specific properties of phospholipids, such as head group composition, and general properties of the hydrophobic bilayer, such as micro viscosity, can have dramatic effects on protein function. This leads to the expectation that if the properties of lipid bilayers have been changed by anesthetics in a comparable way, then protein function should also be altered.

Nash (2002) takes issue with the fact that lipid targets of anesthetic action have fallen from favor. He argues that he knows of no decisive experiment that eliminates lipid targets from contention, particularly if one acknowledges the possibility that subtle alterations of bilayers by volatiles anesthetics might impact on the function of proteins imbedded in them. The function of the ion channel-forming polypeptide gramicidin A is modulated by the lipid environment (Hendry et al. 1978; Pope et al. 1982). Anesthetic changes of membrane parameters have been postulated to directly affect sodium channel and potassium channel function in the squid giant axon (Urban 1993). The lipid environment alters the actions of pentobarbital on purified sodium channels reconstituted in planar lipid bilayers (Rehberg et al. 1995). Studies using site-directed mutations in ligand-gated ion channels combined with molecular modeling suggest that a primary point of action of anesthetics is in the transmembrane domain of these channels (Trudell and Bertaccini 2002). Another example involves certain protein kinases where anesthetics might operate at the protein/lipid interface by changing the lateral pressure profile (Rebecchi and Pentyala 2002).

4.7 *Protein/Protein Interfaces*

The possibility that anesthetics might be able to act at the interface between protein subunits or at the interface between different proteins has not been explored extensively. It has been suggested that anesthetics binding to such sites might disrupt, for example, allosteric transitions at domain/domain interfaces of protein kinases or prevent agonist-induced dissociation of receptor from the heterotrimeric G proteins (Rebecchi and Pentyala 2002).

4.8 Relevant Sites for Anesthetics

Figure 9 summarizes sites of anesthetic action that have been identified in lipid bilayers and in ion channels, the latter representing the best-studied class of membrane proteins in this context. Anesthetics may differ in the spectrum of interaction sites depending on their physicochemical properties and the structures of the biological macromolecules. Within the bilayer, anesthetics may act (1) at the interface between the lipid and the aqueous phase, (2) within the hydrophobic interior of the lipid bilayer itself (Urban et al. 1991; Trudell and Bertaccini 2002), or (3) between the lipid and membrane proteins. Anesthetics may bind to protein binding sites in contact with the aqueous phase, located either (4) inside the channel lumen of ion channels (Dilger 2002; Scholz 2002), or (5) at the water/protein interface. (6) Water-filled crevices or water channels inside or adjacent to membrane proteins have been implicated (Trudell and Bertaccini 2002). Anesthetics may bind (7) within the core of the membrane protein itself, between hydrophobic α-helices (Frenkel et al. 1990) and form hydrophobic or lipophilic pockets (Trudell and Bertaccini 2002). (8) Anesthetics may disturb interactions between subunits of a protein or between different proteins (Trudell and Bertaccini 2002; Rebecchi and Pentyala 2002). In addition, Sandorfy (2002) has pointed out that carbohydrates that are covalently attached to membrane proteins may also constitute sites of anesthetic actions.

Which of the molecular sites are relevant for clinical anesthesia? The answer to this question requires knowledge of the neuronal networks critical to general anesthesia or to one of its essential clinical components. When these relevant neuronal networks will have been identified, it should then become possible to assess which molecular sites contribute to clinical anesthesia.

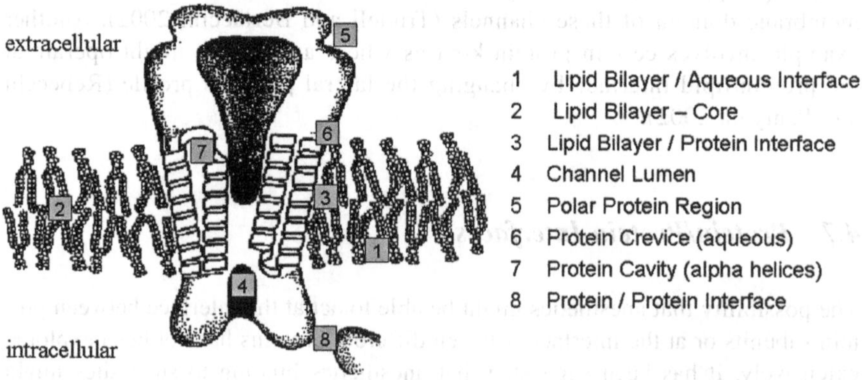

Fig. 9 Summary of identified molecular sites of anesthetic action in membranes and in embedded proteins

References

Abraham MH, Lieb WR, Franks NP (1991) Role of hydrogen bonding in general anesthesia. J Pharm Sci 80:719–724

Adriani J (1962) The chemistry and physics of anesthesia. Charles C Thomas, Springfield

Akabas MH, Horenstein J, Williams DB, Bali M, Bera AK (2002) GABA- and drug-induced conformational changes detected in the GABAA receptor channel-lining segments. In: Urban BW, Barann M (eds) Molecular and basic mechanisms of anesthesia. Pabst Science Publishers, Lengerich, pp 130–142

Andoh T, Blanck TJJ, Nikonorov I, Recio-Pinto E (1997) Volatile anaesthetic effects on calcium conductance of planar lipid bilayers formed with synthetic lipids or extracted lipids from sarcoplasmic reticulum. Br J Anaesth 78:66–74

Antognini JF, Carstens E (2002) In vivo characterization of clinical anaesthesia and its components. Br J Anaesth 89:156–166

Baber J, Ellena JF, Cafiso DS (1995) Distribution of general anesthetics in phospholipid bilayers determined using 2H NMR and 1H-1H NOE spectroscopy. Biochemistry 34:6533–6539

Barchfeld GL, Deamer DW (1985) The effect of general anesthetics on the proton and potassium permeabilities of liposomes. Biochim Biophys Acta 819:161–169

Beene DL, Brandt GS, Zhong W, Zacharias NM, Lester HA, Dougherty DA (2002) Cation-π interactions in ligand recognition by serotonergic (5-HT3A) and nicotinic acetylcholine receptors: the anomalous binding properties of nicotine. Biochemistry 41:10262–10269

Bertaccini EJ, Shapiro J, Brutlag DL, Trudell JR (2005) Homology modeling of a human glycine alpha 1 receptor reveals a plausible anesthetic binding site. J Chem Inf Model 45:128–135

Bhattacharya AA, Curry S, Franks NP (2000) Binding of the general anesthetics propofol and halothane to human serum albumin. High resolution crystal structures. J Biol Chem 275:38731–38738

Butler TC (1950) Theories of general anesthesia. J Pharmacol Exp Ther 98:121–160

Byrem WC, Armstead SC, Kobayashi S, Eckenhoff RG, Eckmann DM (2006) A guest molecule-host cavity fitting algorithm to mine PDB for small molecule targets. Biochim Biophys Acta 1764:1320–1324

Campagna JA, Miller KW, Forman SA (2003) Mechanisms of actions of inhaled anesthetics. N Engl J Med 348:2110–2124

Cantor RS (1997) The lateral pressure profile in membranes: a physical mechanism of general anesthesia. Biochemistry 36:2339–2344

Celie PH, van Rossum-Fikkert SE, van Dijk WJ, Brejc K, Smit AB, Sixma TK (2004) Nicotine and carbamylcholine binding to nicotinic acetylcholine receptors as studied in AChBP crystal structures. Neuron 41:907–914

ChemgaPedia (2006) Chemgapedia. Vernetztes Studium–Chemie. http://www.chemgapedia.de/vsengine/topics/de/vlu/Chemie/index.html. Fachinformationszentrum Chemie GmbH, Berlin. Cited 23 June 2007

Davies RH, Bagnall RD, Jones WGM (1974) A quantitative interpretation of phase effects in anaesthesia. Int J Quant Chem Quant Biol Symp 1:201–212

Davies RH, Bagnall RD, Bell W, Jones WGM (1976) The hydrogen bond proton donor properties of volatile halogenated hydrocarbons and ethers and their mode of action in anaesthesia. Int J Quant Chem Quant Biol Symp 3:171–185

Dilger JP (2002) The effects of general anaesthetics on ligand-gated ion channels. Br J Anaesth 89:41–51

Dubois BW, Evers AS (1992) 19F-NMR spin-spin relaxation (T2) method for characterizing volatile anesthetic binding to proteins. Analysis of isoflurane binding to serum albumin. Biochemistry 31:7069–7076

Dubois BW, Cherian SF, Evers AS (1993) Volatile anesthetics compete for common binding sites on bovine serum albumin: a 19F-NMR study. Proc Natl Acad Sci U S A 90:6478–6482

Eckenhoff RG (1996) An inhalational anesthetic binding domain in the nicotinic acetylcholine receptor. Proc Natl Acad Sci U S A 93:2807–2810

Eckenhoff RG (1998) Do specific or nonspecific interactions with proteins underlie inhalational anesthetic action? Mol Pharmacol 54:610–615

Eckenhoff RG (2001) Promiscuous ligands and attractive cavities: how do the inhaled anesthetics work? Mol Interv 1:258–268

Eckenhoff RG (2002) Promiscuous ligands and attractive cavities. In: Urban BW, Barann M (eds) Molecular and basic mechanisms of anesthesia. Pabst Science Publishers, Lengerich, p 75

Eckenhoff RG, Johansson JS (1997) Molecular interactions between inhaled anesthetics and proteins. Pharmacol Rev 49:343–367

Eckenhoff RG, Shuman H (1993) Halothane binding to soluble proteins determined by photoaffinity labeling. Anesthesiology 79:96–106

Eger EI, Saidman LJ, Brandstater B (1965) Minimum alveolar anesthetic concentration: a standard of anesthetic potency. Anesthesiology 26:756–763

Elliott JR, Needham D, Dilger JP, Haydon DA (1983) The effects of bilayer thickness and tension on gramicidin single-channel lifetime. Biochim Biophys Acta 735:95–103

Enders A (1990) The influence of general, volatile anesthetics on the dynamic properties of model membranes. Biochim Biophys Acta 1029:43–50

Evans JM (1987) Clinical signs and autonomic responses. In: Rosen M, Lunn JN (eds) Consciousness, awareness and pain in general anaesthesia. Butterworth, London, pp 18–34

Evers AS, Crowder CM (2005) Cellular and molecular mechanisms of anesthesia. In: Barash PG, Cullen BF, Stoelting RK (eds) Clinical anesthesia. Lippincott Williams & Wilkins, Philadelphia, pp 111–132

Ferguson J (1939) The use of chemical potentials as indices of toxicity. Proc R Soc Lond B Biol Sci 127:387–404

Fink BR (1975) Molecular mechanisms of anesthesia. Raven Press, New York

Fink BR (1980) Molecular mechanisms of anesthesia 2. Raven Press, New York

Firestone LL, Alifimoff JK, Miller KW (1994) Does general anesthetic-induced desensitization of the Torpedo acetylcholine receptor correlate with lipid disordering? Mol Pharmacol 46:508–515

Franks NP (2006) Molecular targets underlying general anaesthesia. Br J Pharmacol 147 [Suppl 1]:S72–S81

Franks NP, Jenkins A, Conti E, Lieb WR, Brick P (1998) Structural basis for the inhibition of firefly luciferase by a general anesthetic. Biophys J 75:2205–2211

Frazier DT, Murayama K, Abbott NJ, Narahashi T (1975) Comparison of the action of different barbiturates on squid axon membranes. Eur J Pharmacol 32:102–107

Frenkel C, Duch DS, Urban BW (1990) Molecular actions of pentobarbital isomers on sodium channels from human brain cortex. Anesthesiology 72:640–649

Galla HJ, Trudell JR (1980) Asymmetric antagonistic effects of an inhalation anesthetic and high pressure on the phase transition temperature of dipalmitoyl phosphatidic acid bilayers. Biochim Biophys Acta 599:336–340

Glass PS, Shafer SL, Reves JG (2004) Intravenous drug delivery systems. In: Miller RD (ed) Anesthesia. Churchill Livingstone, Philadelphia, pp 439–480

Hardman JG, Limbird LE, Gilman AG (2001) The pharmacological basis of therapeutics. McGraw-Hill, New York

Harris JW, Jones JP, Martin JL, LaRosa AC, Olson MJ, Pohl LR, Anders MW (1992) Pentahaloethane-based chlorofluorocarbon substitutes and halothane: correlation of in vivo hepatic protein trifluoroacetylation and urinary trifluoroacetic acid excretion with calculated enthalpies of activation. Chem Res Toxicol 5:720–725

Harris RA, Mascia MP, Lobo IA (2002) Sites of anesthetic action on a ligand-gated ion channel. In: Urban BW, Barann M (eds) Molecular and basic mechanisms of anesthesia. Pabst Science Publishers, Lengerich, pp 174–178

Haydon DA, Hladky SB (1972) Ion transport across thin lipid membranes: a critical discussion of mechanisms in selected systems. Q Rev Biophys 5:187–282
Haydon DA, Urban BW (1983) The action of alcohols and other non-ionic surface active substances on the sodium current of the squid giant axon. J Physiol 341:411–427
Haydon DA, Hendry BM, Levinson SR, Requena J (1977) Anaesthesia by the *n*-alkanes. A comparative study of nerve impulse blockage and the properties of black lipid bilayer membranes. Biochim Biophys Acta 470:17–34
Hendry BM, Urban BW, Haydon DA (1978) The blockage of the electrical conductance in a pore-containing membrane by the *n*-alkanes. Biochim Biophys Acta 513:106–116
Hildebrand JH, Scott RL (1964) The solubility of non-electrolytes. Dover Publications, New York
Hille B (2001) Ion channels of excitable membranes. Sinauer Assoc., Sunderland
Hug CCJ (1990) Does opioid "anesthesia" exist? Anesthesiology 73:1–4
Husain SS, Forman SA, Kloczewiak MA, Addona GH, Olsen RW, Pratt MB, Cohen JB, Miller KW (1999) Synthesis and properties of 3-(2-hydroxyethyl)-3-*n*-pentyldiazirine, a photoactivable general anesthetic. J Med Chem 42:3300–3307
Jenkins A, Greenblatt EP, Faulkner HJ, Bertaccini E, Light A, Lin A, Andreasen A, Viner A, Trudell JR, Harrison NL (2001) Evidence for a common binding cavity for three general anesthetics within the GABAA receptor. J Neurosci 21:RC136
Johansson JS, Manderson GA (2002) The effect of aromatic amino acid side-chain structure on halothane binding to four-helix bundles. In: Urban BW, Barann M (eds) Molecular and basic mechanisms of anesthesia. Pabst Sciences Publishers, Lengerich, pp 23–28
Johansson JS, Gibney BR, Rabanal F, Reddy KS, Dutton PL (1998) A designed cavity in the hydrophobic core of a four-alpha-helix bundle improves volatile anesthetic binding affinity. Biochemistry 37:1421–1429
Kaufman RD (1977) Biophysical mechanisms of anesthetic action: historical perspective and review of current concepts. Anesthesiology 46:49–62
Kauzmann W (1959) Some factors in the interpretation of protein denaturation. Adv Protein Chem 14:1–63
Kendig JJ (1981) Barbiturates: active form and site of action at node of Ranvier sodium channels. J Pharmacol Exp Ther 218:175–181
Koblin DD (2005) Mechanisms of action. In: Miller RD (ed) Anesthesia. Churchill Livingstone, Philadelphia, pp 105–130
Lins L, Brasseur R (1995) The hydrophobic effect in protein folding. FASEB J 9:535–540
Lipnick RL (1991) Studies of narcosis: Charles Ernest Overton. Chapman and Hall, London
Little HJ (1996) How has molecular pharmacology contributed to our understanding of the mechanism(s) of general anesthesia? Pharmacol Ther 69:37–58
Mashimo T, Ogli K, Uchida I (2005) Basic and systemic mechanisms of anesthesia. Invited papers of the 7th International Conference on Basic and Systematic Mechanisms of Anesthesia, Nara, Japan, 25–27 February 2005. Elsevier, Amsterdam
Miller KW (1985) The nature of the site of general anesthesia. Int Rev Neurobiol 27:1–61
Miller KW (2002) The nature of sites of general anaesthetic action. Br J Anaesth 89:17–31
Miller KW, Paton WD, Smith EB, Smith RA (1972) Physicochemical approaches to the mode of action of general anesthetics. Anesthesiology 36:339–351
Miller RD (2004) Anesthesia, 6th edn. Churchill Livingstone, Philadelphia
Miller SL (1961) A theory of gaseous anesthetics. Proc Natl Acad Sci USA 47:1515–1524
Mullins LJ (1954) Some physical mechanisms in narcosis. Chem Rev 54:289–323
Nash HA (2002) In vivo genetics of anaesthetic action. Br J Anaesth 89:143–155
North C, Cafiso DS (1997) Contrasting membrane localization and behavior of halogenated cyclobutanes that follow or violate the Meyer-Overton hypothesis of general anesthetic potency. Biophys J 72:1754–1761
Overton E (1901) Studien über die Narkose. Verlag Gustav Fischer, Jena
Pauling L (1961) A molecular theory of general anesthesia. Science 134:15–21

Pohorille A, Cieplak P, Wilson MA (1996) Interactions of anesthetics with the membrane-water interface. Chem Phys 204:337–345
Pope CG, Urban BW, Haydon DA (1982) The influence of *n*-alkanols and cholesterol on the duration and conductance of gramicidin single channels in monoolein bilayers. Biochim Biophys Acta 688:279–283
Raines DE (2005) Cation-π interactions modulate the NMDA receptor inhibitory potencies of inhaled aromatic anesthetics. In: Mashimo T, Ogli K, Uchida I (eds) Basic and systemic mechanisms of anesthesia. Elsevier, Amsterdam, pp 85–89
Rebecchi MJ, Pentyala SN (2002) Anaesthetic actions on other targets: protein kinase C and guanine nucleotide-binding proteins. Br J Anaesth 89:62–78
Reeves DC, Sayed MF, Chau PL, Price KL, Lummis SC (2003) Prediction of 5-HT(3) Receptor agonist-binding residues using homology modeling. Biophys J 84:2338–2344
Rehberg B, Urban BW, Duch DS (1995) The membrane lipid cholesterol modulates anesthetic actions on a human brain ion channel. Anesthesiology 82:749–758
Reves JG, Glass PSA, Lubarsky DA (2000) Nonbarbiturate intravenous anesthetics. In: Miller RD, Cuchiara RF, Miller ED, Reves JG, Roizen MF, Savarese JJ (eds) Anesthesia. Churchill Livingstone, Philadelphia, pp 228–272
Reyes J, Latorre R (1979) Effect of the anesthetics benzyl alcohol and chloroform on bilayers made from monolayers. Biophys J 28:259–279
Richards CD (1980) The mechanisms of general anaesthesia. In: Norman J, Whitwam JG (eds) Topical reviews in anaesthesia. John Wright & Sons, Bristol, pp 1–84
Richards CD, Winlow W (1998) Molecular and cellular mechanisms of general anesthesia. Elsevier, New York
Roth SH, Miller KW (1986) Molecular and cellular mechanisms of anesthetics. Plenum Medical Book, New York
Rubin E, Miller KW, Roth SH (1991) Molecular and cellular mechanisms of alcohol and anesthetics. Ann N Y Acad Sci 625:1–848
Rudolph U, Antkowiak B (2004) Molecular and neuronal substrates for general anaesthetics. Nat Rev Neurosci 5:709–720
Sachsenheimer W, Pai EF, Schulz GE, Schirmer RH (1977) Halothane binds in the adenine-specific niche of crystalline adenylate kinase. FEBS Lett 79:310–312
Sandorfy C (2002) Towards a comprehensive theory of general anesthesia. In: Urban BW, Barann M (eds) Molecular and basic mechanisms of anesthesia. Pabst Science Publishers, Lengerich, pp 66–73
Sandorfy C (2004) Hydrogen bonding and anaesthesia. J Mol Struct 708:3–5
Schapira M, Abagyan R, Totrov M (2002) Structural model of nicotinic acetylcholine receptor isotypes bound to acetylcholine and nicotine. BMC Struct Biol 2:1
Schoenborn BP (1967) Binding of cyclopropane to sperm whale myoglobin. Nature 214:1120–1122
Schoenborn BP, Watson HC, Kendrew JC (1965) Binding of xenon to sperm whale myoglobin. Nature 207:28–30
Scholz A (2002) Mechanisms of (local) anaesthetics on voltage-gated sodium and other ion channels. Br J Anaesth 89:52–61
Seeman P (1972) The membrane actions of anesthetics and tranquilizers. Pharmacol Rev 24:583–655
Sonner JM, Antognini JF, Dutton RC, Flood P, Gray AT, Harris RA, Homanics GE, Kendig J, Orser B, Raines DE, Trudell J, Vissel B, Eger EI (2003) Inhaled anesthetics and immobility: mechanisms, mysteries, and minimum alveolar anesthetic concentration. Anesth Analg 97:718–740
Stanski DR, Shafer SL (2004) Monitoring depth of anesthesia. In: Miller RD (ed) Anesthesia. Churchill Livingstone, Philadelphia, pp 1227–1264
Stevens RJ, Rusch D, Davies PA, Raines DE (2005) Molecular properties important for inhaled anesthetic action on human 5-HT3A receptors. Anesth Analg 100:1696–1703
Tanford C (1980) The hydrophobic effect. Wiley, New York
Tanford C (1997) How protein chemists learned about the hydrophobic factor. Protein Sci 6:1358–1366

Tang P, Xu Y (2002) Large-scale molecular dynamics simulations of general anesthetic effects on the ion channel in the fully hydrated membrane: the implication of molecular mechanisms of general anesthesia. Proc Natl Acad Sci U S A 99:16035–16040

Tang P, Yan B, Xu Y (1997) Different distribution of fluorinated anesthetics and nonanesthetics in model membrane: a 19F NMR study. Biophys J 72:1676–1682

Targ AG, Yasuda N, Eger EI, Huang G, Vernice GG, Terrell RC, Koblin DD (1989) Halogenation and anesthetic potency. Anesth Analg 68:599–602

Terrell RC, Speers L, Szur AJ, Treadwell J, Ucciardi TR (1971) General anesthetics. 1. Halogenated methyl ethyl ethers as anesthetic agents. J Med Chem 14:517–519

Thompson AJ, Price KL, Reeves DC, Chan SL, Chau PL, Lummis SC (2005) Locating an antagonist in the 5-HT3 receptor binding site: a modeling and radioligand binding study. J Biol Chem 280:20476–20482

Tikhonov DB, Bruhova I, Zhorov BS (2006) Atomic determinants of state-dependent block of sodium channels by charged local anesthetics and benzocaine. FEBS Lett 580:6027–6032

Tosteson DC (1969) The molecular basis of membrane function. Prentice-Hall, Englewood Cliffs

Trudell JR (1977) A unitary theory of anesthesia based on lateral phase separations in nerve membranes. Anesthesiology 46:5–10

Trudell JR, Bertaccini E (2002) Molecular modelling of specific and non-specific anaesthetic interactions. Br J Anaesth 89:32–40

Tsuchiya H (2001) Structure-specific membrane-fluidizing effect of propofol. Clin Exp Pharmacol Physiol 28:292–299

Ueda I, Hirakawa M, Arakawa K, Kamaya H (1986) Do anesthetics fluidize membranes? Anesthesiology 64:67–71

Unwin N (2005) Refined structure of the nicotinic acetylcholine receptor at 4A resolution. J Mol Biol 346:967–989

Urban BW (1993) Differential effects of gaseous and volatile anaesthetics on sodium and potassium channels. Br J Anaesth 71:25–38

Urban BW (2002) Current assessment of targets and theories of anaesthesia. Br J Anaesth 89:167–183

Urban BW, Barann M (2002) Molecular and basic mechanisms of anesthesia. Pabst Science Publishers, Lengerich

Urban BW, Bleckwenn M (2002) Concepts and correlations relevant to general anaesthesia. Br J Anaesth 89:3–16

Urban BW, Haydon DA (1987) The actions of halogenated ethers on the ionic currents of the squid giant axon. Proc R Soc Lond B Biol Sci 231:13–26

Urban BW, Frenkel C, Duch DS, Kauff AB (1991) Molecular models of anesthetic action on sodium channels, including those from human brain. Ann N Y Acad Sci 625:327–43:327–343

Urban BW, Bleckwenn M, Barann M (2006) Interactions of anesthetics with their targets: non-specific, specific or both? Pharmacol Ther 111:729–770

Valiyaveetil FI, Leonetti M, Muir TW, MacKinnon R (2006) Ion selectivity in a semisynthetic K+ channel locked in the conductive conformation. Science 314:1004–1007

Vanderkooi JM, Landesberg R, Selick H, McDonald GG (1977) Interaction of general anesthetics with phospholipid vesicles and biological membranes. Biochim Biophys Acta 464:1–18

Wartenberg HC, Wang J, Rehberg B, Urban BW, Duch DS (1994) Molecular actions of pentobarbitone on sodium channels in lipid bilayers: role of channel structure. Br J Anaesth 72:668–673

Wick MJ, Mihic SJ, Ueno S, Mascia MP, Trudell JR, Brozowski SJ, Ye Q, Harrison NL, Harris RA (1998) Mutations of gamma-aminobutyric acid and glycine receptors change alcohol cutoff: evidence for an alcohol receptor? Proc Natl Acad Sci U S A 95:6504–6509

Zakim D (1986) Interface between membrane biology and clinical medicine. Am J Med 80:645–657

Inhibitory Ligand-Gated Ion Channels as Substrates for General Anesthetic Actions

A. Zeller, R. Jurd, S. Lambert, M. Arras, B. Drexler, C. Grashoff, B. Antkowiak, and U. Rudolph(✉)

Abstract General anesthetics have been in clinical use for more than 160 years. Nevertheless, their mechanism of action is still only poorly understood. In this review, we describe studies suggesting that inhibitory ligand-gated ion channels are potential targets for general anesthetics in vitro and describe how the involvement of γ-aminobutyric acid $(GABA)_A$ receptor subtypes in anesthetic actions could be demonstrated by genetic studies in vivo.

1 Introduction

In 1846 the first public demonstration of anesthesia with ether by William T. Morton at the Massachusetts General Hospital in Boston heralded a new era in medical practice, in particular enabling the performance of sophisticated surgical operations that would not be possible without general anesthesia. It was soon discovered that a variety of substances have general anesthetic actions. About a century ago, Meyer

U. Rudolph
Laboratory of Genetic Neuropharmacology, McLean Hospital, Department of Psychiatry, Harvard Medical School, Belmont, MA 02478, USA
urudolph@mclean.harvard.edu

J. Schüttler and H. Schwilden (eds.) *Modern Anesthetics.*
Handbook of Experimental Pharmacology 182.

and Overton independently discovered a strong correlation between anesthetic potency and solubility in oil (Meyer-Overton rule). These observations led to the view that general anesthetics act in the lipid bilayer of the neuronal plasma membrane by an unspecific mechanism (lipid theory). However, Franks and Lieb demonstrated that general anesthetics can interact directly with proteins (protein theory), and that the interaction with proteins also fulfills the predictions of the Meyer-Overton rule (Franks and Lieb 1984). The fact that optical isomers of some anesthetics differ in potency also cannot be explained by a nonspecific action (Franks and Lieb 1994). Moreover, substances have been identified that would be predicted by the Meyer-Overton rule to be anesthetic, but they are in fact not ("non-immobilizers"), and the "long chain alcohol cutoff," i.e., the observation that alcohols that exceed a certain size are inactive, also cast doubt on the lipid theory (Koblin et al. 1994). Today there is ample evidence that anesthetics directly modulate ion channels. These interactions can be both specific and unspecific in nature (Urban et al. 2006).

Over time it became apparent that general anesthetics modulate the activity of ion channels in the membrane of nerve cells at clinically relevant concentrations (Krasowski and Harrison 1999; Yamakura and Harris 2000). With respect to the inhibitory ligand-gated ion channels, it is noteworthy that etomidate, propofol, barbiturates, isoflurane, and sevoflurane significantly increase the activity of γ-aminobutyric acid $(GABA)_A$ receptors at clinically relevant concentrations, while ketamine and nitrous oxide apparently do not modulate the activity of $GABA_A$ receptors to a significant degree at these concentrations. At the glycine receptor, isoflurane and sevoflurane significantly increase glycine-induced chloride currents at clinically relevant concentrations, while propofol, etomidate, barbiturates, and nitrous oxide display smaller effects (Belelli et al. 1999). Ketamine does not modulate the glycine receptor (Krasowski and Harrison 1999). However, one should note that the observation that a certain general anesthetic modulates a specific class of ligand-gated ion channels or a subtype thereof in vitro does not tell us whether this ion channel subtype is responsible for mediating any of the effects of this general anesthetic in vivo. Another caveat is that recombinant systems may not contain receptor-associated proteins that may influence anesthetic sensitivity of a particular receptor.

2 Inhibitory Ligand-Gated Ion Channels: $GABA_A$ and Glycine Receptors

$GABA_A$ receptors are involved in the regulation of vigilance, anxiety, memory, and muscle tension. They are pentameric complexes with six α-, three β-, one δ-, one ε-, one π-, one θ-, and three ρ-subunit genes known. Most $GABA_A$ receptors appear to consist of α-, β-, and γ-subunits, believed to be assembled in a 2:2:1 stoichiometry. Preferred combinations include $\alpha_1\beta_2\gamma_2$ (representing ca. 60% of all $GABA_A$ receptors in the brain), $\alpha_2\beta_3\gamma_2$ (15%), and $\alpha_3\beta_n\gamma_2$ (10%–15%). The subunit combinations $\alpha_4\beta_2\gamma$, $\alpha_4\beta_n\delta$, $\alpha_5\beta_{1/3}\gamma_2$, $\alpha_6\beta_{2/3}\gamma_2$, and $\alpha_6\beta_n\delta$ each represent less than 5% of all receptors in the brain (McKernan and Whiting 1996; Mohler et al. 2002). $GABA_A$ receptors can be found in both synaptic and extrasynaptic locations.

For practical purposes, $GABA_A$ receptors are frequently classified on the basis of their α- and β-subunits as α_n-containing $GABA_A$ receptors and β_n-containing $GABA_A$ receptors, respectively.

Glycine receptors also belong to the family of ligand-gated ion channels. They appear to be particularly prevalent in the brain stem and spinal cord. There are four α-subunits and a single β-subunit known, with receptors comprising α-homomers or αβ-heteromers. Most glycine receptors in adult animals are of the $\alpha_1\beta$ type. Volatile anesthetics such as halothane, isoflurane, and sevoflurane strongly potentiate the glycine-induced chloride currents at clinically relevant concentrations in recombinant systems and also in neurons (Harrison et al. 1993; Downie et al. 1996; Mascia et al. 1996; Krasowski and Harrison 1999), while the potentiation by propofol at clinically relevant concentrations is much smaller, suggesting that if glycine receptors play a significant role in clinical anesthesia, this would likely be restricted to volatile anesthetics (Belelli et al. 1999; Grasshoff and Antkowiak 2004). The enflurane- or isoflurane-induced depression of spontaneous action potential firing in ventral horn interneurons in spinal cord cultures has recently been found to be mediated almost equally by $GABA_A$ receptors and glycine receptors (Grasshoff and Antkowiak 2006). Clearcut in vivo data demonstrating that glycine receptors would mediate specific anesthetic actions are currently unavailable.

As pointed out previously, it has been known for some time that most general anesthetics modulate the activity of $GABA_A$ receptors in vivo at clinically relevant concentrations (Krasowski and Harrison 1999). In vitro studies suggest that ketamine and nitrous oxide do not act via $GABA_A$ receptors (Krasowski and Harrison 1999). $GABA_A$ receptor agonistic actions of ketamine have been proposed based on pharmacological in vivo data (Irifune et al. 2000), but other in vivo studies reported that the $GABA_A$ antagonist gabazine did not block ketamine-induced anesthesia (Nelson et al. 2002; Sonner et al. 2003). It has also been reported that nitrous oxide, tested at a concentration (100%, 29.2 mM) that is higher than that used clinically, increases the efficacy of GABA at recombinant $GABA_A$ receptors (Hapfelmeier et al. 2000). At higher concentrations, some general anesthetics also directly activate the $GABA_A$ receptor in the absence of GABA; the pharmacological relevance of this observation is currently unknown. Since most general anesthetics modulate the activity of a variety of neuronal ion channels, in particular ligand-gated ion channels, it is impossible to draw conclusions from in vitro data as to which neuronal ion channels (or other neuronal targets) mediate clinically relevant actions of general anesthetics.

3 Targeted Mutations in $GABA_A$ Receptor Subunit Genes

3.1 $GABA_A$ Receptor Subunit Knockout Mice

Knockout mice with deletions of specific $GABA_A$ receptor subunits potentially provide a valuable tool for assessing physiological or pharmacological functions of the respective $GABA_A$ receptor subunits. For various reasons this approach has met with variable success. Potential problems include compensatory mechanisms, e.g., upregulation of related subunits, and influence on the expression of neighboring genes due to enhancers in the neomycin expression cassette. This is especially problematic for $GABA_A$ receptor subunits since the genes are arranged in clusters (Uusi-Oukari et al. 2000) and multiple impairments may make it difficult to distinguish primary and secondary effects of a knockout. In mice with a knockout of the β_3 subunit (Homanics et al. 1997) the duration of the loss of the righting reflex in response to midazolam and etomidate–but not to pentobarbital, enflurane, halothane, and ethanol–was reduced compared to wildtype mice, and the immobilizing action of halothane and enflurane, as determined in the tail clamp withdrawal test, was decreased (Quinlan et al. 1998). These results point to a role of β_3-containing $GABA_A$ receptors in the hypnotic and immobilizing actions of the drugs mentioned, but it is also worth noting that when the enflurane-induced depression of spinal cord neurotransmission was examined in spinal cord slices of these mice, it was found that other targets substitute for the role that is normally played by β_3-containing $GABA_A$ receptors (Wong et al. 2001).

In δ-subunit knockout mice, the duration of the loss of the righting reflex was significantly decreased in response to the neuroactive steroid alphaxalone and the neurosteroid pregnenolone, but not in response to midazolam, etomidate, propofol, pentobarbital, and ketamine, indicating the potential involvement of δ-containing $GABA_A$ receptors in the actions of neurosteroidal anesthetics (Mihalek et al. 1999).

Another mouse model that has provided valuable information on targets mediating actions of general anesthetics is the α_5 knockout mouse (Collinson et al. 2002). In α_5 knockout mice, the duration of the loss of the righting reflex in response to etomidate was indistinguishable from wildtype mice, indicating that α_5-containing $GABA_A$ receptors do not mediate the hypnotic action of etomidate (Cheng et al. 2006). It was, however, found that the amnestic action of etomidate in a contextual fear conditioning paradigm and in the Morris water maze (a test for hippocampal learning) are absent in α_5 knockout mice, indicating that these actions of etomidate are mediated by α_5-containing $GABA_A$ receptors (Cheng et al. 2006).

3.2 $GABA_A$ Receptor Subunit Knockin Mice

In an attempt to circumvent some of the problems encountered when studying knockout mice, knockin mice carrying point mutations were generated. These point mutations were designed to alter the sensitivity of the respective receptor subtype to CNS-depressant drugs, while largely maintaining the sensitivity for the physiological neurotransmitter GABA. Even if the mutations are not completely "silent," knockin mice offer substantial insights into the functions of defined $GABA_A$ receptors in the actions of general anesthetics (Rudolph and Mohler 2004).

A conserved histidine residue in the extracellular N-terminal domain of α_1, α_2, α_3, and α_5 subunits is required for binding of classical benzodiazepines like diazepam (Wieland et al. 1992; Kleingoor et al. 1993; Benson et al. 1998). In mice with the $\alpha_1(H101R)$ mutation in the α_1 subunit, diazepam does not reduce motor activity, indicating that the sedative action of diazepam is mediated by α_1-containing $GABA_A$ receptors (Rudolph et al. 1999; Crestani et al. 2000; McKernan et al. 2000). It is noteworthy that in α_1 knockout mice diazepam still decreases locomotor activity, even more strongly than in wildtype mice (Kralic et al. 2002b; Reynolds et al. 2003a), so that studies in knockout and knockin mice would apparently lead to opposing conclusions. Interestingly, L-838,417, a benzodiazepine site ligand that is an antagonist at α_1-containing $GABA_A$ receptors but a partial agonist at α_2-, α_3-, and α_5-containing $GABA_A$ receptors, also has no sedative action (McKernan et al. 2000), confirming the conclusion obtained with the $\alpha_1(H101R)$ knockin mice by two independent groups and suggesting that the strong upregulation of the α_2 and α_3 subunits in the α_1 knockout mice (Sur et al. 2001; Kralic et al. 2002a) makes these mice sensitive to diazepam-induced sedation. Furthermore, α_1 knockout mice have been found to display an increased tonic $GABA_A$ receptor-mediated current in cerebellar granule cells, which is likely due to a reduction of GABA transporter (GAT) activity, which thus might represent another adaptive mechanism (Ortinski et al. 2006). Studies with $\alpha_1(H101R)$ knockin mice also suggest that α_1-containing $GABA_A$ receptors mediate the anterograde amnesic action and in part the anticonvulsant actions of diazepam (Rudolph et al. 1999). The anxiolytic-like action of diazepam is absent in $\alpha_2(H101R)$ mice, indicating that sedation and anxiolysis are mediated by distinct receptor subtypes and can be separated pharmacologically (Low et al. 2000). The myorelaxant action of diazepam, determined in the horizontal wire test, is mediated primarily by α_2-, but also by α_3- and α_5-containing $GABA_A$ receptors (Crestani et al. 2001, 2002).

In pioneering studies using recombinant receptors, amino acid residues in the second and third transmembrane domain of α- and β-subunits have been identified that are crucial for the action of many general anesthetic agents on $GABA_A$ receptors. Sites on both α- and β-subunits have been found to be involved in the action of volatile anesthetics such as enflurane and isoflurane. These include (but are not limited to) α_1-S270, α_1-A291, $\beta_{2/3}$-N265, and $\beta_{2/3}$-M286 (Belelli et al. 1997; Mihic et al. 1997; Krasowski et al. 1998; Siegwart et al. 2002, 2003). In contrast, only sites on the β-subunits have been found to be relevant for the actions of the intravenous anesthetics etomidate and propofol (Belelli et al. 1997; Krasowski et al. 1998). The replacement of an asparagine in position 265 of β_2 or β_3 with methionine [the residue found in the homologous position of the *Drosophila melanogaster Rdl* $GABA_A$ receptor, which is insensitive to etomidate (Pistis et al. 1999)] results in a profound decrease of the modulatory and direct (i.e., GABA-independent) actions of etomidate and propofol (Belelli et al. 1997; Siegwart et al. 2002, 2003). The potency of etomidate is roughly ten times smaller at β_1- compared to β_2- and β_3-containing $GABA_A$ receptors (Hill-Venning et al. 1997). The β_1 subunit contains a serine residue at position 265 that is responsible for this property (Belelli et al. 1997; Hill-Venning et al. 1997). Although the β_2- and β_3-containing $GABA_A$ receptors appear to be the prime targets for etomidate, it cannot be formally excluded that β_1-containing $GABA_A$ receptors still may contribute to the clinical actions of etomidate. Moreover, multiple known [e.g., 11β-hydroxylase, α_2B and α_2C adrenoceptors (Paris et al. 2003)] and potentially also unknown targets for etomidate exist. If a mutation e.g., in the $GABA_A$ receptor β_2 subunit renders the respective $GABA_A$ receptor subtype insensitive to etomidate, one should be careful with the conclusion that any remaining etomidate action is mediated by β_3-containing $GABA_A$ receptors, although this is not unlikely. Furthermore it has been shown recently that $GABA_A$ receptor subtypes containing β_1 and rare subunits such as θ may be sensitive to etomidate. Specifically, recombinant $\alpha_3\beta_1\theta$ $GABA_A$ receptors have a higher efficacy for etomidate compared to $\alpha_3\beta_1$ or $\alpha_3\beta_1\gamma_2$ receptors, although the potency for etomidate was apparently unchanged (Ranna et al. 2006).

4 Studies of General Anesthetic Actions In Vivo

4.1 Intravenous Anesthetics: Etomidate and Propofol

4.1.1 Immobilization and Hypnosis

The first knockin mouse model harboring a $GABA_A$ receptor insensitive to a clinically used general anesthetic was the *β_3(N265M)* knockin mouse (Jurd et al. 2003). In vitro, this point mutation completely abolished the modulatory and direct effects of etomidate and propofol and substantially reduced the modulatory action of enflurane. However, the modulatory action of the neuroactive steroid alphaxalone was preserved (Siegwart et al. 2002). In neocortical slices of *β_3(N265M)* knockin mice, etomidate and enflurane were less effective at decreasing spontaneous action potential firing (Jurd et al. 2003). In hippocampal CA1 pyramidal neurons, the modulatory action of etomidate was reduced, consistent with the β_3 subunit being the predominant, but not exclusive, β-subunit in these cells (Jurd et al. 2003). Motor activity and hot plate sensitivity were unchanged in the absence of drugs (Jurd et al. 2003).

As a measure of the immobilizing action of etomidate and propofol, the hindlimb withdrawal reflex, which is lost in response to these drugs, was studied. The absence of this reflex is indicative of surgical tolerance (Arras et al. 2001). In the *β_3(N265M)* knockin mice the loss of the hindlimb reflex in response to etomidate and propofol that is invariably seen in wildtype mice was absent, indicating that the immobilizing action of these agents is apparently completely dependent on β_3-containing $GABA_A$ receptors (Fig. 1; Jurd et al. 2003). To monitor the hypnotic action of etomidate and propofol, the righting reflex was studied. Etomidate and propofol abolished the righting reflex in wildtype mice. In the *β_3(N265M)* knockin mice the duration of the loss of the righting reflex in response to these drugs was significantly reduced, indicating that the hypnotic action of etomidate and propofol is mediated in part by β_3-containing $GABA_A$ receptors (Fig. 1; Jurd et al. 2003). This essential phenotype of the *β_3(N265M)*

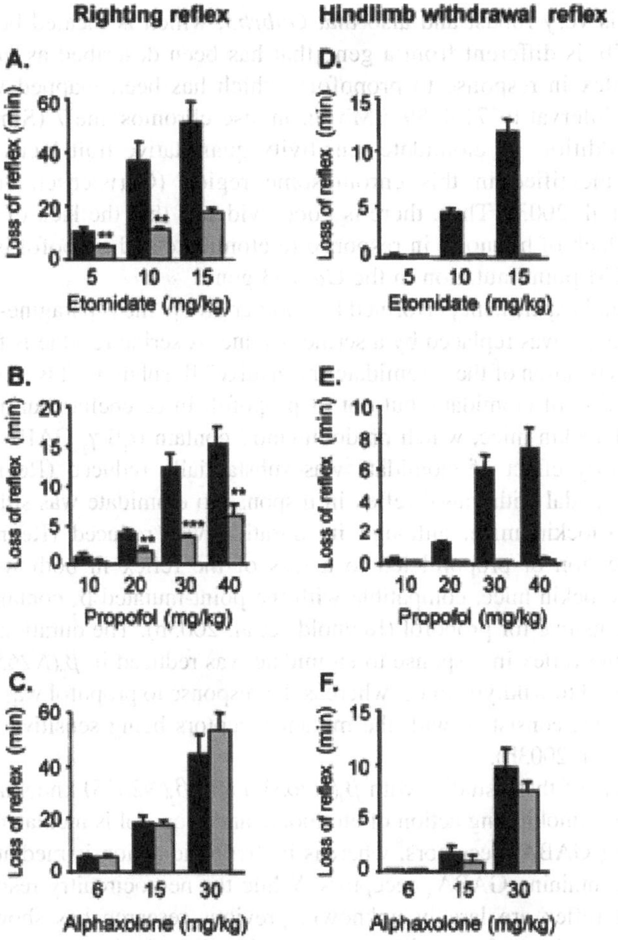

Fig. 1 Behavioral responses to i.v. anesthetics in wildtype and $\beta_3(N265M)$ mice. Reduction in the duration (in minutes) of the loss of righting reflex (LORR) induced by **a** etomidate and **b** propofol in $\beta_3(N265M)$ mice vs wildtype. Etomidate (15 mg/kg) and propofol (40 mg/kg) were lethal for 50% and 58% of the wildtype, respectively, but none of the $\beta_3(N265M)$ mice. **c** Alphaxalone [mixed in a 3:1 ratio with alphadolone, Saffan (Vet Drug, Dunnington, UK)] induced a similar duration (also given in minutes) of LORR in both genotypes. At 30 mg/kg, alphaxalone was lethal in 67% of wildtype mice and 50% of $\beta_3(N265M)$ mice. **d** Etomidate (10, 15 mg/kg) and **e** propofol (20, 30 mg/kg) failed to induce loss of the hind limb withdrawal reflex (LHWR) in $\beta_3(N265M)$ mice in contrast to wildtype mice ($p<0.01$, Fischer's exact test). **f** Alphaxalone (15, 30 mg/kg) induced LHWR with similar duration in $\beta_3(N265M)$ and wildtype mice. All drugs were administered intravenously. Wildtype mice, *black shading*, $\beta_3(N265M)$ mice, *gray shading*. $^{**}p<0.01$, $^{***}p<0.001$, compared with wildtype; median test (n=6–12 per group). (Reprinted with permission from *FASEB Journal*, Jurd et al. 2003)

knockin mice has now been observed on three different genetic backgrounds (129X1/SvJ×129/Sv (87.5%/12.5%) (Jurd et al. 2003), 129X1/SvJ (10 backcrosses), and C57BL/6J (9 backcrosses) (Zeller et al. 2007a), indicating that this phenotype is very robust and also that *Gabrb*3, which is located between 57.4 and 57.7 Mb, is different from a gene that has been described as *lorp*1(loss or righting reflex in response to propofol), which has been mapped with a 99% confidence interval to 71.4–89.7 Mb on mouse chromosome 7 (Simpson et al. 1998); in addition, an etomidate-sensitivity quantitative trait locus (QTL) has also been identified in this chromosome region (Christensen et al. 1996; Downing et al. 2003). Thus, there is good evidence that the lack of immobility and partial lack of hypnosis in response to etomidate and propofol is really due to the N265M point mutation in the *Gabrb*3 gene.

In a parallel experiment performed by another group, the asparagine-265 residue in the β_2 subunit was replaced by a serine residue. A serine residue is found in the homologous position of the "etomidate-insensitive" β_1 subunit. This mutation abolishes the action of etomidate, but not of propofol. In cerebellar Purkinje cells of β_2*(N265S)* knockin mice, which predominantly contain $\alpha_1\beta_2\gamma_2$ $GABA_A$ receptors, the modulatory effect of etomidate was substantially reduced (Reynolds et al. 2003b). The pedal withdrawal reflex in response to etomidate was still present in β_2*(N265S)* knockin mice, although its duration was reduced (Reynolds et al. 2003b). Injection of propofol led to a loss of the reflex in both wildtype and β_2*(N265S)* knockin mice, compatible with the point-mutated β_2-containing receptors being sensitive for propofol (Reynolds et al. 2003b). The duration of the loss of the righting reflex in response to etomidate was reduced in β_2*(N265S)* knockin mice compared to wildtype mice, whereas the response to propofol was identical in both genotypes, consistent with the mutant receptors being sensitive to propofol (Reynolds et al. 2003b).

The results of these studies with β_3*(N265M)* and β_2*(N265S)* knockin mice suggest that the immobilizing action of etomidate and propofol is mediated largely by β_3-containing $GABA_A$ receptors, whereas its hypnotic action is mediated by both β_2- and β_3-containing $GABA_A$ receptors. While the neurocircuitry responsible for the righting reflex are largely unknown, previous research has shown that the immobilizing actions of propofol are mediated at the spinal cord level (Antognini and Schwartz 1993; Rampil et al. 1993; Rampil 1994; Antognini et al. 2000). Thus, it is conceivable that β_3-containing $GABA_A$ receptors in the spinal cord play an important role in mediating the immobilizing action of etomidate and propofol.

Furthermore, the $GABA_A$ receptor antagonists gabazine systemic und picrotoxin increased the ED_{50} for propofol-induced immobilization in rats (Sonner et al. 2003), and the $GABA_A$ receptor antagonist bicuculline antagonized the hypnotic action of propofol (Irifune et al. 2003). While these studies provide strong evidence for an involvement of $GABA_A$ receptors in propofol-induced immobilization, they did not identify which $GABA_A$ receptor subtype would mediate this action. In another study, muscimol (an agonist of the $GABA_A$ receptor at the GABA site), propofol, and pentobarbital, administered intracerebroventricularly, led to a loss of the righting reflex [which these authors termed "sedation" but which in our terminology represents "hypnosis" (see also Rudolph and Antkowiak 2004)]. The actions of these drugs were attenuated by systemic gabazine (Nelson et al. 2002). All three agents were found to increase c-fos staining in the ventrolateral preoptic nucleus (VLPO) and decrease c-fos-staining in the tuberomammillary nucleus (TMN), indicating that they increase neuronal activity in the VLPO and decrease neuronal activity in the TMN, which is an arousal-producing nucleus (Nelson et al. 2002). The VLPO is known to release GABA into the TMN, thus likely causing inhibition of the TMN, which releases histamine in the cortex. Direct injection of muscimol into the TMN results in a loss of the righting reflex, indicating that the action of muscimol in the TMN is sufficient for its hypnotic effect (Nelson et al. 2002). When propofol and gabazine are administered systemically, gabazine, administered into the TMN, reduced the duration of the loss of the righting reflex, indicating that the TMN plays a role in the hypnotic actions of propofol and pentobarbital (Nelson et al. 2002). Since VLPO and TMN are known to be a part of the non-rapid eye movement (REM) sleep-promoting pathway, this work provides an interesting potential connection between anesthesia and sleep.

4.1.2 Sedation

At subanesthetic doses, etomidate decreases motor activity, i.e., exerts a sedative action. This sedative action is observed in *β_3(N265M)* knockin mice (Zeller et al. 2005), but not in *β_2(N265S)* knockin mice (Reynolds et al. 2003b). These results suggest that the sedative action of etomidate is mediated by β_2-containing GABA$_A$ receptors but not by β_3-containing GABA$_A$ receptors. $\alpha_1\beta_2\gamma_2$ is the most abundant GABA$_A$ receptor subtype in the central nervous system (McKernan and Whiting 1996; Mohler et al. 2002). The observations that the sedative action of diazepam is mediated by α_1-containing GABA$_A$ receptors (Rudolph et al. 1999; McKernan et al. 2000) and that the sedative action of etomidate is mediated by β_2-containing GABA$_A$ receptors (Reynolds et al. 2003b) suggest that the $\alpha_1\beta_2\gamma_2$ receptor subtype is the relevant subtype mediating the sedative, i.e., motor depressing actions, of CNS-depressant drugs. It is currently unknown which circuits or neuronal populations are involved in these actions. The observation that general anesthetics reduce activity prominently in cortical networks at sedative concentrations suggests that the cortex might play a prominent role (Hentschke et al. 2005). Etomidate caused impairment of motor performance in a rotating rod test that is indistinguishable between α_5 knockout mice and wildtype mice, which suggests that α_5-containing GABA$_A$ receptors do not mediate the motor impairing action of etomidate in this assay (Cheng et al. 2006).

4.1.3 Hypothermia

At anesthetic doses, etomidate also has a strong hypothermic action. This action is strongly reduced in β_2(N265S) knockin mice (Cirone et al. 2004) and only slightly reduced in β_3(N265M) knockin mice (Zeller et al. 2005), indicating that it is largely mediated by β_2-containing GABA$_A$ receptors and only to a small degree by β_3-containing GABA$_A$ receptors.

4.1.4 Respiratory and Cardiac Depression

When studying the immobilizing actions of etomidate and propofol in *β_3(N265M)* knockin mice and wildtype mice, Jurd and collaborators noticed that high doses of these drugs (etomidate 15 mg/kg i.v., propofol 40 mg/kg i.v.) are lethal for approximately 50% of the wildtype mice but not for *β_3(N265M)* knockin mice. Interestingly, alphaxalone/alphadolone (30/10 mg/kg i.v.) were lethal for approximately 50% of both wildtype and *β_3(N265M)* knockin mice (Jurd et al. 2003). These results suggest that the potentially lethal response is mediated by β_3-containing $GABA_A$ receptors. We hypothesized that either the cardiac depressant action or the respiratory depressant action of these general anesthetics might be responsible for the lethality observed.

In wildtype mice, etomidate and propofol induce a significant decrease in the heart rate. This decrease is also present in *β_3(N265M)* knockin mice, indicating that targets other than β_3-containing $GABA_A$ receptors mediate this effect (Zeller et al. 2005). Heart rate and temperature were determined at the same time. It is possible that the reductions in temperature and heart rate are interrelated and not independent phenomena.

Respiratory depression was assessed by monitoring arterial blood gases (*P*aO_2, *P*aCO_2) and pH values in samples taken from the carotid artery. After application of etomidate or propofol, the *P*aO_2 was significantly higher in *β_3(N265M)* knockin mice and the *P*aCO_2 was significantly lower in *β_3(N265M)* knockin mice compared to wildtype mice (Fig. 2; Zeller et al. 2005). The pH values were significantly higher in *β_3(N265M)* knockin mice compared to wildtype mice (Zeller et al. 2005). In contrast, there was no genotype difference in these parameters after application of a mixture of the neurosteroid anesthetics alphaxalone and alphadolone, demonstrating that *β_3(N265M)* knockin mice respond normally to these agents (Zeller et al. 2005). These results indicate that the respiratory depressant action of etomidate and propofol is largely mediated by β_3-containing $GABA_A$ receptors. Cardiac and respiratory depressant actions of general anesthetics have apparently not been studied in β_2(N265S) mice.

4.1.5 Amnesia

The anterograde amnestic action of propofol was studied in the passive avoidance paradigm and found to be indistinguishable between *β_3(N265M)* knockin mice and wildtype mice, indicating that this effect of propofol is not mediated by β_3-containing $GABA_A$ receptors (Zeller et al. 2007a). Thus, the immobilizing and the anterograde amnestic actions of propofol are mediated by distinct targets. This result is in line with the observation that the anterograde amnestic action of diazepam in the same paradigm is mediated by α_1-containing $GABA_A$ receptors (Rudolph et al. 1999). It is therefore tempting to speculate that the anterograde amnestic action of $GABA_A$ receptor-modulating drugs in

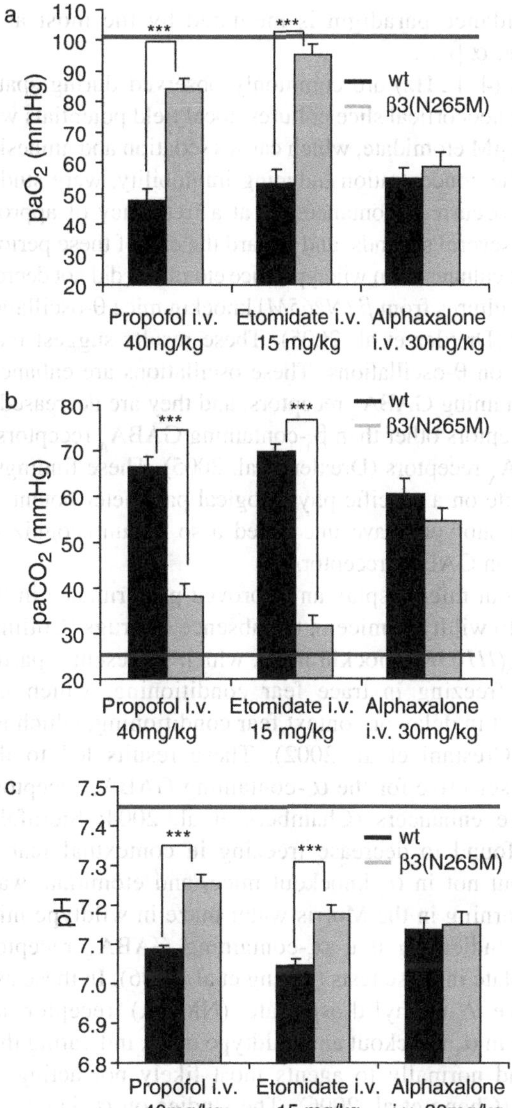

Fig. 2 Assessment of anesthetic-induced respiratory depression by blood gas analysis. **a, b** In *β3(N265M)* mice injected with etomidate and propofol, PaO_2 was higher and $PaCO_2$ was lower compared with wildtype mice, indicating the dependence of the respiratory depressant effects of these anesthetics on β_3-containing $GABA_A$ receptors. The neurosteroid anesthetic alphaxalone (mixed in a 3:1 ration with alphadolone, Saffan), whose action is not affected by the *β_3(N265M)* mutation in vitro, elicits changes in blood gases without a difference between genotypes. **c** Similarly, after etomidate and propofol, but not after alphaxalone, pH was higher in *β_3(N265M)* mice compared with wildtype. The *horizontal bars that span the graphs* indicate normal values. n=10; ***p<0.001. (Reprinted with permission from *FASEB Journal*, Zeller et al. 2005)

the passive avoidance paradigm is mediated by the most abundant $GABA_A$ receptor subtype, $\alpha_1\beta_2\gamma_2$.

θ-Oscillations (4–12 Hz) are commonly observed during spatial learning and memory tasks. In neocortical slice cultures, local field potentials were recorded and the actions of 0.2 μM etomidate, which causes sedation and amnesia and is approximately 15% of the concentration inducing immobility, were studied. Episodes of ongoing activity occurred spontaneously at a frequency of approximately 0.1 Hz and persisted for several seconds, and toward the end of these periods θ-oscillations developed. In slice cultures from wildtype mice etomidate did not depress θ-oscillations, whereas in slice cultures from *β_3(N265M)* knockin mice θ-oscillations were significantly depressed (Drexler et al. 2005). These results suggest that etomidate has opposing actions on θ-oscillations. These oscillations are enhanced by etomidate acting via β_3-containing $GABA_A$ receptors, and they are decreased by the action of etomidate via receptors other than β_3-containing $GABA_A$ receptors, most likely β_2-containing $GABA_A$ receptors (Drexler et al. 2005). These findings of an opposing action of etomidate on a specific physiological parameter potentially via different $GABA_A$ receptor subtypes have uncovered a so far unrecognized complexity of etomidate action on $GABA_A$ receptors.

The α_5 knockout mice display an improved performance in the Morris water maze compared to wildtype mice in the absence of drugs (Collinson et al. 2002). Moreover, the *α_5(H105R)* knockin mice, which represent a partial α_5 knockout, show increased freezing in trace fear conditioning, which is hippocampus-dependent, but not in delay or context fear conditioning, which is not hippocampus-dependent (Crestani et al. 2002). These results led to the concept that inverse agonists selective for the α_5-containing $GABA_A$ receptor would be suitable as cognitive enhancers (Chambers et al. 2004; Sternfeld et al. 2004). Etomidate was found to decrease freezing in contextual fear conditioning in wildtype mice but not in α_5 knockout mice, and etomidate was also found to impair spatial learning in the Morris water maze in wildtype mice but not in α_5 knockout mice, indicating that α_5-containing $GABA_A$ receptors mediate the actions of etomidate in these tests (Cheng et al. 2006). In these assays, ketamine, a noncompetitive *N*-methyl-d-aspartate (NMDA) receptor antagonist, was equally effective in α_5 knockout and wildtype mice, indicating that the α_5 knockout mice respond normally to agents most likely not acting via the $GABA_A$ receptor system (Cheng et al. 2006). The studies on α_5 knockout mice suggest that the amnestic actions of etomidate are mediated at least in part by α_5-containing $GABA_A$ receptors.

4.1.6 Electrocardiography

Etomidate and propofol increased heart rate variability and prolonged intervals in the ECG (RR, PQ, QRS, QT). All these changes are also seen in β_3(N265M) knockin mice, indicating that these are largely independent of β_3-containing $GABA_A$ receptors (Zeller et al. 2007a).

4.2 Barbiturates

In in vitro studies, barbiturates have a wide range of targets, modulating the activity of $GABA_A$ receptors, nicotinic acetylcholine receptors, *S*-alpha-amino-3-hydroxy-5-methyl-4-isoxazolepropionic acid (AMPA) receptors, kainate receptors, and glycine receptors (Krasowski and Harrison 1999), and it is largely unknown which of these ion channels, if any, would mediate the clinical actions of barbiturates. In β_3*(N265M)* knockin mice the barbiturate pentobarbital had no immobilizing action, indicating that the immobilizing action of pentobarbital is mediated by β_3-containing $GABA_A$ receptors (Zeller et al. 2007b). The hypnotic action of pentobarbital is significantly reduced in the β_3*(N265M)* knockin mice, indicating that this action is partially mediated by β_3-containing $GABA_A$ receptors (Zeller et al. 2007b). Thus, with respect to the immobilizing and hypnotic actions, etomidate, propofol, and pentobarbital appear to be dependent on the same drug target, i.e., β_3-containing $GABA_A$ receptors. The respiratory depressant action of pentobarbital was, however, indistinguishable in β_3*(N265M)* knockin mice and wildtype mice, based on the observation that there are no genotypic differences in the PaO_2, $PaCO_2$, and pH values (Zeller et al. 2007b). Thus, the respiratory depressant action of pentobarbital is independent of the β_3-containing $GABA_A$ receptors. How can the observation be explained that while pentobarbital clearly binds to β_3-containing $GABA_A$ receptors and the β_3-containing $GABA_A$ receptors can mediate respiratory depression, pentobarbital is respiratory depressant in β_3*(N265M)* mice? The generation of respiratory rhythms occurs in a network of neurons originating from the pre-Bötzinger complex (Richter et al. 2003). Synaptic interactions involving AMPA, NMDA, $GABA_A$, $GABA_B$, and glycine receptors are thought to play a major role in regulating this network. Etomidate- and propofol-induced respiratory depression is mediated by β_3-containing $GABA_A$ receptors, but it is currently unknown which neurons specifically mediate this effect. The observation that pentobarbital induces respiratory depression in β_3*(N265M)* knockin mice indicates that this effect is not mediated by β_3-containing $GABA_A$ receptors or, if it is to some degree, that pentobarbital can also induce respiratory depression via other, currently unknown targets. Both an increase in the inhibitory GABAergic drive and a decrease in excitatory glutamatergic drive can lead to respiratory depression. It is conceivable that pentobarbital might induce respiratory depression by decreasing the glutamatergic drive. This side effect is thus mediated by different receptors or circuits in etomidate- and propofol-induced anesthesia compared to pentobarbital-induced anesthesia. It is tempting to speculate that this mechanistic difference between etomidate and propofol on one hand and pentobarbital on the other underlies the significantly smaller therapeutic range of barbiturates compared to etomidate and propofol.

The hypothermic action of pentobarbital was slightly but significantly diminished in β_3*(N265M)* knockin mice, indicating that this action is mediated to a small extent by β_3-containing $GABA_A$ receptors, but mostly by other targets (Zeller et al. 2007b). Similarly, the heart rate depressant action of pentobarbital is diminished in β_3*(N265M)* knockin mice, suggesting that this action is mediated both by β_3-containing $GABA_A$ receptors and by other targets (Zeller et al. 2007b). As mentioned previously, we cannot exclude the possibility that the hypothermic action and heart rate depressant action are interdependent.

Pentobarbital increased heart rate variability and ECG intervals (PQ, QT) in both β_3*(N265M)* knockin mice and wildtype mice, suggesting that these actions are largely independent of β_3-containing $GABA_A$ receptors (Zeller et al. 2007b).

4.3 Volatile Anesthetics

The immobilizing action of volatile anesthetics such as isoflurane has been shown to be mediated largely by targets in the spinal cord (Antognini and Schwartz 1993; Rampil et al. 1993; Rampil 1994). The immobilizing response to enflurane, halothane, and isoflurane was moderately decreased in β_3*(N265M)* knockin mice (Jurd et al. 2003; Lambert et al. 2005; Liao et al. 2005) consistent with the hypothesis that the action of these volatile anesthetics are mediated by multiple targets, one of them being β_3-containing $GABA_A$ receptors in the spinal cord. The hypnotic action of these drugs appears to be largely independent of β_3-containing $GABA_A$ receptors (Jurd et al. 2003; Lambert et al. 2005).

A pharmacological study using the $GABA_A$ receptor antagonist picrotoxin suggested that isoflurane-induced immobilization would likely not involve $GABA_A$ receptors (Zhang et al. 2004). This conclusion was largely based on the discrepancy that isoflurane strongly potentiates recombinant $GABA_A$ receptors, in contrast to xenon and cyclopropane, while picrotoxin infusion in the rats increased the EC_{50} for all three anesthetics by approximately 40%. The assumption was that if $GABA_A$ receptors contributed to isoflurane immobilization, picrotoxin should block isoflurane-induced immobilization to a much larger degree than xenon or cyclopropane-induced immobilization. The picrotoxin-induced increase in EC_{50} for xenon and cyclopropane was considered to be unspecific (since the agents apparently do not modulate the $GABA_A$ receptor in vitro), and since the picrotoxin-induced EC_{50} for isoflurane is similar, it was concluded that $GABA_A$ receptors do not mediate isoflurane-induced immobilization. The apparent difference between this study and the study with the knockin mice might be explained by the fact that the pharmacological study may be unable to detect a relatively limited contribution of the $GABA_A$ receptor. Another point to consider is that there is a multitude of $GABA_A$ receptor subtypes, and despite recent advances the exact subunit composition of the $GABA_A$ receptor-mediating immobility is unknown. Thus, the finding that the activity of one or more recombinant $GABA_A$ receptor subtypes is not increased by an anesthetic does not imply that this is true for all $GABA_A$ receptor subtypes expressed in the CNS. Furthermore, recombinant systems lack the natural environment of the $GABA_A$ receptor, and this might have an influence on the responses of this $GABA_A$ receptor to a drug. A recent example of a drug with a discrepancy between its in vitro and in vivo profiles is the anxiolytic ocinaplon, which has no sedative action in humans, but no selectivity for α_2- or α_3-containing $GABA_A$ receptors (which are presumably mediating anxiolysis) over α_1-containing $GABA_A$ receptors (which are mediating sedation) (Lippa et al. 2005).

In neocortical neurons in cultured slices, enflurane at concentrations between minimal alveolar concentration (MAC)-awake and MAC-immobility depresses spontaneous action potential firing. Enflurane blocks inhibitory postsynaptic current decay and decreases peak amplitudes, thus exerting dual prolonging and blocking effects on $GABA_A$ receptors. In slices from *β_3(N265M)* mice, both prolonging and blocking effects were almost absent, indicating that the β_3(N265M) point mutation essentially abolishes both actions and that β_3-containing $GABA_A$ receptors contribute to the depressant action of enflurane (Drexler et al. 2006).

The hypothermic and heart rate depressant actions of isoflurane have also been found to be slightly but significantly inhibited in *β_3(N265M)* knockin mice compared to wildtype mice, suggesting that these actions are mediated mostly by targets other than β_3-containing $GABA_A$ receptors (Zeller et al. 2007a). Isoflurane increased heart rate variability and prolonged ECG intervals (PQ, QRS, QT) in both wildtype and *β_3(N265M)* knockin mice (with the exception that the increase in the QRS interval was not significant in the mutant mice, possibly due to the small number of animals studied), indicating that these effects are mediated by other targets (Zeller et al. 2007a).

4.4 Ethanol

The targets mediating the effects of ethanol at concentrations as they occur after social drinking have not been identified. Attempts are being made to render individual $GABA_A$ receptor subtypes insensitive to ethanol in recombinant systems and in mice.

In recombinant receptors, the *α_1(S270H)* mutation has been shown to convey insensitivity to isoflurane (Borghese et al. 2006b). This mutation also increases the GABA sensitivity (Borghese et al. 2006b). When it is combined with a second point mutation, α_1(L277A), the GABA sensitivity is near normal in heterologous systems, but the maximal current was decreased (Borghese et al. 2006b), with the current decay time constant higher in wildtype than in α_1(S270H:L277A)$\beta_2\gamma_2$ receptors(Borghese et al. 2006b). Recombinant $GABA_A$ receptors containing the double point mutation are essentially insensitive to modulation by high concentrations of ethanol (Borghese et al. 2006b). In hippocampal CA1 pyramidal neurons, 20 mM and 40 mM ethanol (which might be considered to represent concentrations exceeding those seen with "social" drinking with the legal limit for driving in many jurisdictions being 17.4 mM) increased the $GABA_A$ inhibitory postsynaptic current (IPSC) to the same degree in wildtype mice and mutant mice; however, at 80 mM the increase was substantially reduced in the mutant mice compared to wildtype (Werner et al. 2006). Ethanol-induced hypnosis, locomotor stimulation, cognitive impairment, ethanol preference, and ethanol consumption were indistinguishable in mutant and wildtype mice (Werner et al. 2006). *α_1(S270H:L277A)* mice are spontaneously hyperactive (Borghese et al. 2006b). They recover more quickly than wildtype mice from the motor impairing action of ethanol and etomidate, but not pentobarbital (Werner et al. 2006). These studies indicate that α_1-containing $GABA_A$ receptors are involved in only a defined subset of ethanol actions.

In recombinant systems, it has been found that the activity of $GABA_A$ receptors containing α_4(or α_6)β_3(or β_2)δ are enhanced by ethanol concentrations as low as 3 mM, whereas the activity of $\alpha_1\beta_2\gamma_2$ $GABA_A$ receptors are only enhanced by 100 mM ethanol (Sundstrom-Poromaa et al. 2002; Wallner et al. 2003). Other laboratories have been unable to reproduce this finding, suggesting that currently unidentified factors might play a role in ethanol effects at δ-containing $GABA_A$ receptors (Borghese et al. 2006a; Yamashita et al. 2006). Ethanol potently and competitively inhibits binding of the alcohol antagonist Ro15-4513 to $\alpha_4/6\beta_3\delta$ $GABA_A$ receptors (Hanchar et al. 2006), and the low-dose alcohol actions on $\alpha_4\beta_3\delta$ $GABA_A$ receptors are reversed by Ro15-4513 (Wallner et al. 2006), providing further evidence that ethanol might exert some of its effects by interaction with a specific site on a defined $GABA_A$ receptor subtype.

Interestingly, the β_3(N265M) point mutation abolished the effects of high (anesthetic) ethanol concentrations at $\alpha_4\beta_3$(N265M)δ $GABA_A$ receptors, without affecting ethanol enhancement at low doses, suggesting that $\alpha_4\beta_3\delta$ $GABA_A$ receptors have two distinct alcohol modulation sites (Wallner et al. 2006). A R100Q polymorphism in the cerebellar $GABA_A$ receptor α_6 subunit, which increases enhancement of GABA-induced chloride currents in recombinant $\alpha_6\beta_3\delta$ receptors, has been found to enhance granule cell tonic inhibition and to increase alcohol-induced impairment of motor coordination. This suggests that α_6-containing $GABA_A$ receptors in the cerebellum, which are located extrasynaptically, might mediate at least some of the behavioral responses to ethanol (Hanchar et al. 2005).

5 Conclusion

$GABA_A$ receptors have been investigated as molecular targets for the action of a variety of general anesthetics. The intravenous anesthetics etomidate and propofol, as well as pentobarbital, have been shown to exert their immobilizing action and in part their hypnotic action through β_3-containing $GABA_A$ receptors. The proposed roles of β_3-containing $GABA_A$ receptors and other targets for the actions of etomidate and propofol are summarized in Fig. 3. For the immobilizing action of volatile anesthetics, this receptor subtype apparently plays a relatively minor role. While demonstrating a significant role for a specific $GABA_A$ receptors subtype in the action of particular intravenous anesthetics, with respect to volatile anesthetics the data reviewed in this article point to a multisite model of general anesthetic action.

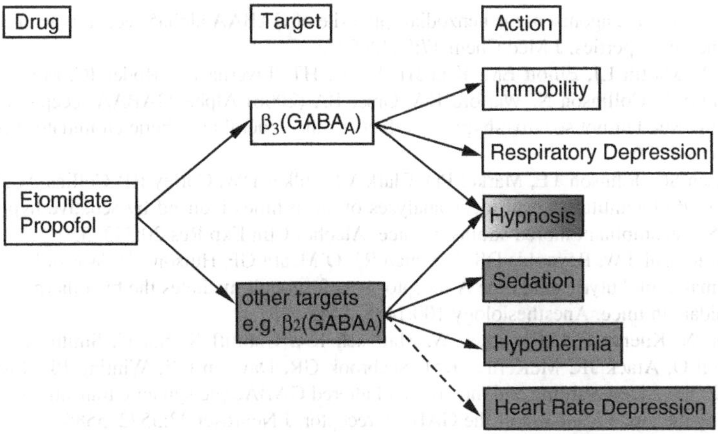

Fig. 3 Proposed roles of etomidate and propofol on $GABA_A$ receptor subtypes. These assignments are based on the following tests: immobility—lost of hind limb withdrawal reflex; respiratory depression—increase in $PaCO_2$ and decrease in PaO_2 and pH; hypnosis—loss of righting reflex; sedation—decrease in motor activity; hypothermia—decrease in core body temperature; cardiac depression—decrease in heart rate. Data are based on this study and previous work. (Reprinted with permission from *FASEB Journal*, Zeller et al. 2005)

References

Antognini JF, Schwartz K (1993) Exaggerated anesthetic requirements in the preferentially anesthetized brain. Anesthesiology 79:1244–1249

Antognini JF, Wang XW, Piercy M, Carstens E (2000) Propofol directly depresses lumbar dorsal horn neuronal responses to noxious stimulation in goats. Can J Anaesth 47:273–279

Arras M, Autenried P, Rettich A, Spaeni D, Rulicke T (2001) Optimization of intraperitoneal injection anesthesia in mice: drugs, dosages, adverse effects, and anesthesia depth. Comp Med 51:443–456

Belelli D, Lambert JJ, Peters JA, Wafford K, Whiting PJ (1997) The interaction of the general anesthetic etomidate with the gamma-aminobutyric acid type A receptor is influenced by a single amino acid. Proc Natl Acad Sci U S A 94:11031–11036

Belelli D, Pistis M, Peters JA, Lambert JJ (1999) General anaesthetic action at transmitter-gated inhibitory amino acid receptors. Trends Pharmacol Sci 20:496–502

Benson JA, Low K, Keist R, Mohler H, Rudolph U (1998) Pharmacology of recombinant gamma-aminobutyric acidA receptors rendered diazepam-insensitive by point-mutated alpha-subunits. FEBS Lett 431:400–404

Borghese CM, Storustovu S, Ebert B, Herd MB, Belelli D, Lambert JJ, Marshall G, Wafford KA, Harris RA (2006a) The delta subunit of gamma-aminobutyric acid type A receptors does not confer sensitivity to low concentrations of ethanol. J Pharmacol Exp Ther 316:1360–1368

Borghese CM, Werner DF, Topf N, Baron NV, Henderson LA, Boehm SL 2nd, Blednov YA, Saad A, Dai S, Pearce RA, Harris RA, Homanics GE, Harrison NL (2006b) An isoflurane- and alcohol-insensitive mutant GABA(A) receptor alpha(1) subunit with near-normal apparent affinity for GABA: characterization in heterologous systems and production of knockin mice. J Pharmacol Exp Ther 319:208–218

Chambers MS, Atack JR, Carling RW, Collinson N, Cook SM, Dawson GR, Ferris P, Hobbs SC, O'Connor D, Marshall G, Rycroft W, Macleod AM (2004) An orally bioavailable, functionally selective inverse agonist at the benzodiazepine site of GABAA alpha5 receptors with cognition enhancing properties. J Med Chem 47:5829–5832

Cheng VY, Martin LJ, Elliott EM, Kim JH, Mount HT, Taverna FA, Roder JC, Macdonald JF, Bhambri A, Collinson N, Wafford KA, Orser BA (2006) Alpha5GABAA receptors mediate the amnestic but not sedative-hypnotic effects of the general anesthetic etomidate. J Neurosci 26:3713–3720

Christensen SC, Johnson TE, Markel PD, Clark VJ, Fulker DW, Corley RP, Collins AC, Wehner JM (1996) Quantitative trait locus analyses of sleep-times induced by sedative-hypnotics in LSXSS recombinant inbred strains of mice. Alcohol Clin Exp Res 20:543–550

Cirone J, Rosahl TW, Reynolds DS, Newman RJ, O'Meara GF, Hutson PH, Wafford KA (2004) Gamma-aminobutyric acid type A receptor beta 2 subunit mediates the hypothermic effect of etomidate in mice. Anesthesiology 100:1438–1445

Collinson N, Kuenzi FM, Jarolimek W, Maubach KA, Cothliff R, Sur C, Smith A, Otu FM, Howell O, Atack JR, McKernan RM, Seabrook GR, Dawson GR, Whiting PJ, Rosahl TW (2002) Enhanced learning and memory and altered GABAergic synaptic transmission in mice lacking the alpha 5 subunit of the GABAA receptor. J Neurosci 22:5572–5580

Crestani F, Martin JR, Mohler H, Rudolph U (2000) Resolving differences in GABAA receptor mutant mouse studies. Nat Neurosci 3:1059

Crestani F, Low K, Keist R, Mandelli M, Mohler H, Rudolph U (2001) Molecular targets for the myorelaxant action of diazepam. Mol Pharmacol 59:442–445

Crestani F, Keist R, Fritschy JM, Benke D, Vogt K, Prut L, Bluthmann H, Mohler H, Rudolph U (2002) Trace fear conditioning involves hippocampal alpha5 GABA(A) receptors. Proc Natl Acad Sci U S A 99:8980–8985

Downie DL, Hall AC, Lieb WR, Franks NP (1996) Effects of inhalational general anaesthetics on native glycine receptors in rat medullary neurones and recombinant glycine receptors in Xenopus oocytes. Br J Pharmacol 118:493–502

Downing C, Shen EH, Simpson VJ, Johnson TE (2003) Mapping quantitative trait loci mediating sensitivity to etomidate. Mamm Genome 14:367–375

Drexler B, Roether CL, Jurd R, Rudolph U, Antkowiak B (2005) Opposing actions of etomidate on cortical theta oscillations are mediated by different gamma-aminobutyric acid type A receptor subtypes. Anesthesiology 102:346–352

Drexler B, Jurd R, Rudolph U, Antkowiak B (2006) Dual actions of enflurane on postsynaptic currents abolished by the gamma-aminobutyric acid type A receptor beta3(N265M) point mutation. Anesthesiology 105:297–304

Franks NP, Lieb WR (1984) Do general anaesthetics act by competitive binding to specific receptors? Nature 310:599–601

Franks NP, Lieb WR (1994) Molecular and cellular mechanisms of general anaesthesia. Nature 367:607–614

Grasshoff C, Antkowiak B (2004) Propofol and sevoflurane depress spinal neurons in vitro via different molecular targets. Anesthesiology 101:1167–1176

Grasshoff C, Antkowiak B (2006) Effects of isoflurane and enflurane on GABAA and glycine receptors contribute equally to the depressant actions on spinal ventral horn neurones in rats. Br J Anaesth 97:687–694

Hanchar HJ, Dodson PD, Olsen RW, Otis TS, Wallner M (2005) Alcohol-induced motor impairment caused by increased extrasynaptic GABA(A) receptor activity. Nat Neurosci 8:339–345

Hanchar HJ, Chutsrinopkun P, Meera P, Supavilai P, Sieghart W, Wallner M, Olsen RW (2006) Ethanol potently and competitively inhibits binding of the alcohol antagonist Ro15-4513 to alpha4/6beta3delta GABAA receptors. Proc Natl Acad Sci U S A 103:8546–8551

Hapfelmeier G, Zieglgansberger W, Haseneder R, Schneck H, Kochs E (2000) Nitrous oxide and xenon increase the efficacy of GABA at recombinant mammalian GABA(A) receptors. Anesth Analg 91:1542–1549

Harrison NL, Kugler JL, Jones MV, Greenblatt EP, Pritchett DB (1993) Positive modulation of human gamma-aminobutyric acid type A and glycine receptors by the inhalation anesthetic isoflurane. Mol Pharmacol 44:628–632

Hentschke H, Schwarz C, Antkowiak B (2005) Neocortex is the major target of sedative concentrations of volatile anaesthetics: strong depression of firing rates and increase of GABAA receptor-mediated inhibition. Eur J Neurosci 21:93–102

Hill-Venning C, Belelli D, Peters JA, Lambert JJ (1997) Subunit-dependent interaction of the general anaesthetic etomidate with the gamma-aminobutyric acid type A receptor. Br J Pharmacol 120:749–756

Homanics GE, DeLorey TM, Firestone LL, Quinlan JJ, Handforth A, Harrison NL, Krasowski MD, Rick CE, Korpi ER, Makela R, Brilliant MH, Hagiwara N, Ferguson C, Snyder K, Olsen RW (1997) Mice devoid of gamma-aminobutyrate type A receptor beta3 subunit have epilepsy, cleft palate, and hypersensitive behavior. Proc Natl Acad Sci U S A 94:4143–4148

Irifune M, Sato T, Kamata Y, Nishikawa T, Dohi T, Kawahara M (2000) Evidence for GABA(A) receptor agonistic properties of ketamine: convulsive and anesthetic behavioral models in mice. Anesth Analg 91:230–236

Irifune M, Takarada T, Shimizu Y, Endo C, Katayama S, Dohi T, Kawahara M (2003) Propofol-induced anesthesia in mice is mediated by gamma-aminobutyric acid-A and excitatory amino acid receptors. Anesth Analg 97:424–429

Jurd R, Arras M, Lambert S, Drexler B, Siegwart R, Crestani F, Zaugg M, Vogt KE, Ledermann B, Antkowiak B, Rudolph U (2003) General anesthetic actions in vivo strongly attenuated by a point mutation in the GABA(A) receptor beta3 subunit. FASEB J 17:250–252

Kleingoor C, Wieland HA, Korpi ER, Seeburg PH, Kettenmann H (1993) Current potentiation by diazepam but not GABA sensitivity is determined by a single histidine residue. Neuroreport 4:187–190

Koblin DD, Chortkoff BS, Laster MJ, Eger EI 2nd, Halsey MJ, Ionescu P (1994) Polyhalogenated and perfluorinated compounds that disobey the Meyer-Overton hypothesis. Anesth Analg 79:1043–1048

Kralic JE, Korpi ER, O'Buckley TK, Homanics GE, Morrow AL (2002a) Molecular and pharmacological characterization of GABA(A) receptor alpha1 subunit knockout mice. J Pharmacol Exp Ther 302:1037–1045

Kralic JE, O'Buckley TK, Khisti RT, Hodge CW, Homanics GE, Morrow AL (2002b) GABA(A) receptor alpha-1 subunit deletion alters receptor subtype assembly, pharmacological and behavioral responses to benzodiazepines and zolpidem. Neuropharmacology 43:685–694

Krasowski MD, Harrison NL (1999) General anaesthetic actions on ligand-gated ion channels. Cell Mol Life Sci 55:1278–1303

Krasowski MD, Koltchine VV, Rick CE, Ye Q, Finn SE, Harrison NL (1998) Propofol and other intravenous anesthetics have sites of action on the gamma-aminobutyric acid type A receptor distinct from that for isoflurane. Mol Pharmacol 53:530–538

Lambert S, Arras M, Vogt KE, Rudolph U (2005) Isoflurane-induced surgical tolerance mediated only in part by beta3-containing GABA(A) receptors. Eur J Pharmacol 516:23–27

Liao M, Sonner JM, Jurd R, Rudolph U, Borghese CM, Harris RA, Laster MJ, Eger EI 2nd (2005) Beta3-containing gamma-aminobutyric acidA receptors are not major targets for the amnesic and immobilizing actions of isoflurane. Anesth Analg 101:412–418

Lippa A, Czobor P, Stark J, Beer B, Kostakis E, Gravielle M, Bandyopadhyay S, Russek SJ, Gibbs TT, Farb DH, Skolnick P (2005) Selective anxiolysis produced by ocinaplon, a GABA(A) receptor modulator. Proc Natl Acad Sci U S A 102:7380–7385

Low K, Crestani F, Keist R, Benke D, Brunig I, Benson JA, Fritschy JM, Rulicke T, Bluethmann H, Mohler H, Rudolph U (2000) Molecular and neuronal substrate for the selective attenuation of anxiety. Science 290:131–134

Mascia MP, Machu TK, Harris RA (1996) Enhancement of homomeric glycine receptor function by long-chain alcohols and anaesthetics. Br J Pharmacol 119:1331–1336

McKernan RM, Whiting PJ (1996) Which GABAA-receptor subtypes really occur in the brain? Trends Neurosci 19:139–143

McKernan RM, Rosahl TW, Reynolds DS, Sur C, Wafford KA, Atack JR, Farrar S, Myers J, Cook G, Ferris P, Garrett L, Bristow L, Marshall G, Macaulay A, Brown N, Howell O, Moore KW, Carling RW, Street LJ, Castro JL, Ragan CI, Dawson GR, Whiting PJ (2000) Sedative but not

anxiolytic properties of benzodiazepines are mediated by the GABA(A) receptor alpha1 subtype. Nat Neurosci 3:587–592
Mihalek RM, Banerjee PK, Korpi ER, Quinlan JJ, Firestone LL, Mi ZP, Lagenaur C, Tretter V, Sieghart W, Anagnostaras SG, Sage JR, Fanselow MS, Guidotti A, Spigelman I, Li Z, DeLorey TM, Olsen RW, Homanics GE (1999) Attenuated sensitivity to neuroactive steroids in gamma-aminobutyrate type A receptor delta subunit knockout mice. Proc Natl Acad Sci U S A 96:12905–12910
Mihic SJ, Ye Q, Wick MJ, Koltchine VV, Krasowski MD, Finn SE, Mascia MP, Valenzuela CF, Hanson KK, Greenblatt EP, Harris RA, Harrison NL (1997) Sites of alcohol and volatile anaesthetic action on GABA(A) and glycine receptors. Nature 389:385–389
Mohler H, Fritschy JM, Rudolph U (2002) A new benzodiazepine pharmacology. J Pharmacol Exp Ther 300:2–8
Nelson LE, Guo TZ, Lu J, Saper CB, Franks NP, Maze M (2002) The sedative component of anesthesia is mediated by GABA(A) receptors in an endogenous sleep pathway. Nat Neurosci 5:979–984
Ortinski PI, Turner JR, Barberis A, Motamedi G, Yasuda RP, Wolfe BB, Kellar KJ, Vicini S (2006) Deletion of the GABA(A) receptor alpha1 subunit increases tonic GABA(A) receptor current: a role for GABA uptake transporters. J Neurosci 26:9323–9331
Paris A, Philipp M, Tonner PH, Steinfath M, Lohse M, Scholz J, Hein L (2003) Activation of alpha 2B-adrenoceptors mediates the cardiovascular effects of etomidate. Anesthesiology 99:889–895
Pistis M, Belelli D, McGurk K, Peters JA, Lambert JJ (1999) Complementary regulation of anaesthetic activation of human (alpha6beta3gamma2L) and Drosophila (RDL) GABA receptors by a single amino acid residue. J Physiol 515:3–18
Quinlan JJ, Homanics GE, Firestone LL (1998) Anesthesia sensitivity in mice that lack the beta3 subunit of the gamma-aminobutyric acid type A receptor. Anesthesiology 88:775–780
Rampil IJ (1994) Anesthetic potency is not altered after hypothermic spinal cord transection in rats. Anesthesiology 80:606–610
Rampil IJ, Mason P, Singh H (1993) Anesthetic potency (MAC) is independent of forebrain structures in the rat. Anesthesiology 78:707–712
Ranna M, Sinkkonen ST, Moykkynen T, Uusi-Oukari M, Korpi ER (2006) Impact of epsilon and theta subunits on pharmacological properties of alpha3beta1 GABAA receptors expressed in Xenopus oocytes. BMC Pharmacol 6:1
Reynolds DS, O'Meara GF, Newman RJ, Bromidge FA, Atack JR, Whiting PJ, Rosahl TW, Dawson GR (2003a) GABA(A) alpha 1 subunit knock-out mice do not show a hyperlocomotor response following amphetamine or cocaine treatment. Neuropharmacology 44:190–198
Reynolds DS, Rosahl TW, Cirone J, O'Meara GF, Haythornthwaite A, Newman RJ, Myers J, Sur C, Howell O, Rutter AR, Atack J, Macaulay AJ, Hadingham KL, Hutson PH, Belelli D, Lambert JJ, Dawson GR, McKernan R, Whiting PJ, Wafford KA (2003b) Sedation and anesthesia mediated by distinct GABA(A) receptor isoforms. J Neurosci 23:8608–8617
Richter DW, Manzke T, Wilken B, Ponimaskin E (2003) Serotonin receptors: guardians of stable breathing. Trends Mol Med 9:542–548
Rudolph U, Antkowiak B (2004) Molecular and neuronal substrates for general anaesthetics. Nat Rev Neurosci 5:709–720
Rudolph U, Mohler H (2004) Analysis of GABAA receptor function and dissection of the pharmacology of benzodiazepines and general anesthetics through mouse genetics. Annu Rev Pharmacol Toxicol 44:475–498
Rudolph U, Crestani F, Benke D, Brunig I, Benson JA, Fritschy JM, Martin JR, Bluethmann H, Mohler H (1999) Benzodiazepine actions mediated by specific gamma-aminobutyric acid(A) receptor subtypes. Nature 401:796–800
Siegwart R, Jurd R, Rudolph U (2002) Molecular determinants for the action of general anesthetics at recombinant alpha(2)beta(3)gamma(2)gamma-aminobutyric acid(A) receptors. J Neurochem 80:140–148

Siegwart R, Krahenbuhl K, Lambert S, Rudolph U (2003) Mutational analysis of molecular requirements for the actions of general anaesthetics at the gamma-aminobutyric acidA receptor subtype, alpha1beta2gamma2. BMC Pharmacol 3:13

Simpson VJ, Rikke BA, Costello JM, Corley R, Johnson TE (1998) Identification of a genetic region in mice that specifies sensitivity to propofol. Anesthesiology 88:379–389

Sonner JM, Zhang Y, Stabernack C, Abaigar W, Xing Y, Laster MJ (2003) GABA(A) receptor blockade antagonizes the immobilizing action of propofol but not ketamine or isoflurane in a dose-related manner. Anesth Analg 96:706–712

Sternfeld F, Carling RW, Jelley RA, Ladduwahetty T, Merchant KJ, Moore KW, Reeve AJ, Street LJ, O'Connor D, Sohal B, Atack JR, Cook S, Seabrook G, Wafford K, Tattersall FD, Collinson N, Dawson GR, Castro JL, MacLeod AM (2004) Selective, orally active gamma-aminobutyric acidA alpha5 receptor inverse agonists as cognition enhancers. J Med Chem 47:2176–2179

Sundstrom-Poromaa I, Smith DH, Gong QH, Sabado TN, Li X, Light A, Wiedmann M, Williams K, Smith SS (2002) Hormonally regulated alpha(4)beta(2)delta GABA(A) receptors are a target for alcohol. Nat Neurosci 5:721–722

Sur C, Wafford KA, Reynolds DS, Hadingham KL, Bromidge F, Macaulay A, Collinson N, O'Meara G, Howell O, Newman R, Myers J, Atack JR, Dawson GR, McKernan RM, Whiting PJ, Rosahl TW (2001) Loss of the major GABA(A) receptor subtype in the brain is not lethal in mice. J Neurosci 21:3409–3418

Urban BW, Bleckwenn M, Barann M (2006) Interactions of anesthetics with their targets: non-specific, specific or both? Pharmacol Ther 111:729–770

Uusi-Oukari M, Heikkila J, Sinkkonen ST, Makela R, Hauer B, Homanics GE, Sieghart W, Wisden W, Korpi ER (2000) Long-range interactions in neuronal gene expression: evidence from gene targeting in the GABA(A) receptor beta2-alpha6-alpha1-gamma2 subunit gene cluster. Mol Cell Neurosci 16:34–41

Wallner M, Hanchar HJ, Olsen RW (2003) Ethanol enhances alpha 4 beta 3 delta and alpha 6 beta 3 delta gamma-aminobutyric acid type A receptors at low concentrations known to affect humans. Proc Natl Acad Sci U S A 100:15218–15223

Wallner M, Hanchar HJ, Olsen RW (2006) Low-dose alcohol actions on alpha4beta3delta GABAA receptors are reversed by the behavioral alcohol antagonist Ro15–4513. Proc Natl Acad Sci U S A 103:8540–8545

Werner DF, Blednov YA, Ariwodola OJ, Silberman Y, Logan E, Berry RB, Borghese CM, Matthews DB, Weiner JL, Harrison NL, Harris RA, Homanics GE (2006) Knockin mice with ethanol-insensitive alpha1-containing gamma-aminobutyric acid type A receptors display selective alterations in behavioral responses to ethanol. J Pharmacol Exp Ther 319:219–227

Wieland HA, Luddens H, Seeburg PH (1992) A single histidine in GABAA receptors is essential for benzodiazepine agonist binding. J Biol Chem 267:1426–1429

Wong SM, Cheng G, Homanics GE, Kendig JJ (2001) Enflurane actions on spinal cords from mice that lack the beta3 subunit of the GABA(A) receptor. Anesthesiology 95:154–164

Yamakura T, Harris RA (2000) Effects of gaseous anesthetics nitrous oxide and xenon on ligand-gated ion channels. Comparison with isoflurane and ethanol. Anesthesiology 93:1095–1101

Yamashita M, Marszalec W, Yeh JZ, Narahashi T (2006) Effects of ethanol on tonic GABA currents in cerebellar granule cells and mammalian cells recombinantly expressing GABA(A) receptors. J Pharmacol Exp Ther 319:431–438

Zeller A, Arras M, Lazaris A, Jurd R, Rudolph U (2005) Distinct molecular targets for the central respiratory and cardiac actions of the general anesthetics etomidate and propofol. FASEB J 19:1677–1679

Zeller A, Arras M, Jurd R, Rudolph U (2007a) Mapping the contribution of beta3-containing GABAA receptors to volatile and intravenous anesthetic actions. BMC Pharmacol 7:2

Zeller A, Arras M, Jurd R, Rudolph U (2007b) Identification of a molecular target mediating the general anesthetic actions of pentobarbital. Mol Pharmacol 71:852–859

Zhang Y, Sonner JM, Eger EI 2nd, Stabernack CR, Laster MJ, Raines DE, Harris RA (2004) Gamma-aminobutyric acidA receptors do not mediate the immobility produced by isoflurane. Anesth Analg 99:85–90

Actions of Anesthetics on Excitatory Transmitter-Gated Channels

G. Akk, S. Mennerick, and J.H. Steinbach(✉)

Abstract Excitatory transmitter-gated receptors are found in three gene families: the glutamate ionotropic receptors, the Cys-loop receptor family (nicotinic and 5HT3), and the purinergic (P2X) receptors. Anesthetic drugs act on many mem-

J.H. Steinbach
Departments of Anesthesiology and Anatomy & Neurobiology and the Neurosciences Program, Washington University School of Medicine, 660 South Euclid Avenue, Saint Louis, MO, 63110 USA
jhs@morpheus.wustl.edu

J. Schüttler and H. Schwilden (eds.) *Modern Anesthetics.*
Handbook of Experimental Pharmacology 182.

bers of these families, but in most cases the effects are unlikely to be related to clinically relevant anesthetic actions. However, the gaseous anesthetics (xenon and nitrous oxide) and the dissociative anesthetics (ketamine) have significant inhibitory activity at one type of glutamate receptor (the NMDA receptor) that is likely to contribute to anesthetic action. It is possible that some actions at neuronal nicotinic receptors may make a smaller contribution to effects of some anesthetics.

1 Introduction and Overview

The overall level of activity in the brain results from the interaction of inhibitory and excitatory inputs, integrated through membrane properties set by voltage-sensitive and intracellular messenger-dependent channels. The transmitter-gated channels whose activation results in excitation in general have channels that allow the passage of monovalent and divalent cations fairly indiscriminately. Both sodium and potassium ions can permeate the open channel so that channel opening results in membrane depolarization, and because calcium ions can often enter there can be a significant calcium flux into the cell. The possible physiological roles for these channels depend on their localization. In the postsynaptic cell, the excitatory transmitter-gated channels can underlie rapid excitatory synaptic transmission and can also mediate longer-term calcium-dependent changes in cell properties. However, the channels are also found on presynaptic boutons. As a result of the high input impedance and small volume of the bouton, the activation of a relatively small number of channels can significantly affect the release of other transmitters. Since either excitatory or inhibitory transmitter release can be modulated, the overall consequences of activation of presynaptically localized excitatory transmitter-gated channels may be complicated and region- (or pathway)-specific.

Overall, clinically used anesthetics affect the function of many excitatory ligand-gated channels. However, the evidence that these effects play an important role in clinically desired effects (including immobility, amnesia, and analgesia) is in most cases equivocal. The clearest example of a clinically relevant effect is the action of some anesthetics on the *N*-methyl-D-aspartate (NMDA) receptor class of glutamate-gated channels. However, the possibility (but not the certainty) exists that other channels are involved in amnesia, analgesia, or some of the significant side effects of anesthetics.

A number of reviews with additional information on this topic have appeared (Franks and Lieb 1998; Dilger 2002; Yamakura et al. 2001; Evers and Maze 2004; Krasowski and Harrison 1999; Sonner et al. 2003).

1.1 Families of Excitatory Transmitter-Gated Channels

There are three gene families containing members that are excitatory transmitter-gated channels: the glutamate receptor family, the Cys-loop receptor family, and the purinergic family. The glutamate receptor family contains the kainate,

S-alpha-amino-3-hydroxy-5-methyl-4-isoxazolepropionic acid (AMPA), and NMDA types of channels. The Cys-loop receptor family contains the excitatory nicotinic receptors and 5HT3 receptors, as well as the major inhibitory transmitter-gated channels (see the chapter by A. Zeller et al., this volume; the $GABA_A$, $GABA_C$, and glycine receptors). The purinergic family contains the P2X ATP-gated channels.

The glutamate receptors are the major class of transmitter-gated channels mediating rapid excitation in the CNS, with AMPA receptors the predominant postsynaptic subtype. Kainate receptors are thought to be critically involved in some brain pathways (e.g., nociception), and may play a role as presynaptic modulators of transmitter release. NMDA receptors mediate many of the relatively long-lived excitatory postsynaptic potentials (EPSPs) (lasting hundreds of milliseconds), which are thought to be important for pattern generation and rhythmic firing. In addition, NMDA receptors are quite permeable to calcium ions, and the influx of calcium is thought to be very important in modulation, including long term potentiation, which may underlie learning and memory in some regions of the brain.

The structure of glutamate receptors is depicted in Fig. 1. The functional receptor is a tetramer of subunits, each of which has an external ligand binding domain and contributes a portion of the channel lining. There are three subtypes of glutamate receptor (AMPA, NMDA, and kainate receptors), and a total of 16 subunits have been identified (AMPA: GluR1–4; NMDA NR1, NR2A–2D, NR3A–3B; kainate: GluR5–7, KA1–2). Not all subunits co-assemble to form receptors; instead there appears to be a set of rules determining which subunits assemble and form hetero-oligomeric receptors that traffic to the surface. Glutamate receptors are expressed on some types of glial cells as well as neurons.

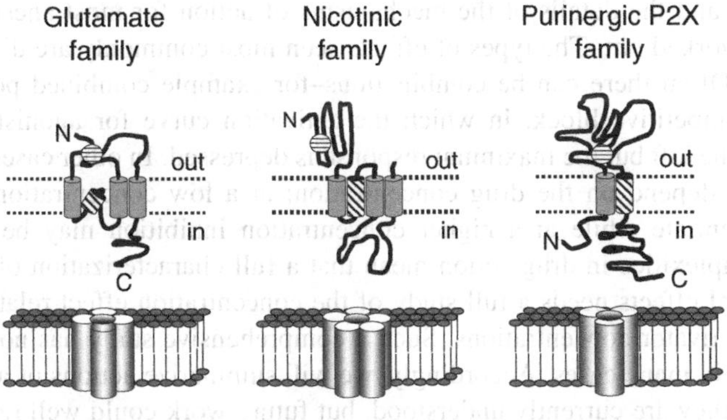

Fig. 1 Cartoon views of the structures of individual subunits (*top row*) and the organization of subunits in a functional receptor (*bottom row*) are shown for the three gene families discussed. In the subunit structures the amino (*N*) and carboxy (*C*) termini are indicated, as well as the approximate membrane location (*dashed lines*; *out* indicates extracellular). The *cylinders* represent helices, and the *diagonally crosshatched helices* indicate the major channel-lining portions. The *hatched circles* indicate the general location of regions important for transmitter binding. In the *lower panels*, note that glutamate receptors form as tetramers of subunits, nicotinic family members as pentamers, and P2X receptors as trimers

Members of the Cys-loop receptor family assemble as pentamers (Fig. 1). It seems that the nicotinic and 5HT3 receptor subunits do not mingle in a receptor. Among nicotinic receptor subunits a variety of combinations has been observed, both in terms of expressed recombinant receptors and in vivo. In the CNS, the α_2–α_6 receptors can assemble with the β_2–β_4 subunits, apparently usually with three α-subunits and two β-subunits. The α_7 subunits form homopentamers. The α_9 and α_{10} receptors co-assemble, particularly in the auditory system (the α_8 subunit has only been described from chicken brain, not mammalian). In the periphery, the muscle fiber expresses a receptor comprising α_1, β_1, δ, and ε (adult type) subunits, while a major type of receptor found postsynaptically on ganglionic neurons contains the α_3, α_5, and β_4 subunits. Nicotinic receptors are also expressed on chromaffin cells and a number of nonexcitable cells, including sperm and cells of the immune system, where they could be involved in some side effects of clinically used drugs. Only two subunits have been identified for 5HT3 receptors, 5HT3A and 5HT3B. In addition to being expressed in the central and peripheral nervous systems, 5HT3 receptors are expressed on enterochromaffin cells of the gut, and so may be involved in some gastrointestinal responses.

The ATP-gated P2X receptors assemble as trimers (Fig. 1). Seven subunits have been identified (P2X1 through P2X7), and it is clear that at least some combine to form heterotrimers. In addition to neurons, P2X receptors are expressed on microglia (where they may play a role in chronic pain), mast cells, and macrophages.

1.2 Pharmacology

Many studies of anesthetic actions involve examination only of whole cell responses, and the details of the mechanisms of action for most anesthetics are not fully worked out. The types of effects seen most commonly are diagrammed in Fig. 2. Often there can be combinations–for example combined potentiation and noncompetitive block, in which the activation curve for agonist action is shifted to the left but the maximum response is depressed. In other cases, the drug action can depend on the drug concentration: at a low concentration the drug might potentiate while at a higher concentration inhibition may be manifest. These complexities in drug action mean that a full characterization of the pharmacological effects needs a full study of the concentration effect relationship at multiple activator concentrations. Such a comprehensive study has not yet been performed in many cases. Accordingly, we will summarize actions of anesthetics insofar as they are currently understood, but future work could well reveal additional effects. Probably the most complete mechanistic analyses have been made for anesthetic actions on the muscle-type nicotinic receptor, although glutamate receptors have also been well studied for some drugs, so more mechanistic detail will be provided for those receptor types.

A nagging question in attempting to relate effects on target proteins, studied in vitro, to clinically relevant actions is relating drug concentrations in vitro to possible

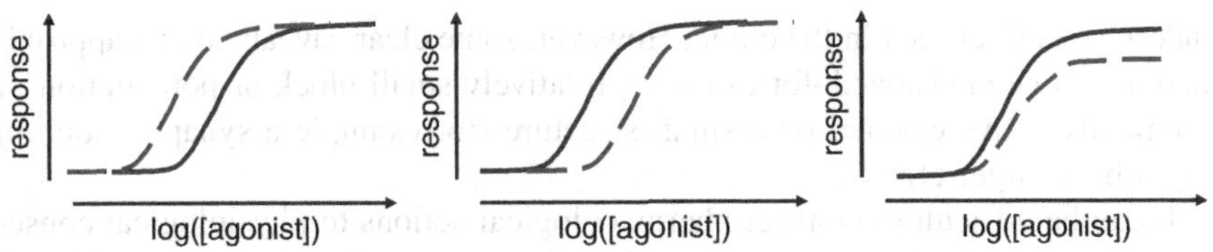

Fig. 2 Three typical patterns of anesthetic action on the agonist concentration-response curve are shown. In the *left panel*, potentiation shows as a left shift in the activation curve, without change in the maximum response for the natural transmitter. In the *middle panel*, (pseudo)-competitive inhibition shows a right shift in the activation curve with no change in the maximum response. In most cases which have been studied, the interaction between agonist and anesthetic does not involve true competitive inhibition of binding of the agonist to the receptor, but appears to reflect negative allosteric interactions. In the *right panel*, noncompetitive inhibition results in a decrease in the maximum response without a change in the position of the activation curve

Table 1 This table gives published estimates for the free concentration of anesthetic at clinically effective doses (the clinically effective concentration, or CEC). These concentrations are assembled from various sources and compiled in the cited references, which should be consulted for details

Anesthetic	CEC	Class	Source
N_2O	105%	Gas	Evers and Crowder 2001
Xenon	71%	Gas	Evers and Crowder 2001
Alphaxalone	0.46 μM	IV	Sewell and Sear 2004
Etomidate R(+)	1.0 μM	IV	Sewell and Sear 2004
Ketamine S(+)	4.3 μM	IV	Sewell and Sear 2004
Pentobarbital	20 μM	IV	Franks and Lieb 1994
Propofol	1.6 μM	IV	Sewell and Sear 2004
Thiopental	25 μM	IV	Franks and Lieb 1994
Enflurane	600 μM	Volatile	Franks and Lieb 1994
Halothane	250 μM	Volatile	Franks and Lieb 1994
Isoflurane	300 μM	Volatile	Franks and Lieb 1994
Sevoflurane	300 μM	Volatile	Violet et al. 1997

concentrations in the effect compartment in vivo. We will use the concentrations shown in Table 1, applied in saline solutions in vitro, as relatively close to estimated effective free concentrations producing surgical levels of anesthesia in vivo. Another question is how to relate an action observed in vitro to a possibly clinically relevant effect (see Eger et al. 2001). For example, a small reduction in voltage-gated sodium current can have a major effect on calcium entry into nerve terminals and so produce a large reduction in evoked release as a result of the very nonlinear relationship between intracellular calcium and release (Wu et al. 2004). However, for the majority of the transmitter-gated channel responses the cellular response is much more linearly related to receptor function. Accordingly, as a first approximation it seems reasonable to assume that a small effect (less than a twofold enhancement or reduction of response) at a clinically appropriate concentration suggests that a particular drug–target interaction is less likely to underlie an effect seen in the clinic. However, some clear caveats to this approximation can be envisioned–for example, relatively small block or potentiation of a tonically active channel on a small structure (for example a synaptic bouton) might have larger effects.

It can be difficult to connect pharmacological actions to physiological consequences because both steady-state and time-dependent actions must be considered. As an example, a drug that inhibited a receptor both when the channel was closed and when it was open would be expected to block rapid synaptic responses and slower responses equally. However, a drug that only blocked receptors with open channels would have a smaller effect on the peak of a rapid response and a larger effect on relatively slow responses. The dissociative anesthetic, ketamine, is an interesting example because it seems to block open channels (and so produces relatively little effect on the first response), but then becomes trapped in the channel. This trapping results in the steady accumulation of blocked channels and a steady increase in inhibition of both rapid and slow responses. Potentiation, in general, is most effective on small responses. This is because, in all examples studied to date, the mechanism for potentiation is to increase the probability a channel is open at a given dose of agonist. For receptors activated by the natural transmitters, at a high agonist concentration the channel already has a very high probability of being open. Hence, even though a drug may potentiate a response to a high concentration from 95% to 96%, the effect will not be observable. However, at a low concentration of transmitter a channel may have a probability of being open of only 3%, and the same concentration of drug may increase that to 30% (a tenfold potentiation).

2 Glutamate Receptors

2.1 Glutamate Receptor Overview

Glutamate receptors are the major excitatory transmitter-gated channels in the CNS. The three classes of ionotropic glutamate receptors serve different functions in the CNS. AMPA receptors (AMPAR) mediate most of the rapid, conventional point-to-point neurotransmission between presynaptic neurons and their postsynaptic targets. NMDA (NMDAR) and kainate (KAR) receptors, in contrast, generally mediate somewhat slower excitatory communication among neurons. These receptors differ from AMPAR in their biophysical properties and cellular localization and thereby sculpt excitatory transmission in ways that AMPAR alone presumably would be incapable of achieving. Extensive reviews of the basic properties of glutamate receptors have been published and should be consulted for more information (Mayer 2005; Mayer and Armstrong 2004; Lerma 2006; Huettner 2003; Dingledine et al. 1999; Palmer et al. 2005). Some of the most exciting work in the glutamate receptor field comes from structural studies of receptors (Madden 2002; Mayer and Armstrong 2004; Wollmuth and Sobolevsky 2004; Mayer 2005). It seems likely that detailed structural models will aid the effort to identify anesthetic binding sites.

AMPAR form as tetramers of GluR1–4 subunits, and native receptors are typically composed of more than one type of subunit. The properties of the receptors depend on the subunit composition, and AMPA receptor subunit transcripts also undergo alternative splicing, with splice variants exhibiting different deactivation and desensitization kinetics (Dingledine et al. 1999). Clusters of AMPAR are located immediately opposite presynaptic active zones of glutamate synapses and are thus reliably and rapidly activated by a vesicle of glutamate. At individual glutamatergic synaptic contacts, a few tens of AMPAR are activated by each glutamate vesicle. The response develops rapidly (~200 μs) and also decays rapidly (2–12 ms), depending heavily on the properties of the particular AMPAR at the synapse. In a typical neuron the peak postsynaptic current produced by a single vesicle of glutamate will be insufficient to depolarize the membrane potential beyond spike threshold, so synchronous release of several glutamate transmitter packets is usually needed to discharge the postsynaptic neuron.

NMDAR share topology and some molecular similarity with AMPAR. NMDAR require the NR1 subunit for a functional channel. The NR1 subunit combines with NR2A, -2B, -2C, or -2D, or with NR3A or -3B subunits. NMDAR exhibit significant permeability for Ca^{2+} and also strong, voltage-dependent block by Mg^{2+}. There are several splice variants of NR1, which can differentially affect trafficking and function of the receptor (Mu et al. 2003), and the subunit composition dictates important properties such as deactivation kinetics and Mg^{2+} sensitivity of the channel (Dingledine et al. 1999). Like AMPAR, NMDAR cluster at synaptic junctions in the CNS and respond to synaptic glutamate. However, because of their strong, voltage-dependent channel block by Mg^{2+}, NMDAR-mediated excitatory postsynaptic currents (EPSCs) are not observed, or are very small, during isolated synaptic activation. Instead, NMDAR channels pass ions only when the postsynaptic cell is strongly depolarized, usually by preceding AMPA receptor-mediated EPSPs. Once activated, NMDAR responses mediate Ca^{2+} influx (in addition to Na^{+} influx). Because Ca^{2+} is an important second messenger, NMDAR activation can result in Ca^{2+}-dependent intracellular biochemical cascades (e.g., protein phosphorylation) that alter cell properties, including function of the synapse itself. A particular case is the NMDAR-dependent induction of long-term potentiation, a phenomenon that is a leading candidate as the cellular substrate for memory formation. NMDAR-mediated EPSCs are also notable for their longevity. After liberation from a synaptic vesicle, glutamate in the synaptic cleft reaches concentrations over 1 mM, but the concentration collapses very quickly (<1 ms) due to diffusion and active uptake. Both AMPAR and NMDAR are activated by this very transient bolus of glutamate. Although AMPA receptor EPSCs decay in a few milliseconds, NMDA receptor currents last for several hundred milliseconds. The difference arises from inherent differences in the deactivation kinetics of the two receptor classes (Lester et al. 1990). The activation and deactivation properties of NMDAR can support cellular bursting properties in some neurons; thus NMDA receptor activation participates in rhythmic behaviors in spinal and other cell types (Dale 1986; however, see Cowley et al. 2005). It is also notable that NMDAR possess a higher equilibrium affinity for glutamate than AMPAR. Therefore, receptors outside the synapses in extrasynaptic regions of the postsynaptic cell can be activated by the levels of glutamate that spill beyond the synaptic borders. Extrasynaptic spillover of glutamate onto NMDAR may therefore influence cell excitability under conditions of high neuronal activity or diminished glutamate transporter activity, which normally helps limit the spread of extrasynaptic glutamate (Kullmann 2000).

KAR assemble from homomeric or heteromeric combinations of GluR5–7. In addition KA1 and KA2 subunits can partner with GluR5–7 subunits but are unable, by themselves, to form channels. RNA splicing again imparts an additional level of diversity (Dingledine et al. 1999). KAR are expressed rather ubiquitously, but understanding of their function has lagged that of other ionotropic glutamate receptors because selective pharmacological tools were lacking. Recently, the use of more selective tools and knockout mice has begun to make KAR function clearer. KAR are found both postsynaptically and presynaptically, and both synaptically and extrasynaptically. KAR can participate in EPSCs at certain synapses, including some pain pathways (Li et al. 1999) and certain retinal visual pathways (DeVries and Schwartz 1999). In most cases the kainate EPSC is small, and its time course is intermediate between fast AMPAR and slow NMDAR EPSCs. KAR on presynaptic terminals and axons can regulate release of both glutamate and γ-aminobutyric acid (GABA) (Huettner 2003). In summary, the function of KAR may be seen as more modulatory than either AMPAR or NMDAR, fine-tuning aspects of synaptic transmission through both presynaptic and postsynaptic mechanisms. Table 2 provides a summary of studies examining anesthetic actions on glutamate receptors.

2.2 Gaseous Anesthetics: N_2O and Xe

Nitrous oxide robustly inhibits NMDAR at concentrations relevant to anesthetic mechanisms (Jevtovic-Todorovic et al. 1998; Mennerick et al. 1998; Yamakura and Harris 2000). The mechanism is noncompetitive with respect to agonist, but little else is known about it. N_2O also mildly inhibits both native (Mennerick et al. 1998) and recombinant GluR2-containing AMPAR (Yamakura and Harris 2000).

Evidence clearly indicates that Xe inhibits NMDAR, but the evidence for its effects on other glutamate receptors is more mixed. Some reports suggest little effect of Xe on AMPAR at concentrations that markedly inhibit NMDAR (Franks et al. 1998). The antagonism of NMDAR by Xe, but not that by N_2O, was diminished by a point mutation in the transmembrane region 3 (abbreviated TM3) of NR1 and a point mutation in TM4 of NR2A (Ogata et al. 2006). These mutations are notable because they also reduce ethanol antagonism of NMDAR.

Even milder inhibition is observed at KAR at these concentrations (Yamakura and Harris 2000). These studies have recently been challenged by a study that found strong effects of Xe on AMPAR and KAR (Dinse et al. 2005). Also, in the invertebrate *Caenorhabditis elegans*, Xe has its major actions through effects on a non-NMDA glutamate receptor (Nagele et al. 2005).

Table 2 Actions of selected anesthetic drugs on glutamate receptors. The top row gives anesthetic and clinically effective concentration (in volume % or in micromolar from Table 1). The first column gives receptor examined, either as cell type or recombinant receptors expressed. The entries give the normalized effect observed (e.g., 1.6 means the current is increased to 1.6 times the control of agonist alone, while 0.6 means it is reduced to 0.6 times control), followed by the concentration of drug (micromolar or volume %). For many blocking drugs a complete concentration–effect curve has been obtained, in which case the concentration producing half maximal block is given in bold. In essentially all cases block was reported or assumed to be complete at high drug concentrations. The notation n.e. indicates that the study found no significant effect of the drug at the concentration given. Where possible, the approximate effective concentration of agonist is given in parentheses (for example EC_{10} means that an agonist concentration eliciting approximately 10% of the maximal response was used). EPSC indicates that the drug was tested against post-synaptic currents, while ukn indicates that the effective concentration is not known. Agonist EC values were taken from previous work (Patneau and Mayer 1990; Yamakura and Harris 2000)

Receptor type	Xe (71%)	N_2O (105%)	Halothane (250 μM)	Isoflurane (300 μM)	Propofol (1.5 μM)	Etomidate (1.5 μM)	Pentobarbital (20 μM)	Ketamine (5 μM)	Reference
Hippocampal AMPA	1.0, 60% (EPSCs)	–	–	**1200** (EPSCs)	–	–	–	–	De Sousa et al. 2000
Cortical AMPA	0.5, 60% (EC_{50}–EC_{90})	–	–	–	–	–	–	–	Dinse et al. 2005
Hippocampal AMPA	–	0.7, 80% (EC_{20}, EPSCs)	–	–	–	–	–	–	Mennerick et al. 1998
GluR1/2	–	0.8, 100% (EC_{50})	–	0.9, 150 (EC_{50})	–	–	–	–	Yamakura and Harris 2000
GluR1/GluR2	–	–	0.8, 500 (ukn)	0.8, 500 (ukn)	–	n.e., 10 (ukn)	–	–	Yamakura et al. 2001
Cortical AMPA	–	–	–	–	–	–	**50**[a] (EC_{20})	–	Marszalec and Narahashi 1993
AMPA w/ GluR2	–	–	–	–	–	–	**200** (EC_{50})	–	Taverna et al. 1994
AMPA w/o GluR2	–	–	–	–	–	–	**1500** (EC_{50})	–	Taverna et al. 1994
AMPA w/ GluR2	–	–	–	–	–	–	**45** (EC_{50})	–	Yamakura et al. 1995b
GluR1–2	–	–	–	–	n.e., 50 (EC_{50})	–	–	–	Yamakura et al. 1995a

(continued)

Table 2 (continued)

Receptor type	Xe (71%)	N_2O (105%)	Halothane (250 µM)	Isoflurane (300 µM)	Propofol (1.5 µM)	Etomidate (1.5 µM)	Pentobarbital (20 µM)	Ketamine (5 µM)	Reference
AMPA GluR 2/3, GluR3	–	–	–	n.e., 600 (EC_{90})	–	–	–	–	Dildy-Mayfield et al. 1996
Neuronal AMPA/KA	–	–	–	–	–	–	–	n.e., 10 (EC_{80})	MacDonald et al. 1987
Hippocampal NMDA	0.3, 60% (EPSC)	–	–	0.75, 310 (EPSC)	–	–	–	–	De Sousa et al. 2000
NR1a/NR2A	0.7, 100% (EC_{50})	0.7, 100% (EC_{50})	–	0.85, 150 (EC_{50})	–	–	–	–	Yamakura and Harris 2000
Hippocampal NMDA	–	0.3, 80% (EC_{50})	–	–	–	–	–	–	Jevtovic-Todorovic et al. 1998
NR1/NR2A	–	–	n.e., 50 (ukn)	0.8, 600 (ukn)	–	n.e., 10 (ukn)	n.e., 100 (ukn)	–	Yamakura et al. 2001
Cortical NMDA	–	–	–	0.5, 300 (EC_{90})	–	–	–	–	Ming et al. 2001
NR1/2A, NR1/2B	–	–	–	–	n.e., 50 (EC_{90})	–	–	–	Yamakura et al. 1995a
Neuronal NMDA	–	–	–	–	–	–	–	**9** (EC_{90})	MacDonald et al. 1987
GluR6	0.5, 60% (EC_{50})	–	–	–	–	–	–	–	Dinse et al. 2005
GluR6/KA2	–	0.82, 60% (EC_{50})	–	1.2, 150 (EC_{50})	–	–	–	–	Yamakura and Harris 2000
GluR5	–	–	3.8, 2000 (EC_{100})	2.5, 2000 (EC_{100})	–	–	0.85, 100 (EC_{100})	–	Minami et al. 1998

GluR6	–	–	2.1, 2000 (EC_{50})	1.5, 2000 (EC_{50})	–	–	0.65, 100 (1 μM KA)	–	Minami et al. 1998
GluR6	–	–	1.4, 250[b] (EC_5)	1.4, 500 (EC_5)	–	–	–	–	Dildy-Mayfield et al. 1996
GluR6	–	–	–	–	1.3, 30 (ukn)	–	–	–	Harris et al. 1995
GluR6/KA2	–	–	–	–	n.e., 50 (EC_{100})	–	–	–	Yamakura et al. 1995a
GluR6/KA2	–	–	–	–		n.e., 10 (ukn)	0.8, 100 (ukn)	n.e., 100 (ukn)	Yamakura et al. 2001

[a]Use-dependent, so the extent of block is dependent on time and agonist concentration

[b]Effects were stronger with pre-incubation

Table 3 Actions of selected anesthetic drugs on nicotinic receptors. The data are presented as in Table 2. Effective concentrations taken from the reference cited

Receptor type	Xe (71%)	N_2O (105%)	Isoflurane (300 μM)	Propofol (1.5 μM)	Etomidate (1.5 μM)	Pentobarbital (20 μM)	Alphaxalone (0.5 μM)	Ketamine (5 μM)	Reference
α2β2, human	–	–	–	–	–	–	–	**92** (~EC_{45})	Yamakura et al. 2000
α2β4, human	–	–	–	–	–	–	–	**29** (~EC_{45})	Yamakura et al. 2000
α3β2, human	–	–	–	–	–	–	–	**50** (~EC_{45})	Yamakura et al. 2000
α3β4, human	–	–	–	–	–	–	–	**9.5** (~EC_{45})	Yamakura et al. 2000
α4β2, chick	–	–	–	–	–	–	–	**50** (EC_{100})	Coates and Flood 2001
α4β2, chick	–	–	**85** (EC_{50})	**19** (EC_{50})	–	–	–	–	Flood et al. 1997
α4β2, human	–	–	–	–	–	–	–	**72** (~EC_{45})	Yamakura et al. 2000
α4β2, human	–	–	**67** (EC_{90})	–	–	–	–	–	Yamashita et al. 2005
α4β2, rat	–	–	**34** (EC_{50})	–	–	–	–	–	Violet et al. 1997
α4β2, rat	0.6, 46% (EC_{50})	0.6, 58% (EC_{50})	–	–	–	–	–	–	Yamakura and Harris 2000
α4β4, chick	–	–	–	–	**33** (EC_{100})	–	–	**0.24** (EC_{100})	Flood and Krasowski 2000
α4β4, human	–	–	–	–	–	–	–	**18** (~EC_{45})	Yamakura et al. 2000
α4β4, rat	0.9, 46% (EC_{50})	0.9, 58% (EC_{50})	–	–	–	–	–	–	Yamakura and Harris 2000
α7, chick	–	–	–	–	–	–	–	**20** (EC_{100})	Coates and Flood 2001
α7, chick	–	–	n.e., 640 (EC_{100})	n.e., 400 (EC_{100})	–	–	–	–	Flood et al. 1997
α7, human	0.5, 100% (EC_{30})	0.7, 100% (EC_{30})	–	–	–	–	–	–	Suzuki et al. 2003
α3,5,7; β4, bovine chromaffin	–	–	–	–	**23** (ukn)	–	–	–	Charlesworth and Richards 1995
α3,5,7; β4, bovine chromaffin	–	–	–	–	–	–	**30** (ukn)	–	Shiraishi et al. 2002

α3,4,7; β2, rat intra–cardiac neurons	–	–	–	–	–	0.6, 50 (ukn)	–	–	Weber et al. 2005
α1β1γδ, chick muscle	–	–	–	–	–	–	**6** (EC_{100})	–	Gillo and Lass 1984
α1β1γδ, mouse muscle	–	–	**1160** (EC_{50})	–	–	–	–	–	Violet et al. 1997
α1β1γδ, BC3H1 mouse	–	–	–	**81** (EC_5)	–	–	**99** (EC_5)	–	Wachtel and Wegrzynowicz 1992
α1β1γδ, BC3H1 mouse	–	IC_{50} for To open is 80% (EC_5)	–	–	–	–	–	–	Wachtel 1995
α1β1γδ, mouse muscle	–	–	–	–	–	**42** (EC_{90})	–	–	Yost and Dodson 1993
α3,5,7; β2,3,4, PC12 rat	–	–	–	Steady-state: **5.4**; peak: **47** (ukn)	–	–	–	steady-state: **2.8**; peak: **21.4** (ukn)	Furuya et al. 1999

2.3 Volatile Anesthetics

Inhalation anesthetics (halothane, isoflurane, enflurane) generally have weak effects on AMPAR (Dildy-Mayfield et al. 1996). At double the concentration needed for clinical effect, these anesthetics either weakly inhibited recombinant AMPAR or had no detectable effect on receptor function.

Halogenated anesthetics are also weak inhibitors of NMDAR (de Sousa et al. 2000; Yamakura and Harris 2000; Yamakura et al. 2001); the effects of isoflurane, halothane, and chloroform ranged from approx. 20%–40% at 1 CEC (clinically effective concentration, see Table 1; Hollmann et al. 2001; Ogata et al. 2006). The combined inhibition of AMPAR and NMDAR by isoflurane is measurable, and possibly functionally significant, when total charge transfer of synaptic events is measured (de Sousa et al. 2000). Fairly robust inhibition of NMDA currents by isoflurane has been reported in cultured cortical neurons (Ming et al. 2001). Inhibition became less robust with time in culture (Ming et al. 2002). This effect was attributed to the lower sensitivity of NR2A subunits, which increase expression with development.

KAR (GluR6) are markedly potentiated by the volatile anesthetics halothane, isoflurane, and enflurane (Dildy-Mayfield et al. 1996; Minami et al. 1998). It may seem unlikely that potentiation of excitatory kainate responses might participate in anesthesia; however, KAR are prominent on GABAergic interneurons (Huettner 2003). It is therefore possible that receptor potentiation could result in enhanced GABA release. Potentiation of KAR was explored with chimeras between GluR3 and GluR6, which localized a single amino acid in TM4 as important for the effects of volatile anesthetics on this receptor.

2.4 Injectable Anesthetics: Propofol, Barbiturates, Etomidate

At clinically relevant concentrations, propofol has only very weak effects on glutamate receptors (Yamakura et al. 1995b; Yamakura et al. 2001; Krampfl et al. 2000). Similarly, etomidate has little effect on glutamate receptor function (Yamakura et al. 2001). It therefore appears unlikely that direct glutamatergic effects are important mechanisms for either drug.

On the other hand, it is clear that barbiturates inhibit AMPAR currents, and these effects are dependent upon the specific subunit composition of the receptor. For instance, GluR1 homomers are not affected by barbiturates, but GluR1/GluR2 heteromers are strongly inhibited (Taverna et al. 1994; Yamakura et al. 1995a; Dildy-Mayfield et al. 1996; Joo et al. 1999). The block of AMPAR by barbiturates may be partly dependent upon the editing of the Q/R site in GluR2 that determines Ca^{2+} permeability and channel rectification properties (Yamakura et al. 1995a). In addition, the inhibition exhibits use-dependence, in that repetitive activation of the receptor appears to facilitate inhibition by barbiturates (Marszalec and Narahashi 1993; Jackson et al. 2003). This latter effect has been attributed to trapping of the receptor in an agonist-bound desensitized state (Jackson et al. 2003).

There is little literature on the effect of barbiturates on NMDAR. Earlier work found no effect on NMDA receptor function (Yamakura et al. 2001), but one recent report suggests that thiopental, at clinically relevant concentrations, inhibits NMDA-gated responses in prefrontal cortex neurons (Liu et al. 2006).

2.5 *Ketamine*

The dissociative anesthetic ketamine is a strong, noncompetitive blocker of NMDAR with little effect on AMPAR or KAR (Anis et al. 1983; Harrison and Simmonds 1985; Thomson et al. 1985; MacDonald et al. 1987; Orser et al. 1997). The mechanism of ketamine action has been proposed to be twofold. First, it appears to act as an open channel blocker (MacDonald et al. 1991), reflected in a concentration-dependent decrease in mean open channel time (Orser et al. 1997). In addition, ketamine exhibits a closed channel block, resulting in decreased channel opening frequency. The latter effect is seen even in cell-attached patches with ketamine applied to bath solution, indicating that to reduce channel opening frequency the drug passes through or laterally within the lipid bilayer to access its site on the receptor (Orser et al. 1997).

Different NMDAR subunit combinations exhibit differing sensitivity to ketamine and other dissociative anesthetics (MK801 and phencyclidine) (Yamakura et al. 1993). Dissociative anesthetic sensitivity is reduced by mutating a critical TM2 arginine residue responsible for Mg^{2+} block of the channel. However, the effect is not one of full abolition, and the mutation affected block by different dissociative anesthetics by different degrees (Yamakura et al. 1993).

2.6 *Ethanol*

The effects of ethanol on excitatory amino acid receptors have been of strong interest. Ethanol noncompetitively and relatively selectively inhibits NMDAR over AMPAR or KAR (Hoffman et al. 1989; Lovinger et al. 1989). Ethanol apparently allosterically reduces channel mean open time and open probability without changing the channel conductance (Lima-Landman and Albuquerque 1989; Wright et al. 1996). However, the actions of ethanol are variable and many factors, including the subunit composition of receptors and the expression system used, influence ethanol sensitivity (Woodward 2000; Smothers et al. 2001). Several domains and amino acid residues have been identified as important in ethanol's antagonism of NMDAR. These include the TM2 region of NR1 (Mirshahi and Woodward 1995) and the C-terminal cytoplasmic domains of the receptor (Mirshahi et al. 1998; Anders et al. 2000). More recent studies have focused on TM3 and TM4 of the NR1 and NR2A subunits, which significantly alter ethanol sensitivity of the receptor (Ronald et al. 2001; Ren et al. 2003; Honse et al. 2004; Smothers and Woodward 2006). Some of these mutations were recently shown to affect the sensitivity of NMDAR to volatile halogenated anesthetics, but not ketamine, N_2O, or benzene (Ogata et al. 2006). The diversity of sites associated with ethanol sensitivity is difficult to interpret but could suggest multiple sites of interaction.

2.7 *Steroids*

A formal publication of studies of anesthetic steroids has not been made, but alphaxalone (Yamakura et al. 2001) and allopregnanolone (Zorumski et al. 2000) are mentioned as having little effect on AMPAR or NMDAR. This is in contrast to the actions of pregnenolone sulfate (a convulsant), which potentiates NMDAR and inhibits AMPAR and KAR at concentrations likely to be present in vivo (Gibbs et al. 2006).

2.8 *Summary*

Most excitatory transmission at all levels of the mature CNS involves glutamatergic signaling. Therefore, it is conceptually attractive that general anesthetic drugs may have as an important target one or more classes of ionotropic glutamate receptors. The best evidence for glutamate receptors serving as clinically relevant anesthetic targets comes from the actions of nitrous oxide, Xe, and ketamine on NMDAR. In contrast, none of these agents acts on AMPAR at relevant concentrations. It is possible that the NMDAR, which serve a more modulatory function, can be inhibited with a larger safety margin than AMPAR, which mediate most rapid excitatory transmission including synapses in the respiratory centers. It is not known whether animals can be anesthetized by inhibition of AMPAR, while ventilation is maintained mechanically.

3 Nicotinic Receptors

3.1 *Nicotinic Receptor Overview*

Despite the multiple classes of subunits and receptor subtypes, the general features of the nicotinic receptor are remarkably uniform. The functional receptor is a pentamer of subunits. Each subunit forms four transmembrane domains with the second membrane-spanning region being the major contributor to the channel pore (Fig. 1). The channel is cation-selective with preference to monovalent inorganic cations, although some receptor subtypes can efficiently conduct divalent cations such as Ca^{2+}. The endogenous activator of the receptor is acetylcholine, with two binding sites per receptor formed at the interfaces between the extracellular domains of the α-subunits and the adjacent (usually non-α) subunit.

In the periphery, nicotinic receptors mediate synaptic transmission in autonomic ganglia and the neuromuscular junction, and are important for catecholamine release from adrenal chromaffin cells. The physiological role of nicotinic receptors in the CNS is debated, as is evident in many review articles. A major proposed role is that presynaptically located receptors modulate the release of other transmitters (Dani and Bertrand 2006; Jensen et al. 2005; Dajas-Bailador and Wonnacott 2004). A particular example is the role of enhanced dopamine release in producing nicotine addiction (Dani and Harris 2005; Wonnacott et al. 2005). However, genetic ablation of subunits expressed in the brain results in relatively subtle consequences (Champtiaux and Changeux 2004) that have not provided clear indications of the possible effects of receptor inhibition. Two major subtypes in the CNS are those containing the α_4 and β_2 subunits ($\alpha_4\beta_2$ receptors) and the homomeric receptor composed of α_7 subunits. The α_7 receptors allow significant Ca^{2+} entry, which can initiate intracellular cascades (Dajas-Bailador and Wonnacott 2004). In addition to the reviews just mentioned, an extensive examination of the possible involvement of nicotinic receptors in anesthesia has appeared (Tassonyi et al. 2002).

3.2 *Gaseous Anesthetics: Xe and N_2O*

Both Xe and N_2O inhibit the activity of nicotinic receptors (Yamakura and Harris 2000; Suzuki et al. 2003; Wachtel 1995). The effect has been described as a reversible, voltage-independent reduction of peak current. Although the two gasses can act on a wide variety of nicotinic receptor types, receptors containing the β_2 subunit are markedly more sensitive to either Xe or N_2O than receptors containing the β_4 subunit (Yamakura and Harris 2000). Xe and N_2O reduce the response from the rat $\alpha_4\beta_2$ receptor by approx. 40% at doses corresponding to approximately half of MAC. In contrast, the same doses of Xe and N_2O inhibit the $\alpha_4\beta_4$ receptor by only about 10%. The sensitivity of α_7 receptors is intermediate between the two α_4 subunit-containing receptors (Suzuki et al. 2003).

In agonist dose-response measurements, the presence of N_2O reduces the maximal response to acetylcholine (ACh) but does not affect the EC_{50} value or the slope of the dose-response curve, suggesting that N_2O noncompetitively interferes with activation (Yamakura and Harris 2000; Suzuki et al. 2003). The findings are qualitatively similar for $\alpha_4\beta_2$ and $\alpha_4\beta_4$ receptors, and the α_7 homooligomeric receptor. Little, however, is known of the molecular mechanism of inhibition. Studies on nicotinic receptors expressed in BC3H1 cells (muscle, embryonic-type) have shown that N_2O leads to a reduction in the mean open duration without affecting the number of events per burst (Wachtel 1995).

3.3 Volatile Anesthetics

Isoflurane is among the best-studied halogenated volatile anesthetics. It is extraordinarily effective at inhibiting the $\alpha_4\beta_2$ receptor with IC_{50} values at 10%–25% of the MAC value (Flood et al. 1997; Violet et al. 1997; Yamashita et al. 2005). The muscle-type nicotinic receptor is less sensitive to isoflurane. Violet et al. (1997) reported an IC_{50} of over 1 mM (~3 MAC) for muscle-type receptors expressed in oocytes, although in single-channel recordings isoflurane affected several kinetic parameters at concentrations corresponding to 1 MAC or below (Dilger et al. 1992). Finally, the least sensitive nicotinic receptor subtype is one composed of α_7 subunits (Flood et al. 1997).

Single-channel experiments on muscle-type receptors from BC3H1 cells have provided a mechanistic picture of isoflurane-mediated block (Dilger et al. 1992). Coapplication of isoflurane with ACh transforms the isolated openings into groups or bursts of openings, a pattern suggestive of open channel block (Neher and Steinbach 1978). As expected for such a mechanism, the presence of isoflurane reduces the mean open duration in a dose-dependent manner. However, the number of openings per burst did not increase as much as expected, and the burst duration actually decreased in the presence of isoflurane instead of increasing as simple open channel block would predict. Accordingly, the effect of isoflurane was described as open channel block with a caveat that blocked receptors can close, and that the closing rate of blocked channels is higher than that of unblocked channels.

Although isoflurane inhibition of the muscle-type ACh receptor does not contribute to its sedative effects, it should be kept in mind that isoflurane at its typical clinical concentrations reduces the peak current from muscle receptors by 10% or more, and may thus contribute to the side effects of isoflurane, or act in concert with neuromuscular blockers as a muscle relaxant.

Isoflurane-mediated inhibition of currents from neuronal $\alpha_4\beta_2$ receptors shows no flickering behavior (Yamashita et al. 2005). Isoflurane slightly reduces the mean open duration and the channel burst duration but affects most strongly channel closed times by increasing the duration of the longest closed time component. Macroscopic studies in which the solution was rapidly switched from ACh to one containing ACh and isoflurane and then back to ACh showed that the recovery from block was relatively slow (~50 s^{-1}). Such a slow dissociation rate for isoflurane likely explains the absence of rapid flickering in single-channel currents from $\alpha_4\beta_2$ receptors exposed to isoflurane.

Many other halogenated anesthetics, such as sevoflurane or halothane, act in a manner similar to isoflurane and inhibit the activation of the nicotinic receptor. Again, sensitivity to sevoflurane and halothane is the greatest in $\alpha_4\beta_2$ receptors, which are inhibited at concentrations several-fold less than MAC (Violet et al. 1997; Yamashita et al. 2005). In contrast, α_7-containing receptors and the muscle-type nicotinic receptor are less sensitive to halothane or sevoflurane, and have IC_{50} values at several MAC.

However, a role of the $\alpha_4\beta_2$ receptor in the actions of volatile anesthetics is unlikely, as the ability of isoflurane to anesthetize mice genetically modified to lack the β_2 subunit is unaltered from controls (Flood et al. 2002).

3.4 *Anesthetic Steroids*

Anesthetic steroids, best known for their potentiating actions on the related $GABA_A$ receptor, can also inhibit the nicotinic receptor (Gillo and Lass 1984; Paradiso et al. 2000). However, the concentrations required to produce inhibition of nicotinic receptors are several-fold higher than those producing potentiation of the $GABA_A$ receptor or loss of righting reflex (LRR) in *Xenopus* tadpoles (Paradiso et al. 2000). For example, allopregnanolone potentiates $GABA_A$ receptor-mediated currents with an EC_{50} at or below 0.5 μM and produces LRR with an EC_{50} of 0.5 μM, while the IC_{50} value for inhibition of the $\alpha_4\beta_2$ nicotinic receptor is greater than 10 μM. On the other hand, there is a correlation between the ability of a steroid anesthetic to cause LRR and inhibition of the $\alpha_4\beta_2$ nicotinic receptor, and it is possible that this receptor is a secondary site of action involved in anesthesia.

Alphaxalone, an erstwhile clinical anesthetic, inhibits nicotinic receptor-mediated currents in bovine adrenal chromaffin cells with an IC_{50} of approximately 30 μM (Shiraishi et al. 2002). The steroid is more potent at blocking whole cell currents from chick embryonic muscle-type receptors [IC_{50} of 6 μM (Gillo and Lass 1984)]. However, a much lower sensitivity to alphaxalone (IC_{50}=99 μM) was reported for single-channel open times from muscle-type receptors in BC3H1 cells (Wachtel and Wegrzynowicz 1992). These findings suggest that alphaxalone administration can result in inhibition of nicotinic receptors, although the IC_{50} values are much higher than clinical concentrations.

A synthetic steroid (3α,5α,17β)-3-hydroxyandrostane-17-carbonitrile (ACN) blocks the rat $\alpha_4\beta_2$ receptor with an IC_{50} of 1.5 μM and a Hill slope of greater than 1, indicating that block can involve the binding of more than one steroid molecule (Paradiso et al. 2000). Inhibition is the same at low and high ACh concentrations, and ACN appears to be without effect on the binding of radiolabeled cytisine, indicating that the steroid does not occlude the agonist binding site (Sabey et al. 1999). In addition, block develops at a similar rate in the absence and presence of ACh, and steroid does not interfere with desensitization, suggesting that steroid interactions with the receptor do not depend on the functional status of the receptor.

3.5 *Propofol*

Propofol acts as a nicotinic receptor blocker at concentrations far exceeding those clinically relevant. ACh-elicited currents from muscle-type receptors are blocked with an IC_{50} of approx. 50–100 μM (Wachtel and Wegrzynowicz 1992; Dilger et al. 1994; Violet et al. 1997). Although the blocking mechanism has been proposed to be similar to that of halogenated volatile anesthetics, e.g., isoflurane, and mediated by shortened channel open durations, flickering between conducting and nonconducting states is not seen, presumably due to slow dissociation of propofol from the receptor (Dilger et al. 1994).

The ability of propofol to inhibit neuronal nicotinic receptor activation is similarly weak. Neuronal-type chicken $\alpha_4\beta_2$ receptors are inhibited by propofol with an IC_{50} of 19 μM (Flood et al. 1997). The effect is pseudocompetitive in that the drug is more potent at lower concentrations of ACh. In rat pheochromocytoma (PC12) cells [which express $\alpha_{3,5,7}$ and $\beta_{2,3,4}$ subunits (Rogers et al. 1992)], propofol blocks peak current elicited by 30 μM nicotine with an IC_{50} of 47 μM, and the steady-state current with an IC_{50} of 5.4 μM (Furuya et al. 1999). The effect was reversible and voltage-independent, and increasing the ACh concentration to 300 μM did not affect the magnitude of the depression of steady-state or peak current. Preincubation with propofol did not increase the magnitude of inhibition, suggesting little effect of propofol on closed channels (or that the effect on open channels is very rapid). Finally, α_7 receptors from chicken have been found to be insensitive to 400 μM propofol (Flood et al. 1997).

3.6 Barbiturates

Barbiturates at clinically relevant concentrations inhibit the nicotinic receptor (Flood and Krasowski 2000; Weber et al. 2005). The IC_{50} values of pentobarbital and thiopental for most nicotinic receptor types are estimated to be less than 100 μM. The presence of barbiturates results in a reduction in peak current and a more rapid desensitization (Krampfl et al. 2000). In oocytes expressing human α_7 receptors, thiopental is a competitive inhibitor with IC_{50} values at 41 μM and 285 μM for 0.1 mM and 1 mM ACh, respectively (Coates et al. 2001). In contrast, Kamiya et al. (2001) found that in rat medial habenula neurons, inhibition of the peak current by thiopental was unchanged when 10 μM (~EC_{30}) or 100 μM (EC_{100}) of nicotine were used to activate the receptors. Thiopental block of steady-state current was actually more potent at higher nicotine concentrations.

In single-channel recordings, the presence of pentobarbital leads to shorter open time durations (Gage and McKinnon 1985; Dilger et al. 1997), although a bimodal effect with prolongation of open durations at low pentobarbital concentrations and block at higher concentrations has also been reported (Liu and Madsen 1996). In addition to an effect on open durations, the presence of high concentrations of barbiturates introduces a novel gap closed state. The duration of the gap is 1–3 ms for pentobarbital but much shorter (50 μs) for barbital, probably reflecting difference in dissociation rates (Dilger et al. 1997). The binding of pentobarbital appears to be state-specific; for muscle-type receptors, pentobarbital binds more tightly to open channels but allows closing of open-blocked channels. Dilger et al. (1997) found that pentobarbital and barbital interacted with distinct sites but the binding of one destabilized the binding of the other.

The number of sites for barbiturates in unclear. Dodson et al. (1987) reported two sites per receptor from *Torpedo*. Binding of radiolabeled amobarbital was completely inhibited by other barbiturates, and partly inhibited by nicotinic ligands in the absence but not in the presence of α-bungarotoxin, a nicotinic site antagonist. This suggests a negative interaction between the barbiturate site and the ACh site in *Torpedo* receptor. In contrast, Arias et al. (2001) reported a single high-affinity site for amobarbital on the resting receptor. Interestingly, the data suggested that a desensitized receptor contains several (11, on average) low-affinity sites for amobarbital.

Despite the ability of barbiturates to act on nicotinic receptors at clinically relevant concentrations, their role in anesthesia is unlikely, as studies on stereoisomers suggest. Although both stereoisomers of 1-methyl-5-phenyl-5-propyl barbituric acid suppress nicotinic receptor currents in PC12 cells and rat medial habenula neurons (Watanabe et al. 1999; Kamiya et al. 2001), only the R(−) isomer induces LRR. The S(+) isomer, in contrast, is a convulsant (Buch et al. 1973). Similarly, there is lack of correlation between the ability of stereoisomers of thiopental to inhibit the $\alpha_4\beta_2$ and α_7 receptors and their anesthetic potencies in mouse (Downie et al. 2000).

3.7 *Etomidate*

Etomidate also inhibits nicotinic receptor function. In bovine adrenal chromaffin cells, etomidate results in shorter open duration and an excess number of brief closures within bursts. However, the burst durations are shortened rather than prolonged, suggesting that blocked open channels maintain the ability to close (Charlesworth and Richards 1995). Etomidate also inhibits the peak response from the chick $\alpha_4\beta_4$ receptor (Flood and Krasowski 2000). This, however, is likely to be without clinical consequence as the IC_{50} values for both muscle and neuronal receptors (23 μM and 33 μM, respectively) are far outside the clinically relevant concentration range.

3.8 *Ketamine*

Both neuronal-type and neuromuscular nicotinic receptors are blocked by ketamine, although the IC_{50} values are generally above the clinically relevant range (Wachtel and Wegrzynowicz 1992; Yamakura et al. 2000; Coates and Flood 2001; but see Flood and Krasowski 2000). There appears to be little subunit-specificity, although β_4-containing receptors are more sensitive than receptors containing the β_2 subunit (Yamakura et al. 2000). In macroscopic recordings, block manifests as a reduction of peak and steady-state currents. In PC12 cells, the steady-state current is more sensitive than peak current to ketamine with IC_{50} values of 3 μM and 21 μM, respectively (Furuya et al. 1999). In clinical practice, S-ketamine is several times more potent than R-ketamine at producing anesthetic effects. Stereoselectivity of ketamine-mediated inhibition of nicotinic receptors in vitro has been observed in some studies (Friederich et al. 2000) but not in others (Sasaki et al. 2000).

In single-channel recordings, exposure to ketamine results in a reduction in open time duration accompanied by a new, prominent closed time component (Wachtel and Wegrzynowicz 1992; Scheller et al. 1996). In addition to the open channel block, ketamine can interact with closed channels (Scheller et al. 1996).

3.9 *Summary*

Among nicotinic receptors, the $\alpha_4\beta_2$ subtype seems most sensitive to anesthetic drugs, especially volatile anesthetics. However, studies of transgenic mice lacking the β_2 subunit have shown no difference in the anesthetic actions of isoflurane. Accordingly, it seems unlikely that nicotinic receptors play a major role. On the other hand, actions in the periphery may be important for some side effects, including reductions in the safety factor for neuromuscular transmission, reduction of catecholamine release from chromaffin cells, and inhibition of transmission at ganglionic synapses.

4 Serotonin-Activated Channels

The channels activated by extracellular serotonin (5HT3 receptors) have been less studied than glutamate or nicotinic receptors. 5HT3 receptors have received some attention as possible targets involved in the actions of ethanol and as possible factors in post-operative nausea and vomiting (PONV). The 5HT3 receptor is a member of the gene family including $GABA_A$, $GABA_C$, nicotinic, and glycine receptors, and shares the pentameric structure and basic subunit topology (Fig. 1). Two subunits have been identified for the 5HT3 receptor, designated A and B. The subunit composition of receptors in the brain is not well characterized. Reeves and Lummis (2002) and Peters et al. (2005) provide some recent reviews on 5HT3 receptors. The physiological roles for 5HT3 receptors are not clearly understood, at present.

The summary statement is that 5HT3 receptors are not likely to be major targets for the clinically relevant actions of anesthetic drugs, although Xe may be an effective blocker (see Table 4). Even in the case of PONV, it seems more likely that system effects, for example indirect stimulation of the emesis center in the brain, are more likely than a direct effect of anesthetics on the 5HT3 receptor. For example, although all volatile anesthetics increase the risk of PONV (Apfel et al. 2002), some potentiate 5HT3 responses (e.g., halothane) while others inhibit them (e.g., sevoflurane) (Suzuki et al. 2002; Stevens et al. 2005a).

In addition to a lack of consistent effect, most effects are relatively small at concentrations near the clinical range. In one study of the binding of a radiolabeled antagonist, several intravenous anesthetics could reduce binding but only at concentrations several-fold higher than concentrations producing functional effects, and much higher than clinically used (Appadu and Lambert 1996). Accordingly, it seems unlikely that drug interactions with the transmitter binding site could underlie the functional effects.

Table 4 Actions of selected anesthetic drugs on 5HT3 receptors. Data are presented as in Table 3. N1E115 are mouse neuroblastoma cells, likely expressing 5HT3A receptors

Receptor type	Xe (71%)	N_2O (105%)	Halothane (250)	Isoflurane (300)	Propofol (1.5)	Etomidate (1.5)	Pentobarbital (20)	Thiopental (25)	Ketamine (5)	Reference
5HT3A	–	–	2.0, 1250 (EC_5)	2.0, 5000 (EC_5)	n.e., 20 (EC_5)	–	–	–	–	Machu and Harris 1994
5HT3A	–	–	3.0, 5000 (EC_5)	3.5, 5000 (EC_5)	–	–	–	–	–	Zhang et al. 1997
N1E115	–	–	–	–	**10** (EC_{90})	–	–	–	–	Barann et al. 2000a
5HT3A	–	0.85, 58% (EC_{50})	–	1.15, 150 (EC_{50})	–	–	–	–	–	Yamakura and Harris 2000
h5HT3A	0.5, 35% (EC_{15})	0.6, 100% (EC_{15})	1.5, 210 (EC_{15})	1.2, 230 (EC_{15})	–	–	–	–	–	Suzuki et al. 2002
N1E115	–	–	1.5, 210 (EC_{20})	1.5, 600 (EC_{20})	–	–	–	**100** (EC_{20})	–	Jenkins et al. 1996
5HT3A	–	–	–	–	–	–	**300** (EC_{90})	–	–	Barann et al. 2000b
h5HT3A	–	–	2.3, 430 (EC_{10})	1.9, 550 (EC_{10})	–	–	–	–	–	Stevens et al. 2005b
N1E115	–	–	–	–	–	–	**400** (EC_{90})	–	–	Barann et al. 1997
N1E115	–	–	–	–	**10** (EC_{100})	**12** (EC_{100})	–	**70** (EC_{100})	**180** (EC_{100})	Barann et al. 1993
5HT3A	–	–	–	–	–	–	–	–	Competitive **400**, non competitive **900**	Yamakura et al. 2000

Ethanol and short chain alcohols potentiate the responses of 5HT3 receptors, at concentrations below anesthetic concentrations (c.f. Machu and Harris 1994), which has suggested that at least some of the intoxication might reflect actions at this receptor. Two studies have provided evidence that potentiation of responses by ethanol (Lovinger et al. 2000) and halothane or isoflurane (Solt et al. 2005) is the result of increased gating efficacy rather than a change in the binding of agonist.

In general, coexpression of the 5HT3A and -B subunits reduces the ability of volatile anesthetics (Stevens et al. 2005a) and short chain alcohols (Hayrapetyan et al. 2005) to potentiate responses, while not affecting the ability of some volatile anesthetics or longer chain alcohols to inhibit (Stevens et al. 2005a).

Morphine has been reported to potently inhibit receptors composed of recombinant 5HT3A subunits expressed in human embryonic kidney (HEK)-293 cells (Wittmann et al. 2006), so opiate anesthetics might also inhibit them. Alphaxalone is a weak inhibitor (Barann et al. 1999), but 17β-estradiol inhibits 5HT3A receptors at low micromolar concentrations (Barann et al. 1999; Wetzel et al. 1998).

5 ATP-Activated Channels

The P2X receptors belong to a different gene family than the glutamate receptors and nicotinic receptors. The P2X receptor family comprises seven identified subunits, named P2X1 through P2X7. Each subunit has only two membrane-spanning regions, with a long extracellularly located loop between them, and a functional receptor is composed of three subunits (Fig. 1). At least some receptors contain more than one type of subunit (e.g., P2X3 and P2X4), but the rules for assembly and the native receptor subunit composition are not worked out. P2X receptors are expressed in nonneural tissues as well as neurons, and are thought to be involved in some inflammatory responses, and when expressed in microglial cells may mediate some aspects of chronic pain. Some recent reviews of various aspects of P2X receptor structure and function are Khakh and North (2006), Khakh et al. (2001), and Chizh and Illes (2001).

Relatively few studies were found to examine the actions of anesthetics on P2X receptors. Among volatile anesthetics, sevoflurane is a weak blocker [reduction to 0.6×control at 500 μM (Masaki et al. 2001)], while others have not been studied. Inhibition by sevoflurane is more profound at higher concentrations of ATP, suggesting a noncompetitive mechanism for block (Masaki et al. 2001). In one study of the binding of radiolabeled α,β-methylene ATP to rat brain synaptic membranes, neither isoflurane nor sevoflurane inhibited binding [maximal concentration 1 mM, (Masaki et al. 2004)]. P2X receptors are blocked at high concentrations (>100 μM) of barbiturates (Andoh et al. 1997; Kitahara et al. 2003). Propofol potentiates responses from P2X4 receptors, although only weakly [1.4× at concentrations of 50 μM or more (Tomioka et al. 2000; Davies et al. 2005b)], but has no effect on P2X2 receptors (Tomioka et al. 2000).

The effects of ethanol depend on the subunit composition of the P2X receptor (Davies et al. 2005a)–ethanol inhibits P2X4 and potentiates P2X3. Propofol may show a reversed subunit sensitivity (Davies et al. 2005b; Tomioka et al. 2000).

Opioids inhibit P2X receptors in rat sensory ganglia, apparently not by a direct effect but through a guanosine triphosphate (GTP)-binding protein (Chizhmakov et al. 2005). Anesthetic steroids have not been studied, but 17β-estradiol inhibits recombinant P2X7 (Cario-Toumaniantz et al. 1998) and P2X receptors in rat sensory neurons (Ma et al. 2005) at high nanomolar to micromolar concentrations.

6 Summary

General anesthetics have the reputation of being "dirty" drugs, and they do, indeed, act on multiple classes of excitatory transmitter-gated channels. However, the effects in the clinically relevant range are more restricted. Inhibition of NMDA-type glutamate receptors by gaseous and dissociative anesthetics is the most compelling case for clinical relevance. A number of other channels can be affected by anesthetics at low concentrations, including AMPAR, KAR, and nicotinic $\alpha_4\beta_2$ receptors, but it is difficult to argue for relevance to clinically desired effects.

References

Anders DL, Blevins T, Smothers CT, Woodward JJ (2000) Reduced ethanol inhibition of *N*-methyl-d-aspartate receptors by deletion of the NR1 C0 domain or overexpression of alpha-actinin-2 proteins. J Biol Chem 275:15019–15024

Andoh T, Furuya R, Oka K, Hattori S, Watanabe I, Kamiya Y, Okumura F (1997) Differential effects of thiopental on neuronal nicotinic acetylcholine receptors and P2X purinergic receptors in PC12 cells. Anesthesiology 87:1199–1209

Anis NA, Berry SC, Burton NR, Lodge D (1983) The dissociative anaesthetics, ketamine and phencyclidine, selectively reduce excitation of central mammalian neurones by N-methyl-aspartate. Br J Pharmacol 79:565–575

Apfel CC, Kranke P, Katz MH, Goepfert C, Papenfuss T, Rauch S, Heineck R, Greim CA, Roewer N (2002) Volatile anaesthetics may be the main cause of early but not delayed postoperative vomiting: a randomized controlled trial of factorial design. Br J Anaesth 88:659–668

Appadu BL, Lambert DG (1996) Interaction of i.v. anaesthetic agents with 5-HT3 receptors. Br J Anaesth 76:271–273

Arias HR, McCardy EA, Gallagher MJ, Blanton MP (2001) Interaction of barbiturate analogs with the Torpedo californica nicotinic acetylcholine receptor ion channel. Mol Pharmacol 60:497–506

Barann M, Gothert M, Fink K, Bonisch H (1993) Inhibition by anaesthetics of 14C-guanidinium flux through the voltage-gated sodium channel and the cation channel of the 5-HT3 receptor of N1E-115 neuroblastoma cells. Naunyn Schmiedebergs Arch Pharmacol 347:125–132

Barann M, Gothert M, Bonisch H, Dybek A, Urban BW (1997) 5-HT3 receptors in outside-out patches of N1E-115 neuroblastoma cells: basic properties and effects of pentobarbital. Neuropharmacology 36:655–664

Barann M, Gothert M, Bruss M, Bonisch H (1999) Inhibition by steroids of [14C]-guanidinium flux through the voltage-gated sodium channel and the cation channel of the 5-HT3 receptor of N1E-115 neuroblastoma cells. Naunyn Schmiedebergs Arch Pharmacol 360:234–241

Barann M, Dilger JP, Bonisch H, Gothert M, Dybek A, Urban BW (2000a) Inhibition of 5-HT(3) receptors by propofol: equilibrium and kinetic measurements. Neuropharmacology 39:1064–1074

Barann M, Meder W, Dorner Z, Bruss M, Bonisch H, Gothert M, Urban BW (2000b) Recombinant human 5-HT3A receptors in outside-out patches of HEK 293 cells: basic properties and barbiturate effects. Naunyn Schmiedebergs Arch Pharmacol 362:255–265

Buch HP, Schneider-Affeld F, Rummel W (1973) Stereochemical dependence of pharmacological activity in a series of optically active N-methylated barbiturates. Naunyn Schmiedebergs Arch Pharmacol 277:191–198

Cario-Toumaniantz C, Loirand G, Ferrier L, Pacaud P (1998) Non-genomic inhibition of human P2X7 purinoceptor by 17beta-oestradiol. J Physiol 508:659–666

Champtiaux N, Changeux JP (2004) Knockout and knockin mice to investigate the role of nicotinic receptors in the central nervous system. Prog Brain Res 145:235–251

Charlesworth P, Richards CD (1995) Anaesthetic modulation of nicotinic ion channel kinetics in bovine chromaffin cells. Br J Pharmacol 114:909–917

Chizh BA, Illes P (2001) P2X receptors and nociception. Pharmacol Rev 53:553–568

Chizhmakov I, Yudin Y, Mamenko N, Prudnikov I, Tamarova Z, Krishtal O (2005) Opioids inhibit purinergic nociceptors in the sensory neurons and fibres of rat via a G protein-dependent mechanism. Neuropharmacology 48:639–647

Coates KM, Flood P (2001) Ketamine and its preservative, benzethonium chloride, both inhibit human recombinant alpha7 and alpha4beta2 neuronal nicotinic acetylcholine receptors in Xenopus oocytes. Br J Pharmacol 134:871–879

Coates KM, Mather LE, Johnson R, Flood P (2001) Thiopental is a competitive inhibitor at the human alpha7 nicotinic acetylcholine receptor. Anesth Analg 92:930–933

Cowley KC, Zaporozhets E, Maclean JN, Schmidt BJ (2005) Is NMDA receptor activation essential for the production of locomotor-like activity in the neonatal rat spinal cord? J Neurophysiol 94:3805–3814

Dajas-Bailador F, Wonnacott S (2004) Nicotinic acetylcholine receptors and the regulation of neuronal signalling. Trends Pharmacol Sci 25:317–324

Dale N (1986) Excitatory synaptic drive for swimming mediated by amino acid receptors in the lamprey. J Neurosci 6:2662–2675

Dani JA, Bertrand D (2006) Nicotinic acetylcholine receptors and nicotinic cholinergic mechanisms of the central nervous system. Annu Rev Pharmacol Toxicol 47:699–729

Dani JA, Harris RA (2005) Nicotine addiction and comorbidity with alcohol abuse and mental illness. Nat Neurosci 8:1465–1470

Davies DL, Kochegarov AA, Kuo ST, Kulkarni AA, Woodward JJ, King BF, Alkana RL (2005a) Ethanol differentially affects ATP-gated P2X(3) and P2X(4) receptor subtypes expressed in Xenopus oocytes. Neuropharmacology 49:243–253

Davies DL, Kuo ST, Alkana RL (2005b) Differential effects of propofol and ethanol on P2X4 receptors expressed in Xenopus oocytes. Int Congr Ser 1283:285–287

de Sousa SL, Dickinson R, Lieb WR, Franks NP (2000) Contrasting synaptic actions of the inhalational general anesthetics isoflurane and xenon. Anesthesiology 92:1055–1066

DeVries SH, Schwartz EA (1999) Kainate receptors mediate synaptic transmission between cones and 'Off' bipolar cells in a mammalian retina. Nature 397:157–160

Dildy-Mayfield JE, Eger EI 2nd, Harris RA (1996) Anesthetics produce subunit-selective actions on glutamate receptors. J Pharmacol Exp Ther 276:1058–1065

Dilger JP (2002) The effects of general anaesthetics on ligand-gated ion channels. Br J Anaesth 89:41–51

Dilger JP, Brett RS, Lesko LA (1992) Effects of isoflurane on acetylcholine receptor channels. 1. Single-channel currents. Mol Pharmacol 41:127–133

Dilger JP, Vidal AM, Mody HI, Liu Y (1994) Evidence for direct actions of general anesthetics on an ion channel protein. A new look at a unified mechanism of action. Anesthesiology 81:431–442

Dilger JP, Boguslavsky R, Barann M, Katz T, Vidal AM (1997) Mechanisms of barbiturate inhibition of acetylcholine receptor channels. J Gen Physiol 109:401–414

Dingledine R, Borges K, Bowie D, Traynelis SF (1999) The glutamate receptor ion channels. Pharmacol Rev 51:7–61

Dinse A, Fohr KJ, Georgieff M, Beyer C, Bulling A, Weigt HU (2005) Xenon reduces glutamate-, AMPA-, and kainate-induced membrane currents in cortical neurones. Br J Anaesth 94:479–485

Dodson BA, Braswell LM, Miller KW (1987) Barbiturates bind to an allosteric regulatory site on nicotinic acetylcholine receptor-rich membranes. Mol Pharmacol 32:119–126

Downie DL, Franks NP, Lieb WR (2000) Effects of thiopental and its optical isomers on nicotinic acetylcholine receptors. Anesthesiology 93:774–783

Eger EI 2nd, Fisher DM, Dilger JP, Sonner JM, Evers A, Franks NP, Harris RA, Kendig JJ, Lieb WR, Yamakura T (2001) Relevant concentrations of inhaled anesthetics for in vitro studies of anesthetic mechanisms. Anesthesiology 94:915–921

Evers A, Crowder C (2001) General anesthetics. In: Hardman J, Limbird L, Gilman A (eds) Goodman and Gilman's The Pharmacological Basis of Therapeutics. McGraw-Hill, New York, pp 337–365

Evers AS, Maze M (2004) Anesthetic pharmacology: physiologic principles and clinical practice. Churchill Livingstone, Philadelphia

Flood P, Krasowski MD (2000) Intravenous anesthetics differentially modulate ligand-gated ion channels. Anesthesiology 92:1418–1425

Flood P, Ramirez-Latorre J, Role L (1997) Alpha 4 beta 2 neuronal nicotinic acetylcholine receptors in the central nervous system are inhibited by isoflurane and propofol, but alpha 7-type nicotinic acetylcholine receptors are unaffected [see comments]. Anesthesiology 86:859–865

Flood P, Sonner JM, Gong D, Coates KM (2002) Heteromeric nicotinic inhibition by isoflurane does not mediate MAC or loss of righting reflex. Anesthesiology 97:902–905

Franks NP, Lieb WR (1994) Molecular and cellular mechanisms of general anaesthesia. Nature 367:607–614

Franks NP, Lieb WR (1998) Which molecular targets are most relevant to general anaesthesia? Toxicol Lett 100–101:1–8

Franks NP, Dickinson R, de Sousa SL, Hall AC, Lieb WR (1998) How does xenon produce anaesthesia? Nature 396:324

Friederich P, Dybek A, Urban BW (2000) Stereospecific interaction of ketamine with nicotinic acetylcholine receptors in human sympathetic ganglion-like SH-SY5Y cells. Anesthesiology 93:818–824

Furuya R, Oka K, Watanabe I, Kamiya Y, Itoh H, Andoh T (1999) The effects of ketamine and propofol on neuronal nicotinic acetylcholine receptors and P2x purinoceptors in PC12 cells. Anesth Analg 88:174–180

Gage PW, McKinnon D (1985) Effects of pentobarbitone on acetylcholine-activated channels in mammalian muscle. Br J Pharmacol 85:229–235

Gibbs TT, Russek SJ, Farb DH (2006) Sulfated steroids as endogenous neuromodulators. Pharmacol Biochem Behav 84:555–567

Gillo B, Lass Y (1984) The mechanism of steroid anaesthetic (alphaxolone) block of acetylcholine-induced ionic currents. Br J Pharmacol 82:783–789

Harris RA, Mihic SJ, Dildy-Mayfield JE, Machu TK (1995) Actions of anesthetics on ligand-gated ion channels: role of receptor subunit composition. FASEB J 9:1454–1462

Harrison NL, Simmonds MA (1985) Quantitative studies on some antagonists of N-methyl D-aspartate in slices of rat cerebral cortex. Br J Pharmacol 84:381–391

Hayrapetyan V, Jenschke M, Dillon GH, Machu TK (2005) Co-expression of the 5-HT(3B) subunit with the 5-HT(3A) receptor reduces alcohol sensitivity. Brain Res Mol Brain Res 142:146–150

Hoffman PL, Rabe CS, Moses F, Tabakoff B (1989) N-methyl-D-aspartate receptors and ethanol: inhibition of calcium flux and cyclic GMP production. J Neurochem 52:1937–1940
Hollmann M, Liu H, Hoenemann C, Liu W, Durieux M (2001) Modulation of NMDA receptor function by ketamine and magnesium. Part II: interactions with volatile anesthetics. Anesth Analg 92:1182–1191
Honse Y, Ren H, Lipsky RH, Peoples RW (2004) Sites in the fourth membrane-associated domain regulate alcohol sensitivity of the NMDA receptor. Neuropharmacology 46:647–654
Huettner JE (2003) Kainate receptors and synaptic transmission. Prog Neurobiol 70:387–407
Jackson MF, Joo DT, Al-Mahrouki AA, Orser BA, Macdonald JF (2003) Desensitization of alpha-amino-3-hydroxy-5-methyl-4-isoxazolepropionic acid (AMPA) receptors facilitates use-dependent inhibition by pentobarbital. Mol Pharmacol 64:395–406
Jenkins A, Franks NP, Lieb WR (1996) Actions of general anaesthetics on 5-HT3 receptors in N1E-115 neuroblastoma cells. Br J Pharmacol 117:1507–1515
Jensen AA, Frolund B, Liljefors T, Krogsgaard-Larsen P (2005) Neuronal nicotinic acetylcholine receptors: structural revelations, target identifications, and therapeutic inspirations. J Med Chem 48:4705–4745
Jevtovic-Todorovic V, Todorovic SM, Mennerick S, Powell S, Dikranian K, Benshoff N, Zorumski CF, Olney JW (1998) Nitrous oxide (laughing gas) is an NMDA antagonist, neuroprotectant and neurotoxin. Nat Med 4:460–463
Joo DT, Xiong Z, MacDonald JF, Jia Z, Roder J, Sonner J, Orser BA (1999) Blockade of glutamate receptors and barbiturate anesthesia: increased sensitivity to pentobarbital-induced anesthesia despite reduced inhibition of AMPA receptors in GluR2 null mutant mice. Anesthesiology 91:1329–1341
Kamiya Y, Andoh T, Watanabe I, Higashi T, Itoh H (2001) Inhibitory effects of barbiturates on nicotinic acetylcholine receptors in rat central nervous system neurons. Anesthesiology 94:694–704
Khakh BS, North RA (2006) P2X receptors as cell-surface ATP sensors in health and disease. Nature 442:527–532
Khakh BS, Burnstock G, Kennedy C, King BF, North RA, Seguela P, Voigt M, Humphrey PP (2001) International union of pharmacology. XXIV. Current status of the nomenclature and properties of P2X receptors and their subunits. Pharmacol Rev 53:107–118
Kitahara S, Yamashita M, Ikemoto Y (2003) Effects of pentobarbital on purinergic P2X receptors of rat dorsal root ganglion neurons. Can J Physiol Pharmacol 81:1085–1091
Krampfl K, Schlesinger F, Dengler R, Bufler J, Klaus K, Friedrich S, Reinhardt D (2000) Pentobarbital has curare-like effects on adult-type nicotinic acetylcholine receptor channel currents. Anesth Analg 90:970–974
Krasowski MD, Harrison NL (1999) General anaesthetic actions on ligand-gated ion channels. Cell Mol Life Sci 55:1278–1303
Kullmann DM (2000) Spillover and synaptic cross talk mediated by glutamate and GABA in the mammalian brain. Prog Brain Res 125:339–351
Lerma J (2006) Kainate receptor physiology. Curr Opin Pharmacol 6:89–97
Lester RA, Clements JD, Westbrook GL, Jahr CE (1990) Channel kinetics determine the time course of NMDA receptor-mediated synaptic currents. Nature 346:565–567
Li P, Wilding TJ, Kim SJ, Calejesan AA, Huettner JE, Zhuo M (1999) Kainate-receptor-mediated sensory synaptic transmission in mammalian spinal cord. Nature 397:161–164
Lima-Landman MT, Albuquerque EX (1989) Ethanol potentiates and blocks NMDA-activated single-channel currents in rat hippocampal pyramidal cells. FEBS Lett 247:61–67
Liu GJ, Madsen BW (1996) Biphasic effect of pentobarbitone on chick myotube nicotinic receptor channel kinetics. Br J Pharmacol 118:1385–1388
Liu H, Dai T, Yao S (2006) Effect of thiopental sodium on N-methyl-D-aspartate-gated currents. Can J Anaesth 53:442–448
Lovinger DM, White G, Weight FF (1989) Ethanol inhibits NMDA-activated ion current in hippocampal neurons. Science 243:1721–1724

Lovinger DM, Sung KW, Zhou Q (2000) Ethanol and trichloroethanol alter gating of 5-HT3 receptor-channels in NCB-20 neuroblastoma cells. Neuropharmacology 39:561–570

Ma B, Rong W, Dunn PM, Burnstock G (2005) 17beta-estradiol attenuates alpha, beta-meATP-induced currents in rat dorsal root ganglion neurons. Life Sci 76:2547–2558

MacDonald JF, Miljkovic Z, Pennefather P (1987) Use-dependent block of excitatory amino acid currents in cultured neurons by ketamine. J Neurophysiol 58:251–266

MacDonald JF, Bartlett MC, Mody I, Pahapill P, Reynolds JN, Salter MW, Schneiderman JH, Pennefather PS (1991) Actions of ketamine, phencyclidine and MK-801 on NMDA receptor currents in cultured mouse hippocampal neurones. J Physiol 432:483–508

Machu TK, Harris RA (1994) Alcohols and anesthetics enhance the function of 5-hydroxytryptamine3 receptors expressed in Xenopus laevis oocytes. J Pharmacol Exp Ther 271:898–905

Madden D (2002) The structure and function of glutamate receptor ion channels. Nat Rev Neurosci 3:91–101

Marszalec W, Narahashi T (1993) Use-dependent pentobarbital block of kainate and quisqualate currents. Brain Res 608:7–15

Masaki E, Kawamura M, Kato F (2001) Reduction by sevoflurane of adenosine 5'-triphosphate-activated inward current of locus coeruleus neurons in pontine slices of rats. Brain Res 921:226–232

Masaki E, Yamazaki K, Hori S, Kawamura M (2004) [3H]alpha,beta-methylene ATP binding to P2X purinoceptor is unaffected by volatile anaesthetics. Eur J Anaesthesiol 21:221–225

Mayer ML (2005) Glutamate receptor ion channels. Curr Opin Neurobiol 15:282–288

Mayer ML, Armstrong N (2004) Structure and function of glutamate receptor ion channels. Annu Rev Physiol 66:161–181

Mennerick S, Jevtovic-Todorovic V, Todorovic SM, Shen W, Olney JW, Zorumski CF (1998) Effect of nitrous oxide on excitatory and inhibitory synaptic transmission in hippocampal cultures. J Neurosci 18:9716–9726

Minami K, Wick MJ, Stern-Bach Y, Dildy-Mayfield JE, Brozowski SJ, Gonzales EL, Trudell JR, Harris RA (1998) Sites of volatile anesthetic action on kainate (Glutamate receptor 6) receptors. J Biol Chem 273:8248–8255

Ming Z, Knapp DJ, Mueller RA, Breese GR, Criswell HE (2001) Differential modulation of GABA- and NMDA-gated currents by ethanol and isoflurane in cultured rat cerebral cortical neurons. Brain Res 920:117–124

Ming Z, Griffith BL, Breese GR, Mueller RA, Criswell HE (2002) Changes in the effect of isoflurane on N-methyl-D-aspartic acid-gated currents in cultured cerebral cortical neurons with time in culture: evidence for subunit specificity. Anesthesiology 97:856–867

Mirshahi T, Woodward JJ (1995) Ethanol sensitivity of heteromeric NMDA receptors: effects of subunit assembly, glycine and NMDAR1 Mg(2+)-insensitive mutants. Neuropharmacology 34:347–355

Mirshahi T, Anders DL, Ronald KM, Woodward JJ (1998) Intracellular calcium enhances the ethanol sensitivity of NMDA receptors through an interaction with the C0 domain of the NR1 subunit. J Neurochem 71:1095–1107

Mu Y, Otsuka T, Horton AC, Scott DB, Ehlers MD (2003) Activity-dependent mRNA splicing controls ER export and synaptic delivery of NMDA receptors. Neuron 40:581–594

Nagele P, Metz LB, Crowder CM (2005) Xenon acts by inhibition of non-N-methyl-D-aspartate receptor-mediated glutamatergic neurotransmission in Caenorhabditis elegans. Anesthesiology 103:508–513

Neher E, Steinbach JH (1978) Local anaesthetics transiently block currents through single acetylcholine-receptor channels. J Physiol 277:153–176

Ogata J, Shiraishi M, Namba T, Smothers CT, Woodward JJ, Harris RA (2006) Effects of anesthetics on mutant N-methyl-D-aspartate receptors expressed in Xenopus oocytes. J Pharmacol Exp Ther 318:434–443

Orser BA, Pennefather PS, MacDonald JF (1997) Multiple mechanisms of ketamine blockade of N-methyl-D-aspartate receptors. Anesthesiology 86:903–917

Palmer CL, Cotton L, Henley JM (2005) The molecular pharmacology and cell biology of alpha-amino-3-hydroxy-5-methyl-4-isoxazolepropionic acid receptors. Pharmacol Rev 57: 253–277

Paradiso K, Sabey K, Evers AS, Zorumski CF, Covey DF, Steinbach JH (2000) Steroid inhibition of rat neuronal nicotinic alpha 4 beta 2 receptors expressed in HEK 293 cells. Mol Pharmacol 58:341–351

Patneau DK, Mayer ML (1990) Structure-activity relationships for amino acid transmitter candidates acting at N-methyl-D-aspartate and quisqualate receptors. J Neurosci 10: 2385–2399

Peters JA, Hales TG, Lambert JJ (2005) Molecular determinants of single-channel conductance and ion selectivity in the Cys-loop family: insights from the 5-HT3 receptor. Trends Pharmacol Sci 26:587–594

Reeves DC, Lummis SC (2002) The molecular basis of the structure and function of the 5-HT3 receptor: a model ligand-gated ion channel (review). Mol Membr Biol 19:11–26

Ren H, Honse Y, Peoples RW (2003) A site of alcohol action in the fourth membrane-associated domain of the N-methyl-D-aspartate receptor. J Biol Chem 278:48815–48820

Rogers SW, Mandelzys A, Deneris ES, Cooper E, Heinemann S (1992) The expression of nicotinic acetylcholine receptors by PC12 cells treated with NGF. J Neurosci 12:4611–4623

Ronald KM, Mirshahi T, Woodward JJ (2001) Ethanol inhibition of N-methyl-D-aspartate receptors is reduced by site-directed mutagenesis of a transmembrane domain phenylalanine residue. J Biol Chem 276:44729–44735

Sabey K, Paradiso K, Zhang J, Steinbach JH (1999) Ligand binding and activation of rat nicotinic alpha 4 beta 2 receptors stably expressed in HEK293 cells. Mol Pharmacol 55:58–66

Sasaki T, Andoh T, Watanabe I, Kamiya Y, Itoh H, Higashi T, Matsuura T (2000) Nonsteroselective inhibition of neuronal nicotinic acetylcholine receptors by ketamine isomers. Anesth Analg 91:741–748

Scheller M, Bufler J, Hertle I, Schneck HJ, Franke C, Kochs E (1996) Ketamine blocks currents through mammalian nicotinic acetylcholine receptor channels by interaction with both the open and the closed state. Anesth Analg 83:830–836

Sewell JC, Sear JW (2004) Derivation of preliminary three-dimensional pharmacophoric maps for chemically diverse intravenous general anaesthetics. Br J Anaesth 92:45–53

Shiraishi M, Shibuya I, Minami K, Uezono Y, Okamoto T, Yanagihara N, Ueno S, Ueta Y, Shigematsu A (2002) A neurosteroid anesthetic, alphaxalone, inhibits nicotinic acetylcholine receptors in cultured bovine adrenal chromaffin cells. Anesth Analg 95:900–906

Smothers CT, Woodward JJ (2006) Effects of amino acid substitutions in transmembrane domains of the NR1 subunit on the ethanol inhibition of recombinant N-methyl-D-aspartate receptors. Alcohol Clin Exp Res 30:523–530

Smothers CT, Clayton R, Blevins T, Woodward JJ (2001) Ethanol sensitivity of recombinant human N-methyl-D-aspartate receptors. Neurochem Int 38:333–340

Solt K, Stevens RJ, Davies PA, Raines DE (2005) General anesthetic-induced channel gating enhancement of 5-hydroxytryptamine type 3 receptors depends on receptor subunit composition. J Pharmacol Exp Ther 315:771–776

Sonner JM, Antognini JF, Dutton RC, Flood P, Gray AT, Harris RA, Homanics GE, Kendig J, Orser B, Raines DE, Rampil IJ, Trudell J, Vissel B, Eger EI 2nd (2003) Inhaled anesthetics and immobility: mechanisms, mysteries, and minimum alveolar anesthetic concentration. Anesth Analg 97:718–740

Stevens R, Rusch D, Solt K, Raines DE, Davies PA (2005a) Modulation of human 5-hydroxytryptamine type 3AB receptors by volatile anesthetics and n-alcohols. J Pharmacol Exp Ther 314:338–345

Stevens RJ, Rusch D, Davies PA, Raines DE (2005b) Molecular properties important for inhaled anesthetic action on human 5-HT3A receptors. Anesth Analg 100:1696–1703

Suzuki T, Koyama H, Sugimoto M, Uchida I, Mashimo T (2002) The diverse actions of volatile and gaseous anesthetics on human-cloned 5-hydroxytryptamine3 receptors expressed in Xenopus oocytes. Anesthesiology 96:699–704

Suzuki T, Ueta K, Sugimoto M, Uchida I, Mashimo T (2003) Nitrous oxide and xenon inhibit the human (alpha 7)5 nicotinic acetylcholine receptor expressed in Xenopus oocyte. Anesth Analg 96:443–448

Tassonyi E, Charpantier E, Muller D, Dumont L, Bertrand D (2002) The role of nicotinic acetylcholine receptors in the mechanisms of anesthesia. Brain Res Bull 57:133–150

Taverna FA, Cameron BR, Hampson DL, Wang LY, MacDonald JF (1994) Sensitivity of AMPA receptors to pentobarbital. Eur J Pharmacol 267:R3–R5

Thomson AM, West DC, Lodge D (1985) An N-methylaspartate receptor-mediated synapse in rat cerebral cortex: a site of action of ketamine? Nature 313:479–481

Tomioka A, Ueno S, Kohama K, Goto F, Inoue K (2000) Propofol potentiates ATP-activated currents of recombinant P2X(4) receptor channels expressed in human embryonic kidney 293 cells. Neurosci Lett 284:167–170

Violet JM, Downie DL, Nakisa RC, Lieb WR, Franks NP (1997) Differential sensitivities of mammalian neuronal and muscle nicotinic acetylcholine receptors to general anesthetics [see comments]. Anesthesiology 86:866–874

Wachtel RE (1995) Relative potencies of volatile anesthetics in altering the kinetics of ion channels in BC3H1 cells. J Pharmacol Exp Ther 274:1355–1361

Wachtel RE, Wegrzynowicz ES (1992) Kinetics of nicotinic acetylcholine ion channels in the presence of intravenous anaesthetics and induction agents. Br J Pharmacol 106:623–627

Watanabe I, Andoh T, Furuya R, Sasaki T, Kamiya Y, Itoh H (1999) Depressant and convulsant barbiturates both inhibit neuronal nicotinic acetylcholine receptors. Anesth Analg 88: 1406–1411

Weaver CE Jr, Park-Chung M, Gibbs TT, Farb DH (1997) 17beta-Estradiol protects against NMDA-induced excitotoxicity by direct inhibition of NMDA receptors. Brain Res 761:338–341

Weber M, Motin L, Gaul S, Beker F, Fink RH, Adams DJ (2005) Intravenous anaesthetics inhibit nicotinic acetylcholine receptor-mediated currents and Ca2+ transients in rat intracardiac ganglion neurons. Br J Pharmacol 144:98–107

Wetzel CH, Hermann B, Behl C, Pestel E, Rammes G, Zieglgansberger W, Holsboer F, Rupprecht R (1998) Functional antagonism of gonadal steroids at the 5-hydroxytryptamine type 3 receptor. Mol Endocrinol 12:1441–1451

Wittmann M, Peters I, Schaaf T, Wartenberg HC, Wirz S, Nadstawek J, Urban BW, Barann M (2006) The effects of morphine on human 5-HT3A receptors. Anesth Analg 103: 747–752

Wollmuth LP, Sobolevsky AI (2004) Structure and gating of the glutamate receptor ion channel. Trends Neurosci 27:321–328

Wonnacott S, Sidhpura N, Balfour DJ (2005) Nicotine: from molecular mechanisms to behaviour. Curr Opin Pharmacol 5:53–59

Woodward JJ (2000) Ethanol and NMDA receptor signaling. Crit Rev Neurobiol 14:69–89

Wright JM, Peoples RW, Weight FF (1996) Single-channel and whole-cell analysis of ethanol inhibition of NMDA-activated currents in cultured mouse cortical and hippocampal neurons. Brain Res 738:249–256

Wu XS, Sun JY, Evers AS, Crowder M, Wu LG (2004) Isoflurane inhibits transmitter release and the presynaptic action potential. Anesthesiology 100:663–670

Yamakura T, Harris RA (2000) Effects of gaseous anesthetics nitrous oxide and xenon on ligand-gated ion channels. Comparison with isoflurane and ethanol. Anesthesiology 93:1095–1101

Yamakura T, Mori H, Masaki H, Shimoji K, Mishina M (1993) Different sensitivities of NMDA receptor channel subtypes to non-competitive antagonists. Neuroreport 4:687–690

Yamakura T, Sakimura K, Mishina M, Shimoji K (1995a) The sensitivity of AMPA-selective glutamate receptor channels to pentobarbital is determined by a single amino acid residue of the alpha 2 subunit. FEBS Lett 374:412–414

Yamakura T, Sakimura K, Shimoji K, Mishina M (1995b) Effects of propofol on various AMPA-, kainate- and NMDA-selective glutamate receptor channels expressed in Xenopus oocytes. Neurosci Lett 188:187–190

Yamakura T, Chavez-Noriega LE, Harris RA (2000) Subunit-dependent inhibition of human neuronal nicotinic acetylcholine receptors and other ligand-gated ion channels by dissociative anesthetics ketamine and dizocilpine. Anesthesiology 92:1144–1153

Yamakura T, Bertaccini E, Trudell JR, Harris RA (2001) Anesthetics and ion channels: molecular models and sites of action. Annu Rev Pharmacol Toxicol 41:23–51

Yamashita M, Mori T, Nagata K, Yeh JZ, Narahashi T (2005) Isoflurane modulation of neuronal nicotinic acetylcholine receptors expressed in human embryonic kidney cells. Anesthesiology 102:76–84

Yost CS, Dodson BA (1993) Inhibition of the nicotinic acetylcholine receptor by barbiturates and by procaine: do they act at different sites? Cell Mol Neurobiol 13:159–172

Zhang L, Oz M, Stewart RR, Peoples RW, Weight FF (1997) Volatile general anaesthetic actions on recombinant nACh alpha 7, 5-HT3 and chimeric nACh alpha 7–5-HT3 receptors expressed in Xenopus oocytes. Br J Pharmacol 120:353–355

Zorumski CF, Mennerick S, Isenberg KE, Covey DF (2000) Potential clinical uses of neuroactive steroids. IDrugs 3:1053–1063

Voltage-Gated Ion Channels

C. Nau

Abstract How and where simple volatile organic molecules act in the central nervous system to cause loss of consciousness and insensitivity to pain has eluded investigation; yet remarkable progress has been made recently towards identifying possible molecular targets through which the mechanism of anesthesia is transduced. It is likely that anesthetics act by binding directly to protein targets; several possible candidates have been identified and the debate now focuses on whether general anesthesia is due to large effects at a relatively small number of critical molecular sites or due to the combined effects of small perturbations at a very large number of sites; voltage-gated ion channels are contenders for either possibility and are the subject of this review.

1 Introduction

The superfamily of voltage-gated ion channels and structural relatives, also termed the voltage-gated-like (VGL) ion channel superfamily, is one of the largest superfamilies of signal transduction proteins, only exceeded by G protein-coupled receptors and protein kinases. Many members of this superfamily are common drug targets.

C. Nau
Klinik für Anästhesiologie, Universität Erlangen-Nürnberg, Krankenhausstr. 12, 91054 Erlangen, Germany
carla.nau@kfa.imed.uni-erlangen.de

J. Schüttler and H. Schwilden (eds.) *Modern Anesthetics.*
Handbook of Experimental Pharmacology 182.

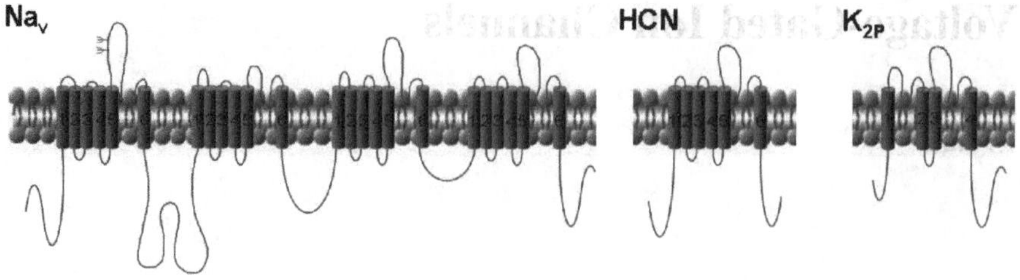

Fig. 1 Schematic representation of the membrane topology of voltage-gated Na^+ (*Na_v*), hyperpolarization-activated cyclic nucleotide-gated (*HCN*), and two-pore K^+ (*K_{2P}*) channels

The VGL ion channel superfamily comprises the following ion channel families: the four-domain voltage-gated Na^+ (Na_v) and Ca^{2+} (Ca_v) channels; the one-domain voltage-gated K^+ channels, including K_v channels, Ca^{2+}-activated K^+ (K_{Ca}) channels, and cyclic nucleotide-gated (CNG) and hyperpolarization-activated cyclic nucleotide-gated (HCN) channels; the TRP channels; the inwardly rectifying K^+ (K_{ir}) channels; and the two-pore K^+ (K_{2P}) channels (Yu et al. 2005). Among these ion channel families, Na_v, Ca_v, and K_v channels are directly and rapidly gated by voltage. For K_{Ca} and HCN channels, ligand binding and voltage together gate the pore. The other ion channel families are not voltage-gated in the strict sense of the word; however, all of these ion channel families are related in molecular and evolutionary terms.

The following chapter will present and discuss the evidence for three of these ion channel families as potential targets for anesthetics, based on their ability to regulate neuronal activity, their expression pattern, and their sensitivity to anesthetics in clinically relevant concentrations. These are the Na_v, HCN, and K_{2P} channel families (Fig. 1).

2 Voltage-Gated Na^+ Channels

Voltage-gated Na^+ channels are dynamic transmembrane proteins that govern action potential initiation and propagation in excitable membranes. Nine mammalian Na^+ channel isoforms have been identified and functionally expressed thus far. Their amino acid sequences in the transmembrane and extracellular domains are more than 50% identical (Catterall et al. 2005).

All Na^+ channel isoforms show the same overall structure: They consist of a large α-subunit and one or more of four auxiliary β-subunits. The primary functional properties of Na^+ channels reside in the α-subunit. Associated β-subunits modify kinetics and voltage-dependence of channel gating. The α-subunit comprises four homologous domains (D1–D4), each containing six α-helical transmembrane segments (S1–S6). The linkers between segments S5 and S6 form pore loops from the extracellular side and line the narrow outer part of the channel's pore. The S5 and S6 segments of each domain line the inner part of the channel's pore. The highly positively charged S4 segments in each domain serve as voltage sensors. Their outward movements upon depolarization induce conformational changes in the pore resulting in channel activation (Catterall 2000).

The structural determinants of Na^+ channel fast inactivation are hydrophobic residues in the intracellular D3–D4 loop that may form an inactivation gate. Several residues at the intracellular end of D4–S6 and within intracellular S4–S5 loops of D3 and D4 may function as receptors for the inactivation gate (Catterall 2000).

Among the nine mammalian Na^+ channel isoforms, three isoforms—$Na_v1.7$, $Na_v1.8$, and $Na_v1.9$—are predominantly expressed in the peripheral nervous system and critically contribute to nociception. $Na_v1.4$ is predominantly expressed in adult skeletal muscle, $Na_v1.5$ in cardiac myocytes, and $Na_v1.3$ in embryonic and prenatal life central neurons. $Na_v1.1$, $Na_v1.2$, and $Na_v1.6$ are predominantly expressed in central neurons (Catterall et al. 2005) and are thus potential targets for general anesthetics.

There is evidence that recombinant and native voltage-gated Na^+ channels are indeed sensitive to clinically relevant concentrations of volatile anesthetics. Isoflurane, but not propofol, in a clinically relevant concentration inhibited currents of $Na_v1.2$, $Na_v1.4$, and $Na_v1.6$ heterologously expressed in *Xenopus* oocytes (Shiraishi and Harris 2004). A detailed analysis of the effect of inhalation anesthetics on $Na_v1.2$ heterologously expressed in Chinese hamster ovary cells demonstrated a voltage-dependent interaction resulting in depression of peak Na^+ current and in significant frequency-dependent inhibition (Rehberg et al. 1996). Subtype-specific effects of anesthetics have never been shown unequivocally and are considered to be unlikely. Accordingly, inhalation anesthetics inhibit Na^+ channels in various in vitro preparations including dorsal root ganglion neurons and isolated nerve terminals (Ouyang and Hemmings 2005). Comprehensive attempts to map the binding region for general anesthetics in voltage-gated Na^+ channels, in contrast to local anesthetics (Nau and Wang 2004), have not been documented to date.

There is controversy about the relevance of Na^+ channel block for anesthetic action. Two findings, however, might be of significance in this respect. First, axonal conduction is depressed by clinically relevant concentrations of halothane in thin, lightly myelinated hippocampal axons in an in vitro brain slice preparation (Mikulec et al. 1998). Second and more importantly, just a small reduction in presynaptic action potential amplitude without any direct effect on Ca^{2+} currents elicited by isoflurane was sufficient to significantly depress action potential-evoked synaptic vesicle exocytosis and excitatory postsynaptic current in a large, glutamatergic calyx-type synapse in the medial nucleus of the trapezoid body in rat brainstem (calyx of Held) (Wu et al. 2004). This finding suggests that depression of synaptic transmission by general anesthetics might be secondary to effects on the action potential, a hypothesis in stark contrast to a long-standing concept (Perouansky et al. 2004).

3 Hyperpolarization-Activated Cyclic Nucleotide-Gated Channels

In contrast to most other voltage-gated channels, the HCN channels are activated by hyperpolarization and close at positive potentials. The cyclic nucleotides cyclic guanosine monophosphate (cGMP) and cyclic adenosine monophosphate (cAMP) directly bind to the channel protein and enhance HCN channel activity by shifting activation to more positive voltages.

Structurally, HCN channels comprise six transmembrane helical segments, with a pore loop between segment 5 and 6, and assemble in tetramers. Like in Na_v channels, the S4 segments are positively charged and serve as voltage sensors. HCN channels govern cation currents termed I_h, I_f, or I_q, depending on the tissue. They are found in neurons, cardiac pacemakers, and photoreceptors. In neurons, I_h contributes to generation of pacemaker potentials, determination of resting potential, transduction of sour taste, dendritic integration, control of synaptic transmission, and plasticity (Hofmann et al. 2005). In mammals, the HCN family comprises four members (HCN1–HCN4). These channels differ in their speed of activation and the extent of modulation by cAMP. All four subunits are found in brain. HCN2 is found almost ubiquitously in the brain, HCN4 is concentrated in the thalamus, HCN1 in the hippocampus, and HCN3 in some hypothalamic nuclei, but is also expressed at low levels in most other brain areas.

Inhalation anesthetics were demonstrated to act directly on rat brainstem motoneurons at clinically relevant concentrations to cause membrane hyperpolarization and decreased excitability via inhibition of I_h (Sirois et al. 2002; Sirois et al. 1998). Anesthetic inhibition of I_h involves a hyperpolarizing shift in voltage dependence of activation and decrease in maximal current amplitude. These effects could be ascribed to HCN1 and HCN2 subunits (Chen et al. 2005). Among intravenous anesthetics, pentobarbital inhibits I_h in thalamic neurons (Wan et al. 2003), and propofol block of I_h was demonstrated to contribute to the suppression of neuronal excitability and rhythmic burst firing in thalamocortical neurons (Ying et al. 2006). Deficits of anesthetic action in genetically engineered animals that lack HCN subunits have not been documented to date.

HCN channels might well represent a yet under-appreciated anesthetic target-site.

4 Two-Pore K^+ Channels

Background leak K^+ currents control cellular excitability. The molecular correlates governing these background leak currents are the K_{2P} channels. Structurally, they comprise two pore-forming loops in tandem in each subunit and four transmembrane domains. Both amino and carboxy termini are intracellular. Unlike the channel families with six transmembrane segments, Na_v and HCN, K_{2P} subunits most likely dimerize to form a functional channel.

The human K_{2P} family consists of 15 known members (Goldstein et al. 2005). K_{2P} channels are potassium-selective, active at the resting membrane potential, and controlled by various chemical and physical stimuli.

A reduction of neuronal excitability by the activation of K^+ channels has long been considered a conceivable concept for a mechanism of general anesthesia (Franks and Lieb 1999; Nicoll and Madison 1982). That inhalation anesthetics indeed activate leak K^+ currents was first discovered in the mollusc *Lymnaea stagnalis* (Franks and Lieb 1988). Sequence analysis and functional properties revealed recently the molecular entity to be a member of the TASK family of channels with approx. 47% sequence identity when compared with human TASK-1 (K_{2p}3.1) and TASK-3 (K_{2p}9.1) (Andres-Enguix et al. 2007) (TASK: Twik related acid-sensitive K^- channel: TWIK: Tandem of P domain in a weak inward rectifying K^+ channel). Other neuronal human K_{2p} channels to be selectively opened by inhalation anesthetics are TREK-1 (K_{2p}2.1), TREK-2 (K_{2p}10.1), and TASK-2 (K_{2p}5.1) (Patel and Honore 2001a) (TREK: TWIK-related K^+ channel). Local anesthetics, in contrast, reversibly block K_{2P} channels. Reports of genetically engineered animals that lack TREK-1 or TASK-1 and exhibit diminished anesthetic sensitivity (Heurteaux et al. 2004; Linden et al. 2006) have substantiated a possible role of these two channels for general anesthesia. In contrast, TASK-2 knockout mice did not show any significant alteration in anesthetic sensitivity (Gerstin et al. 2003).

Human TREK-1 in the CNS has the highest levels of expression in GABA-containing interneurons of the caudate nucleus and putamen and in hippocampal glutamate-containing neurons. TREK-1 is also expressed in spinal cord and dorsal root ganglion neurons (Hervieu et al. 2001; Medhurst et al. 2001). TREK-1 is gated by membrane stretch and modulated in whole-cell analyses by cellular volume, with hyperosmolarity closing the channel. Heat reversibly opens TREK-1. Low intracellular pH enables channel opening at atmospheric pressure due to a right-shift in the pressure–activation relationship and essentially converts TREK-1 in a constitutively active background channel. Among the chemical substances activating TREK-1 are polyunsaturated fatty acids including arachidonic acids, lysophospholipids, and the neuroprotective drug riluzole. TREK-1 is modulated via various intracellular signaling cascades (Franks and Honore 2004).

Heterologously expressed TREK-1 channels are opened by the inhalation anesthetics chloroform, diethyl ether, halothane, and isoflurane. Channel opening leads to cell hyperpolarization. Human TREK-1 is most sensitive to chloroform and is opened by inhalation anesthetics in clinically relevant concentrations (Patel et al. 1998, 1999). Clinically relevant concentrations of nitrous oxide, xenon, and the chloral hydrate metabolite trichloroethanol also open TREK-1 (Gruss et al. 2004; Harinath and Sikdar 2004). Most anesthetics require the C-terminal domain for channel activation.

Knockout mice provided more direct evidence for a role of TREK-1 in anesthesia. These mice reportedly did not display any abnormal phenotype, showing normal reflex and cognitive function. However, the sensitivity of these mice toward the inhalation anesthetics chloroform, halothane, sevoflurane, and desflurane was significantly decreased (Franks and Honore 2004; Heurteaux et al. 2004). This applied to both latency for anesthesia (which was longer) and the concentrations required to reach the common anesthetic endpoints loss of righting reflex and failure to respond to a painful stimulus (which were significantly higher). In these experiments, Halothane in a concentration that was sufficient to anesthetize all wild-type mice was essentially without effect in the knockout mice. These experiments, however, also suggested the recruitment of further targets at higher concentrations of anesthetics. Importantly, the effect of pentobarbital, which does not open TREK-1, was similar in wild-type and knockout mice, suggesting that there was no general increase in excitability in knockout mice.

Human TASK-1 in the CNS has the highest expression in the cerebellum, thalamus, and pituitary gland (Medhurst et al. 2001). TASK-1 is also abundant in human dorsal root ganglion neurons and in rat carotid body. TASK-1 is sensitive to external pH changes in a narrow range near physiological pH and might be involved in both oxygen- and acid-sensing in peripheral chemoreceptors (Patel and Honore 2001b). TASK-1 is modulated by G protein-coupled receptors. Inhibition of TASK-1 leads to membrane depolarization; activation induces hyperpolarization. TASK-1 heterodimerizes with TASK-3 in cell types expressing both genes.

TASK-1 is opened by halothane and isoflurane but is insensitive to chloroform (Patel et al. 1999; Sirois et al. 2000). At higher concentrations, isoflurane slightly inhibits TASK-1 homodimeric channels (Berg et al. 2004). A defined region within the C-terminal domain seems to be required for channel activation by anesthetics. A study employing chimeric channel constructs and site-directed mutagenesis has identified a specific amino acid located at the cytosolic interface of transmembrane segment 3 to be a critical determinant of anesthetic sensitivity and a putative part of an anesthetic binding site (Andres-Enguix et al. 2007).

TASK-1 knockout mice displayed a largely normal behavioral phenotype; however, they exhibited significantly shorter latencies in the hot-plate test, suggesting enhanced thermal nociception. In low concentrations of halothane, the loss of righting reflex was similar in wild-type and knockout mice. However, the concentration at which mice lost their tail-withdrawal reflex was significantly higher in knockout than in wild-type mice. In the case of isoflurane, knockout mice required a higher concentration for the loss of righting reflex; however, no significant difference was found for the loss of tail-withdrawal (Linden et al. 2006). The less clear effect in TASK-1 knockout mice with respect to anesthetic effects might be due to a compensatory action of TASK-3 in TASK-1 knockout mice and/or the biphasic effect of some anesthetics on TASK-1.

Altogether, there is strong evidence for an important role of TREK-1 and possibly TASK-1 in general anesthesia by inhalation anesthetics.

Whether or not the effects of anesthetics on Na_v, HCN, or K_{2P} channels indeed contribute to any endpoint of the anesthetic state in humans remains a challenging question for future research of mechanisms of anesthesia.

References

Andres-Enguix I, Caley A, Yustos R, Schumacher MA, Spanu PD, Dickinson R, Maze M, Franks NP (2007) Determinants of the anesthetic sensitivity of two-pore domain acid-sensitive potassium channels: molecular cloning of an anesthetic-activated potassium channel from Lymnaea stagnalis. J Biol Chem 282:20977–20990

Berg AP, Talley EM, Manger JP, Bayliss DA (2004) Motoneurons express heteromeric TWIK-related acid-sensitive K+ (TASK) channels containing TASK-1 (KCNK3) and TASK-3 (KCNK9) subunits. J Neurosci 24:6693–6702

Catterall WA (2000) From ionic currents to molecular mechanisms: the structure and function of voltage-gated sodium channels. Neuron 26:13–25

Catterall WA, Goldin AL, Waxman SG (2005) International Union of Pharmacology. XLVII. Nomenclature and structure-function relationships of voltage-gated sodium channels. Pharmacol Rev 57:397–409

Chen X, Sirois JE, Lei Q, Talley EM, Lynch C, Bayliss DA 3rd (2005) HCN subunit-specific and cAMP-modulated effects of anesthetics on neuronal pacemaker currents. J Neurosci 25:5803–5814

Franks NP, Honore E (2004) The TREK K2P channels and their role in general anaesthesia and neuroprotection. Trends Pharmacol Sci 25:601–608

Franks NP, Lieb WR (1988) Volatile general anaesthetics activate a novel neuronal K+ current. Nature 333:662–664

Franks NP, Lieb WR (1999) Background K+ channels: an important target for volatile anesthetics? Nat Neurosci 2:395–396

Gerstin KM, Gong DH, Abdallah M, Winegar BD, Eger EI 2nd, Gray AT (2003) Mutation of KCNK5 or Kir3.2 potassium channels in mice does not change minimum alveolar anesthetic concentration. Anesth Analg 96:1345–1349

Goldstein SA, Bayliss DA, Kim D, Lesage F, Plant LD, Rajan S (2005) International Union of Pharmacology. LV. Nomenclature and molecular relationships of two-P potassium channels. Pharmacol Rev 57:527–540

Gruss M, Bushell TJ, Bright DP, Lieb WR, Mathie A, Franks NP (2004) Two-pore-domain K+ channels are a novel target for the anesthetic gases xenon, nitrous oxide, and cyclopropane. Mol Pharmacol 65:443–452

Harinath S, Sikdar SK (2004) Trichloroethanol enhances the activity of recombinant human TREK-1 and TRAAK channels. Neuropharmacology 46:750–760

Hervieu GJ, Cluderay JE, Gray CW, Green PJ, Ranson JL, Randall AD, Meadows HJ (2001) Distribution and expression of TREK-1, a two-pore-domain potassium channel, in the adult rat CNS. Neuroscience 103:899–919

Heurteaux C, Guy N, Laigle C, Blondeau N, Duprat F, Mazzuca M, Lang-Lazdunski L, Widmann C, Zanzouri M, Romey G, Lazdunski M (2004) TREK-1, a K+ channel involved in neuroprotection and general anesthesia. EMBO J 23:2684–2695

Hofmann F, Biel M, Kaupp UB (2005) International Union of Pharmacology. LI. Nomenclature and structure-function relationships of cyclic nucleotide-regulated channels. Pharmacol Rev 57:455–462

Linden AM, Aller MI, Leppa E, Vekovischeva O, Aitta-Aho T, Veale EL, Mathie A, Rosenberg P, Wisden W, Korpi ER (2006) The in vivo contributions of TASK-1-containing channels to the actions of inhalation anesthetics, the alpha(2) adrenergic sedative dexmedetomidine, and cannabinoid agonists. J Pharmacol Exp Ther 317:615–626

Medhurst AD, Rennie G, Chapman CG, Meadows H, Duckworth MD, Kelsell RE, Gloger II, Pangalos MN (2001) Distribution analysis of human two pore domain potassium channels in tissues of the central nervous system and periphery. Brain Res Mol Brain Res 86:101–114

Mikulec AA, Pittson S, Amagasu SM, Monroe FA, MacIver MB (1998) Halothane depresses action potential conduction in hippocampal axons. Brain Res 796:231–238

Nau C, Wang GK (2004) Interactions of local anesthetics with voltage-gated Na+ channels. J Membr Biol 201:1–8

Nicoll RA, Madison DV (1982) General anesthetics hyperpolarize neurons in the vertebrate central nervous system. Science 217:1055–1057

Ouyang W, Hemmings HC Jr (2005) Depression by isoflurane of the action potential and underlying voltage-gated ion currents in isolated rat neurohypophysial nerve terminals. J Pharmacol Exp Ther 312:801–808

Patel AJ, Honore E (2001a) Anesthetic-sensitive 2P domain K+ channels. Anesthesiology 95:1013–1021

Patel AJ, Honore E (2001b) Molecular physiology of oxygen-sensitive potassium channels. Eur Respir J 18:221–227

Patel AJ, Honore E, Maingret F, Lesage F, Fink M, Duprat F, Lazdunski M (1998) A mammalian two pore domain mechano-gated S-like K+ channel. EMBO J 17:4283–4290

Patel AJ, Honore E, Lesage F, Fink M, Romey G, Lazdunski M (1999) Inhalational anesthetics activate two-pore-domain background K+ channels. Nat Neurosci 2:422–426

Perouansky M, Hemmings HC, Pearce R (2004) Anesthetic effects on glutamatergic neurotransmission: lessons learned from a large synapse. Anesthesiology 100:470–472

Rehberg B, Xiao YH, Duch DS (1996) Central nervous system sodium channels are significantly suppressed at clinical concentrations of volatile anesthetics. Anesthesiology 84:1223–1233

Shiraishi M, Harris RA (2004) Effects of alcohols and anesthetics on recombinant voltage-gated Na+ channels. J Pharmacol Exp Ther 309:987–994

Sirois JE, Pancrazio JJ, Iii CL, Bayliss DA (1998) Multiple ionic mechanisms mediate inhibition of rat motoneurones by inhalation anaesthetics. J Physiol 512:851–862

Sirois JE, Lei Q, Talley EM, Lynch C, Bayliss DA 3rd (2000) The TASK-1 two-pore domain K+ channel is a molecular substrate for neuronal effects of inhalation anesthetics. J Neurosci 20:6347–6354

Sirois JE, Lynch C, Bayliss DA 3rd (2002) Convergent and reciprocal modulation of a leak K+ current and I(h) by an inhalational anaesthetic and neurotransmitters in rat brainstem motoneurones. J Physiol 541:717–729

Wan X, Mathers DA, Puil E (2003) Pentobarbital modulates intrinsic and GABA-receptor conductances in thalamocortical inhibition. Neuroscience 121:947–958

Wu XS, Sun JY, Evers AS, Crowder M, Wu LG (2004) Isoflurane inhibits transmitter release and the presynaptic action potential. Anesthesiology 100:663–670

Ying SW, Abbas SY, Harrison NL, Goldstein PA (2006) Propofol block of I(h) contributes to the suppression of neuronal excitability and rhythmic burst firing in thalamocortical neurons. Eur J Neurosci 23:465–480

Yu FH, Yarov-Yarovoy V, Gutman GA, Catterall WA (2005) Overview of molecular relationships in the voltage-gated ion channel superfamily. Pharmacol Rev 57:387–395

G-Protein-Coupled Receptors

R.D. Sanders, D. Brian, and M. Maze(✉)

Abstract G-Protein-coupled receptors mediate many of the hypnotic and analgesic actions of the drugs employed in anesthesia. Notably, opioid agonists represent the most successful and efficacious class of analgesic agents employed over the last century. Also, major clinical advances have been made by the study of α_2 adrenoceptor agonists, which possess both hypnotic and analgesic qualities that are being increasingly exploited in both anesthetic and critical care settings. Furthermore

M. Maze
Academic Anaesthetics, Imperial College, Chelsea & Westminster Hospital,
369 Fulham Road, London SW10 9NH, UK
m.maze@ic.ac.uk

J. Schüttler and H. Schwilden (eds.) *Modern Anesthetics.*
Handbook of Experimental Pharmacology 182.

orexin, γ-aminobutyric acid $(GABA)_B$, and muscarinic cholinergic receptors have been identified as potential anesthetic targets; clinical exploitation of ligands at these receptors may lead to important advances in anesthetic pharmacology. In this review we discuss the relevant molecular and neural network pharmacology of anesthetic agents acting at G-protein-coupled receptors.

1 Introduction

Guanine nucleotide-binding protein (G-protein)-coupled receptors (GPCRs) are the largest and most versatile group of cell surface receptors, and represent a conserved mechanism for extracellular signal perception in eukaryotic organisms (Pierce et al. 2002). Various stimuli (e.g., photons and odors) and ligands (e.g., neurotransmitters, cytokines, hormones, and drugs) can activate intracellular signaling cascades via G-proteins. Indeed, GPCRs mediate many anesthetic and analgesics effects of the drugs we employ.

1.1 Structure of G-Protein-Coupled Receptors

GPCRs are a superfamily of integral membrane proteins, and possess seven transmembrane helices (I–VII), three extracellular loops (II–III, IV–V, and VI–VII), and three cytosolic loops (I–II, III–IV, and V–VI). They have a periplasmic N-terminal domain (N), and a cytosolic C-terminal (C) domain; domain VIII is also contained in the C-terminal and runs parallel to the cytosolic membrane surface (Palczewski et al. 2000; see Fig. 1). Signal transduction through membrane-bound GPCRs enables diverse intracellular responses to a wide array of chemical ligands in a highly selective fashion. To date, 616 functionally diverse members (2.3% of total genes) have been described (Hemmings and Girault 2004), facilitated by a shift from ligand-based to sequence-based discovery (Lee et al. 2001). Perhaps surprisingly, current evidence suggests that of all drugs targeting GPCRs, the majority exert their effect predominantly on a group of only approximately 30 of these (Wise et al. 2004).

1.2 G-Protein-Coupled Receptor Subtypes

In 1971, Rodbell first outlined how a guanine-nucleotide binding regulatory protein linked receptors with downstream cellular effectors, in the context of hormonal modulation of the adenylyl cyclase system (Rodbell et al. 1971). Subsequent purification led to the identification of a heterotrimeric G-protein, composed of α-, β-, and γ-subunits, and molecular cloning has now defined 35 genes encoding

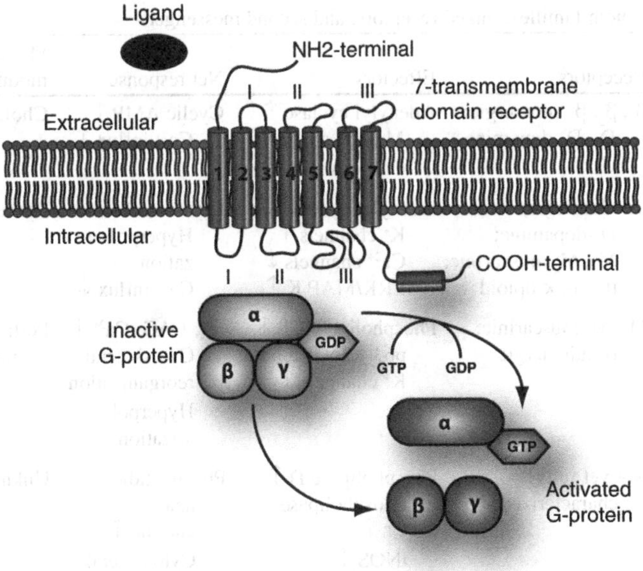

Fig. 1 Illustration of a G-protein-coupled receptor (GPCR), consisting of seven membrane spanning domains (*1–7*), an extracellular N-terminal and intracellular C-terminal. The three extracellular and three intracellular loops (*I–III*) are also indicated. Upon ligand binding, the GPCR activates the coupled G-protein, causing it to exchange bound GDP for GTP and dissociate into an α-subunit and β/γ-dimer and stimulate downstream effectors. The GTP bound to the α-subunit is then hydrolyzed to GDP (not shown), allowing re-association of the α- and β/γ-subunits, returning the GPCR to its original resting state

G-proteins in humans, 16 encoding α-, 5 encoding β-, and 14 encoding γ-subunits. The α-subunit is responsible for binding of guanosine diphosphate (GDP) or guanosine triphosphate (GTP), depending on its conformational state.

Heterotrimeric G-proteins are classified based on their function and α-subunit; for example, the $G_s\alpha$ protein (abbreviated G_s) couples to a stimulatory α-subunit activating adenylyl cyclase, leading to increased cAMP. The G_i and G_o proteins (known as $G_{i/o}$) and G_z proteins activate an inhibitory α-subunit that blocks adenylyl cyclase, but activates G-protein-coupled inwardly rectifying potassium (GIRK) channels (Milligan and Kostenis 2006; see Table 1). Agonists of receptors coupled to $G_{i/o}$ proteins are of importance in anesthesia as they mediate the analgesic and sedative/hypnotic actions of many important anesthetic drugs. Other families include the $G_{q/11}$ proteins, causing the activation of phospholipase Cβ and its downstream effectors, and G_{12} proteins, which cause activation of the Rho small G-proteins, which are involved in cytoskeletal organization (Sah et al. 2000).

Table 1 G-protein families, linked receptors, and second messengers

Family	Receptors	Effectors	Net response	Pharmacological modulation
$G_s\alpha$	β_1, β_2, β_3 adrenergic; D_1, D_5-dopamine	Adenylyl cyclase ↑ Maxi K channel ↑ Ca^{2+} channels ↑	Cyclic AMP ↑ Ca^{2+} influx ↑	Cholera toxin
$G_{i/o}\alpha/G_z\alpha$	α_2 adrenergic; D_2-dopamine; M_2, M_4 muscarinic; μ-, δ-, κ-opioid	Adenylyl cyclase ↓ K^+ channels ↑ Ca^{2+} channels ↓ ERK/MAP K ↑	Cyclic AMP ↓ Hyperpolarization Ca^{2+} influx ↓	Pertussis toxin
$G_{q/11}\alpha/G_{14-16}\alpha$	M_1, M_3 muscarinic; α_1 adrenergic	Phospholipase Cβ ↑ p63-RhoGEF ↑ K^+ channels ↑	IP_3, DAG, Ca^{2+} ↑ Cytoskeletal reorganization Hyperpolarization	Pertussis toxin-insensitive
$G_{12/13}\alpha$	Not yet fully characterized	Phospholipase D ↑ Phospholipase Cε ↑ iNOS ↑ p115-RhoGEF ↑	Phosphatidic acid, choline ↑ Cytoskeletal reorganization	Unknown
Gβ/γ	Numerous, dependent on α-subunit	Phospholipase Cβ ↑ Adenylyl cyclase I ↓ Adenylyl cyclases II, IV, VII↑ PI-3 kinases ↑ K^+ channels (GIRK1,2,4) ↑ Ca^{2+} (N-, P/Q-, R-type) channels Protein kinase D ↑ p114-RhoGEF ↑	IP_3, DAG, Ca^{2+} ↑ Cyclic AMP ↑↓ PIP_3 ↑ Hyperpolarization Cytoskeletal reorganization	Unknown

1.3 Overview of G-Protein-Coupled Receptor Function

Functionally, GPCRs transduce a signal in response to agonist binding by undergoing a conformational change in transmembrane and cytosolic regions of the receptor, leading to exposure of the linked G-protein α-subunit and subsequent exchange of bound GDP for GTP (see Fig. 1). The α- and β/γ-subunits dissociate and both the α-subunit and the β/γ-dimer have the capacity to then independently regulate separate cellular effectors (Gilman 1987), depending on the type of GPCR. The GTP bound to the α-subunit is then hydrolyzed to GDP, returning the GPCR to its original resting state with re-association of the α- and β/γ-subunits.

1.4 *Scope of this Chapter*

In this article we review the molecular mechanisms of the most important analgesic drugs in medicine, opioids, and share insights from the molecular mechanisms of α_2 adrenoceptor agonists, concerning both their sedative/hypnotic and analgesic effects. Having reviewed the drugs in widespread use that have clear evidence for GPCR-related mechanisms of action, we will then address the new developments in this field, notably the potential for drugs that modulate orexinergic, cholinergic, and $GABA_B$ signaling to affect anesthetic practice.

2 Opioid Receptor Signaling

The existence of opioid receptors was originally proposed in the mid 1950s by Beckett and Casy (1954) but not demonstrated until the 1970s by Pert and Snyder (1973). Martin and colleagues subsequently began to classify opioid receptors based upon their response patterns to three different opioid compounds in the chronic spinal dog model (Martin et al. 1976). Receptors were named after their prototypic agonists; namely mu (μ), morphine; kappa (κ), ketocyclazocine; and sigma (σ), after the compound SKF 10047. σ, however, is no longer considered an opioid receptor. Subsequently a delta (δ) opioid receptor was discovered in and named after the mouse vas deferens, exhibiting high affinity for enkephalins (Lord et al. 1977).

2.1 *Nomenclature*

Current views support the presence of these three major classes of opioid receptor within the CNS, but acknowledge the existence of various subgroups within each class (Pasternak 1993). When the genes encoding the different receptors were cloned in 1992, they were renamed accordingly as *MOR* (μ), *DOR* (δ), and *KOR* (κ) receptors and in 1997 they became known as OP_1 (δ), OP_2 (κ), and OP_3 (μ) opioid receptors after the International Union of Pharmacology (IUPHAR) reclassified them in their order of cloning. Later, a fourth, opioid receptor-like receptor 1 (ORL_1) or "orphan" receptor was discovered, and was subsequently found to react with the endogenous peptide "nociceptin", and is thus also referred to as the nociceptin/orphanin FQ (N/OFQ) receptor (Henderson and McKnight 1997).

However, as many authors have failed to adopt the new names, the most recent guidelines (in 2005) of the IUPHAR are to revert to the use of the well-defined Greek terminology, with the currently recommended names being μ or MOP, δ or DOP, κ or KOP receptors and ORL_1 or N/OFQ being referred to as the NOP receptor (IUPHAR 2005).

2.2 *Morphology*

Opioid receptors show about 60% homology with one another, greatest within the transmembrane helices, and most diverse in the N- and C-termini and extracellular loops (Chen et al. 1993). Numerous ligands act promiscuously on μ, δ, and κ receptors, though selective ligands also exist for each receptor subtype. Evidence suggests that all opioid receptors share a common opioid-binding pocket situated within transmembrane helices 3–7, but divergent extracellular loops play a role in ligand selectivity (Waldhoer et al. 2004).

The opioid receptors all are members of the Rhodopsin class of GPCRs, principally, although not exclusively, mediating their effects via the $G_{i/o}$ pertussis toxin (PTX)-sensitive heterotrimeric G-protein family (Waldhoer et al. 2004). Additionally, the μ- and δ-receptors also interact with PTX-insensitive inhibitors of adenylyl cyclase, namely the G_z and G_{16} proteins (Garzon et al. 1998; Hendry et al. 2000), but none of the opioid receptors interact substantially with the stimulatory G_s proteins (Connor and Christie 1999). As discussed previously, each specific G-protein is able to modulate a diverse range of cellular effects.

2.3 *Pharmacology*

On receptor binding, opiates may act as agonists, neutral antagonists, or inverse agonists; activating, having no effect upon, or inhibiting the coupled G-protein, respectively. Compared to full agonists, partial agonists must occupy a greater fraction of an available pool of functional receptors than full agonists to induce an equivalent response (Cox 1999). Mixed agonists/antagonists (e.g., buprenorphine, butorphanol, nalbuphine, pentazocine) may act as agonists at low doses and as antagonists (at the same or a different receptor) at greater doses (Stein and Rosow 2004). Typically, such compounds exhibit ceiling effects for analgesia.

Many G-protein-linked receptors exist as dimers (Cvejic and Devi 1997), and the formation of opioid receptor heterodimers is a possible mechanism underlying the cross communication between different opioid ligands and the variety of downstream effects a given ligand can produce. In the case of δ- and κ-receptors, heterodimerization has been proved to enhance agonist-induced inhibition of adenylyl cyclase as well as alter receptor pharmacology (Jordan and Devi 1999). Interestingly, opioid receptors have also been shown to form heterodimers with certain non-opioid receptors, for example μ-opioid with α_{2A} adrenoceptors (Milligan 2004), although the functional significance of this is currently unclear.

2.4 *Molecular Mechanisms of Action*

2.4.1 Action on Potassium Conductances

The phenomenon of opioid-mediated inhibition of neuronal excitability is believed to result largely from potassium-mediated membrane hyperpolarization (Corbett et al. 2006), as opioid receptors have been shown to cause activation of a variety of different potassium channels. The most important of these is the GIRK (or K_{IR3}), which is opened by the G-protein β/γ-subunit (see Table 1). These are widely expressed in the brain and are stimulated by all three types of opioid receptor, as well as several other receptors. Mutations and knockout studies have demonstrated GIRK to be important in mediating analgesic responses to opioids (Ikeda et al. 2002), and that mutated forms show reduced coupling to G-proteins (Navarro et al. 1996). In addition, opioids have also been shown to activate delayed rectifier potassium channels, voltage-dependent potassium channels, the BK calcium-sensitive potassium channel (Williams et al. 2001), as well as dendrotoxin-sensitive and M-type channels (Corbett et al. 2006).

2.4.2 Action on Adenylyl Cyclase

Physiological studies of opioid effects on neurons have delineated several downstream effects of G-protein-mediated adenylyl cyclase inhibition and the consequent reduction in cyclic AMP (cAMP). First, decreased cAMP increases the threshold for opening of the hyperpolarization-activated cation channels (I_h), and in lowering cAMP, opioids effectively inhibit I_h (Ingram and Williams 1994; Svoboda and Lupica 1998). This results in reduced pacemaker activity and a lowering of the rate of firing of action potentials and thus the flow of nociceptive information to the CNS (Corbett et al. 2006). Second, decreased cAMP results in an inhibition of protein kinase A (PKA)-activated neurotransmitter release at certain synapses (Williams et al. 2001). The role of opioids in modulating this system is supported by the finding that in hyperalgesia, PKA-activated neurotransmitter release is enhanced (Willis 2001), and that the μ-opioid agonist morphine has, via a PKA-dependent pathway, been shown to inhibit the pronociceptive responses of vanilloid receptor 1 (TRPV1), which is critical in the development of inflammatory hyperalgesia (Vetter et al. 2006).

2.4.3 Action on Neurotransmitter Release

Inhibition of neurotransmitter release by opioids was originally observed in 1917 in the peripheral nervous system by Trendelenburg, who reported that morphine inhibited the peristaltic reflex in guinea pig ileum. It was not until the 1950s, however, that this finding was discovered to be due to the inhibition of acetylcholine release. Subsequently, morphine was shown to inhibit the release of noradrenaline from postganglionic sympathetic nerve endings in animal studies. It is now clear that, throughout the CNS, stimulation of μ-, δ-, κ- or NOP receptors is able to inhibit the release of many neurotransmitters, such as glutamate, GABA, and glycine (Williams et al. 2001), and at least two mechanisms exist by which neurotransmitter release is inhibited in this fashion. Previously, the activation of potassium conductance and/or the inhibition of calcium conductance was thought to account for this effect (Williams et al. 2001). More recently however it has been suggested that inhibition of adenylyl cyclase plays a role in downregulating release of transmitters, although it has been reported that opioid receptors may somehow inhibit neurotransmitter vesicle-release machinery directly, independent of any effect on potassium and calcium conductance (Williams et al. 2001; Capogna et al. 1993).

2.4.4 Action on Phospholipase C and Calcium Currents

In addition to the action of opioid receptors on adenylyl cyclase and membrane conductances, opioid receptors also modulate phospholipase Cβ (PLCβ) via $G_{i/o}$ and G_q proteins (Ueda et al. 1995; Lee et al. 1998; see Table 1). The exact role of PLCβ in opioid responses is less clear but has been studied in animals (Murthy and Makhlouf 1996; Lee et al. 1998) and of note, PLCβ3 knockout mice exhibit enhanced morphine-induced analgesia (Xie et al. 1999). Because presynaptic calcium ion influx is essential for neurotransmitter release, the role of calcium channels in mediating opioid analgesia has also been investigated. In particular, N-, P/Q-, and R-type voltage-dependent calcium channels (VDCCs) have been studied, as these are directly inhibited by the G_i family protein β/γ-subunits (Herlitze et al. 1996; Ikeda et al. 2002). Although, there is currently no direct evidence for the inhibition of VDCCs in opioid-induced analgesia, in VDCC knockout mice, nociceptive responses are generally reduced (Saegusa et al. 2000; Hatakeyama et al. 2001). However, many studies have demonstrated a transient increase in intracellular calcium following opioid receptor activation (Williams et al. 2001). This effect of opioids on intracellular calcium is sensitive to pertussis toxin and partly results from release of calcium from intracellular stores but also from enhanced dihydropyridine-sensitive entry of calcium. This release of calcium from internal stores appears to be depend on PLC (Jin et al. 1994) and its downstream effectors, inositol triphosphate (IP_3) and diacyl-glycerol (DAG), which effect stored calcium release and protein kinase C (PKC) activation, respectively.

2.5 *Receptor Effects and Localization*

Opioid receptors are located throughout the body, in both the CNS and peripheral nervous system, and are found in primary afferent neurons, dorsal root ganglia, spinal cord, brainstem, midbrain, and cortex (Stein 1995; Millan 1993). In addition, they are expressed by neuroendocrine, immune, and ectodermal tissues (Slominski et al. 2000; Sharp 2001). Undoubtedly, the multitude of receptor locations and their numerous downstream effector mechanisms underpin the efficacy of opioid agonists in clinical practice. Opioid receptors modulate responses to pain within the normal nociceptive pathway, at both presynaptic and postsynaptic terminals, and activate descending inhibition of spinal cord nociceptive responses. Importantly, the different responses associated with a given receptor—for example μ (euphoria) vs κ (dysphoria) or μ (supraspinal analgesia) vs NOP (supraspinal antagonism of opioid analgesia)—result from the anatomical distribution of receptors, rather than receptor subtype alone (Corbett et al. 2006).

2.5.1 Supraspinal Effects

Within the brain, the highest densities of opioid receptors are found within the brainstem, specifically in the midbrain periaqueductal gray matter (PAG), the locus coeruleus (LC), and the rostral ventral medulla (RVM). The PAG plays a major role in descending inhibition, and in both the PAG and RVM, μ- and δ-receptors presynaptically inhibit interneuron release of GABA (Christie et al. 2000). The resulting disinhibition causes activation of descending monoaminergic pathways in the dorsolateral funiculus, with a net inhibitory effect on nociceptive processing in the spine (Heinricher and Morgan 1999). Conversely, postsynaptic NOP-receptor stimulation results in pronociception via inhibition of descending neuronal output (Corbett et al. 2006). Other supraspinal sites mediating opioid analgesia include the ventral tegmental area, globus pallidus, hypothalamus, and insular cortex. Additionally, the amygdala has reciprocal connections with the PAG and contains high levels of μ-, δ-, and κ-receptors (Stein and Rosow 2004). μ-Receptors present in the respiratory center of the medulla are responsible for the dose-dependent depression of the ventilatory response to hypercapnia and hypoxia resulting from opioid administration (Weil et al. 1975).

2.5.2 Pronociceptive Effects

Unexpectedly, a large number of clinical studies have demonstrated that opioids can elicit hyperalgesia (enhanced responses to noxious stimulation) and allodynia (pain elicited by normal innocuous stimuli) (Simonnet and Rivat 2003). In evolutionary terms, opioid-induced hyperalgesia may have had biological utility in conditioning behavioral responses serving to avoid noxious stimuli (Simonnet and

Rivat 2003). A possible mechanism for this is that opioids can selectively potentiate excitatory postsynaptic *N*-methyl-d-aspartate (NMDA) receptor-mediated glutamate responses in a PKC-dependent manner (Chen and Huang 1991). However, more recent research has demonstrated that opioid-mediated excitatory glutamate responses appear to be dependent on a specific NMDA receptor subunit or PKC isoform (Williams et al. 2001), as although this effect was reaffirmed in the neurons of the nucleus accumbens and hippocampus (Martin et al. 1997, 1999; Przewlocki et al. 1999), it was not seen in the LC (Oleskevich et al. 1993).

2.5.3 Sedation and Considerations During Co-administration with Other Anesthetic Drugs

Opioid administration leads to sedation, but when given as a single agent the opioids do not induce anesthesia. Notably, however, at subanalgesic doses, the κ-agonist butorphanol has a marked sedative effect, and has been used clinically for this purpose (Dershwitz et al. 1991). Furthermore, many opioids can interact synergistically with other agents, such as midazolam and propofol (Short et al. 1992), to increase their hypnotic effect. In clinical anesthesia, opioids are widely known to cause a considerable reduction in the minimum alveolar concentration (MAC) of inhalational anesthetics, such as isoflurane, that is required to produce immobility in 50% of subjects given a noxious stimulus (McEwan et al. 1993). However, numerous studies have demonstrated that it is not opioid receptors that mediate the capacity of inhaled anesthetics to produce immobility in the face of noxious stimulation, because administration of naloxone (a nonspecific opioid receptor antagonist) does not increase the MAC of inhaled anesthetics (Liao et al. 2006).

2.5.4 Spinal Effects

Within the dorsal horn of the spinal cord all three types of opioid receptors exist, and numerous studies indicate that opioid receptors are also located on terminals of primary afferents originating in the dorsal root ganglion as well as intrinsic spinal cord neurons (Cesselin et al. 1999). In the dorsal horn it appears that enkephalins act to suppress noxious input by acting on μ- and κ-receptors, (Stein and Rosow 2004) and when applied directly to the spinal cord, μ-, δ-, and κ-agonists all produce profound analgesia (Yaksh 1997). Postsynaptically, opioids, in particular μ-agonists, hyperpolarize ascending projection neurons by increasing potassium conductance (Stein and Rosow 2004). One possible mechanism involved in this opioid-induced spinal anesthesia is the suppression of the release of pronociceptive peptides, such as substance P, glutamate, and calcitonin gene-related peptide (CGRP), from peripheral terminals of primary afferent sensory neurons in the spinal cord (Stein 1995). This has been reported to be modulated by μ- and δ-receptor-linked inhibition of Ca^{2+} influx (Yaksh 1997), although the significance of this effect has also been questioned (Trafton et al. 1999).

2.5.6 Peripheral Effects

It was only in the last 20 years that the existence of opioid receptors outside the CNS has been widely acknowledged, but all three type of receptor have now been shown to also mediate analgesia peripherally, especially in inflamed tissue, in both animals and humans (Schäfer 1999). In addition, the μ- and δ-receptor-mediated inhibition of voltage-dependent calcium channels of primary afferent neurons is also an important mechanism decreasing release of substance P into peripheral tissues, with resultant analgesic as well as potent antiinflammatory effects in response to peripheral opioid administration being revealed recently (Stein et al. 2001).

2.6 Summary of Opioid Receptors

The characterization of opioid receptor morphology, signaling mechanisms, and subtypes of receptor, as well as their tissue distribution and cellular localization, has greatly elucidated the manner by which opioid analgesics mediate their effects, both desirable and adverse. However, in spite of ongoing work there has been a lack of significant progress toward the development of a powerful new opioid analgesic that is free from the undesirable effects associated with current agents. Continuing research into the effects of opioids in neuronal and nonneuronal systems, as well as the availability of novel peptides, will bring new insight to the application of these drugs. In future, greater understanding of the role played by phenomena such as opioid-induced hyperalgesia and the contribution of opioid receptor heterodimerization to the pharmacology of analgesia will allow us to refine clinical practice.

3 α_2 Adrenoceptor Agonists

Activation of α_2 adrenoceptors plays a prominent role in the endogenous hypnotic and antinociceptive systems. There are three known receptor subtypes: $\alpha_{2A,}$ α_{2B}, and α_{2C} adrenoceptors (Maze and Fujinaga 2000). These receptors couple to G_i and G_s (notably α_{2B} adrenoceptors; Pohjanoksa et al. 1997) proteins; however, it is predominantly the pertussis toxin-sensitive G_i α_{2A} adrenoceptors that mediate the anesthetic actions of this group of agents. Using D79N mice that express dysfunctional α_{2A} adrenoceptors, Lakhlani and colleagues showed that α_2 adrenoceptor agonist antinociception (assessed by the hot plate test) and sedation were dependent on this receptor subtype (Lakhlani et al. 1997). In the absence of functional α_{2A} adrenoceptors, the agents could not suppress voltage-gated calcium or activate potassium currents. This mutation did not affect morphine analgesia but inhibited dexmedetomidine sedation and analgesia. We have also subsequently shown that the neuroprotective effects of dexmedetomidine are mediated by the α_{2A} adrenoceptor (Ma et al. 2004).

3.1 Molecular Mechanisms of Action

In the fifth transmembrane domain of the adrenergic receptors are three critical amino acid residues which modulate agonist binding to adrenoceptors (Peltonen et al. 2003). Human α_{2A} adrenoceptors have one cysteine and two serine residues while rodent α_{2A} adrenoceptors have three serine residues, thus explaining some species-dependent ligand-binding differences (Blaxall et al. 1993). Using sophisticated mutant receptor techniques, the impact of exchanging these serine and cysteine residues has been studied, revealing separate binding and activation roles of differing residues (Peltonen et al. 2003). While imidazoline compounds generally retained their efficacy at mutant receptors, the efficacy of phenethylamine compounds varied. Furthermore while both cysteine 201 and serine 204 are important for receptor binding of catecholamines, only serine 204 is important for receptor activation (Peltonen et al. 2003). These studies will be critical to the development of novel ligands to improve both affinity and efficacy at particular receptor subtypes and to clarify the coupled effectors of G-protein-related signaling.

When stimulated, α_{2A} adrenoceptors inhibit adenylyl cyclase through G_i protein coupling, with subsequent effects on ligand-gated ion channels. These include inhibition of N-type calcium channels (Adamson et al. 1989) and P/Q-type calcium channels (Ishibashi and Akaike 1995) and activation of I_A potassium channels (North et al. 1987), calcium-activated potassium channels (Ryan et al. 1998), the ATP sensitive potassium channel, voltage-dependent potassium channels (Galeotti et al. 1999) and the Na^+/H^+ antiporter (Ryan et al. 1998). Furthermore, recent work has highlighted the association of α_2 adrenoceptors with GIRK channels (Blednov et al. 2003; Mitrovic et al. 2003) and potentially TASK-1 channels (Linden et al. 2006). Two separate studies investigated the effects of clonidine in GIRK-2-null mutant mice using the hot plate and tail flick latency tests (Blednov et al. 2003; Mitrovic et al. 2003); the mutation reduced clonidine antinociception almost to baseline indicating primarily a postsynaptic action of clonidine. It is also noteworthy that pharmacogenetic analysis of different inbred mouse strains showed significant correlation between strain dependence of morphine and clonidine analgesia (in hot plate and formalin tests; Wilson et al. 2003). Therefore mutual dependency on GIRK channel signaling may account for this effect. The inhibition of adenylyl cyclase by α_2 adrenoceptor activation may also hinder the development of hyperalgesia, as cAMP is a key mediator of this process (Hoeger-Bement and Sluka 2003). The net effect is reduced neuronal excitability and hyperpolarization in key populations of neurons that contribute to hypnosis/sedation and analgesia.

3.2 Hypnotic Mechanisms of Action

The neural networks underlying the effects of exogenous α_2 adrenoceptor agonists have recently been identified. The hypnotic pathway involves activation of the nonrapid eye movement (NREM) pathway, with the primary site of action the noradrenergic nucleus, the LC. Coupled with lesioning, antagonist, and pharmacogenetic studies, we have used immunohistochemical techniques to sequentially map the neuronal activation and inhibition provoked by the α_2 adrenoceptor agonist dexmedetomidine to elucidate the pathway. The interesting discovery that the $GABA_A$ antagonist gabazine could reduce dexmedetomidine's sedative effect combined with evidence of activated inhibitory neurons in the ventrolateral preoptic (VLPO) nucleus in the anterior hypothalamus suggested that α_2 adrenoceptor agonist sedation converged on the NREM sleep system. Indeed lesioning of the VLPO reduced dexmedetomidine's hypnotic efficacy. Therefore α_2 adrenoceptor activation inhibited norepinephrine release within the LC, leading to disinhibition of GABAergic neurons in the VLPO nucleus in the anterior hypothalamus, which controls sleep and its maintenance (Nelson et al.; Fig. 2). The resultant effect is release of the inhibitory neurotransmitter

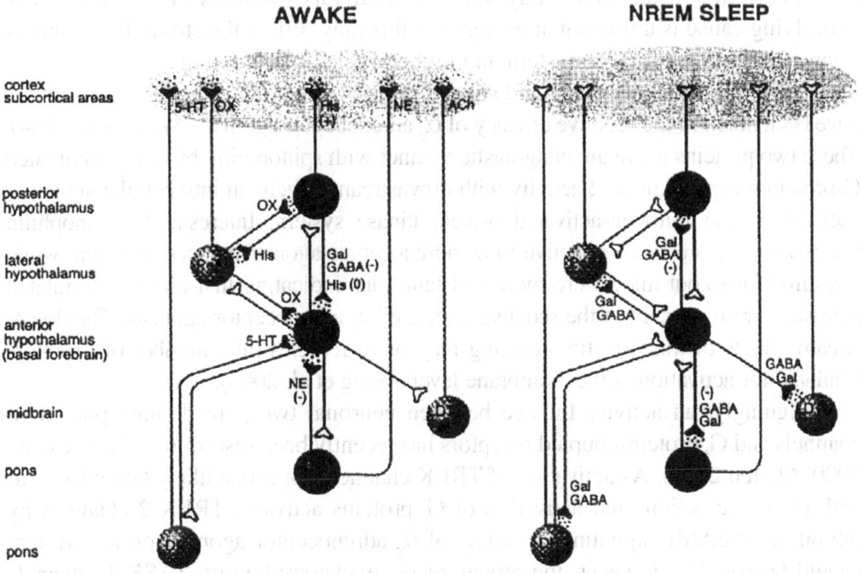

Fig. 2 Diagram depicting a simplified nonrapid eye movement (NREM) sleep-promoting pathway activated by dexmedetomidine. An inhibition of firing of noradrenergic neurons in the locus coeruleus (LC), which accompanies endogenous NREM sleep and is the site of initiation of dexmedetomidine-induced hypnosis, releases a tonic noradrenergic inhibition of the ventrolateral preoptic nucleus (VLPO). The activated VLPO is believed to release γ-aminobutyric acid (GABA) into the tuberomammillary nucleus (TMN), which inhibits its release of arousal-promoting histamine into the cortex and forebrain to induce loss of consciousness. A number of pathways are involved in NREM sleep; the sleep-active VLPO projects to all the ascending monoaminergic, cholinergic, and orexinergic arousal nuclei, which in turn project to the cortex, forebrain, and subcortical areas where they release neurotransmitters of arousal to promote wakefulness. The LC widely innervates the brain, but only projections associated with NREM sleep are shown here. A simplified version of this circuitry, the portion of the pathway highlighted in *black*, is the focus of this investigation. *Ach*, acetylcholine; *DR*, dorsal raphe nuclei; *His*, histamine; *5-HT*, serotonin; *LDTg*, laterodorsal tegmental nuclei; *NE*, norepinephrine; *OX*, orexin (hypocretin); *PeF*, perifornical area; *PPTg*, pedunculopontine tegmental nuclei. (Reproduced with permission from Nelson et al. 2003)

GABA leading to the inhibition of excitatory pathways notably the histaminergic (tuberomammillary nucleus; TMN), serotonergic (dorsal raphe nucleus; DRN) and cholinergic (basal forebrain; BF) systems. Again these effects were not observed in D79N mutant mice, indicating this effect was mediated by α_{2A} adrenoceptors. It is of course of interest that gabazine can attenuate both α_2 adrenoceptor agonist and GABAergic drug (e.g., propofol)-induced sedation/hypnosis yet α_2 adrenoceptor antagonists can only reduce α_2 adrenoceptor agonist-induced sedation/hypnosis (not that induced by GABAergic drugs; Segal et al. 1988). This is because these GABAergic drugs act downstream of the LC at the VLPO to potentiate the inhibitory neurotransmission from this nucleus.

A further interesting discovery has been the profound sensitivity of the young to anesthetic agents; however, they appear particularly sensitive to α_2 adrenoceptor agonists with a greater than tenfold difference in the hypnotic potency of dexmedetomidine noted between 7-day-old and adult rats (Sanders et al. 2005). The underlying cause is unknown at present but this may reflect the strength of connections of the LC to other brainstem and higher nuclei in the young.

Critical roles for spinophilin and arrestin proteins, which regulate GPCR signaling, have been noted in the sedative efficacy of α_2 adrenoceptor agonists (Wang et al. 2004). These two proteins act in an antagonistic manner with spinophilin, blocking stimulated G-protein receptor kinase 2 activity with downstream effects on intracellular signaling such as by the mitogen-activated protein kinase system. Interestingly, spinophilin knockout mice are more sensitive to α_2 adrenoceptor agonist-induced sedation, while arrestin-3 knockout mice were more resistant, thus indicating that arrestin-stimulated pathways are important in the sedative effects of α_2 adrenoceptor agonists. The downstream effects of this arrestin signaling may be to replenish the number of receptors available for activation at the membrane level (Wang et al. 2004).

Intriguingly, an activity linkage between neuronal two-pore domain potassium channels and G_i protein-coupled receptors has recently been discovered (Lesage et al. 2000; Mathie 2007). As activation of TREK channels appears a likely target for general anesthetic action, and activation of G_i proteins activates TREK-2 channels by inhibition of cAMP signaling, an effect of α_2 adrenoceptor agonists on this system should be sought. However, the effects of dexmedetomidine on TASK-1 channels have already been approached with TASK-1 knockout mice less sensitive to the sedative effects of dexmedetomidine (Linden et al. 2006), which is likely due to a reduced effect in the LC where TASK1/3 channels are particularly abundant. As TASK-1 knockout mice exhibit increased pain sensitivity, activation of TASK-1 receptors by α_2 adrenoceptor agonists may also be involved in their antinociceptive effects.

3.3 *Analgesic Mechanisms of Action*

Both spinal and supraspinal sites are activated by α_2 adrenoceptor agonists (or norepinephrine release) to produce analgesia (Sanders and Maze 2007). The supraspinal sites, provoked primarily by disinhibition of brainstem noradrenergic nuclei, provide analgesia mediated by descending inhibitory neurons (DINs). The LC tonically inhibits the brainstem nuclei; the A5 and A7 are then coupled to DINs. Activation of α_2 adrenoceptors in the LC inhibits neuronal firing in this region (Guo et al. 1996). Inhibition of the LC by discrete administration of α_2 adrenoceptor agonists leads to "disinhibition" (i.e., activation) of the A5 and A7 and therefore DINs.

These DINs inhibit nociceptive responses in the dorsal horn of the spinal cord via release of norepinephrine, enkephalins, and acetylcholine (Li and Zhuo 2001; Eisenach et al. 1996). In the dorsal horn, norepinephrine or exogenous α_2 adrenoceptor agonists depress wide-dynamic-range neuron responses after Aδ and C nociceptive fiber activation by stimulation of α_2 adrenoceptors (Jones and Gebhart 1986). The subtype of α_2 adrenoceptor mediating the spinal antinociceptive effects of adrenergic compounds is not entirely clear in humans despite the strong pharmacogenomic evidence in mice (Lakhlani et al. 1997). Roles for α_{2A}, α_{2B}, and α_{2C} adrenoceptors have been suggested to potentially mediate the differences between endogenously and exogenously stimulated pathways (Maze and Fujinaga 2000); further evaluation of the different receptor subtypes involved would help design future analgesic and hypnotic therapies.

3.4 *Summary of α_2 Adrenoceptor Agonists*

Activation of α_{2A} adrenoceptors represents the most likely molecular target underlying the hypnotic and analgesic effects of the α_2 adrenoceptor agonists. Further understanding of both the molecular and neural network systems involved will contribute to the targeting of future pharmacological strategies to improve clinical anesthesia. The development of more efficacious and subtype-selective agonists (and antagonists) would also significantly enhance the utility of this class of agents.

4 Muscarinic Cholinergic Agents

Cholinergic signaling is involved in a multitude of actions including arousal, cognition, learning and memory, and the modulation of pain responses. In addition, acetylcholine plays a critical role in the autonomic nervous system (ANS), and anticholinergic drugs such as atropine and the neuromuscular blocking agents have indisputable importance in anesthesia. The G-protein-coupled muscarinic acetylcholine receptors (mAChR) are either excitatory (odd numbered, M_1, M_3, M_5) or inhibitory (even numbered, M_2, M_4) in nature. Even numbered channels inhibit adenylyl cyclase via G_i/G_o and activate TREK-2 channels while odd numbered channels, coupled to G_q/G_{11}, activate phospholipase C (Caulfield and Birdsall 1998) and inhibit TREK-2 channels (Lesage et al. 2000; Mathie 2007). Similar to opioid and α_2 adrenoceptors, M_2 receptor activation also activates GIRK channels (Fernandez-Fernandez et al. 1999).

4.1 Role in the Mechanism of Anesthesia

In terms of anesthetic actions (beyond effects on the ANS), mAChR primarily have a role in antinociception; for example, morphine antinociception is reduced in M_4 and M_4/M_2 knockout mice (Duttaroy et al. 2000). Furthermore, activation of muscarinic receptors induces antinociception in various pain paradigms including thermal, inflammatory, and neuropathic pain (Wess et al. 2003; Shannon et al. 1997). M_2 and M_4 receptors couple to G_i proteins, with dual knockout of both these receptors abolishing the antinociception induced by oxotremorine (Duttaroy et al. 2002). Sole knockout of the M_2 receptor reduced antinociception (but to a lesser extent than dual knockout) and also reduced the inhibitory action of muscarine on CGRP release from peripheral nerve endings (Bernardini et al. 2002). The antinociceptive action of oxotremorine is reduced in mice with a GIRK-2 null mutation, indicating primarily a postsynaptic action of this drug via GIRK channels. As M_2 receptors are known to activate GIRK channels it is likely that M_2 and GIRK channels mediate muscarinic antinociception, at least in mice.

Muscarinic antinociception is also reduced in the presence of the $GABA_B$ receptor antagonist CGP55845. This effect is reasoned to be a presynaptic effect of augmented endogenous GABA release inhibiting other neurotransmitter release (Li et al. 2002). Antagonists of the M_2, M_3, and M_4 receptor subtypes inhibit this GABA release (Zhang et al. 2005). However, M_2 receptor activation has also been associated with reduced thalamic GABA release and increased arousal, which would likely affect the anesthetic state (Rowell et al. 2003). Further investigation is required.

Anesthetic actions at muscarinic receptors in the CNS are of unknown significance; however, halothane (Durieux 1995), desflurane (Nietgen et al. 1998), and propofol (Murasaki et al. 2003) all inhibit M_1 receptor signaling, though isoflurane does not (but does inhibit the M_3 receptor). Furthermore, the local anesthetics have been shown to inhibit M_1 receptor signaling likely via interaction with the extracellular domain of the G-protein (Hollmann et al. 2000). This effect on $G_q\alpha$ proteins has subsequently been shown to be time dependent and reversible and independent of PKC, protein phosphatases, and increased guanosine triphosphatase activity (Hollmann et al. 2004). These effects may also involve further protein expression. How these effects interact in the short term with anesthetic action is still unclear, though they may contribute significantly to the antiinflammatory and antithrombotic effects of local anesthetics. Due to the putative role of muscarinic signaling in Alzheimer's dementia, antagonism of M_1 receptors (Eglen 2006) may also play a role in the development of postoperative cognitive dysfunction (POCD), if the parallels drawn between Alzheimer's and POCD hold.

5 Orexin Signaling

Orexinergic signaling plays a key role in the arousal/waking system, and therefore a role in the state of anesthesia has been proposed. The orexins were identified as endogenous ligands for two orphan GPCRs [now named orexin 1 (OX_1R) and orexin 2 (OX_2R)] and showed no significant homology with previously described peptides (Sakurai 2007; Sakurai et al. 1998; Huang et al. 2001). OX_1R couples to $G_{11}\alpha$ and activates phospholipase C with subsequent phosphatidylinositol and Ca^{2+} signaling, while OX_2R couples to both $G_{11}\alpha$ and G_i proteins. In the lateral hypothalamus there is a dense nucleus of orexinergic neurons that project widely throughout the cerebrum but notably innervate the thalamic paraventricular nucleus, arcuate nucleus, DRN, BF, LC, and TMN. The latter two nuclei contain the highest density of orexin receptors consistent with the orexins' role as arousal-promoting neuropeptides (Marcus et al. 2001; Huang et al. 2001). Indeed orexins have been shown to activate the DRN, BF, LC, and TMN, which are integral parts of the arousal promoting system. Knockout of the OX_2R produces a narcoleptic phenotype with abnormal attacks of NREM sleep (Willie et al. 2003) and show abnormal activity of the TMN which, at least in part, mediates the hypnotic effects of anesthetics (Nelson et al. 2002, 2003). Interestingly the VLPO sends inhibitory GABAergic connections to the lateral hypothalamus, and functional inhibition of this area has been achieved with GABAergic drugs such as anesthetics (Nelson et al. 2002).

5.1 *Role in the Mechanism of Anesthesia*

Functional investigations of the orexin system are underway to analyze their potential therapeutic effects in narcolepsy (agonists), sleep medicine (antagonists), and anesthetic applications (agonists and antagonists). Indeed in anesthesia, inhibition of orexin signaling likely contributes to the anesthetic state (Nelson et al. 2002; Kushikata et al. 2003; Dong et al. 2006) and conceivably activation of the orexin system may prove useful as a pharmacological stimulant to enhance emergence from anesthesia. Furthermore, orexin signaling is associated with antinociceptive effects and therefore may be useful in the post-anesthesia care unit for maintaining arousal and analgesia.

In a series of experiments, Kushikata and colleagues showed that an OX_1R agonist could reduce barbiturate-induced anesthesia time (assessed by loss of righting reflex; Kushikata et al. 2003). Furthermore in two studies from Japan, the excitatory effects of intracerebroventricularly administered orexins on the electroencephalogram (EEG) under isoflurane anesthesia have been established (Dong et al. 2006; Yasuda et al. 2003). Exogenous orexin-stimulated basal forebrain acetylcholine release correlated with a change in the EEG pattern from burst suppression to arousal, an effect reversed with an OX_1R antagonist. It is of interest that while an arousal EEG was obtained the rats did not move, an intriguing set of possibilities may explain this: (1) Cholinergic stimulation may have been insufficient itself to overcome the anesthetic state; (2) the arousal EEG may have reflected a more REM than NREM type of hypnotic state, with arousal EEG and muscle atonia; or (3) activation/inhibition of brainstem nuclei such as the mesopontine tegmental area may play a greater role in the anesthetic state. Nonetheless, further research is required in this area to elucidate the impact of orexin signaling on the anesthetic state.

6 $GABA_B$ Signaling

The role of $GABA_A$ receptor signaling in the mechanism of anesthesia is well established with sophisticated in vitro and in vivo work demonstrating the critical involvement of this receptor (Franks and Lieb 1994; Nelson et al. 2002). However the role of the G_i protein-coupled $GABA_B$ receptor is less clear. With only two receptor subtypes known, they can be located both pre- and postsynaptically and generate inhibitory postsynaptic potentials via interaction with potassium channels of the $G\beta/\gamma$ subunit (Ulrich and Bettler 2007); $G_{i/o}\alpha$ subunits also act to inhibit adenylyl cyclase. Therefore a biologically plausible interaction could occur; in addition, sevoflurane has been reported to potentiate both $GABA_A$ and $GABA_B$ receptors (Hirota and Roth 1997). However, at present there are conflicting reports in the literature on whether this interaction is significant to the mechanism of anesthesia. Manson and colleagues showed no effect on halothane anesthesia (using nocifensive behavior as the outcome) of $GABA_B$ receptor antagonists administered intrathecally in rats (Mason et al. 1996). In contrast the $GABA_B$ receptor agonist baclofen augmented the time to induction and duration of anesthesia (assessed by loss of righting reflex) in mice (Sugimura et al. 2002). The conflict in these results may merely represent different methods of testing anesthesia (analgesia vs hypnosis) and therefore may indicate that $GABA_B$ receptor signaling is more important in hypnotic rather than analgesic actions of anesthetics. This conflict, however, requires further investigation to clarify whether $GABA_B$ receptor signaling contributes to the anesthetic state.

7 Conclusion

GPCRs mediate many actions of analgesic and anesthetic drugs; it is clear, however, that the downstream effectors beyond the receptor are becoming increasingly understood at least for opioid and α_2 adrenoceptor agonists. This increased understanding may precipitate the development of new anesthetic agents in the near future. Knowledge of the roles of other GPCRs including the orexin, $GABA_B$, and cholinergic system may similarly contribute to the development of anesthetic pharmacology. Finally understanding the neural networks transducing the anesthetic effect may yield further targets for future drug development.

References

Adamson P, Xiang JZ, Mantzourides T, Brammer MJ, Campbell IC (1989) Presynaptic alpha2-adrenoceptor and kappa-opiate receptor occupancy promotes closure of neuronal (N-type) calcium channels. Eur J Pharmacol 174:63–70

Beckett AH, Casy AF (1954) Synthetic analgesics: stereochemical considerations. J Pharm Pharmacol 6:986–1001

Bernardini N, Roza C, Sauer SK, Gomeza J, Wess J, Reeh PW (2002) Muscarinic M2 receptors on peripheral nerve endings: a molecular target of antinociception. J Neurosci 22:RC229

Blaxall HS, Heck DA, Bylund DB (1993) Molecular determinants of the alpha-2D adrenergic receptor subtype. Life Sci 53:PL255–PL259

Blednov YA, Stoffel M, Alva H, Harris RA (2003) A pervasive mechanism for analgesia: activation of GIRK2 channels. Proc Natl Acad Sci U S A 100:277–282

Capogna M, Gahwiler BH, Thompson SM (1993) Mechanism of mu-opioid receptor-mediated presynaptic inhibition in the rat hippocampus in vitro. J Physiol 470:539–558

Caulfield MP, Birdsall NJ (1998) International Union of Pharmacology. XVII Classification of muscarinic acetylcholine receptors. Pharmacol Rev 50:279–290

Cesselin F, Benoliel JJ, Bourgoin S, Collin E, Pohl M, Hamon M (1999) Spinal mechanisms of opioid analgesia. In: Stein C (ed) Opioids in pain control: basic and clinical aspects. Cambridge University Press, Cambridge, pp 70–95

Chen L, Huang LY (1991) Sustained potentiation of NMDA receptor-mediated glutamate responses through activation of protein kinase C by a mu opioid. Neuron 7:319–326

Chen SR, Pan HL (2001) Spinal endogenous acetylcholine contributes to the analgesic effect of systemic morphine in rats. Anesthesiology 95:525–530

Chen SR, Wess J, Pan HL (2005) Functional activity of the m2 and m4 receptor subtypes in the spinal cord studied with muscarinic acetylcholine receptor knockout mice. J Pharmacol Exp Ther 313:765–770

Chen Y, Mestek A, Liu J, Yu L (1993) Molecular cloning of a rat kappa opioid receptor reveals sequence similarities to the mu and delta opioid receptors. Biochem J 295:625–628

Christie MJ, Connor M, Vaughan CW, Ingram SL, Bagley EE (2000) Cellular actions of opioids and other analgesics: implications for synergism in pain relief. Clin Exp Pharmacol Physiol 7:520–523

Connor M, Christie MD (1999) "Opioid receptor signalling mechanisms". Clin Exp Pharmacol Physiol 26:493–499

Corbett AD, Henderson G, McKnight AT, Paterson SJ (2006) 75 years of opioid research: the exciting but vain quest for the Holy Grail. Br J Pharmacol 147[Suppl 1]:S153–S162

Cox BM (1999) Mechanisms of tolerance. In: Stein C (ed) Opioids in pain control: basic and clinical aspects. Cambridge University Press, Cambridge, pp 109–130

Cvejic S, Devi LA (1997) Dimerization of the delta opioid receptor: implication for a role in receptor internalization. J Biol Chem 272:26959–26964

Dershwitz M, Rosow CE, DiBiase PM, Zaslavsky A (1991) Comparison of the sedative effects of butorphanol and midazolam. Anesthesiology 74:717–724

Detweiler DJ, Eisenach JC, Tong C, Jackson C (1993) A cholinergic interaction in alpha2 adrenoreceptor-mediated antinociception in sheep. J Pharmacol Exp Ther 265:536–542

Dong HL, Fukuda S, Murata E, Zhu Z, Higuchi T (2006) Orexins increase cortical acetylcholine release and electroencephalographic activation through orexin-1 receptor in the rat basal forebrain during isoflurane anesthesia. Anesthesiology 104:1023–1032

Durieux ME (1995) Halothane inhibits signaling through m1 muscarinic receptors expressed in Xenopus oocytes. Anesthesiology 82:174–182

Duttaroy A, Gomeza J, Gan JW, Basile AS, Harman WD, Smith PL, Felder CC, Wess J (2000) Analysis of muscarinic agonist-induced analgesia by the use of receptor knockout mice (abstract). Neurosci Abstr 26:616–618

Duttaroy A, Gomeza J, Gan JW, Siddiqui N, Basile AS, Harman WD, Smith PL, Felder CC, Levey AI, Wess J (2002) Evaluation of muscarinic agonist-induced analgesia in muscarinic acetylcholine receptor knockout mice. Mol Pharmacol 62:1084–1093

Eglen RM (2006) Muscarinic receptor subtypes in neuronal and non-neuronal cholinergic function. Auton Autacoid Pharmacol 26:219–233

Eisenach JC, Detweiler DJ, Tong C, D'Angelo R, Hood DD (1996) Cerebrospinal fluid norepinephrine and acetylcholine concentrations during acute pain. Anesth Analg 82:621–626

Fernandez-Fernandez JM, Wanaverbecq N, Halley P, Caulfield MP, Brown DA (1999) Selective activation of heterologously expressed G protein-gated K+ channels by M2 muscarinic receptors in rat sympathetic neurones. J Physiol 515:631–637

Franks NP (2006) Molecular targets underlying general anaesthesia. Br J Pharmacol 147: S72–81

Franks NP, Lieb WR (1994) Molecular and cellular mechanisms of general anaesthesia. Nature 367:607–614

Galeotti N, Ghelardini C, Vinci MC, Bartolini A (1999) Role of potassium channels in the antinociception induced by agonists of alpha2-adrenoceptors. Br J Pharmacol 126:1214–1220

Garzon J, Castro M, Sanchez-Blazquez P (1998) Influence of Gz and Gi2 transducer proteins in the affinity of opioid agonists to mu receptors. Eur J Neurosci 10:2557–2564

Gilman AG (1987) G proteins: transducers of receptor-generated signals. Annu Rev Biochem 56:615–649

Guo TZ, Jiang JY, Buttermann AE, Maze M (1996) Dexmedetomidine injection into the locus ceruleus produces antinociception. Anesthesiology 84:873–881

Hatakeyama S, Wakamori M, Ino M, Miyamoto N, Takahashi E, Yoshinaga T, Sawada K, Imoto K, Tanaka I, Yoshizawa T, Nishizawa Y, Mori Y, Niidome T, Shoji S (2001) Differential nociceptive responses in mice lacking the alpha(1B) subunit of N-type Ca(2+) channels. Neuroreport 12:2423–2427

Heinricher MM, Morgan MM (1999) Supraspinal mechanisms of opioid analgesia. In: Stein C (ed) Opioids in pain control: basic and clinical aspects University Press, Cambridge, pp 46–69

Hemmings HC Jr, Girault JA (2004) Signal transduction mechanisms: receptor-effector coupling. In: Evers AS, Maze M (eds) Anesthetic pharmacology, physiologic principles and clinical practice. Churchill Livingstone, Philadelphia, pp 21–39

Henderson G, McKnight AT (1997) The orphan opioid receptor and its endogenous ligand—nociceptin/orphanin FQ. Trends Pharmacol Sci 18:293–300

Hendry IA, Kelleher KL, Bartlett SE, Leck KJ, Reynolds AJ, Heydon K, Mellick A, Megirian D, Matthaei KI (2000) Hypertolerance to morphine in G(z alpha)-deficient mice. Brain Res 870:10–19

Herlitze S, Garcia DE, Mackie K, Hille B, Scheuer T, Catterall WA (1996) Modulation of Ca2+ channels by G protein beta gamma subunits. Nature 380:258–262

Hirota K, Roth SH (1997) Sevoflurane modulates both GABAA and GABAB receptors in area CA1 of rat hippocampus. Br J Anaesth 78:60–65

Hoeger-Bement MK, Sluka KA (2003) Phosphorylation of CREB, mechanical hyperalgesia is reversed by blockade of the cAMP pathway in a time-dependent manner after repeated intramuscular acid injections. J Neurosci 23:5437–5445

Hollmann MW, Ritter CH, Henle P, de Klaver M, Kamatchi GL, Durieux ME (2001) Inhibition of m3 muscarinic acetylcholine receptors by local anaesthetics. Br J Pharmacol 133:207–216

Hollmann MW, Herroeder S, Kurz KS, Hoenemann CW, Struemper D, Hahnenkamp K, Durieux ME (2004) Time-dependent inhibition of G protein-coupled receptor signaling by local anesthetics. Anesthesiology 100:852–860

Hood DD, Mallak KA, James RL, Tuttle R, Eisenach JC (1997) Enhancement of analgesia from systemic opioid in humans by spinal cholinesterase inhibition. J Pharmacol Exp Ther 282:86–92

Huang ZL, Qu WM, Li WD, Mochizuki T, Eguchi N, Watanabe T, Urade Y, Hayaishi O (2001) Arousal effect of orexin A depends on activation of the histaminergic system. Proc Natl Acad Sci U S A 98:9965–9970

Ikeda K, Kobayashi T, Kumanishi T, Yano R, Sora I, Niki H (2002) Molecular mechanisms of analgesia induced by opioids and ethanol: is the GIRK channel one of the keys? Neurosci Res 44:121–131

Ingram SL, Williams JT (1994) Opioid inhibition of Ih via adenylyl cyclase. Neuron 13:179–186

Ishibashi H, Akaike N (1995) Norepinephrine modulates high voltage-activated calcium channels in freshly dissociated rat nucleus tractus solitarii neurons. Neuroscience 68:1139–1146
IUPHAR (2005) International Union of Basic and Clinical Pharmacology database website. http://www.iuphar-db.org/. Cited 12 Jul 2007
Iwasaki H, Collins JG, Saito Y, Uchida H, Kerman-Hinds A (1991) Low dose clonidine enhances pregnancy-induced analgesia to visceral but not somatic stimuli in rats. Anesth Analg 72:325–329
Jin W, Lee NM, Loh HH, Thayer SA (1994) Opioids mobilize calcium from inositol 1,4,5-trisphosphate-sensitive stores in NG108–15 cells. J Neurosci 14:1920–1929
Jones SL, Gebhart GF (1986) Characterization of coerulospinal inhibition of the nociceptive tail-flick reflex in the rat: mediation by spinal a2-adrenoreceptors. Brain Res 364:315–330
Jordan BA, Devi LA (1999) G-protein-coupled receptor heterodimerization modulates receptor function. Nature 399:697–700
Kushikata T, Hirota K, Yoshida H, Kudo M, Lambert DG, Smart D, Jerman JC, Matsuki A (2003) Orexinergic neurons and barbiturate anesthesia. Neuroscience 121:855–863
Lakhlani PP, MacMillan LB, Guo TZ, McCool BA, Lovinger DM, Maze M, Limbird LE (1997) Substitution of a mutant alpha2a-adrenergic receptor via hit and run gene targeting reveals the role of this subtype in sedative, analgesic, and anesthetic-sparing responses in vivo. Proc Natl Acad Sci U S A 94:9950–9955
Lee DK, George SR, Evans JF, Lynch KR, O'Dowd BF (2001) Orphan G protein-coupled receptors in the CNS. Curr Opin Pharmacol 1:31–39
Lee JW, Joshi S, Chan JS, Wong YH (1998) Differential coupling of mu-, delta-, and kappa-opioid receptors to G alpha16-mediated stimulation of phospholipase C. J Neurochem 70:2203–2211
Lesage F, Terrenoire C, Romey G, Lazdunski M (2000) Human TREK2, a 2P domain mechano-sensitive K+ channel with multiple regulations by polyunsaturated fatty acids, lysophospholipids, and Gs, Gi, and Gq protein-coupled receptors. J Biol Chem 275:28398–28405
Li DP, Chen SR, Pan YZ, Levey AI, Pan HL (2002) Role of presynaptic muscarinic and GABA(B) receptors in spinal glutamate release and cholinergic analgesia in rats. J Physiol 543:807–818
Li P, Zhuo M (2001) Cholinergic, noradrenergic, and serotonergic inhibition of fast synaptic transmission in spinal lumbar dorsal horn of rat. Brain Res Bull 54:639–647
Li X, Eisenach JC (2001) alpha2A-adrenoceptor stimulation reduces capsaicin-induced glutamate release from spinal cord synaptosomes. J Pharmacol Exp Ther 299:939–944
Liao M, Laster MJ, Eger EI, Tang M, Sonner JM (2006) Naloxone does not increase the minimum alveolar anesthetic concentration of sevoflurane in mice. Anesth Analg 102:1452–1455
Linden AM, Aller MI, Leppa E, Vekovischeva O, Aitta-Aho T, Veale EL, Mathie A, Rosenberg P, Wisden W, Korpi ER (2006) The in vivo contributions of TASK-1-containing channels to the actions of inhalation anesthetics, the alpha(2) adrenergic sedative dexmedetomidine, and cannabinoid agonists. J Pharmacol Exp Ther 317:615–626
Lord JA, Waterfield AA, Hughes J, Kosterlitz HW (1977) Endogenous opioid peptides: multiple agonists and receptors. Nature 267:495–499
Ma D, Hossain M, Rajakumaraswamy N, Arshad M, Sanders RD, Franks NP, Maze M (2004) Dexmedetomidine produces its neuroprotective effect via the alpha 2A-adrenoceptor subtype. Eur J Pharmacol 502:87–97
Marcus JN, Aschkenasi CJ, Lee CE, Chemelli RM, Saper CB, Yanagisawa M, Elmquist JK (2001) Differential expression of orexin receptors 1 and 2 in the rat brain. J Comp Neurol 435:6–25
Martin G, Nie Z, Siggins GR (1997) mu-Opioid receptors modulate NMDA receptor-mediated responses in nucleus accumbens neurons. J Neurosci 17:11–22
Martin G, Ahmed SH, Blank T, Spiess J, Koob GF, Siggins GR (1999) Chronic morphine treatment alters NMDA receptor-mediated synaptic transmission in the nucleus accumbens. J Neurosci 19:9081–9089

Martin WR, Eades CG, Thompson JA, Huppler RE, Gilbert PE (1976) The effects of morphine- and nalorphine-like drugs in the nondependent and morphine-dependent chronic spinal dog. J Pharmacol Exp Ther 197:517–532

Mason P, Owens CA, Hammond DL (1996) Antagonism of the antinocifensive action of halothane by intrathecal administration of GABAA receptor antagonists. Anesthesiology 84:1205–1214

Mathie A (2007) Neuronal two-pore-domain potassium channels and their regulation by G protein-coupled receptors. J Physiol 578:377–385

Maze M, Fujinaga M (2000) Alpha2 adrenoceptors in pain modulation: which subtype should be targeted to produce analgesia? Anesthesiology 92:934–936

McEwan AI, Smith C, Dyar O, Goodman D, Smith LR, Glass PS (1993) Isoflurane minimum alveolar concentration reduction by fentanyl. Anesthesiology 78:864–869

Millan MJ (1993) Multiple opioid systems and chronic pain. In: Herz A (ed) Opioids II, Springer-Verlag, Berlin Heidelberg New York

Milligan G (2004) G protein-coupled receptor dimerization: function and ligand pharmacology. Mol Pharmacol 66:1–7

Milligan G, Kostenis E (2006) Heterotrimeric G-proteins: a short history. Br J Pharmacol 147[Suppl 1]:S46–S55

Mitrovic I, Margeta-Mitrovic M, Bader S, Stoffel M, Jan LY, Basbaum AI (2003) Contribution of GIRK2-mediated postsynaptic signaling to opiate and alpha 2-adrenergic analgesia and analgesic sex differences. Proc Natl Acad Sci U S A 100:271–276

Murasaki O, Kaibara M, Nagase Y, Mitarai S, Doi Y, Sumikawa K, Taniyama K (2003) Site of action of the general anesthetic propofol in muscarinic M1 receptor-mediated signal transduction. J Pharmacol Exp Ther 307:995–1000

Murthy KS, Makhlouf GM (1996) Opioid mu, delta, and kappa receptor-induced activation of phospholipase C-beta 3 and inhibition of adenylyl cyclase is mediated by Gi2 and G(o) in smooth muscle. Mol Pharmacol 50:870–877

Nakamura M, Ferreira SH (1998) Peripheral analgesic action of clonidine: mediation by enkephalin-like substances. Eur J Pharmacol 146:223–228

Navarro B, Kennedy ME, Velimirovic B, Bhat D, Peterson AS, Clapham DE (1996) Nonselective and G betagamma-insensitive weaver K+ channels. Science 272:1950–1953

Nelson LE, Guo TZ, Lu J, Saper CB, Franks NP, Maze M (2002) The sedative component of anesthesia is mediated by GABA(A) receptors in an endogenous sleep pathway. Nat Neurosci 5:979–984

Nelson LE, Lu J, Guo T, Saper CB, Franks NP, Maze M (2003) The alpha2-adrenoceptor agonist dexmedetomidine converges on an endogenous sleep-promoting pathway to exert its sedative effects. Anesthesiology 98:428–436

Nietgen GW, Honemann CW, Chan CK, Kamatchi GL, Durieux ME (1998) Volatile anaesthetics have differential effects on recombinant m1 and m3 muscarinic acetylcholine receptor function. Br J Anaesth 81:569–577

North RA, Williams JT, Surprenant A, Christie MJ (1987) Mu and delta opioid receptors belong to a family of receptors that are coupled to potassium channels. Proc Natl Acad Sci U S A 84:5487–5491

Oleskevich S, Clements JD, Williams JT (1993) Opioid-glutamate interactions in rat locus coeruleus neurons. J Neurophysiol 70:931–937

Palczewski K, Kumasaka T, Hori T, Behnke CA, Motoshima H, Fox BA, Le Trong I, Teller DC, Okada T, Stenkamp RE, Yamamoto M, Miyano M (2000) Crystal structure of rhodopsin: a G protein-coupled receptor. Science 289:739–745

Pan HL, Chen SR, Eisenach JC (1999) Intrathecal clonidine alleviates allodynia in neuropathic rats: interaction with spinal muscarinic and nicotinic receptors. Anesthesiology 90: 509–514

Pan PM, Huang CT, Wei TT, Mok MS (1998) Enhancement of analgesic effect of intrathecal neostigmine and clonidine on bupivacaine spinal anesthesia. Reg Anesth Pain Med 23: 49–56

Paqueron X, Li X, Bantel C, Tobin JR, Voytko ML, Eisenach JC (2001) An obligatory role for spinal cholinergic neurons in the antiallodynic effects of clonidine after peripheral nerve injury. Anesthesiology 94:1074–1081

Pasternak GW (1993) Pharmacological mechanisms of opioid analgesics. Clin Neuropharmacol 16:1–18

Peltonen JM, Nyronen T, Wurster S, Pihlavisto M, Hoffren AM, Marjamaki A, Xhaard H, Kanerva L, Savola JM, Johnson MS, Scheinin M (2003) Molecular mechanisms of ligand-receptor interactions in transmembrane domain V of the alpha2A-adrenoceptor. Br J Pharmacol 140:347–358

Pert CB, Snyder SH (1973) Opiate receptor: demonstration in nervous tissue. Science 179:1011–1014

Pierce KL, Premont RT, Lefkowitz RJ (2002) Seven-transmembrane receptors. Nat Rev Mol Cell Biol 3:639–650

Pogozheva ID, Lomize AL, Mosberg HI (1998) Opioid receptor three-dimensional structures from distance geometry calculations with hydrogen bonding constraints. Biophys J 75:612–634

Pohjanoksa K, Jansson CC, Luomala K, Marjamaki A, Savola JM, Scheinin M (1997) Alpha2-adrenoceptor regulation of adenylyl cyclase in CHO cells: dependence on receptor density, receptor subtype and current activity of adenylyl cyclase. Eur J Pharmacol 335:53–63

Poree LR, Guo TZ, Kingery WS, Maze M (1998) The analgesic potency of dexmedetomidine is enhanced after nerve injury: a possible role for peripheral a2-adrenoreceptors. Anesth Analg 87:941–948

Przewlocki R, Parsons KL, Sweeney DD, Trotter C, Netzeband JG, Siggins GR, Gruol DL (1999) Opioid enhancement of calcium oscillations and burst events involving NMDA receptors and L-type calcium channels in cultured hippocampal neurons. J Neurosci 19:9705–9715

Puke MJ, Wiesenfeld-Hallin Z (1993) The differential effects of morphine and the [alpha]2-adrenoceptor agonists clonidine and dexmedetomidine on the prevention and treatment of experimental neuropathic pain. Anesth Analg 77:104–109

Rodbell M, Birnbaumer L, Pohl SL (1971) Characteristics of glucagon action on the hepatic adenylate cyclase system. Biochem J 125:58P–59P

Rowell PP, Volk KA, Li J, Bickford ME (2003) Investigations of the cholinergic modulation of GABA release in rat thalamus slices. Neuroscience 116:447–453

Rueter LE, Meyer MD, Decker MW (2000) Spinal mechanisms underlying A-85380-induced effects on acute thermal pain. Brain Res 872:93–101

Ryan JS, Tao QP, Kelly ME (1998) Adrenergic regulation of calcium-activated potassium current in cultured rabbit pigmented ciliary epithelial cells. J Physiol 511:145–157

Sabbe MB, Penning JP, Ozaki GT, Yaksh TL (1994) Spinal and systemic action of the alpha 2 receptor agonist dexmedetomidine in dogs. Anesthesiology 80:1057–1072

Saegusa H, Kurihara T, Zong S, Minowa O, Kazuno A, Han W, Matsuda Y, Yamanaka H, Osanai M, Noda T, Tanabe T (2000) Altered pain responses in mice lacking alpha 1E subunit of the voltage-dependent Ca2+ channel. Proc Natl Acad Sci U S A 97:6132–6137

Sah VP, Seasholtz TM, Sagi SA, Brown JH (2000) The role of Rho in G protein-coupled receptor signal transduction. Annu Rev Pharmacol Toxicol 40:459–489

Sakurai T (2007) The neural circuit of orexin (hypocretin): maintaining sleep and wakefulness. Nat Rev Neurosci 8:171–181

Sakurai T, Amemiya A, Ishii M, Matsuzaki I, Chemelli RM, Tanaka H, Williams SC, Richardson JA, Kozlowski GP, Wilson S, Arch JR, Buckingham RE, Haynes AC, Carr SA, Annan RS, McNulty DE, Liu WS, Terrett JA, Elshourbagy NA, Bergsma DJ, Yanagisawa M (1998) Orexins and orexin receptors: a family of hypothalamic neuropeptides and G protein-coupled receptors that regulate feeding behavior. Cell 92:573–585

Sanders RD, Maze M (2007) Adrenergic and cholinergic compounds. In: Stein C (ed) Analgesia. (Handbook of Experimental Pharmacology, vol 177) Springer, Berlin Heidelberg New York, pp 251–264

Sanders RD, Giombini M, Ma D, Ohashi Y, Hossain M, Fujinaga M, Maze M (2005) Dexmedetomidine exerts dose-dependent age-independent antinociception but age-dependent hypnosis in Fischer rats. Anesth Analg 100:1295–1302

Schäfer M (1999) Peripheral opioid analgesia: from experimental to clinical studies. Curr Opin Anaesthesiol 12:603–607

Segal IS, Vickery RG, Walton JK, Doze VA, Maze M (1988) Dexmedetomidine diminishes halothane anesthetic requirements in rats through a postsynaptic alpha 2 adrenergic receptor. Anesthesiology 69:818–823

Shannon HE, Sheardown MJ, Bymaster FP, Calligaro DO, Delapp NW, Gidda J, Mitch CH, Sawyer BD, Stengel PW, Ward JS, Wong DT, Olesen PH, Suzdak PD, Sauerberg P, Swedberg MD (1997) Pharmacology of butylthio[2. 2 2] (LY297802/NNC11-1053): a novel analgesic with mixed muscarinic receptor agonist and antagonist activity. J Pharmacol Exp Ther 281:884–894

Sharp BM (2001) Opioid receptor expression and intracellular signalling by cells involved in host defence and immunity. In: Machelska H, Stein C (eds) Immune mechanisms of pain and analgesia. Landes Bioscience, Georgetown, pp 98–105

Sheardown MJ, Shannon HE, Swedberg MD, Suzdak PD, Bymaster FP, Olesen PH, Mitch CH, Ward JS, Sauerberg P (1997) M1 receptor agonist activity is not a requirement for muscarinic antinociception. J Pharmacol Exp Ther 281:868–875

Short TG, Plummer JL, Chui PT (1992) Hypnotic and anaesthetic interactions between midazolam, propofol and alfentanil. Br J Anaesth 69:162–167

Simonnet G, Rivat C (2003) Opioid-induced hyperalgesia: abnormal or normal pain? Neuroreport 14:1–7

Slominski A, Wortsman J, Luger T, Paus R, Solomon S (2000) Corticotropin releasing hormone and proopiomelanocortin involvement in the cutaneous response to stress. Physiol Rev 80:979–1020

Stein C (1995) The control of pain in peripheral tissue by opioids. N Engl J Med 332:1685–1690

Stein C, Rosow CE (2004) Analgesics: receptor ligands and opiate narcotics. In: Evers AS, Maze M (eds) Anesthetic pharmacology, physiologic principles and clinical practice. Churchill Livingstone, Philadelphia, pp 457–471

Stein C, Machelska H, Schäfer M (2001) Peripheral analgesic and antiinflammatory effects of opioids. Z Rheumatol 60:416–424

Sugimura M, Kitayama S, Morita K, Imai Y, Irifune M, Takarada T, Kawahara M, Dohi T (2002) Effects of GABAergic agents on anesthesia induced by halothane, isoflurane, and thiamylal in mice. Pharmacol Biochem Behav 72:111–116

Svoboda KR, Lupica CR (1998) Opioid inhibition of hippocampal interneurons via modulation of potassium and hyperpolarization-activated cation (Ih) currents. J Neurosci 18: 7084–7098

Swedberg MD, Sheardown MJ, Sauerberg P, Olesen PH, Suzdak PD, Hansen KT, Bymaster FP, Ward JS, Mitch CH, Calligaro DO, Delapp NW, Shannon HE (1997) Butylthio[2. 2 2] (NNC 11-1053/LY297802): an orally active muscarinic agonist analgesic. J Pharmacol Exp Ther 281:876–883

Takano Y, Yaksh TL (1998) Release of calcitonin gene-related peptide (CGRP) substance P (SP) and vasoactive intestinal polypeptide (VIP) from rat spinal cord: modulation by alpha 2 agonists. Peptides 14:371–378

Tassonyi E, Charpantier E, Muller D, Dumont L, Bertrand D (2002) The role of nicotinic acetylcholine receptors in the mechanisms of anesthesia. Brain Res Bull 57:133–150

Thomas T, Robinson C, Champion D, McKell M, Pell M (1998) Prediction and assessment of the severity of postoperative pain and of satisfaction with management. Pain 75:177–185

Tjolsen A, Lund A, Hole K (1990) The role of descending noradrenergic systems in regulation of nociception: the effects of intrathecally administered alphaadrenoreceptor antagonists and clonidine. Pain 43:113–120

Trafton JA, Abbadie C, Marchand S, Mantyh PW, Basbaum AI (1999) Spinal opioid analgesia: how critical is the regulation of substance P signaling? J Neurosci 19:9642–9653
Traynor JR (1998) Epibatidine and pain. Br J Anaesth 81:69–76
Ueda H, Miyamae T, Hayashi C, Watanabe S, Fukushima N, Sasaki Y, Iwamura T, Misu Y (1995) Protein kinase C involvement in homologous desensitization of delta-opioid receptor coupled to Gi1-phospholipase C activation in Xenopus oocytes. J Neurosci 15:7485–7499
Ulrich D, Bettler B (2007) GABA(B) receptors: synaptic functions and mechanisms of diversity. Curr Opin Neurobiol 17:298–303
Vetter I, Wyse BD, Monteith GR, Roberts-Thomson SJ, Cabot PJ (2006) The mu opioid agonist morphine modulates potentiation of capsaicin-evoked TRPV1 responses through a cyclic AMP-dependent protein kinase A pathway. Mol Pain 2:22
Waldhoer M, Bartlett SE, Whistler JL (2004) Opioid receptors. Annu Rev Biochem 73:953–990
Wang Q, Zhao J, Brady AE, Feng J, Allen PB, Lefkowitz RJ, Greengard P, Limbird LE (2004) Spinophilin blocks arrestin actions in vitro and in vivo at G protein-coupled receptors. Science 304:1940–1944
Weil JV, McCullough RE, Kline JS, Sodal IE (1975) Diminished ventilatory response to hypoxia and hypercapnia after morphine in normal man. N Engl J Med 292:1103–1106
Wess J, Duttaroy A, Gomeza J, Zhang W, Yamada M, Felder CC, Bernardini N, Reeh PW (2003) Muscarinic receptor subtypes mediating central and peripheral antinociception studied with muscarinic receptor knockout mice: a review. Life Sci 72:2047–2054
Wilcox GL, Carlsson KH, Jochim A, Jurna I (1987) Mutual potentiation of antinociceptive effects of morphine and clonidine on motor and sensory responses in rat spinal cord. Brain Res 405:84–93
Williams JT, Christie MJ, Manzoni O (2001) Cellular and synaptic adaptations mediating opioid dependence. Physiol Rev 81:299–343
Willie JT, Chemelli RM, Sinton CM, Tokita S, Williams SC, Kisanuki YY, Marcus JN, Lee C, Elmquist JK, Kohlmeier KA, Leonard CS, Richardson JA, Hammer RE, Yanagisawa M (2003) Distinct narcolepsy syndromes in Orexin receptor-2 and Orexin null mice: molecular genetic dissection of Non-REM and REM sleep regulatory processes. Neuron 38:715–730
Willis WD (2001) Role of neurotransmitters in sensitization of pain responses. Ann N Y Acad Sci 933:142–156
Wilson SG, Smith SB, Chesler EJ, Melton KA, Haas JJ, Mitton B, Strasburg K, Hubert L, Rodriguez-Zas SL, Mogil JS (2003) The heritability of antinociception: common pharmacogenetic mediation of five neurochemically distinct analgesics. J Pharmacol Exp Ther 304:547–559
Wise A, Jupe SC, Rees S (2004) The identification of ligands at orphan G-protein coupled receptors. Annu Rev Pharmacol Toxicol 44:43–66
Xie W, Samoriski GM, McLaughlin JP, Romoser VA, Smrcka A, Hinkle PM, Bidlack JM, Gross RA, Jiang H, Wu D (1999) Genetic alteration of phospholipase C beta3 expression modulates behavioral and cellular responses to mu opioids. Proc Natl Acad Sci U S A 96:10385–10390
Yaksh TL (1997) Pharmacology and mechanisms of opioid analgesic activity. Acta Anaesthesiol Scand 41:94–111
Yasuda Y, Takeda A, Fukuda S, Suzuki H, Ishimoto M, Mori Y, Eguchi H, Saitoh R, Fujihara H, Honda K, Higuchi T (2003) Orexin a elicits arousal electroencephalography without sympathetic cardiovascular activation in isoflurane-anesthetized rats. Anesth Analg 97:1663–1666
Zhang HM, Li DP, Chen SR, Pan HL (2005) M2, m3, and m4 receptor subtypes contribute to muscarinic potentiation of GABAergic inputs to spinal dorsal horn neurons. J Pharmacol Exp Ther 313:697–704

Part II
Modern Inhalation Anesthetics

Section Editor: J.G. Bovill

Inhalation Anaesthesia: From Diethyl Ether to Xenon

J.G. Bovill

Abstract Modern anaesthesia is said to have began with the successful demonstration of ether anaesthesia by William Morton in October 1846, even though anaesthesia with nitrous oxide had been used in dentistry 2 years before. Anaesthesia with ether, nitrous oxide and chloroform (introduced in 1847) rapidly became commonplace for surgery. Of these, only nitrous oxide remains in use today. All modern volatile anaesthetics, with the exception of halothane (a fluorinated alkane), are halogenated methyl ethyl ethers. Methyl ethyl ethers are more potent, stable and better anaesthetics than diethyl ethers. They all cause myocardial depression, most markedly halothane, while isoflurane and sevoflurane cause minimal cardiovascular depression. The halogenated ethers also depress the normal respiratory response to carbon dioxide and to hypoxia. Other adverse effects include hepatic and renal damage. Hepatitis

J.G. Bovill
Department of Anaesthesiology, Leiden University Medical Centre, Leiden, The Netherlands
j.g.bovill@lumc.nl

J. Schüttler and H. Schwilden (eds.) *Modern Anesthetics.*
Handbook of Experimental Pharmacology 182.

occurs most frequently with halothane, although rare cases have been reported with the other agents. Liver damage is not caused by the anaesthetics themselves, but by reactive metabolites. Type I hepatitis occurs fairly commonly and takes the form of a minor disturbance of liver enzymes, which usually resolves without treatment. Type II, thought to be immune-mediated, is rare, unpredictable and results in a severe fulminant hepatitis with a high mortality. Renal damage is rare, and was most often associated with methoxyflurane because of excessive plasma fluoride concentrations resulting from its metabolism. Methoxyflurane was withdrawn from the market because of the high incidence of nephrotoxicity. Among the contemporary anaesthetics, the highest fluoride concentrations have been reported with sevoflurane, but there are no reports of renal dysfunction associated with its use. Recently there has been a renewed interest in xenon, one of the noble gases. Xenon has many of the properties of an ideal anaesthetic. The major factor limiting its more widespread is the high cost, about 2,000 times the cost of nitrous oxide.

1 Introduction

On the morning of Friday 16th October 1846, in front of an invited audience in the Bullfinch operating theatre of the Massachusetts General Hospital in Boston, the dentist William Morton administered diethyl ether to Edward Abbott for the excision of a tumour from his neck. This was the first successful demonstration of anaesthesia with ether in man, although anaesthesia with nitrous oxide had been used in dentistry 2 years before. Although the patient subsequently admitted being conscious during the procedure, he had experienced no pain. A newspaper reporter was present in the audience, and the discovery of surgical anaesthesia soon spread worldwide, and ether anaesthesia soon became commonplace. Chloroform was introduced as an anaesthetic almost simultaneously with ether (1847) and for a time largely replaced it in popularity. It was not until the introduction of halothane in 1956 that the popularity of ether waned.

The first half of the twentieth century saw the introduction of a variety of volatile liquids and gases as anaesthetics, most of which are now only of historical interest. Developments in organic fluorine chemistry in the 1950s paved the way for the synthesis of the fluorinated anaesthetic alkanes and ethers used in modern anaesthesia.

2 Physical Properties

2.1 Vapour Pressure

Inhalational anaesthetics are either gases or the vapours of volatile liquids. A substance is a gas when above its critical temperature (the temperature above which it cannot be liquefied irrespective of how much pressure is applied), and a vapour when below the critical temperature. Thus nitrous oxide (N_2O), which has a critical temperature of +36.4°C, is a vapour when inhaled at 20°C, but a gas when exhaled at 37°C.

In the gaseous phase, vapours exert a measurable pressure, the vapour pressure. When a vapour is in equilibrium with the liquid agent, the vapour pressure is referred to as the saturated vapour pressure or SVP. The lower the SVP the more volatile is the anaesthetic. In the early days of anaesthesia ether and chloroform were commonly administered using a Schimmelbusch mask, a wire frame covered with gauze on to which the liquid was dropped from a suitable bottle. This technique relied on high volatility for its success. An advance on the Schimmelbusch mask was the draw-over vaporiser, in which the anaesthetic was vaporised in a glass container by a flow of air or oxygen. A major drawback of these devices was that the process of vaporisation cooled the liquid (latent heat of vaporisation). Since SVP decreases with temperature, with time the concentration of anaesthetic being delivered decreased, necessitating frequent adjustments to the vaporiser to maintain a constant inspired concentration. Modern vaporisers are designed to compensate for changes in the temperature of the liquid, so that for any setting of the device the concentration delivered to the patient remains constant.

2.2 *Solubility and Anaesthetic Properties*

Solubility in blood and brain is important if anaesthetics are to cross the alveolar–capillary membrane and the blood–brain barrier. Solubility is quantified by the partition coefficient, 'the ratio of the concentration of dissolved gas/vapour in the blood or tissue to the concentration in the gaseous phase at equilibrium'. There is a good correlation between the oil/gas partition coefficient of an anaesthetic and its potency (Fig. 1).

The blood/gas solubility values for modern anaesthetic drugs vary fourfold (Table 1) from the least soluble (N_2O, 0.47) to the most soluble (halothane, 2.4). The most soluble drugs have the slowest induction and recovery characteristics. This seeming paradox occurs because the speed of induction and recovery are not related to the mass of drug absorbed by or removed from the blood but to its relative partial pressure (tension) in the alveoli and the brain. The anaesthetic delivered to the lungs diffuses into the blood until its partial pressure in the alveoli and blood are in equilibrium. Likewise the transfer to the tissues (including the brain) also proceeds towards equilibrium of the partial pressures. For agents with high blood/gas solubility, the blood has a tremendous capacity for absorbing the agent so that it is constantly being removed from the alveoli. Consequently it takes a long time for the alveolar tension to approach the inspired tension (Fig. 2). As alveolar tension is virtually synonymous with brain tension, both induction of and recovery from anaesthesia with these drugs will be slow. Because the partial pressures of inhaled anaesthetics equilibrate throughout the body, monitoring their alveolar concentration provides a reliable way of monitoring their effect on the brain.

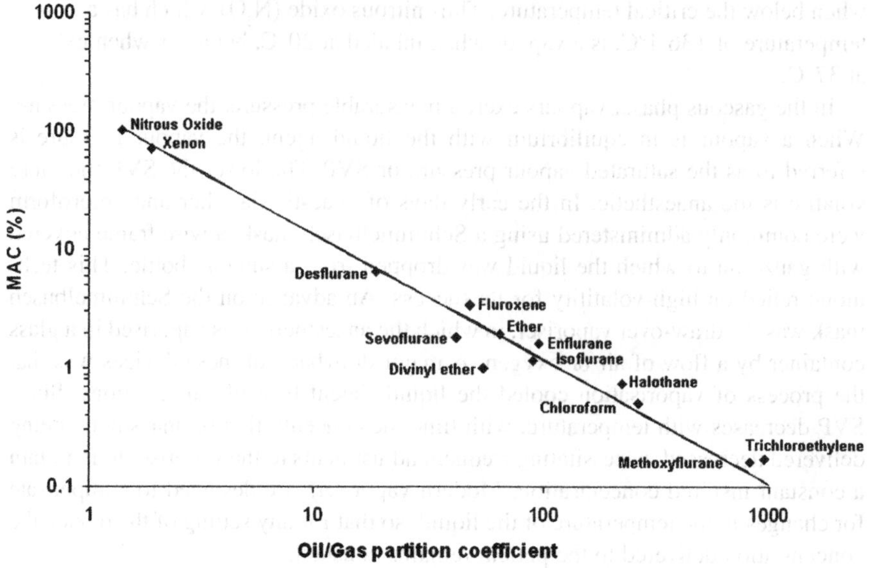

Fig. 1 Correlation between the potencies of a wide variety of inhalational anaesthetics and their oil/gas solubility

Table 1 Physical properties of inhalational anaesthetics

Agent	MW	Boiling point (°C)	SVP (kP_a) at 20°C	$\lambda_{B/G}$	$\lambda_{O/G}$	Metabolism %	Inflammable	MAC in O_2	Airway irritability
Nitrous oxide	44.02	−88.5	5,200	0.47	1.4	None	No	105%	No
Xenon	131.3	−108.1		0.114		None	No	60%–70%	No
Diethyl ether	74.1	34.6	58.6	12.1	65	6	Yes	12%	Very marked
Chloroform	113.4	62	21.15	10.3	265	Low	No	0.5%	No
Cyclopropane				0.415	11.2		Yes	10%	No
Trichlorethylene		87.5	57 mmHg	9.15	960		No	0.17%	No
Fluroxene			286 mmHg	1.37	47.7		Yes	3.4%	No
Halothane	197.4	50.2	32.3	2.4	224	20–50	No	0.8%	Minimal
Methoxyflurane	164.97	104.97		13.0	825		No	0.16%	None
Isoflurane	184.5	48.5	33.2	1.46	90.8	0.2	No	1.2%	Marked
Enflurane	184.5	56.5	22.9	1.9	96.5	2	No	2–8%	Some
Sevoflurane	200.5	58.5	21.3	0.65	42	3	No	1.8%	Minimal
Desflurane	168	23.5	88.3	0.42	18.7	0.02	No	6.5%	Marked

The rate of induction of anaesthesia is influenced by other factors in addition to the physical characteristics of the anaesthetic. The higher the inspired concentration, the more rapid the rise in alveolar concentration and hence the more quickly equilibrium is attained between tensions in the alveoli and the brain. An increase in alveolar ventilation will also increase the alveolar concentration of the inhaled

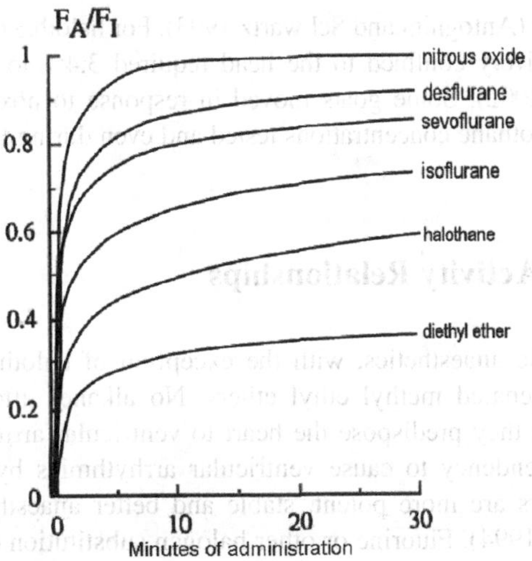

Fig. 2 Graph showing how the ratio between the inspired (F_I) and alveolar (F_A) concentrations of inhalational anaesthetics changes with time of administration. The least soluble drugs approach equilibrium (F_A/F_I) the fastest

agent. A decrease in cardiac output, by slowing the transit time through the pulmonary circulation, will allow the tension of the inhaled agent in the blood to increase more rapidly, and consequently induction of anaesthesia will be faster. In contrast, an increase in cardiac output will slow induction, as in patients who are anxious.

3 Potency: Minimum Alveolar Concentration

The 'minimum alveolar concentration' (MAC) has become accepted as the standard measure of clinical potency of the inhaled anaesthetics. MAC is defined as the minimum alveolar concentration of an anaesthetic at one atmosphere ambient pressure that suppresses gross movement in response to a defined painful stimulus in 50% of subjects. It is thus the equivalent of the EC_{50} for intravenous drugs. It is important to note that MAC only measures the potency of an anaesthetic to suppress the motor response to a noxious stimulus, which is mediated by the spinal cord, not the brain (Sonner et al. 2003).

Rampil and Laster (1992) showed that there was no correlation between immobility during noxious stimulation and electroencephalographic (EEG) activity, suggesting that the cortex is not the site at which anaesthetics act to block motor responses to noxious stimulation. In rats, precollicular decerebration (Rampil et al. 1993) or complete section of the upper thoracic spinal cord (Rampil 1994) minimally affected the capacity of isoflurane to suppress movement. In goats, the MAC for isoflurane delivered to the whole body was 1.2%, but delivery only to the brain increased

MAC to nearly 3% (Antognini and Schwartz 1993). For halothane whole body MAC was 0.9%, but delivery confined to the head required 3.4% to abolish movement (Antognini et al. 2002). Some goats moved in response to noxious stimuli at the largest cerebral halothane concentrations tested and even during EEG silence.

4 Structure–Activity Relationships

All modern volatile anaesthetics, with the exception of halothane (a fluorinated alkane), are halogenated methyl ethyl ethers. No alkanes after halothane were developed because they predispose the heart to ventricular arrhythmias. An ether link reduces the tendency to cause ventricular arrhythmias by a factor of four. Methyl ethyl ethers are more potent, stable and better anaesthetics than diethyl ethers (Eger et al. 1994). Fluorine or other halogen substitution on the ether molecule lowers the boiling point, increases chemical stability and generally decreases toxicity and flammability. Addition of halogens also decreases blood/gas solubility (compare isoflurane and ether). However, the presence of at least one hydrogen atom is necessary for anaesthetic potency, and full halogenation results in compounds that are convulsive (Targ et al. 1989).

Fluorine atoms form a strong chemical bond with carbon atoms, which contributes to the stability of fluorinated anaesthetics. However, among structurally similar compounds, an increase in molecular weight is associated with an increase in anaesthetic potency. The potency of isoflurane is four times that of desflurane as a result of replacing one fluoride atom in desflurane by a chloride atom. Compared to other halogens, fluorine is also extremely electronegative, and this confers a strong polarity to the carbon-fluorine bond. This may contribute to the ability of fluorinated agents to interact with proteins that mediate their anaesthetic activity.

5 Non-anaesthetic Effects of Inhalational Anaesthetics

5.1 Cardiovascular System

All the volatile anaesthetics cause a concentration-dependent myocardial depression. The main mechanisms are a decrease in transsarcolemmal calcium entry and changes in sarcoplasmic reticulum function (Wheeler et al. 1994; Connelly and Coronado 1994). Halothane has the most negative inotropic effect of the currently used volatile agents. It also inhibits muscarinic receptor regulation of myocardial adenylyl cyclase activity and stimulates G protein-dependent adenylyl cyclase activity (Vulliemoz and Verosky 1988; Bohm et al. 1994). Increased adenylyl cyclase activity may explain why halothane sensitises the myocardium to catecholamine-induced arrhythmias. Low concentrations of enflurane cause less myocardial depression than halothane, although this advantage is lost at higher concentrations. Isoflurane causes minimal cardiovascular depression at concentrations below 2 MAC, but decreases systemic vascular resistance more than the other agents. It also causes more coronary arterial vasodilatation, which has led to the suggestion that it might cause a "coronary steal" in patients with coronary artery disease. This arises from the inability of diseased coronary arteries to dilate further during isoflurane anaesthesia while at the same time normal, non-diseased vessels in other areas dilate. In this way normal vascular beds could 'steal' blood from diseased beds, thereby worsening oxygen lack and ischaemia in those areas of myocardium. There is no evidence, however, that the risks associated with the careful administration of isoflurane to patients with coronary artery disease exceed those of other volatile agents.

Sevoflurane causes myocardial depression and a reduction in vascular resistance similar to isoflurane, but has minimal effects on heart rate. A rapid increase in the inspired concentration of desflurane causes an increase in heart rate and blood pressure. This is associated with an increase in sympathetic activity, possibly mediated by receptors in the upper airways, lungs and systemic receptors (Muzi et al. 1996). Although similar responses do occur with isoflurane, the increases in heart rate and blood pressure are less prominent.

Anaesthetics may have various effects on the duration of the QT interval in the electrocardiogram (ECG). Prolongation of the QT interval may result in polymorphous ventricular tachycardia of the 'torsades de pointes' type and ventricular fibrillation. Sevoflurane, isoflurane and desflurane prolong QT, whereas the influence of halothane is controversial (Booker et al. 2003).

Currently there is considerable interest in the ability of volatile anaesthetics to protect the myocardium form ischaemic insults, in a manner similar to ischaemic preconditioning. This is a phenomenon whereby brief episodes of sublethal cardiac ischaemia protect against subsequent prolonged ischaemia. While the mechanism by which this effect is produced is not fully understood, broadly similar mechanisms appear to be involved in both ischaemic and anaesthetic-induced preconditioning. Myocardial preconditioning by volatile anaesthetics is discussed in detail in the chapter by N.C. Weber and W. Schlack, this volume.

5.2 *Respiratory System*

All the halogenated ethers cause a dose-dependent respiratory depression. The normal ventilatory response to carbon dioxide is depressed, as is the response to hypoxia, even at sub-anaesthetic concentrations (van den Elsen et al. 1998). The greatest effect occurs with enflurane and the least with desflurane. Depression of ventilation results from a general depression of the respiratory centres in the central nervous system, loss of wakefulness drive and suppression of the function of motor neurones, intercostal muscles and the diaphragm. The peripheral drive of ventilation from the chemoreceptors in the carotid bodies is also abolished. Isoflurane and desflurane are irritants to the respiratory tract. This can result in breath holding and laryngospasm, and makes them unsuitable for induction of anaesthesia. Sevoflurane produces little respiratory tract irritation, and high concentrations are well tolerated. This, combined with low blood solubility, makes it highly suitable for induction of anaesthesia, particularly in children.

A rapid increase in pulmonary ventilation (time constant 2–10 s) in response to acute hypoxaemia (acute hypoxic response) is a physiological response initiated by oxygen-sensitive glomus type I cells in the carotid bodies. Volatile anaesthetics suppress or abolish the acute hypoxic response at concentrations that can be found in patients up to several hours after discontinuation of anaesthesia (Dahan and Teppema 2003). The end-tidal C_{50} concentrations for reduction of the response vary from 0.08% for halothane to 0.27% for sevoflurane. The mechanism of volatile anaesthetic-induced impairment of oxygen sensing in the carotid bodies is not completely understood. A decrease in arterial oxygen tension in the blood leads to closure of TASK-1 and K_V potassium channels in the membrane of carotid body type I cells, followed by membrane depolarisation, an influx of Ca^{2+} ions and activation of afferent fibres in the carotid sinus nerve (López-Barneo et al. 2001). While hypoxia closes potassium channels, volatile anaesthetics open them (Patel and Honoré 2001).

Volatile anaesthetics, with the possible exception of desflurane, also cause the formation of reactive oxygen species (ROS) during hypoxia. Probably because desflurane undergoes minimal metabolism, it produces few ROS and causes minimal depression of the acute hypoxic response (Dahan et al. 1996). There is a good correlation between the extent of metabolism of volatile anaesthetics and their suppression of the acute hypoxic response. Administration of the anti-oxidants ascorbic acid and α-tocopherol completely reversed the reduction in the acute hypoxic response by halothane (Teppema et al. 2002) and isoflurane (Teppema et al. 2005). In the case of isoflurane, the acute hypoxic response decreased from the control value of 0.82±0.41 (mean±SD) $l\ min^{-1}\ \%^{-1}$ to 0.49±0.23 $l\ min^{-1}\ \%^{-1}$ (p=0.0013) during isoflurane. This reduction of the acute hypoxic response was completely reversed when isoflurane was combined with anti-oxidants.

5.3 *Malignant Hyperthermia*

Malignant hyperthermia is an uncommon inherited genetic disorder of skeletal muscle affecting humans and certain strains of swine, dogs, horses and other animals (Brandon 2005). In susceptible individuals, triggering agents induce a hypermetabolic state characterised by increased CO_2 production, elevated O_2 consumption, acid-base disturbances, muscle rigidity and muscle breakdown. This cascade is set in motion by excessive release of calcium from intracellular stores. Among the common triggering agents are the depolarising muscle relaxant suxamethonium, and the halogenated volatile anaesthetics. Halothane is a particularly potent trigger, although none of the volatile agents is safe. With early recognition and treatment (the specific treatment is dantrolene) the mortality is about 10%. Before the use of dantrolene mortality was about 80%.

5.4 *Genotoxicity and Mutagenic Potential of Volatile Anaesthetics*

Inhalation anaesthetics have the potential to be mutagenic or carcinogenic, raising concerns about health risks to patients and to operating theatre personnel through occupational exposure (Horeauf et al. 1999). They may increase the frequency of spontaneous abortion among female operating room personnel or affect human reproduction in other ways (Boivin 1997). Genetic damage, with changes in DNA structure or increases in sister chromatid exchanges, have been demonstrated for all inhalational anaesthetics (Karelova et al. 1992; Akin et al 2005). However, Krause et al. (2003) investigated the formation of sister chromatid exchanges in mitogen-stimulated T lymphocytes of 40 children undergoing sevoflurane anaesthesia for minor surgical procedures and did not observe any genotoxic effects. Xenon can halt cell division by blocking mitosis at the metaphase–anaphase stage, although this is reversible on withdrawing xenon (Petzelt et al 1999)

5.5 *Liver Damage*

Hepatotoxicity caused by inhalational anaesthetics was recognised in the 1850s in patients anaesthetised with chloroform, but did not occur in patients given ether. Liver damage is not caused by the anaesthetics themselves, but rather by reactive metabolites produced by their biotransformation by cytochrome P450 (Kenna and van Pelt 1994). Concerning the modern anaesthetics, hepatitis occurs most frequently with halothane, although rare cases have been reported with the other agents. Halothane-related hepatitis was first reported in 1958 just 2 years after the drug's introduction. There are two types of halothane-related hepatotoxicity.

5.5.1 Type I Halothane Hepatitis

Type I halothane hepatitis occurs fairly commonly (estimates vary from 1 in 20 to perhaps as often as 1 in 3 patients) and takes the form of a minor disturbance of liver enzymes. There is an asymptomatic rise in serum transaminases 1–2 weeks after exposure, which resolves without treatment. Repeat exposure is not a requirement and the clinical significance of the biochemical changes is uncertain. The cause of type I hepatitis is not fully understood. It is thought to result either directly from the toxic effects of halothane or indirectly after covalent bonding of halothane with cellular components. The latter reaction is more likely to occur under hypoxic condition, e.g. global reduction in hepatic perfusion or localised hypoxia during periods of hypotension. The first step in the reductive pathway of halothane metabolism is the insertion of a single electron into the halothane molecule to produce a highly reactive metabolite, which then undergoes debromination to another free radical intermediate. Liver macromolecules may interact with these free radicals or other metabolic intermediates, causing an autocatalytic peroxidative chain reaction in the liver, with breakdown and necrosis of cell membranes.

5.5.2 Type II Halothane Hepatitis

The second form of hepatitis is rare (1 in 35,000 halothane anaesthetics), unpredictable and results in a severe fulminant hepatitis with a high mortality. Previous exposure to halothane is usual and there may be a history of delayed onset postoperative pyrexia or jaundice. The first signs of fulminant injury (pyrexia, rash and/or joint pains) can precede jaundice that may be delayed for up to a month after halothane anaesthesia. Without liver transplantation, fulminant halothane hepatitis has a very high mortality rate. Reports of liver damage after halothane exposure in children are rare and the overall incidence has been estimated at 1 in 82,000 halothane anaesthetics.

It is now accepted that type II halothane hepatitis is immune mediated, with the immune response directed against hepatocytes. Cytochrome P450 2E1 (CYP2E1)-mediated oxidation of halothane to a reactive intermediate (trifluoroacetyl chloride) that covalently binds to hepatic proteins forming trifluoroacetylated neoantigens is believed to be the initiating event in a complex immunologic cascade culminating in antibody formation and severe hepatic necrosis in susceptible patients. Oxidative metabolism of sevoflurane produces no reactive intermediaries and therefore is not associated with immune-mediated hepatotoxicity.

Serum from patients with type II halothane hepatitis contains antibodies that react with an acyl halide that is covalently bounded to liver cell membranes. This acyl halide (CF_3COCl) acts as an epitope or hapten that is presented to the immunocompetent cells, setting up an antibody reaction. This form of immune sensitisation is specific to patients with halothane hepatitis (Neuberger et al 1983).

Patients suffering from halothane hepatitis develop auto-antibodies specifically targeting CYP2E1, the cytochrome P450 enzyme responsible for the biotransformation of halogenated hydrocarbons such as halothane (Bourdi et al. 1996). Similar auto-antibodies in high titres have also been detected in paediatric anaesthesiologists exposed to halogenated anaesthetics (Njoku et al. 2002). However, since few of these individuals develop hepatitis the pathogenetic role of auto-antibodies in anaesthetic-induced hepatitis remains questionable.

5.6 Renal Toxicity

5.6.1 Fluoride-Induced

Inorganic fluoride nephrotoxicity was first recognised in 1960 with the introduction of methoxyflurane (2-2 dichlorofluroethyl methyl ether). Methoxyflurane was withdrawn from the market because of the high incidence of nephrotoxicity, with a high output renal failure unresponsive to vasopressin. This was associated with plasma fluoride concentrations exceeding 50 μmol l^{-1}. Among the contemporary anaesthetics, the highest fluoride concentrations have been reported with sevoflurane. After only two MAC-hours of sevoflurane, anaesthesia concentrations of fluoride exceeding 50 μmol l^{-1} have been documented. However, no reports of renal dysfunction associated with prolonged exposure to sevoflurane have been published. The important difference between methoxyflurane and sevoflurane is that the fluoride liberated during methoxyflurane anaesthesia is produced in the kidney causing direct renal damage (Kharasch et al. 1995). This is in part related to the presence in the kidneys of multiple cytochrome P450 enzymes (CYP2A6, CYP3A, CYP2E1) responsible for the metabolism of methoxyflurane. Renal metabolism of sevoflurane is four times lower, so that much lower fluoride levels are reached within the kidney.

5.6.2 Degradation Products

Sevoflurane (2-(fluoromethoxy)-1,1,1,3,3,3-hexafluoropropane) undergoes spontaneous degradation when exposed to temperatures in excess of 50°C in the presence of carbon dioxide absorbents to produce fluoromethyl-2,2-difluoro-1-(trifluoromethyl)vinyl ether (FDVE), also known as compound A (Fig. 3), and trace amounts of 2-(fluoromethoxy)-3-methoxy-1,1,1,3,3-pentafluoropropane (compound B). These degradation products result from the extraction of the

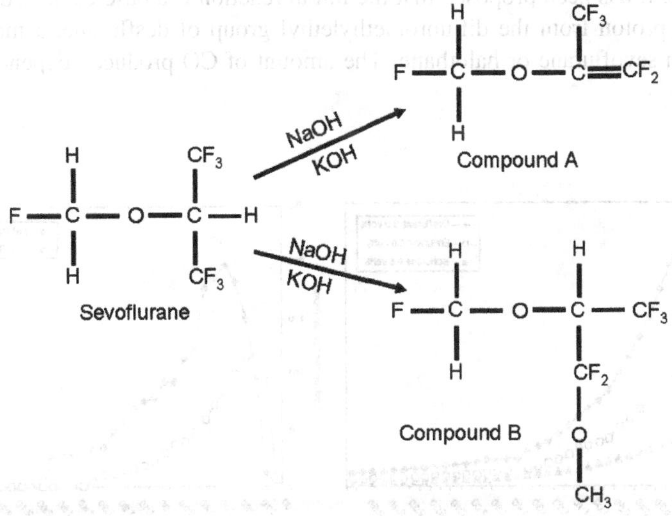

Fig. 3 The formation of compounds A and B from exposure of sevoflurane at temperatures above 60°C to the strong bases, NaOH and KOH, present in soda lime and Baralyme (Allied Healthcare Products, St. Louis)

acidic proton from sevoflurane in the presence of a strong base (KOH and/or NaOH). Baralyme (Allied Healthcare Products, St. Louis) causes more FDVE production than does soda lime. FDVE is metabolised in rats and humans to glutathione *S*-conjugates that are hydrolysed to the corresponding cysteine *S*-conjugates. Uptake of these *S*-conjugates by the kidneys and their subsequent metabolism by β-lyase is thought to be responsible for the renal tubular necrosis caused by FDVE in rats (Kharasch and Spracklin 1996).

In contrast to rats, patient exposure to FDVE during sevoflurane anaesthesia has no clinically significant renal effects. In humans, renal function was unaffected by low-flow sevoflurane, in which compound A concentrations averaged 8–32 ppm, and exposures were as high as 400 ppm·h (Kharasch et al. 2003). The differences between rats and humans may be the result of an inherent susceptibility to FDVE nephrotoxicity in rats, since human renal β-lyase activity is much lower than the rat's.

6 Carbon Monoxide Production

When volatile anaesthetics are passed through dry CO_2 absorbents, carbon monoxide (CO) may be produced in potentially life-threatening concentrations (Fang et al. 1995; Wissing et al. 2001). CO production is highest with desflurane and enflurane, less with isoflurane, and insignificant with sevoflurane and halothane (Fig. 4) (Keijzer et al. 2006). For all anaesthetics CO production is higher with Baralyme than with soda lime. The exact mechanism of CO production is uncertain. For desflurane it has been proposed that the initial reaction is a base-catalysed abstraction of a proton from the difluoromethylethyl group of desflurane, a moiety not present in sevoflurane or halothane. The amount of CO produced depends on the

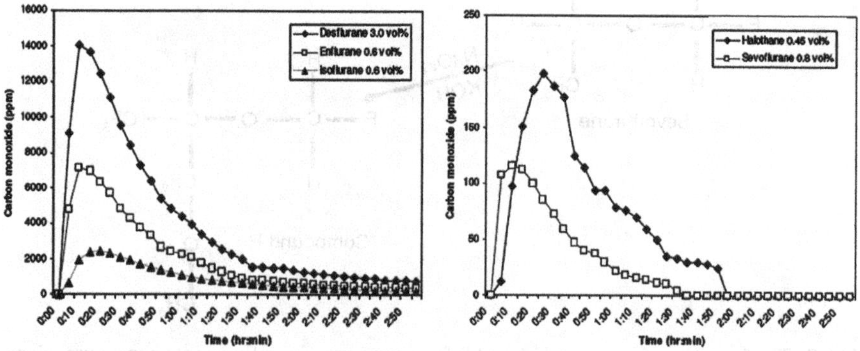

Fig. 4 CO production in dry soda lime by inhalational anaesthetics: Note the different scales in the two graphs. (From Keijzer et al. 2006, with permission)

quantity of dry absorbent with which desflurane makes contact, the water content of the absorbent and the fresh gas flow. The water content needed to prevent CO production is approximately 4.8% for soda lime and 9.7% for Baralyme.

7 Individual Agents

7.1 *Of Historical Interest Only*

7.1.1 Diethyl Ether $(CH_5)_2O$

Ether is a colourless, volatile and highly inflammable liquid with a characteristic pungent smell. Low concentrations of ether burn whereas, in the presence of oxygen, high concentrations of ether vapour can explode with potentially devastating consequences.

Ether has a high blood/gas solubility (Table 1), slowing both induction of and recovery from anaesthesia. Its low potency and the fact that it is an irritant to the respiratory tract further slowed inhalational uptake, resulting in prolonged induction times (15–25 min to achieve deep anaesthesia). Despite its many disadvantages, ether is a relatively safe anaesthetic largely because, with overdose, respiratory depression occurs before serious cardiac depression. This is advantageous as, with progressive respiratory depression, the amount of ether taken up by the lungs falls, thereby reducing the depth of anaesthesia.

7.1.2 Chloroform $(CHCl_3)$

Chloroform is a highly volatile, non-flammable liquid with a sweet-smelling odour. Induction and recovery were more rapid than with ether. Because of the lack of airway irritation induction was also much more pleasant than that with ether. In 1847, the Edinburgh obstetrician James Young Simpson first used chloroform for general anaesthesia during childbirth. John Snow set the seal of propriety on anaesthesia in obstetrics when in 1853 he administered chloroform to Queen Victoria during the birth of Prince Leopold, and again in 1857 at the birth of Princess Beatrice. The use of chloroform during surgery expanded rapidly thereafter, and began to replace ether as an anaesthetic. However, it later lost favour because of fears about its toxicity, especially liver damage, and its tendency to cause fatal cardiac arrhythmia.

7.1.3 Cyclopropane (C_3H_6)

Cyclopropane was introduced into clinical anaesthesia in 1933. It is a pleasant, sweet-smelling gas, irritating to the respiratory tract in concentrations over 40%

(20%–30% was required for deep anaesthesia). It was stored as a liquid at a pressure of 505 kP_a in light metal cylinders. The low blood–gas solubility coefficient resulted in rapid induction and recovery. Cyclopropane is explosive when mixed with air, oxygen or nitrous oxide.

7.2 Agents Currently Used in Anaesthesia

7.2.1 Nitrous Oxide

Nitrous oxide (N_2O) is a stable, colourless gas used as an inhalation anaesthetic. Of the three pillars of early anaesthetic practice—nitrous oxide, chloroform and ether—only nitrous oxide remains in regular use, although its popularity has waned in recent years, and it is no longer used in a number of hospitals.

Due to its low blood gas solubility (Table 1), equilibrium between alveoli and blood, and across the blood–brain barrier is rapidly established. The vast majority of N_2O is exhaled unchanged although a small amount may defuse through the skin or be excreted in the urine. Because it is 34 times more soluble in blood than nitrogen it will diffuse into and out of air-containing cavities more rapidly than nitrogen. Thus, during nitrous oxide anaesthesia, air-filled cavities, e.g. lung bullae, middle ear cavity, will tend to expand with the risk of rupture and pneumothorax.

Nitrous oxide is a potent analgesic; 20% N_2O is equivalent to 15 mg subcutaneous morphine. Entonox (BOC Gases, Wiesbaden, Germany) is a gas mixture containing 50% N_2O in oxygen, is widely used to provide analgesia during labour, for trauma victims or other emergencies. It is manufactured by bubbling O_2 through liquid N_2O, with vaporisation of the liquid to form a gaseous O_2/N_2O mixture. Entonox is supplied in cylinders at a pressure of 137 bar and must be stored above −6°C. Below this temperature the N_2O liquefies and the two gases separate in a process called lamination. If this occurs, a high concentration of O_2 will be delivered first, but as the cylinder empties the mixture will become progressively more hypoxic as it approaches 100% N_2O.

Toxicity

Monovalent cobalamin is essential for the synthesis of methionine and tetrahydrofolate, and necessary for the synthesis of DNA in rapidly proliferating tissues. The activated form of methionine, *S*-adenosylmethionine, is also the principal substrate for methylation in many other biochemical reactions, including assembly of the myelin sheath and methyl substitutions in neurotransmitters. Nitrous oxide within 2–4 h of exposure irreversibly oxidises the cobalt atom of vitamin B_{12}, converting monovalent cobalamin to a bivalent form which cannot participate in these reactions. As a result, the activity of the cobalamin-dependent enzyme, methionine synthase (5-methyltetrahydrofolate-homocysteine *S*-methyltransferase) is completely and irreversibly inhibited. Recovery of methionine synthase activity requires synthesis of new enzymes, which in humans takes 3–4 days, although full recovery may need several weeks.

Chronic exposure to nitrous oxide can cause megaloblastic erythropoiesis, neurone death and damage to the spinal cord. Reversible megaloblastic changes can be detected in the bone marrow after 12- to 24-h exposure. Patients have developed severe myelopathy or neurological impairment following nitrous oxide anaesthesia (McNeely et al. 2000; Lacassie et al. 2006).

Nitrous oxide toxicity may affect staff as well as patients. However, after extensive investigation there is still no evidence linking low-level occupational exposure with an increased incidence of spontaneous abortion. Although nitrous oxide does not appear to be fetotoxic in humans, it is prudent to avoid exposures in the first trimester of pregnancy, given its effects on DNA synthesis.

7.2.2 Xenon

Xenon, one of the four noble gases, is colourless, odourless, tasteless and four times denser than air. Both its density and viscosity are substantially higher than those of other inhalational anaesthetics. It occurs in extremely low concentrations (0.0875 ppm) in the atmosphere, hence its name from the Greek 'xenos' meaning 'stranger'. Xenon has been used experimentally as an anaesthetic for more than 50 years (Cullen and Gross 1951). Recently there has been a renewed interest in xenon as a safe, effective and more environmentally friendly substitute for nitrous oxide (Sanders et al. 2003). It is manufactured by fractional distillation of liquefied air, currently at a cost of US $10 per litre (i.e. about 2,000 times the cost of producing N_2O). This high cost is the major factor limiting its more widespread use, even when used in low-flow delivery systems. At the time of writing, xenon is only approved for clinical use in Russia and Germany.

Xenon has many of the properties of an ideal anaesthetic. Its blood/gas partition coefficient (0.12) is lower than that of any other anaesthetic, giving rapid induction and emergence. It is unlikely to be involved in any biochemical events in the body, and is not metabolised. Xenon causes no significant changes in myocardial contractility, blood pressure or systemic vascular resistance, even in the presence of severe cardiac disease (Sanders et al. 2005). The unique combination of analgesia, hypnosis, and lack of haemodynamic depression in one agent would make xenon a very attractive choice for patients with limited cardiovascular reserve and under some circumstances may compensate for its high cost.

In contrast to other inhaled anaesthetic agents, xenon slows the respiratory rate and increases the tidal volume, thereby maintaining minute ventilation constant. Airway pressure is increased during xenon anaesthesia, due to its higher density and viscosity rather than direct changes in airway resistance (Baumert et al 2002).

Because of its high cost xenon must be used in low-flow closed circuits. Crucial to this method of administration is accurate measurement of the concentration of xenon in the circuit. This measurement is generally difficult as xenon is diamagnetic and does not absorb infrared radiation (commonly used to measure the concentrations of other agents), and its low reactivity precludes the use of specific fuel cell or electrode-type devices. Xenon conducts heat better than other gases, and a technique based on thermal conductivity has proved to be effective (Luginbuhl et al 2002). Because xenon is heavier than air, the speed of sound is slower in xenon than that in air, and this difference has been also been used to measure xenon concentration.

Because xenon is a normal constituent of the atmosphere, it does not add to atmospheric pollution when emitted from the anaesthesia circuit. This is in contrast to the other inhalational anaesthetics, which have ozone-depleting potential and pollute the atmosphere when released from the anaesthesia system (Marx et al. 2001). On a molecular basis, N_2O is 230 times more potent as a greenhouse gas than carbon dioxide. N_2O released as a waste anaesthetic contributes roughly 0.1% of total global warming. The lifetime of N_2O in the atmosphere is long—approximately 120 years.

The anaesthetic actions of xenon are thought to result primarily from non-competitive inhibition of *N*-methyl-d-aspartate (NMDA) receptors (De Sousa et al. 2000), a property it shares with nitrous oxide. In common with other NMDA receptor antagonists, xenon appears to have neuroprotective properties (Sanders et al. 2003). Xenon is also an excellent analgesic, an action mediated by NMDA receptors (De Sousa et al. 2000). Xenon also inhibits the plasma membrane Ca^{2+} pump, altering neuronal excitability and inhibiting the nociceptive responsiveness of spinal dorsal horn neurones.

7.2.3 The Fluorinated Hydrocarbons

In fluorinated hydrocarbons (Fig. 5) the fluorine atoms form a strong chemical bond with the carbon atoms. The result is that the fluorine atom is quite non-reactive, particularly when the compound contains a CF_2 or CF_3 grouping. As a result this group is highly stable, volatile and non-inflammable under clinical conditions

Halothane

Halothane (2-bromo-2-chloro-1,1,1-trifluoroethane) was introduced into clinical anaesthesia in 1956. It was not the first fluorinated anaesthetic—fluroxene holds that distinction—but it was the first to achieve widespread acceptability. It is the most potent of the currently used volatile anaesthetics. Halothane is non-inflammable and non-irritating to the respiratory tract. Despite its molecular stability, due to the CF_3 group, halothane oxidises spontaneously and is decomposed by UV light to HCI, HBr, free chlorine and bromine ions and phosgene ($COCl_2$). To prevent decomposition it is stored in amber-coloured bottles, with thymol added as a preservative and to help prevent the liberation of free bromine. Between 20% and 50% of halothane undergoes metabolism, much higher than other currently available volatile anaesthetics.

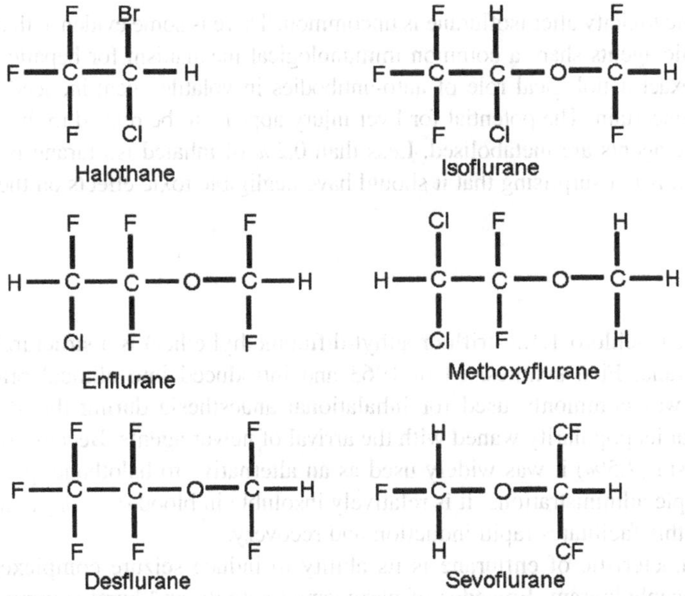

Fig. 5 Molecular structure of the fluorinated hydrocarbon anaesthetics

Halothane is readily soluble in rubber and less so in polyethylene. When halothane was first introduced large amounts of rubber were commonly used in anaesthetic systems, and uptake in the anaesthetic circuit was often significant. Nowadays rubber tubing has been universally replaced by plastic tubing that does not absorb halothane or other anaesthetics.

The most prominent effect of halothane on the circulation is a dose-related decrease in arterial blood pressure. This is due mainly to reduced myocardial contractility and ventricular slowing. Systemic vascular resistance also falls but this is less pronounced than with some other agents. Halothane sensitises the myocardium to the effects of catecholamines, and this can result in the development of ventricular arrhythmias.

Isoflurane

Isoflurane, a halogenated methyl ethyl ether (1-chloro-2,2,2-trifluoroethyl difluoromethyl ether), is a structural isomer of enflurane. It is a clear, colourless liquid with a slightly pungent smell. Isoflurane is non-flammable in oxygen, air and nitrous oxide under all normal conditions. It does not require a preservative and is stable in the presence of UV light. With a blood/gas solubility coefficient of 1.4 it occupies an intermediate position between the highly insoluble agents desflurane and sevoflurane and the more soluble enflurane and halothane.

Hepatic toxicity after isoflurane is uncommon. There is some evidence that volatile anaesthetic agents share a common immunological mechanism for hepatic damage, but the exact aetiological role of auto-antibodies in volatile agent-induced hepatitis remains uncertain. The potential for liver injury appears to be related to the extent to which the agents are metabolised. Less than 0.2% of inhaled isoflurane is metabolised, so it is not surprising that it should have negligible toxic effects on the liver.

Enflurane

Enflurane (2-chloro-1,1,2,-trifluoroethyl-difluomethyl ether) is a structural isomer of isoflurane. First synthesised in 1963 and introduced into clinical practice in 1966, it was commonly used for inhalational anaesthesia during the 1970s and 1980s, but its popularity waned with the arrival of newer agents. Because of its low metabolism (2.5%) it was widely used as an alternative to halothane, particularly for multiple administrations. It is relatively insoluble in blood (blood/gas solubility 1.8) and this facilitates rapid induction and recovery.

A characteristic of enflurane is its ability to induce seizure complexes in the electroencephalogram. Episodes of paroxysmal activity and burst suppression are most marked during deep anaesthesia in the presence of hypocarbia. However, patients with epilepsy are not thought to be at increased risk of seizures during or after enflurane anaesthesia.

Enflurane is metabolised by the cytochrome P450 series, specifically P450 2E1, but the agent is much less extensively metabolised than halothane (see Sect. 7.2.3.1). Metabolites include trifluoroacetic acid (TFA) and inorganic fluoride ion. A small number of cases of 'enflurane hepatitis' have been reported. However, the overall incidence of liver damage following enflurane anaesthesia is low, estimated to be only 1 in 800,000. In normal clinical use the peak plasma fluoride concentration rarely exceeds 25 $\mu mol\ l^{-1}$ and is well within the threshold for renal toxicity.

Desflurane

Desflurane (1,2,2,2-tetrafluoroethyl-difluoromethylether) was synthesised in the early 1960s and was the 653rd of a series of compounds evaluated for their anaesthetic potential. It is the least soluble of all the volatile anaesthetics with the same blood–gas solubility as nitrous oxide (0.42). Desflurane differs from isoflurane by just one atom; a fluorine atom is substituted for chlorine on the α-ethyl group. This replacement decreases blood and tissue solubility and potency (Table 1). Further, the complete fluorination of the methyl ether molecule results in a higher vapour pressure, and this together with the low boiling point of desflurane necessitates the use of a special vaporiser. The desflurane vaporiser is heated, thus requiring electrical power,

Desflurane undergoes the least metabolism of the halogenated hydrocarbons (Table 1). Because of its very low metabolism desflurane is generally not considered to be associated with liver injury. However, there are three case reports of patients who developed acute hepatotoxicity after desflurane anaesthesia (Martin et al. 1995; Berghaus et al. 1999, Tung et al. 2005). Although desflurane resists degradation by soda lime, carbon monoxide can be generated under certain conditions and may accumulate in the breathing system (see Sect. 6).

Sevoflurane

Sevoflurane is a fluorinated methyl isopropyl ether. Its low solubility (blood gas solubility coefficient, 0.68), lack of airway irritability and moderate potency make it particularly useful for induction in children.

Approximately 5% of a given dose of sevoflurane is metabolised, a higher proportion than with isoflurane or enflurane. As with other volatile agents, cytochrome P450 2E1 appears to be the specific enzyme involved. Sevoflurane is broken down to organic and inorganic fluorides and hexafluoroisopropanol. These compounds are excreted as fluoride ions in the urine and as conjugates in the bile. Despite the relatively high proportion of drug metabolised, hepatitis is unlikely since the putative metabolic pathway does not include a reactive metabolite with potential to bind to lipid or protein.

8 Intravenous Volatile Anaesthetics

Although the primary route of administration of volatile anaesthetics is through the lungs, attempts have been made to circumvent the anaesthesia circuitry and the lung's functional residual capacity by giving these drugs directly intravenously. Unfortunately direct intravenous administration of liquid volatile anaesthetics is usually lethal. There are a number of case reports of self-administered or accidental administration of IV halothane that resulted in the production of an acute respiratory distress-like syndrome and often death (Berman and Tattersall 1982; Dwyer and Coppel 1989). Less than 9 ml of IV liquid halothane resulted in immediate tachycardia, apnoea, and loss of consciousness. In addition, these patients experienced hypotension, right bundle branch block, pulmonary oedema, cyanosis, hypoxia, and acidosis within 30 min of administration. In contrast, the intravenous administration of volatile anaesthetics dissolved in fat or as emulsions was without adverse effects in animals (Johannesson et al. 1984; Eger and MacLeod 1995; Musser et al. 1999). Haynes and Kirkpatrick (1985) injected a lecithin-coated methoxyflurane preparation into the tails of rats without the toxicity observed with the injection of liquid methoxyflurane. Zhou et al. (2006) successfully induced anaesthesia in rats by IV emulsified isoflurane. Recovery of anaesthesia after IV emulsified isoflurane was faster than with propofol. Intravenous infusions of lipid emulsions of isoflurane, enflurane or sevoflurane had no haemodynamic effects in rabbits, but produced acute and delayed preconditioning against myocardial infarction, similar to that seen with inhalation of the same anaesthetics (Chiari et al. 2004).

References

Akin A, Ugur F, Ozkul Y, Esmaoglu A, Gunes I, Ergul H (2005) Desflurane anaesthesia increases sister chromatid exchanges in human lymphocytes. Acta Anaesthesiol Scand 49:1559–1561

Antognini JF, Schwartz K (1993) Exaggerated anesthetic requirements in the preferentially anesthetized brain. Anesthesiology 79:1244–1249

Antognini JF, Carstens E, Atherley R (2002) Does the immobilizing effect of thiopental in brain exceed that of halothane? Anesthesiology 96:980–986

Baumert JH, Reyle-Hahn M, Hecker K, Tenbrinck T, Kuhlen R, Rossaint R (2002) Increased airway resistance during xenon anaesthesia in pigs is attributed to physical properties of the gas. Br J Anaesth 88:540–545

Berghaus TM, Baron A, Geier A, Lamerz R, Paumgartner G (1999) Hepatotoxicity following desflurane anesthesia. Hepatology 29:613–614

Berman P, Tattersall M (1982) Self-poisoning with intravenous halothane. Lancet 1:340

Bohm M, Schmidt U, Gierschik P, Schwinger RHG, Bohm S, Erdmann E (1994) Sensitization of adenylate cyclase by halothane in human myocardium and S49 lymphoma wild-type and cyccells: evidence for an inactivation of the inhibitory G protein (Gi alpha). Mol Pharmacol 45:380–389

Boivin JF (1997) Risk of spontaneous abortion in women occupationally exposed to anaesthetic gases: a meta-analysis. Occup Environ Med 54:541–548

Booker PD, Whyte SD, Ladusans EJ (2003) Long QT syndrome and anaesthesia. Br J Anaesth 90:349–366

Bourdi M, Chen W, Peter RM, Martin JL, Buters JTM, Nelson SD, Pohl LR (1996) Human cytochrome P450 2E1 is a major autoantigen associated with halothane hepatitis. Chem Res Toxicol 9:1159–1166

Brandon BW (2005) The genetics of malignant hyperthermia. Anesthesiol Clin North America 23:615–619

Chiari PC, Pagel PS, Tanaka K, et al (2004) Intravenous emulsified halogenated anesthetics produce acute and delayed preconditioning against myocardial infarction in rabbits. Anesthesiology 101:1160–1166

Connelly TJ, Coronado R (1994) Activation of the calcium release channel of cardiac sarcoplasmic reticulum by volatile anesthetics. Anesthesiology 81:459–469

Cullen SC, Gross EG (1951) The anaesthetic properties of xenon in animals and human beings, with additional observations on krypton. Science 113:580–582

Dahan A, Teppema LJ (2003) Influence of anaesthesia and analgesia on the control of breathing. Br J Anaesth 91:40–49

Dahan A, Sarton E, van den Elsen M, van Kleef J, Teppema L, Berkenbosch A (1996) Ventilatory response to hypoxia: influences of subanesthetic desflurane. Anesthesiology 85:60–68

De Sousa SLM, Dickinson R, Lieb WR, Franks NP (2000) Contrasting synaptic actions of the inhalational general anesthetics isoflurane and xenon. Anesthesiology 92:1055–1066

Dwyer R, Coppel DL (1989) Intravenous injection of liquid halothane. Anesth Analg 69:250–255

Eger EI 2nd, Liu J, Koblin DD, et al (1994) Molecular properties of the "ideal" inhaled anesthetic: studies of fluorinated methanes, ethanes, propanes, and butanes. Anesth Analg 79:245–251

Eger RP, MacLeod BA (1995) Anaesthesia by intravenous emulsified isoflurane in mice. Can J Anaesth 42:173–176

Fang ZX, Eger EI 2nd, Laster MJ, Chortkoff BS, Kandel L, Ionescu P (1995) Carbon monoxide production from degradation of desflurane, enflurane, isoflurane, halothane and sevoflurane by soda lime and Baralyme. Anesth Analg 80:1187–1193

Haynes DH, Kirkpatrick AF (1985) Ultra-long-duration local anesthesia produced by injection of lecithin-coated methoxyflurane microdroplets. Anesthesiology 63:490–499

Horeauf K, Lierz M, Wiesner G, Schroegendorfer K, Lierz P, Spacek A, et al (1999) Genetic damage in operating room personnel exposed to isoflurane and nitrous oxide. Occup Environ Med 56:433–437

Johannesson G, Alm P, Biber B, et al (1984) Halothane dissolved in fat as an intravenous anaesthetic to rats. Acta Anaesthesiol Scand 28:381–384

Karelova J, Jablonicka A, Gavora J, Hano L (1992) Chromosome and sister-chromatid exchange analysis in peripheral lymphocytes, and mutagenicity of urine in anesthesiology personnel. Int Arch Occup Environ Health 64:303–306

Keijzer C, Perez RS, De Lange JJ (2005) Carbon monoxide production from five volatile anesthetics in dry sodalime in a patient model: halothane and sevoflurane do produce carbon monoxide; temperature is a poor predictor of carbon monoxide production. BMC Anesthesiol 5:1–11

Kenna JG, van Pelt FN (1994) The metabolism and toxicity of inhaled anaesthetic agents. Anaesth Pharmacol Rev 2:29–42

Kharasch ED, Spracklin DK (1996) Evidence for metabolism of fluoromethyl 2,2-difluoro-1-(trifluoromethyl)vinyl ether (compound A), a sevoflurane degradation product, by cysteine conjugate β-lyase. Chem Res Toxicol 9:696–702

Kharasch ED, Hankins DC, Thummel KE (1995) Human kidney methoxyflurane and sevoflurane metabolism: intrarenal fluoride production as a possible mechanism of methoxyflurane nephrotoxicity. Anesthesiology 82:689–699

Kharasch ED, Conzen PF, Michalowski P, Weiss BM, Rooke GA, Artru AA, Ebert TJ, Czerner SF, Reichle FM (2003) Safety of low-flow sevoflurane anesthesia in patients. Anesthesiology 99:752–754

Krause T, Scholz J, Jansen L, Boettcher H, Koch C, Wappler F (2003) Sevoflurane anaesthesia does not induce the formation of sister chromatid exchanges in peripheral blood lymphocytes of children. Br J Anaesth 90:233–235

Lacassie HJ, Nazar C, Yonish B, et al (2006) Reversible nitrous oxide myelopathy and a polymorphism in the gene encoding 5,10-methylenetetrahydrofolate reductase. Br J Anaesth 96:222–225

López-Barneo J, Pardal R, Ortega-Sáenz P (2001) Cellular mechanisms of oxygen sensing. Annu Rev Physiol 63:259–287

Luginbuhl M, Lauber R, Feigenwinter P, Zbinden AM (2002) Monitoring xenon in the breathing circuit with a thermal conductivity sensor. Comparison with a mass spectrometer and implications on monitoring other gases. J Clin Monit Comput 17:23–30

Martin JL, Plevak DJ, Flannery KD, et al (1995) Hepatotoxicity after desflurane anesthesia. Anesthesiology 83:1125–1129

Marx T, Schmidt M, Schirmer U, Reinelt H (2001) Pollution of the environment and the workplace with anesthetic gases. Int Anesthesiol Clin 39:15–27

McNeely JK, Buczulinski B, Rosner DR (2000) Severe neurological impairment in an infant after nitrous oxide anesthesia. Anesthesiology 93:1549–1550

Musser JB, Fontana JL, Mongan PD (1999) The anesthetic and physiologic effects of intravenous administration of halothane lipid emulsion (5% vol/vol). Anesth Analg 88:671–675

Muzi M, Ebert TJ, Hope WG, Robinson BJ, Bell LB (1996) Site(s) mediating sympathetic activation with desflurane. Anesthesiology 85:737–747

Neuberger J, Gimson AES, Davis M, Williams R (1983) Specific serological markers in the diagnosis of fulminant hepatic failure associated with halothane anaesthesia. Br J Anaesth 55:15–19

Njoku DB, Greenberg RS, Bourdi M, Borkowf CB, Dake EM, Martin JL, Pohl LR (2002) Autoantibodies associated with volatile anesthetic hepatitis found in the sera of a large cohort of pediatric anesthesiologists. Anesth Analg 94:239–240

Patel AJ, Honoré E (2001) Anesthetic-sensitive 2P domain K+ channels. Anesthesiology 95:1013–1021

Petzelt C, Taschenberger G, Schmehl W, Hafner M, Kox WJ (1999) Xenon induces metaphase arrest in rat astrocytes. Life Sci 65:901–913

Rampil IJ (1994) Anesthetic potency is not altered after hypothermic spinal cord transection in rats. Anesthesiology 80:606–610

Rampil IJ, Laster MJ (1992) No correlation between quantitative electroencephalographic measurements and movement response to noxious stimuli during isoflurane anesthesia in rats. Anesthesiology 77:920–925

Rampil IJ, Mason P, Singh H (1993) Anesthetic potency (MAC) is independent of forebrain structures in the rat. Anesthesiology 78:707–712

Sanders RD, Franks NP, Maze M (2003) Xenon: no stranger to anaesthesia. Br J Anaesth 91:709–717

Sanders RD, Ma D, Maze M (2005) Xenon: elemental anaesthesia in clinical practice. Br Med Bull 71:115–135

Sonner JM, Antognini JF, Dutton RC, et al (2003) Inhaled anesthetics and immobility: mechanisms, mysteries, and minimum alveolar anesthetic concentration. Anesth Analg 97:718–740

Targ AG, Yasuda N, Eger EI, et al (1989) Halogenation and anesthetic potency. Anesth Analg 68:599–602

Teppema LJ, Nieuwenhuijs D, Sarton E, Romberg R, Olievier CN, Ward DS, Dahan A (2002) Antioxidants prevent depression of the acute hypoxic ventilatory response by subanaesthetic halothane in men. J Physiol 544:931–938

Teppema LJ, Romberg RR, Dahan A (2005) Antioxidants reverse reduction of the human hypoxic ventilatory response by subanesthetic isoflurane. Anesthesiology 102:747–753

Tung D, Yoshida EM, Wang CSK, Steinbrecher US (2005) Severe desflurane hepatotoxicity after colon surgery in an elderly patient. Can J Anaesth 52:133–136

van den Elsen M, Sarton E, Teppema L, Berkenbosch A, Dahan A (1998) Influence of 0.1 minimum alveolar concentration of sevoflurane, desflurane and isoflurane on dynamic ventilatory response to hypercapnia in humans. Br J Anaesth 80:174–182

Vulliemoz Y, Verosky M (1988) Halothane interaction with guanine nucleotide binding proteins in mouse heart. Anesthesiology 69:876–880

Wheeler DM, Katz A, Rice RT, Hansford RG (1994) Volatile anesthetic effects on sarcoplasmic reticulum calcium content and sarcolemmal calcium flux in isolated rat cardiac cell suspensions. Anesthesiology 80:372–382

Wissing H, Kuhn I, Warnken U, Dudziak R (2001) Carbon monoxide production from desflurane, enflurane, halothane, isoflurane, and sevoflurane with dry soda lime. Anesthesiology 95:1205–1212

Zhou JX, Luo NF, Liang XM, Liu J (2006) The efficacy and safety of intravenous emulsified isoflurane in rats. Anesth Analg 102:129–134

General Anesthetics and Long-Term Neurotoxicity

M. Perouansky

Abstract We do not know how general anesthetics cause their desired effects. Contrary to what has been thought until relatively recently, the clinical state of anesthesia consists of multiple components that are mediated via interaction of the anesthetic drugs with different targets on the molecular–cellular, the network, and the structural–anatomical levels. The molecular targets by which some of these drugs induce the different components of "anesthesia" may be rather specific: discrete mutations of single amino acids in specific proteins profoundly affect the ability of certain anesthetics to achieve specific endpoints. Despite this potential specificity, inhalational anesthetics are present in the body at very high concentrations during surgical anesthesia. Due to their lipid solubility, general anesthetics dissolve in every membrane, penetrate into every organelle, and can interact with numerous cellular structures in multiple ways. A priori, it is therefore not unreasonable to assume that these drugs have the potential to cause insidious changes in the body other than those acute and readily apparent ones that we routinely monitor. Some changes may wane within a short time after

M. Perouansky
Department of Anesthesiology, University of Wisconsin School of Medicine,
B6/319 Clinical Science Center, 600 Highland Ave., Madison, WI, USA
mperouansky@wisc.edu

J. Schüttler and H. Schwilden (eds.) *Modern Anesthetics.*
Handbook of Experimental Pharmacology 182.

removal of the drug (e.g., the suppression of immune cell function). Others may persist after complete removal of the drug and even become self-propagating [e.g., β-oligomerization of proteins (Eckenhoff et al. 2004)], still others may be irreversible [e.g., the induction of apoptosis in the CNS (Jevtovic-Todorovic et al. 2003)] but of unclear significance. This article will focus on evidence for anesthetic toxicity in the central nervous system (CNS). The CNS appears to be susceptible to anesthetic neurotoxicity primarily at the extremes of ages, possibly via different pathways: in the neonate, during the period of most intense synaptogenesis, anesthetics can induce excessive apoptosis; in the aging CNS subtle cognitive dysfunction can persist long after clearance of the drug, and processes reminiscent of neurodegenerative disorders may be accelerated (Eckenhoff et al. 2004). At all ages, anesthetics affect gene expression-regulating protein synthesis in poorly understood ways. While it seems reasonable to assume that the vast majority of our patients completely restore homeostasis after general anesthesia, it is also time to acknowledge that exposure to these drugs has more profound and longer lasting effects on the brain than heretofore imagined.

1 Introduction

Anesthetic agents are some of the most potent and fastest acting drugs available in clinical medicine. The speed of onset of most drugs is limited only by the body's ability to deliver them to their targets, leading to almost immediate profound changes in fundamental physiological parameters. Conversely, it is also generally assumed that the effects of these pharmacological interventions dissipate almost as quickly as they arise and without long-term sequelae. Nowhere is the change of state as profound as in the organ that is most closely associated with our identity—the brain: deep coma, gives way to normal consciousness. Unresponsiveness is followed by alertness. Complete amnesia is gradually replaced by normal memory function.

The belief that general anesthetics are drugs with profound, instantaneous but fully reversible effects on the most critical organs is shared by the majority of healthcare professionals. Implicit in this belief is also the notion that once the drugs have been cleared, the body returns to the same state that it occupied before anesthesia (except for the effects of surgery).

Recent laboratory data indicate that it is time for a cautious reassessment of this assumption. It appears that the drugs that brought about a revolution in medical practice more than 150 years ago may, in addition to their profound immediate effects, also have subtle but measurable long-term consequences. The purpose of this review is to provide an overview of the current research into effects of anesthetics on the brain that appear to have consequences that persist beyond the complete removal of the drugs. I would also like to acknowledge that this direction in anesthesia-related research is only in its infancy; some of the data presented are only preliminary and our understanding of this topic is likely to change dramatically within the foreseeable future.

2 The Altered Brain

2.1 Anesthetics and Brain Genomics

More than a decade ago the capacity of general anesthetics to induce changes in gene expression in the brain was noted. Initially, only changes in the highly reactive acute early genes *c-fos* and *c-jun* were reported (Marota et al. 1992). These acute, anesthetic-induced changes were primarily considered to be a confounding problem for investigators, and recommendations for the use of the optimal anesthesia protocol for experimental purposes were based on the findings of differential anesthetic drug effects on the expression of these genes (Takayama et al. 1994). Since then, effects on gene expression during and/or immediately following anesthesia have been observed with newer anesthetic agents, in other vital organs, and with genes other than the immediate early genes (Hamaya et al. 2000). Recent preliminary results indicate that changes in gene expression may also persist long beyond the time frame required to clear the anesthetic drug. In the hippocampus of aged rats the expression of dozens of genes was affected 48 h after an inhalational anesthetic (Culley et al. 2004a). The significance of the majority of observed changes on the gene expression level remains, however, unclear. Changes in RNA expression are common and do not necessarily imply quantitative or qualitative changes in protein synthesis. Therefore changes in gene expression do not in themselves prove that the organism underwent "constitutive" changes and do not answer the question whether or not the organism that emerges from general anesthesia without any apparent insult to its homeostasis is "identical" to the organism that was anesthetized.

2.2 Anesthetics and Brain Proteomics

This question has been recently addressed for the first time using the proteomic approach. The proteome is defined as the complement of proteins expressed by a genome at a certain point in time. Proteomics refers to the quantitative and qualitative analysis of this complement of proteins over time and under varying conditions. The purpose of such an analysis is to gain insight into the functional state at a certain point in time of the biological unit whose proteome is under scrutiny. It is a task of staggering complexity: the human genome contains 30,000–40,000 genes. The number of proteins, however, is thought to exceed one million. Many factors account for the difference between gene number and protein diversity. Two important ones are alternate splicing of the transcriptional unit and posttranslational modifications of the assembled protein. Thus, multiple proteins can be synthesized from a single gene template e.g., more than 1,000 different proteins could originate from the three *neurexin* genes (Ullrich et al. 1995). Not all proteins are present in detectable amounts at every single point in time. The proteome therefore resembles a snapshot out of the constantly changing movie of life. Detailed analysis of large numbers of proteins (including isoforms and modifications) was made possible by the advent of high-throughput methodologies such as two-dimensional polyacrylamide gel electrophoresis and mass spectrometry. These methods are now being used to analyze the effect of anesthesia on the mammalian proteome. Fütterer et al. (2004) exposed rats to 3 h of 5.7% desflurane in air and prepared whole-brain homogenates immediately after the exposure as well as 24 and 72 h thereafter. The cytosolic proteins obtained at these time points were compared with proteins obtained from rats that were not anesthetized (except very briefly for sacrifice). Out of the thousands of proteins that are present simultaneously in a living rat brain, 263 "spots" representing individual proteins met the inclusion criteria for further analysis. Even within this limited sample, the researchers found that the abundance of a number of proteins was changed (either decreased or increased) for up to 72 h after exposure. The change ranged from a decrease to 60% to an increase to 179% of control. The authors controlled a number of experimental variables (hypotension, hypoxia, hypoventilation, gender) in order to increase the likelihood that the observed changes could be attributed to the tested drug. Although no firm conclusions about the long-term consequences or functional implications of these changes can be drawn from this work—single doses for single durations of single agents do not support firm or generalizable deductions—they do warrant attention as they indicate that "constitutive" changes are indeed induced by anesthetics. In the coming years it will be possible to extend these investigations using alternatives to gel-based detection methods with increased sensitivity and reduced variation and this may allow the analysis of the functional consequences of the reported fluctuations in protein expression. Nevertheless, the results of these experiments indicate that on the molecular level, general anesthesia is not as reversible a condition as the phenotype suggests. Under certain conditions, these lasting changes may be used to the advantage of the anesthetized subject: protection of the myocardium from ischemia by anesthetic preconditioning was an unexpected benefit derived from a class of drugs used to achieve completely unrelated endpoints. Recent data suggest that the benefits of anesthetic preconditioning may also extend to nervous tissue (Xiong et al. 2003). However, these discoveries should remind us that familiar drugs can have unexpected side effects and that not all of them are bound to be beneficial.

2.3 *Anesthetic Neurotoxicity: Fact or Fiction?*

2.3.1 Clinical Evidence

The existing evidence pointing toward the existence of anesthetic neurotoxicity is diametrically opposite in the two age groups that are under scrutiny. In the aged population, the International Study of Post-Operative Cognitive Dysfunction (ISPOCD) has convincingly demonstrated the existence of POCD in the clinical setting (Moller et al. 1998). Animal models replicating this clinical entity are in the process of being established and the available data will be reviewed. One possibility, proposed more than a decade ago but never substantiated (Houx et al. 1991), linking age and anesthesia with cognitive dysfunction is that exposure to (surgery and) anesthesia accelerates preexisting but heretofore latent neurodegenerative disorders, e.g., Alzheimer's disease (AD), that then become manifest sometime in the postoperative period as POCD or mild cognitive impairment (MCI; a prelude to AD). Could anesthetic drugs affect the progression of neurodegenerative disorders? Where in the pathogenetic chain of cognitive dysfunction could these small and relatively inert molecules play a role?

By contrast, no human data suggest that brief exposure to clinically used general anesthetics causes neurotoxicity at the other extreme of age, the neonate. Here, however, there is solid laboratory evidence suggesting that the immature central nervous system (CNS) might be susceptible to deleterious effects induced by commonly used anesthetic drugs, and that evidence for such an effect in humans might (I repeat *might*) simply await a concerted effort, on the scale of the ISPOCD studies, at identifying it.

2.3.2 Oligomerization and Neurodegeneration

One proposed mechanism of AD (and possibly of other neurodegenerative disorders) that is supported by extensive experimental data is that uncontrolled oligomerization (microaggregation) of peptides or proteins that are normally present in the brain leads to neurotoxic effects. The suspected peptide in AD is the amyloid β peptide (Aβ), 35 to 42 amino acids in length (e.g., Aβ42), that is constitutively released after proteolytic cleavage of the amyloid precursor protein (APP). Amorphous deposits of Aβ, i.e., the nonfibrillar form, can be found in large amounts in the brains of AD patients but also, to a lesser extent, in normal aged humans, and their toxic potential is unknown. Under certain environmental circumstances, however, these peptides are capable of changing their secondary structure from α-helix to β-sheet and self-assemble to oligomers of varying and increasing sizes. The oligomers produce the characteristic fibrils, the building blocks of the pathognomonic AD plaques. The other typical AD lesion, the neurofibrillary tangle, is composed of bundles of the microtubule-associated protein τ. While it is not entirely clear how and what products of oligomerization cause neurodegeneration, the following lines of evidence bolster the "amyloid (or more precisely Aβ) hypothesis of AD" (reviewed by Hardy and Selkoe 2002; Walsh and Selkoe 2004):

- Mutations of the APP that increase its cleavage to Aβ peptide are associated with AD
- Some inherited mutations in the presenilin genes (*PS1* and *PS2*, which code for the active site of the APP cleaving enzyme) increase the formation of Aβ and cause extremely early and aggressive forms of AD
- Aβ is the subunit of amyloid that is progressively deposited in innumerable neuritic plaques in the limbic and association cortices of all AD patients

- Synthetic Aβ peptides are toxic to hippocampal and cortical neurons
- Similarities in the neuropathology of Down's syndrome and AD point to a pathogenetic role of the APP gene, congruent with the Aβ hypothesis

The following evidence provides direct links between the Ab protein, particularly in its oligomerized form, and impairment of learning and memory:

- Injection of Aβ protein into the cerebral ventricles prevented the induction of long-term potentiation (LTP, a cellular form of learning and memory), while wash-out of Aβ protein restored inducibility of LTP (Walsh et al. 2002).
- Inhibitors of Aβ oligomerization rescue LTP (Klyubin et al. 2005)
- Neutralization of Aβ prevents some manifestations of AD in some models (Klyubin et al. 2005)

Current thinking within the framework of the Aβ hypothesis envisages the neurotoxic element to be the intermediate-sized oligomer and not the mature fibril. Therefore, the possibility that the physicochemical nature of inhalational anesthetics could favor oligomerization of Aβ as they have been shown to do for other proteins is intriguing.

3 Anesthetic Neurotoxicity In Vitro

The interaction of anesthetic molecules and Aβ peptides was tested recently by Eckenhoff and colleagues in a cell-free experimental system (Eckenhoff et al. 2004). The presence of halothane and isoflurane in the protein suspension significantly accelerated the oligomerization of Aβ42 and led to an increase in the total amount of oligomerized peptide (note, however, that the lowest concentration tested was 1 mM, i.e., more than three times the "minimal alveolar concentration" or MAC that is necessary to achieve a surgical plane of anesthesia). This effect was specific for the substrate (human serum albumin, a hydrophobic protein used as control, was not affected) and for inhalational drugs: Propofol and alcohol, when tested at "clinical" concentrations, mildly inhibited oligomerization (but enhanced oligomerization at very high concentrations). Removal of halothane from the protein suspension after 1 h of incubation did not reverse this process immediately: Enhanced amounts of oligomers were detectable for up to 3 days thereafter. In a second series of experiments, the authors examined the toxicity of the oligomer-anesthetic combination in rat pheochromocytoma cells, a cell type that, being of neural crest origin, is frequently used as a model for nerve cells. Toxicity was assayed by measuring the release of lactate dehydrogenase (LDH) from cultured pheochromocytoma cells incubated with 15 μM Aβ42 for 72 h with or without different anesthetic drugs. Neither isoflurane nor halothane, when given alone, increased LDH release, indicating lack of toxicity in this model. By contrast, incubation of pheochromocytoma cells with Aβ42 increased LDH release above control levels. Addition of the equivalent of 1 MAC of the volatile agents to

Aβ42 increased its toxicity while addition of propofol or ethanol did not. The researchers concluded that under their experimental conditions volatile anesthetics enhanced the formation of amyloid and its toxicity in cell culture. If similar processes occurred in vivo, volatile anesthetics could lead to long-lasting increases of Aβ42, a neurotoxic form of amyloid in the brain of susceptible subjects. Recently, this same group presented preliminary data indicating that the AD-promoting PS-1 mutation, transfected into pheochromocytoma cells, rendered these cells more susceptible to isoflurane-induced toxicity (Wei et al. 2005). Recently, the apoptogenic potential of isoflurane was confirmed in cultured human neuroglioma cells and was found to be reinforced by increased levels of APP C-terminal fragments (Xie 2006).

4 Anesthetic Neurotoxicity In Vivo

The most extensive clinical trials published to date (Rasmussen et al. 2003) has neither proved nor excluded a direct causal link between general anesthetic drugs and cognitive impairment. Therefore, some investigators have turned to animal models to test the hypothesis that general anesthetics can induce changes in the brain that outlast their physical presence there and that these changes lead to long-lasting, measurable functional consequences.

4.1 The Mature Brain: Adult vs Aged

General anesthetics affect learning and memory. Temporary amnesia is a highly desirable component of the anesthetic state that can be reliably achieved with general anesthetics. Prolonged memory impairment, by contrast, is one essential component of POCD.

In the early 1990s, laboratory studies of anesthetic interaction with memory reported a seemingly paradoxical improvement of memory consolidation. Adult mice anesthetized with halothane, isoflurane, or enflurane immediately after aversive conditioning had improved performance when tested on the same task 24 h later compared to unanesthetized controls (Komatsu et al. 1993). The mechanisms underlying the observed memory improvement by anesthesia were not further investigated, but it was noted that in these experiments anesthetic drugs were present in the brain at anesthetic concentrations during a time window that might be important for memory consolidation on the cellular-molecular level. Improvement of memory by anesthetics not explainable by the same mechanism was observed in Crosby's laboratory, where researchers have worked to establish an animal model of long-term anesthetic effects on cognitive performance (Culley et al. 2003). The prototypical experiment consisted of evaluating the effects of a standardized anesthetic (2 h of 1.2% isoflurane/70% N_2O/30% oxygen) on performance in a 12-arm radial-arm maze (RAM, a standard test to evaluate spatial orientation skills). The animals were either adult (6 months old) or aged (18–20 months old) Fischer 344 rats (median life expectancy 26 months) and were randomly assigned to either the test or the age-matched control group. The experimental protocols differed in the relative timing of anesthesia (before or after training), the degree of training, and the duration of the observation period after anesthesia. In contrast to the work by Komatsu et al. (1993), when training followed anesthesia, it was separated from anesthesia by a time interval sufficient to eliminate the drugs. In their initial publication, Culley et al. reported that anesthesia administered 24 h after the training had differential effects in adult vs aged rats: it improved performance in the former and impaired it in the latter. These effects remained measurable for 3 weeks and were undetectable by 8 weeks after anesthesia (Culley et al. 2003). However, at the time of anesthesia the adult animals (who learned faster) were overtrained compared to the old animals and learning continued to take place during the post-anesthesia testing sessions. Therefore, this experimental protocol did not allow for a separation between effects on acquisition of new information (learning) vs retrieval of stored information (memory). When, by contrast, the effect of anesthesia was tested on the ability to acquire new memories (training/testing took place only after anesthesia), the same investigators found that learning was impaired in both adult and aged animals even when the training began for up to 2 weeks after anesthesia, i.e., the impairment lasted for considerably longer than predicted by the pharmacokinetics of the drugs used (Crosby et al. 2005; Culley et al. 2004b). Interestingly, the researchers were not able to demonstrate any age-by-anesthesia interactions, i.e., both age groups were equally impaired. The authors attributed this apparent inconsistency with their earlier study to differences in the protocol: retrieval of stored information in the first study vs acquisition of new memory (arguably more susceptible to disruption and therefore affected in both age groups) in the later ones. In summary, this group of investigators concluded that inhalational anesthetics had effects on spatial learning and memory that outlasted their physical presence in the body. The mechanism(s) of these protracted memory effects and whether or not they are related in any way to either in vitro or to clinical observations is unclear, and the results have not yet been replicated in other laboratories or using other memory paradigms. The reported cognitive impairment was not accompanied by an identifiable reduction of life expectancy (based on a sample of 16 aged rats; Culley et al. 2006).

In summary, the establishment of an experimental model for long-term cognitive effects of volatile anesthetics is just beginning. The aged rodent may prove to be useful, but the most useful experimental paradigms have yet to be defined. The intriguing Aβ-neurodegenerative hypothesis provides a potential link between anesthetics and long-term cognitive consequences in the aged brain, but other mechanisms interlinking anesthetic drugs and persistent neurological impairment should be explored, e.g., a possible link between the effects of anesthetics on mitochondrial function (Miro et al. 1999; Kayser et al. 1999) and CNS dysfunction (Morgan et al. 2002).

4.2 *The Immature Brain*

4.2.1 Neurotoxicity, Apoptosis, Alcohol

Among the proteins expressed in the brain whose function is affected by anesthetic drugs at concentrations achieved during clinical anesthesia are receptors for the most abundant excitatory and inhibitory neurotransmitters in the mammalian CNS: l-glutamate and γ-aminobutyric acid (GABA). Both transmitter systems play important roles also in the developing brain. All clinically used general anesthetics enhance $GABA_A$ receptors, block *N*-methyl-d-aspartate (NMDA) receptors, or do both (it is not known with certainty, however, to what degree these effects contribute to the clinical phenomenon of general anesthesia). In the adult and the developing brain, excessive activation of l-glutamate receptors, primarily of the NMDA type, is associated with neurotoxicity. In contrast to the mature brain, however, it has been recently discovered that transient pharmacological blockade of NMDA receptors in the developing rodent brain causes excessive neuronal apoptosis. This excess is seen only in brain areas that undergo physiological apoptosis in normal development and only if NMDA receptors are blocked at specific time points within a period of accelerated synaptogenesis (Ikonomidou et al. 1999). It appears that during this brain growth spurt, neurons that do not receive sufficient excitation are doomed to apoptotic degeneration (Mennerick and Zorumski 2000).

Ethanol, in the same model, caused neuronal degeneration that is even wider spread than that caused by selective NMDA receptor blockade (Fig. 1). While

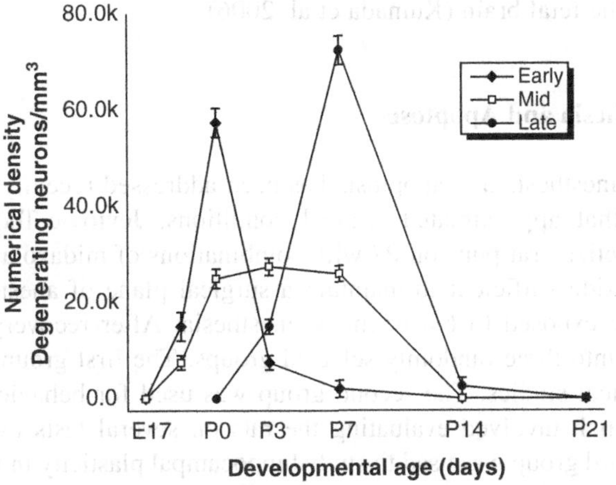

Fig. 1 Induction of apoptosis by ethanol depends on developmental stage and is brain region-specific. Brain regions were categorized as developing either at an early, intermediate, or a late stage. The lines are individual brain regions that are representative of the different temporal profiles: ventromedial hypothalamus, *early*; laterodorsal thalamus, *intermediate*; frontal cortex, *late*. The window of maximum sensitivity to apoptosis induction by alcohol changed with development from *P0* (early), to *P3* (intermediate), to *P7* (late). (Redrawn with permission from Ikonomidou et al. 2000)

alcohol is not used clinically as an anesthetic drug, it is important to note that alcohols are model anesthetics that share targets and mechanisms with clinically used anesthetics. An apoptogenic potential of alcohol on the developing human brain (synaptogenesis in humans lasts throughout the last trimester of pregnancy and continues postnatally) would be therefore clinically relevant. The widespread alcohol-induced apoptosis could be attributed to the fact that alcohol in addition to blocking NMDA receptors also enhances $GABA_A$ receptors, i.e., developing neurons are "silenced" via two pathways and are therefore more likely to commit to apoptosis. Similarly to the NMDA blockers, alcoholic neurotoxicity was only observed when the alcohol was administered during the critical developmental period of intense synaptogenesis (Ikonomidou et al. 2000). In the rat, synaptogenesis is most intense in the last 2 days of pregnancy (gestation lasts 21 days in the rat) and the first two postnatal weeks. Within this time window, different brain regions show peak sensitivity to alcohol's proapoptotic effects at different times. When administered on the seventh postnatal day (P7), alcohol caused a approximately 20-fold increase in the density of degenerating cells in the CA1 area of the hippocampus, and increases of the same order of magnitude were found in the thalamus, the septum, basal ganglia, and some cortical areas (Ikonomidou et al. 2000).

Alcoholic neurodegeneration was also associated with a decreased brain mass, leading the authors to conclude that neurodegeneration mediated by alcohol's effects on NMDA and $GABA_A$ receptors could explain some aspects of the clinical presentation of fetal alcohol syndrome. It should be noted, however, that alcohol also affects other aspects of neuronal development in detrimental ways, e.g., interference with second messenger signaling leading to aberrant neuronal migration in the fetal brain (Kumada et al. 2006).

4.2.2 Anesthesia and Apoptosis

The issue of anesthesia and apoptosis has been addressed recently in a series of experiments that approximated clinical conditions. Jevtovic-Todorovic et al. (2003) anesthetized rat pups on P7 with combinations of midazolam, isoflurane, and nitrous oxide sufficient to maintain a surgical plane of anesthesia for 6 h. Controls were exposed to 6 h of mock anesthesia. After recovery the animals were divided into three randomly selected groups. The first group was used for histopathological studies. The second group was used for behavioral studies in adulthood, which involved evaluating the rats on several tests over a 160-day period. The third group was used to study hippocampal plasticity in vitro (a model for learning and memory) at P29–P33. Daily inspection and weighing was performed on the latter two groups at P6–P21 to evaluate general health and development. Histopathology revealed that isoflurane (0.75%–1.5%) caused a dose-dependent increase in apoptotic neurodegeneration. Midazolam (3–9 mg/kg) and N_2O (50%–150% in a hyperbaric chamber) when given alone did not cause increased rates of apoptosis compared to control animals. However, when midazolam was followed by maintenance with isoflurane (double cocktail) the damage caused by the latter was increased primarily in the thalamus and the parietal cortex. The damage was further augmented by adding N_2O to the maintenance phase of anesthesia (triple cocktail: midazolam 9 mg/kg, isoflurane 0.75%, N_2O 75%). The triple cocktail caused widespread, more than 15-fold increases in the number of apoptotic neurons. When the hippocampi (a structure important for memory formation) from rats treated with the triple cocktail at P7 were evaluated electrophysiologically at P29–P33, it was found that the ability of neuronal connections to express long-term potentiation was severely reduced, suggesting that learning and memory may also be impaired. This deficit was confirmed in behavioral tests: animals exposed to the triple cocktail as neonates had measurable deficits in spatial memory tests when tested in the water maze and the radial arms maze as adults.

Recently, this group of researchers proposed that anesthetics activate both the intrinsic and the extrinsic apoptotic pathways, depending on the length of the exposure (Yon et al. 2005). In neonatal rats the intrinsic pathway is activated within 2 h of anesthesia exposure, while activation of the extrinsic pathway occurs later—within 6 h. It was also noted that the susceptibility to induction of apoptosis decreased dramatically from the 7th to the 14th postnatal day, coinciding with reduced rate of synaptogenesis.

4.2.3 Are Anesthetics to Blame?

It has been suggested that the reported histopathological damage and neurological deficits could be attributed to factors other than the anesthetic drugs (e.g., hypoxia or malnutrition; Anand and Soriano 2004). A recent investigation directly addressed the issue of metabolic homeostasis in anesthetized neonatal mice. Loepke et al. found that mouse pups anesthetized with 1.8% isoflurane developed marked hypoglycemia within 90 min (to below 40 mg% in 50% of animals), while control pups separated from the dam for the same amount of time did not (Loepke et al. 2006). Hypoglycemia of this severity has been shown to cause neuronal damage in adult rodents in some models, although primarily of the necrotic (Auer 2004) as opposed to the apoptotic type described by Jevtovic-Todorovic. Moreover, the neonate brain is more adept at using alternate fuel sources and therefore may be more resistant to hypoglycemia-induced damage (Belik et al. 1989). In addition to posing the interesting question of how isoflurane induces hypoglycemia in neonates (hyperglycemia is seen in adult rodents under isoflurane), this finding also offers an additional potential mechanism for the neurodegeneration attributed solely to anesthetics by Jevtovic-Todorovic et al. (2003). However, preliminary results indicate that neurodegeneration is also observed when guinea pig fetuses are exposed to anesthetics in utero, when they should be far less susceptible to developing hypoglycemia, as the dam remains normoglycemic throughout the experiment (Rizzi et al. 2005). Moreover, isoflurane neurotoxicity has been also tested in cultured slices from rat hippocampi harvested at 3, 7, and 14 days postnatally. This "in vitro" model has the advantage of eliminating homeostatic confounding factors present in vivo (hypoxemia, acidosis, hypoglycemia etc.). The results were in general agreement with the in vivo findings, even though in vivo the hippocampus is not the structure most affected by excessive induction of apoptosis. Isoflurane 1.5% for 5 h, caused a significant increase in the number of apoptotic neurons in slices obtained from 7-day-old animals. Cultures obtained from either younger or older animals or exposed to isoflurane for shorter time periods were less affected (Wise-Faberowski et al. 2005). A conclusion that can be drawn from this study is that hypoglycemia is not the sole mechanism by which anesthetics can induce neuronal apoptosis. Nevertheless, the role of hypoglycemia in the anesthetic-induced apoptotic neurodegeneration requires further clarification.

The other major problem for extrapolations from rodent data is the different developmental stages and life spans. In other words, are 6 h of drug exposure during synaptogenesis such an extreme insult to the rodent brain that it may not be appropriate to extrapolate these findings to clinical anesthesia in humans? Or are some of the developmental problems in the pup, secondary to behavioral changes in the mother, induced by separation, which has an effect on epigenetic imprinting (Meaney and Szyf 2005)?

While detailed dose-response data for the anesthetic cocktail of predominantly $GABA_A$-enhancing drugs is not available, it appears that ketamine (a potent NMDA receptor blocker) induce dose-dependent incremental apoptosis and identifiable toxicity occurs even at subanesthetic doses in rodents (Olney et al. 2004). Recently the neurotoxic potential of a single "mildly" anesthetic dose (defined as preservation of pain response and righting reflex) of both ketamine and midazolam (individually and combined) in rat pups has been demonstrated (Young et al. 2005). Before conclusions for clinical practice can be drawn, however, the hypothesis that anesthetic agents cause excessive neurodegeneration that has measurable long-term consequences requires testing in species with different patterns of synaptogenesis. Preliminary results from guinea pig (synaptogenesis in this species takes place prenatally and over a much longer time period than in rats; Rizzi et al. 2005) and piglet (synaptogenesis is prolonged and spans pre- and postnatal time periods; Rizzi et al. 2005) models indicate that these animals are also susceptible to anesthetic neurotoxicity if exposed to midazolam, isoflurane, and nitrous oxide pre- (guinea pigs) and postnatally (piglets). Whether the neurotoxicity has long-term consequences in models other then rodents remains to be established. A nonhuman primate model may provide particularly useful information but is also the most difficult to establish.

5 Summary

Laboratory evidence of anesthetic-induced lasting changes in, or potentially affecting, the CNS include

- Increased β-oligomerization of proteins after exposure to volatile anesthetics (Eckenhoff et al. 2004)

- Increased cytotoxicity of β-oligomers if combined with anesthetics in cultured cells (Eckenhoff et al. 2004)
- Brief exposure to desflurane, causing changes in protein expression in the brain that far outlast the presence of the drug (Futterer et al. 2004)
- Neuronal degeneration in the developing brain, with the effect of combined application of drugs acting via different mechanisms having more than additive effects (Jevtovic-Todorovic et al. 2003)
- Neurodegeneration in the developing brain caused by activation of both the intrinsic and the extrinsic apoptotic pathways (Yon et al. 2005)
- Neonatal exposure to anesthetic drugs that has measurable effects on learning in adulthood (Jevtovic-Todorovic et al. 2003)
- Exposure of aged rats to inhalational anesthetics causing lasting impairment of spatial memory performance (Culley et al. 2004c)

In light of the existing evidence, the question is not so much whether long-lasting, anesthetic-induced changes in the CNS do occur but whether they have any identifiable or preventable deleterious impact. Convincing clinical evidence attesting to such changes is lacking but may not be obtainable due to the methodological constraints of studies in human subjects. Therefore, more evidence will have to be gathered from animal models for whom the neurodevelopmental profile better matches that of humans. Until proved otherwise, however, it may be prudent to assume that there are no side effect-free pharmacological interventions. The ideal of stress-free surgery may be more difficult to achieve then expected, especially in the most vulnerable patient populations.

References

Anand KJ, Soriano SG (2004) Anesthetic agents and the immature brain: are these toxic or therapeutic? Anesthesiology 101:527–530

Auer RN (2004) Hypoglycemic brain damage. Metab Brain Dis 19:169–175

Belik J, Wagerle LC, Stanley CA, Sacks LM, Herbert DW, Delivoriapapadopoulos M (1989) Cerebral metabolic response and mitochondrial activity following insulin-induced hypoglycemia in newborn lambs. Biol Neonate 55:281–289

Crosby C, Culley DJ, Baxter MG, Yukhananov R, Crosby G (2005) Spatial memory performance 2 weeks after general anesthesia in adult rats. Anesth Analg 101:1389–1392

Culley DJ, Baxter M, Yukhananov R, Crosby G (2003) The memory effects of general anesthesia persist for weeks in young and aged rats. Anesth Analg 96:1004–1009

Culley DJ, Yukhananov RY, Crosby G (2004a) Hippocampal gene expression is altered 48 hours after general anesthesia in aged rats. Anesthesiology 101:A64

Culley DJ, Baxter MG, Crosby CA, Yukhananov R, Crosby G (2004b) Impaired acquisition of spatial memory 2 weeks after isoflurane and isoflurane-nitrous oxide anesthesia in aged rats. Anesth Analg 99:1393–1397

Culley DJ, Baxter MG, Yukhananov R, Crosby G (2004c) Long-term impairment of acquisition of a spatial memory task following isoflurane-nitrous oxide anesthesia in rats. Anesthesiology 100:309–314

Culley DJ, Loguinov A, Yukhananov R, Crosby G (2006) General anesthesia does not reduce life expectancy in aged rats. Anesth Analg 102:956–959

Eckenhoff RG, Johansson JS, Wei HF, Carnini A, Kang BB, Wei WL, Pidikiti R, Keller JM, Eckenhoff MF (2004) Inhaled anesthetic enhancement of amyloid-beta oligomerization and cytotoxicity. Anesthesiology 101:703–709

Fütterer CD, Maurer MH, Schmitt A, Feldmann RE, Kuschinsky W, Waschke KF (2004) Alterations in rat brain proteins after desflurane anesthesia. Anesthesiology 100:302–308

Hamaya Y, Takeda T, Dohi S, Nakashima S, Nozawa Y (2000) The effects of pentobarbital, isoflurane, and propofol on immediate-early gene expression in the vital organs of the rat. Anesth Analg 90:1177–1183

Hardy J, Selkoe DJ (2002) The amyloid hypothesis of Alzheimer's disease: progress and problems on the road to therapeutics. Science 297:353–356

Houx PJ, Vreeling FW, Jolles J (1991) Age-associated cognitive decline is related to biological life events. In: Iqbal K, McLachlan DRC, Winblad B, Wisniewski HS (eds) Alzheimer's disease: basic mechanisms, diagnosis, and therapeutic strategies. John Wiley & Sons, Chichester, pp 353–358

Ikonomidou C, Bosch F, Miksa M, Bittigau P, Vockler J, Dikranian K, Tenkova TI, Stefovska V, Turski L, Olney JW (1999) Blockade of NMDA receptors and apoptotic neurodegeneration in the developing brain. Science 283:70–74

Ikonomidou C, Bittigau P, Ishimaru MJ, Wozniak DF, Koch C, Genz K, Price MT, Stefovska V, Horster F, Tenkova T, Dikranian K, Olney JW (2000) Ethanol-induced apoptotic neurodegeneration and fetal alcohol syndrome. Science 287:1056–1060

Jevtovic-Todorovic V, Hartman RE, Izumi Y, Benshoff ND, Dikranian K, Zorumski CF, Olney JW, Wozniak DF (2003) Early exposure to common anesthetic agents causes widespread neurodegeneration in the developing rat brain and persistent learning deficits. J Neurosci 23:876–882

Kayser EB, Morgan PG, Sedensky MM (1999) GAS-1: a mitochondrial protein controls sensitivity to volatile anesthetics in the nematode Caenorhabditis elegans. Anesthesiology 90:545–554

Klyubin I, Walsh DM, Lemere CA, Cullen WK, Shankar GM, Betts V, Spooner ET, Jiang L, Anwyl R, Selkoe DJ, Rowan MJ (2005) Amyloid beta protein immunotherapy neutralizes Abeta oligomers that disrupt synaptic plasticity in vivo. Nat Med 11:556–561

Komatsu H, Nogaya J, Anabuki D, Yokono S, Kinoshita H, Shirakawa Y, Ogli K (1993) Memory facilitation by posttraining exposure to halothane, enflurane, and isoflurane in ddN mice. Anesth Analg 76:609–612

Kumada T, Lakshmana MK, Komuro H (2006) Reversal of neuronal migration in a mouse model of fetal alcohol syndrome by controlling second-messenger signalings. J Neurosci 26:742–756

Loepke AW, McCann JC, Kurth D, McAuliffe JJ (2006) The physiologic effects of isoflurane anesthesia in neonatal mice. Anesth Analg 102:75–80

Marota JJ, Crosby G, Uhl GR (1992) Selective effects of pentobarbital and halothane on c-fos and jun-B gene expression in rat brain. Anesthesiology 77:365–371

Meaney MJ, Szyf M (2005) Maternal care as a model for experience-dependent chromatin plasticity? Trends Neurosci 28:456–463

Mennerick S, Zorumski CF (2000) Neural activity and survival in the developing nervous system. Mol Neurobiol 22:41–54

Miro O, Barrientos A, Alonso JR, Casademont J, Jarreta D, Urbano-Marquez A, Cardellach F (1999) Effects of general anaesthetic procedures on mitochondrial function of human skeletal muscle. Eur J Clin Pharmacol 55:35–41

Moller JT, Cluitmans P, Rasmussen LS, Houx P, Rasmussen H, Canet J, Rabbitt P, Jolles J, Larsen K, Hanning CD, Langeron O, Johnson T, Lauven PM, Kristensen PA, Biedler A, van Beem H, Fraidakis O, Silverstein JH, Beneken JEW, Gravenstein JS (1998) Long-term postoperative cognitive dysfunction in the elderly: ISPOCD1 study. Lancet 351:857–861

Morgan PG, Hoppel CL, Sedensky MM (2002) Mitochondrial defects and anesthetic sensitivity. Anesthesiology 96:1268–1270

Olney JW, Young C, Wozniak DF, Ikonomidou C, Jevtovic-Todorovic V (2004) Anesthesia-induced developmental neuroapoptosis. Does it happen in humans? Anesthesiology 101:273–275

Rasmussen LS, Johnson T, Kuipers HM, Kristensen D, Siersma VD, Vila P, Jolles J, Papaioannou A, Abildstrom H, Silverstein JH, Bonal JA, Raeder J, Nielsen IK, Korttila K, Munoz L, Dodds C, Hanning CD, Moller JT (2003) Does anaesthesia cause postoperative cognitive dysfunction? A randomised study of regional versus general anaesthesia in 438 elderly patients. Acta Anaesthesiologica Scandinavica 47:260–266

Rizzi S, Carter LB, Jevtovic-Todorovic V (2005) Clinically used general anesthetics induce neuroapoptosis in the developing piglet brain. Society for Neuroscience Program No. 251.7

Rizzi S, Yon JH, Carter LB, Jevtovic-Todorovic V (2005) Short exposure to general anesthesia caused widespread neuronal suicide in the developing guinea pig brain. Society for Neuroscience Program No. 241.6

Takayama K, Suzuki T, Miura M (1994) The comparison of effects of various anesthetics on expression of Fos protein in the rat-brain. Neurosci Lett 176:59–62

Ullrich B, Ushkaryov YA, Sudhof TC (1995) Cartography of neurexins—more than 1000 isoforms generated by alternative splicing and expressed in distinct subsets of neurons. Neuron 14:497–507

Walsh DM, Selkoe DJ (2004) Deciphering the molecular basis of memory failure in Alzheimer's disease. Neuron 44:181–193

Walsh DM, Klyubin I, Fadeeva JV, Cullen WK, Anwyl R, Wolfe MS, Rowan MJ, Selkoe DJ (2002) Naturally secreted oligomers of amyloid beta protein potently inhibit hippocampal long-term potentiation in vivo. Nature 416:535–539

Wei H, Liang G, Wei W, Li Y, Eckenhoff RG (2005) Volatile anesthetics induce neurotoxicity differently in PC12 cells featured with Alzheimer's disease. Anesthesiology 103:A121

Wise-Faberowski L, Zhang H, Ing R, Pearlstein RD, Warner DS (2005) Isoflurane-induced neuronal degeneration: an evaluation in organotypic hippocampal slice cultures. Anesth Analg 101:651–657

Xie Z, Dong Y, Maeda U, Alfille P, Culley DJ, Crosby G, Tanzi RE (2006) Anesthetic isoflurane induces apoptosis and increases Abeta levels in H4 human neuroglioma cells overexpressing APP. J Am Geriatr Soc 54:S7

Xiong L, Zheng Y, Wu M, Hou L, Zhu Z, Zhang X, Lu Z (2003) Preconditioning with isoflurane produces dose-dependent neuroprotection via activation of adenosine triphosphate-regulated potassium channels after focal cerebral ischemia in rats. Anesth Analg 96:233–237

Yon JH, Daniel-Johnson J, Carter LB, Jevtovic-Todorovic V (2005) Anesthesia induces neuronal cell death in the developing rat brain via the intrinsic and extrinsic apoptotic pathways. Neuroscience 135:815–827

Young C, Jevtovic-Todorovic V, Qin YQ, Tenkova T, Wang H, Labruyere J, Olney JW (2005) Potential of ketamine and midazolam, individually or in combination, to induce apoptotic neurodegeneration in the infant mouse brain. Br J Pharmacol 146:189–197

Special Aspects of Pharmacokinetics of Inhalation Anesthesia*

J.F.A. Hendrickx(✉) and A. De Wolf

Safe anesthesia requires the dedicated attention to the patient by a safe anesthesiologist no matter which method, device, or kind of apparatus is in vogue.
Lucien Morris, inventor of the copper kettle (Morris 1994)

Abstract Recent interest in the use of low-flow or closed circuit anesthesia has rekindled interest in the pharmacokinetics of inhaled anesthetics. The kinetic properties of inhaled anesthetics are most often modeled by physiologic models because of the abundant information that is available on tissue solubilities and organ perfusion. These models are intuitively attractive because they can be easily understood in terms of the underlying anatomy and physiology. The use of classical compartment modeling, on the other hand, allows modeling of data that are routinely available to the anesthesiologist, and eliminates the need to account for every possible confounding factor at each step of the partial pressure cascade of potent inhaled agents. Concepts used to describe IV kinetics can readily be applied to inhaled agents (e.g., context-sensitive half-time and effect site concentrations).

J.F.A. Hendrickx
Department of Anesthesiology and Intensive Care, OLV Hospital, Moorselbaan 164, 9300 Aalst, Belgium
jcnwahendrickx@yahoo.com

* Parts of this chapter appeared in Dr. Jan Hendrickx's doctoral thesis (Hendrickx 2004).

J. Schüttler and H. Schwilden (eds.) *Modern Anesthetics. Handbook of Experimental Pharmacology 182.*

The interpretation of the F_A/F_I vs time curve is expanded by reintroducing the concept of the general anesthetic equation—the focus is shifted from "how F_A approaches F_I" to "what combination of delivered concentration and fresh gas flow (FGF) can be used to attain the desired F_A." When the desired F_A is maintained with a FGF that is lower than minute ventilation, rebreathing causes a discrepancy between the concentration delivered by the anesthesia machine (=selected by the anesthesiologist on the vaporizer, F_D) and that inspired by the patient. This F_D–F_I discrepancy may be perceived as "lack of control" and has been the rationale to use a high FGF to ensure the delivered matched the inspired concentration. Also, with low FGF there is larger variability in F_D because of interpatient variability in uptake. The F_D–F_I discrepancy increases with lower FGF because of more rebreathing, and as a consequence the uptake pattern *seems* to be more reflected in the F_D required to keep F_A constant. The clinical implication for the anesthesiologist is that with high FGF few F_D adjustments have to be made, while with a low FGF F_D has to be adjusted according to a pattern that follows the decreasing uptake pattern in the body. The ability to model and predict the uptake pattern of the individual patient and the resulting kinetics in a circle system could therefore help guide the anesthesiologist in the use of low-flow anesthesia with conventional anesthesia machines. Several authors have developed model-based low FGF administration schedules, but biologic variability limits the performance of any model, and therefore end-expired gas analysis is obligatory. Because some fine-tuning based on end-expired gas analysis will always be needed, some clinicians may not be inclined to use very low FGF in a busy operating room, considering the perceived increase in complexity. This practice may be facilitated by the development of anesthesia machines that use closed circuit anesthesia (CCA) with end-expired feedback control—they "black box" these issues (see Chapter 21).

In this chapter, we first explore how and why the kinetic properties of intravenous and inhaled anesthetics have been modeled differently. Next, we will review the method most commonly used to describe the kinetics of inhaled agents, the F_A/F_I vs time curve that describes how the alveolar (F_A) approaches the inspired (F_I) fraction (in the gas phase, either "fraction," "concentration," or "partial pressure" can be used). Finally, we will reintroduce the concept of the general anesthetic equation to explain why the use of low-flow or closed circuit anesthesia has rekindled interest in the modeling of pharmacokinetics of inhaled anesthetics. Clinical applications of some of these models are reviewed. A basic understanding of the circle system is required, and will be provided in the introduction.

1 Introduction: Nuts and Bolts of the Circle System

The circle system is the anesthesia breathing system most widely used with adults. The kinetic properties of inhaled vapors and carrier gases are significantly affected by the manner in which the anesthesiologist uses the system. A sound understanding

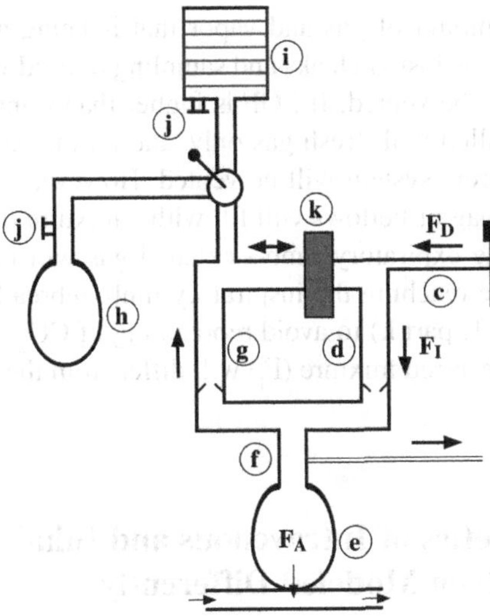

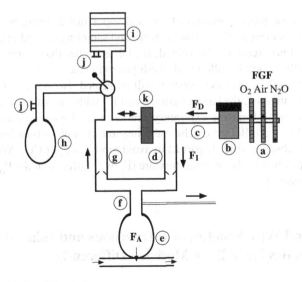

Fig. 1 Nuts and bolts of the circle system

of its composition is essential to understand the remainder of this chapter. We describe the circle system (Fig. 1) by following gases and vapors along their partial pressure cascade. The fresh gas flow rate (FGF) of a carrier gas or gases (O_2, N_2O, and/or air) is selected by adjusting the knobs of the rotameter(s) (Fig. 1, part a). By turning the wheel of the vaporizer (Fig. 1, part b) of the agent of choice, the appropriate amount of anesthetic vapor is added. The concentration of gases and vapors entering the circle system via the common gas outlet (Fig. 1, part c) is referred to as the delivered concentration (F_D). Once these gases enter the inspiratory limb (Fig. 1, part d) they are labeled "inspired mixture" (with concentrations F_I). The composition of the mixture may match that of the delivered gas F_D, or it may be a mixture of delivered gas and some gas that is returning from the previously exhaled tidal volume(s) (see the next section). During inspiration, gases enter the lungs (Fig. 1, part e) from where they are taken up by the body (during wash-in and maintenance). The composition of the exhaled gas is a complex mixture of alveolar gas (F_A) and dead space gas (F_I, since by definition no gas exchange has occurred), and the correct term to describe its concentration is the mixed-expired concentration. Anesthesiologists measure the end-expired or end-tidal concentration, which is the concentration of anesthetic gas in the alveolar part of the exhaled gas, F_A. The sampling port of the gas analyzer is located at the Y-piece (Fig. 1, part f) connecting the circle system to the patient's airway. Exhaled gas then moves along the expiratory limb (Fig. 1, part g) toward either the breathing bag (Fig. 1, part h) when the patient is breathing spontaneously, or toward the bellows of the ventilator (Fig. 1, part i) when ventilation is controlled. Once the breathing bag or the bellows are full, the remainder of the gas still flowing through the expiratory limb is vented to the atmosphere (Fig. 1, part j).

Only when the precise amount of gas and vapor that is being administered is taken up by the patient and/or is lost via leaks and sampling (closed-circuit anesthesia, CCA) will no excess gas be vented. If FGF is higher than minute ventilation, the bag or bellows will be filled with fresh gas only, and all the gas coming from the expiratory limb of the circle system will be vented. However, if FGF is lower than minute ventilation, the bag or bellows will fill with a mixture of fresh gas and exhaled gas coming form the expiratory limb—exhaled gas will therefore be re-inhaled or rebreathed. Before reaching the inspiratory limb, rebreathed gases pass though a CO_2 absorber (Fig. 1, part k) to avoid rebreathing of CO_2. With rebreathing, the composition of the inspired mixture (F_I) will differ from the F_D selected by the anesthesiologist.

2 How and Why Kinetics of Intravenous and Inhaled Anesthetics Have Been Modeled Differently

During general anesthesia, the goal of an anesthesiologist is to attain and maintain those concentrations of anesthetic drugs in the blood (and ultimately the effect site) to ensure hypnosis and immobility (suppression of movement after noxious stimulation) (Eger and Sonner 2006). Kinetic models attempt to describe and predict these concentrations, and can be broadly categorized as either physiologic or classic compartmental ("empiric"). With a physiologic model the investigator incorporates the underlying physiologic processes that may affect drug kinetics into the model—the model describes the data as well as the processes by which the observations came to be. With the empiric approach, the only goal is to describe the data.

Because blood concentrations of intravenous anesthetics cannot be measured continuously in the operating room, kinetic models are very useful to optimize maintenance of the desired blood concentration; kinetic models are incorporated in the software that steers syringe pumps (target-controlled infusion, TCI). Pharmacokinetic models for intravenous agents have most often been built empirically because frequently not enough information is available to build physiologic models. Programs like NONMEM fit (multi)exponential curves to the course of the concentrations of the agent of interest using dose history and covariates (e.g., age, gender, weight) as inputs (NONMEM Project Group 1992). The parameters of the model equations are intuitively most accessible when they are expressed as volumes of distributions and clearances because they have a physiologic flavor to it. Nevertheless, these volumes of distribution and clearances are fictitious entities that are not directly related to any underlying anatomic compartments or physiologic processes. The model most often consists of one central and one or two peripheral compartments. The concentration in the central compartment (which matches the blood concentrations which the model predicts) is considered to be the result of drug input into and elimination from a central compartment and drug transfer between compartments (distribution). After the model is derived, it is prospectively tested in a *different* group of patients using performance criteria such as those developed by Varvel et al.—performance error (PE), median PE (MDPE), median absolute PE, (MDAPE), divergence, and wobble (Varvel et al. 1992). The kinetic models can be incorporated into more complex pharmacokinetic/pharmacodynamic (PK/PD) models that use the effect site concentration to link blood concentrations to a desired clinical end-point, e.g., an EEG derivative such as Bispectral Index (BIS; Aspect Medical Systems, Norwood, MA) when the end-point is hypnosis, or the degree of neuromuscular blockade when muscle relaxants are used. These models can be incorporated in closed-loop systems.

If enough physiologic information *is* available (such as tissue solubilities, tissue volumes, and perfusion), a physiologic model can also be used to describe the kinetics of intravenous agents. For example, a physiologic model predicted lidocaine (Benowitz et al. 1974) and propofol (Levitt and Schnider 2005) plasma concentrations well. The latter study is one of the few quantitative comparisons of physiologic and compartment models available.

The uptake and distribution of inhaled anesthetics have most often been modeled by physiologic models such as Eger's four compartment (4C) model (Eger 1974). Plenty of information is available to build a physiologic model. The parameters needed to calculate the course of tissue partial pressures (tissue volumes, tissue solubilities, and tissue blood flows) can be readily retrieved from the literature (Eger and Saidman 2005). The models assume uptake of anesthetic gases is perfusion limited. Organ vapor capacity depends on the size of the organ and the solubility of the agent in that particular organ. The rate at which the partial pressure in the organ increases, and eventually saturates toward the partial pressure in blood, depends both on the organ's capacity and organ blood flow. This rate is described by a time constant (tissue storage capacity divided by blood flow). Based on both tissue storage capacity and blood flow, Eger grouped organs and tissues into the vessel rich group (VRG), muscle group (MG), fat group (FG), and vessel poor group (VPG) (Eger 1974). Uptake according to the 4C model is presented in Fig. 2, where it is compared with uptake according to the square root of time model (SqRT; see below) and with clinical uptake data. In Eger's five-compartment (5C) model the VRG, MG, and FG from the 4C model are retained; the VPG is deleted because its contribution to uptake is considered insignificant, but a lung and an "intertissue diffusion" compartment are added (Carpenter et al. 1986). The intertissue diffusion group is hypothesized to be fat adjacent to well-perfused tissues. The model has recently been reviewed by Eger and Saidman (2005). The SqRT model was developed by Lowe and Ernst specifically to facilitate the practice of CCA in an era when multigas analyzers were not available (Lowe and Ernst 1981). The sum of uptake by the individual organs was found to increase according to the square root of time, an observation first made by Severinghaus for N_2O (Severinghaus 1954). When the arterial concentration is maintained, the same amount of agent is taken up by the tissues during each subsequent "square root of time" interval (0–1 min, 1–4 min, 4–9 min, 9–16 min, etc.). This amount is called the "unit dose," and is calculated based on patient weight. At the start, a "prime dose" is given to prime the circuit, functional residual capacity, and blood pool. Uptake according to the SqRT model is presented in Fig. 2.

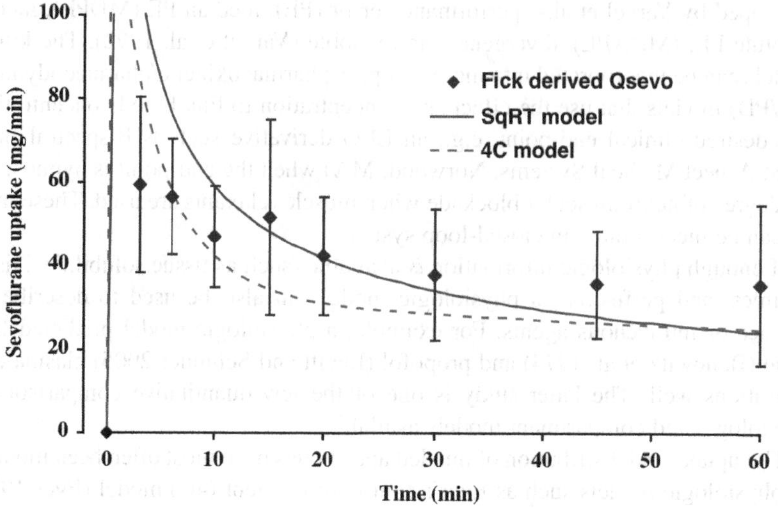

Fig. 2 Comparison of the sevoflurane uptake rate (mg.min^{-1}) determined by Fick's method (mean ± standard deviation) with that predicted by the 4C model and the square root of time model (SqRT) model. F_A was maintained at 1.3% (Frietman et al. 2001)

Using modern computer technology, the number of differential equations that can be solved simultaneously is enormous, spurring the development of models with ever-increasing numbers of compartments (Fukui and Smith 1981; Heffernan et al. 1982; Lerou et al. 1991; Vermeulen et al. 1995; Lerou and Booij 2001a). An 18-compartment model by Fukui and Smith (1981), for example, carries over 88 equations and 124 parameter settings. Some of the models simulate how a drug affects its own uptake by, e.g., altering cardiac output (i.e., nonlinear pharmacokinetics).

How complex a model needs to be depends on the goal of the investigator. The more complex models should only be used if they better represent what actually happens or when more sophistication is required, such as when there is the need to study the effect of changes in physiologic parameters on uptake (Vermeulen 2000). The 4C model is intuitive and didactic, and is incorporated in GasMan (Med Man Simulations, Chestnut Hill, MA).The SqRT model by Lowe and Ernst is useful to provide dosing guidelines during CCA. Both models tend to overestimate initial uptake and underestimate it after 30–45 min (Fig. 2 ; Hendrickx et al. 1997, 1998a, 2003; Frietman et al. 2001). Interest in Heffernan's 10-compartment model (Heffernan et al. 1982), first described more than 20 years ago, has rekindled recently in a series of studies by Kennedy to help predict concentrations of inhaled anesthetics during reduced FGF (Kennedy et al. 2002) (see Sect. 5). Sophisticated physiologic models offer advantages over simpler models for the study of interactions among ventilation, circulation, and the uptake and distribution of inhaled agents, and provide the basis for training simulators. Especially with the multicompartment physiologic models, it is important "not to be carried away with uncritical enthusiasm, because these models require an

Table 1 Parameters of the classic two-compartment model of inhaled anesthetics derived from inspired and expired tidal volumes and concentrations of desflurane, isoflurane, and sevoflurane in O_2/N_2O by Wissing et al. (2000). The estimated pharmacokinetic variables and extrapolated parameters are given as median and range (in parentheses)

	Isoflurane		Sevoflurane		Desflurane	
k_{12} (min^{-1})	0.158	(0.065–0.583)	0.117	(0.070–0.344)	0.078	(0.029–0.186)
k_{21} (min^{-1})	0.007	(0.001–0.014)	0.007	(0.001–0.019)	0.011	(0.003–0.022)
Cl_{12} (ml_{vapor} kg^{-1} min^{-1})	30.7	(15.9–38.7)	13	(9.8–22.4)	7	(4.4–11.1)
V_1 (ml_{vapor} kg_{bw}^{-1})	196	(37–332)	106	(57–171)	75	(49–140)
V_2 (ml_{vapor} kg_{bw}^{-1})	4,112	(1,472–9,396)	1,634	(762–8,842)	612	(343–1,850)
V_{ss} (ml_{vapor} kg_{bw}^{-1})	4,285	(1,509–9,640)	1,748	(819–8,997)	698	(408–1,917)

Cl_{12}, transport clearance from central to peripheral compartment; k_{12}, microconstant for transport from central to peripheral compartment; k_{21}, microconstant for transport from peripheral to central compartment; V_1, volume of distribution of the central compartment; V_2, volume of distribution of the peripheral compartment; V_{ss}, volume of distribution during steady state. V_1, V_2, and V_{ss} are given as milliliters of inhaled anesthetic in relation to body weight

immense amount of detailed information, much of which must be assumed, estimated, or simply guessed" (Hull 1997). Even with simple physiologic models many assumptions are made (Hendrickx et al. 1997). Tissue solubilities vary up to 150% between authors (Yasuda et al. 1989), and the tissue homogenates used to determine these coefficients may not represent in vivo conditions. Arterial to end-expired gradients exist that may not be explained by ventilation/perfusion mismatching alone (Landon et al. 1993; Doolette et al. 1998; Doolette et al. 2001). Brain time constants in vivo may be longer than the theoretically calculated values (Lockhart et al. 1991). In addition, from a more practical point, physiologic models are not well suited for the analysis of the F_A vs time curves that are available in a clinical setting (Bouillon and Shafer 2000). One of the strengths of classic compartment modeling is that it can be used without having to take into account these confounding factors, and that they are well suited for the analysis of the F_A vs time curves. Wissing describes classic compartmental parameters for isoflurane, sevoflurane, and desflurane based on inspired and expired concentrations and tidal volumes (Table 1; Rietbrock et al. 2000; Wissing et al. 2000). Yasuda et al. also used classic compartment modeling to describe the kinetics of inhaled anesthetics (Yasuda et al. 1991a, b). The exhaled concentrations of sevoflurane, desflurane, isoflurane, and halothane were measured using chromatography up to a week after these agents had been concomitantly administered for 30 min, and a five-compartment model was derived. In more recent work, arterial and mixed venous blood concentration profiles were linked to uptake derived from inspired and expired tidal volumes and partial pressures using compartment modeling (Ishibashi et al. 2006). Using lung uptake as the input function, the time course profiles of the arterial and the mixed venous blood concentrations were best described by a two- and one-compartment model, respectively. The use of compartment modeling of inhaled agents is currently being applied to derive dosing guidelines for the liquid infusion rate of sevoflurane with a commercially available device AnaConDa® (Hudson RCI, Upplands Väsby, Sweden) (Enlund et al. 2006).

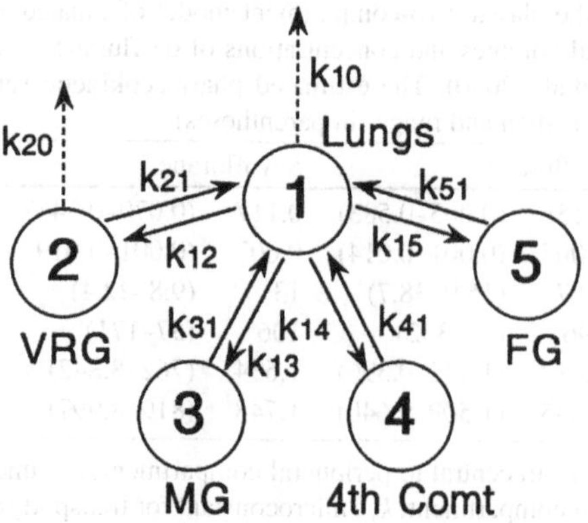

Fig. 3 Five-compartment model derived from end-expired wash-out data (Yasuda et al. 1991a, b)

Can distribution volumes and clearances, the parameters of compartment models, be interpreted in terms of tissue volumes and blood flows? Yasuda et al. (1991a, b; see above) tried to relate the distribution volumes and clearances with tissue volumes and tissue blood flows of a physiologic model. Thus, the first, second, third, fourth, and fifth compartment were interpreted as representing lungs, VRG, MG, intertissue diffusion, and the FG (Fig. 3). In a model developed by Ishibashi et al. (2006) that links arterial and mixed venous blood concentrations to uptake derived from inspired and expired tidal volumes and partial pressures, the relationship between distribution volumes and clearances (the parameters of compartment models) and covariates cardiac output and patient demographic data was not a straightforward one, suggesting that correlating clearances and distribution volumes with tissue volumes and blood flows should be done with care, if at all. Hull also argues that "[while] it is often suggested that some particular tissue or organ (such as the brain) be 'in' one compartment or another, such suggestions are ill-founded because parameters of the fit to the uptake data contain no information that might support such assumptions" (Hull 1997; Shafer 1998). Similarly, Wissing argues that a precise allocation of several hypothetical peripheral compartments to anatomically defined tissues is hardly feasible (Rietbrock et al. 2000). In a theoretical analysis, we documented that both classic compartment modeling and physiologic modeling describe the course of the anesthetic concentrations equally well, but the relationship between the parameters of the two models was complex (Hendrickx et al. 2006a). However, because both physiologic and compartment modeling described the course of the anesthetic concentrations equally well, concepts applied to IV anesthetics such as context-sensitive half-times (Bailey 1997; Eger and Shafer 2005) or k_{eo} (the plasma-effect site equilibration rate constant; Kennedy 2005) can equally well be applied to inhaled agents.

In contrast to the clinical requirement for kinetic models when a specific target concentration of an intravenous agent is aimed for, some authors have suggested that there is no clinical need for kinetic models of potent inhaled anesthetics

(Vermeulen 2000). First, F_A can be continuously measured. Second, F_A defines the concentrations needed to ensure the relevant clinical endpoints of hypnosis and immobility (mediated at the spinal and supraspinal level respectively) through the concepts of MAC_{awake} and MAC (Eger et al. 1965; Stoelting et al. 1970). This dose-response curve for suppression of movement and hypnosis is steep—within a population, MAC varies by not more than 10%–15% among individuals (Sani and Shafer 2003; de Jong and Eger 1975; Eger et al. 2001). Third, the partial pressure in the brain lags behind that in the alveoli with only a modest delay for modern agents—the equilibration half-time of this process (determined using EEG power spectrum) is 2.4 min for isoflurane and sevoflurane and 1.1 min for desflurane (Rehberg et al. 1999). We would therefore argue that the MAC and MAC_{awake} concepts by definition make any kinetic model for inhaled agents also a PK/PD model for the end-points immobility and hypnosis. Some authors prefer to incorporate this delay in their model by introducing an effect site concentration in their model (see Sect. 5) (Kennedy 2005). And finally, automated closed-loop administration of inhaled agents has now enabled the anesthesiologist to select an F_A without having to bother about uptake or delivered or inspired partial pressure to achieve that particular F_A (see Chapter 21). While we concur that inhaled anesthetics can be and are being administered safely without the use of any model, we will show in the remainder of this chapter that models remain of clinical value. Models can help the interested anesthesiologist understand the kinetics of inhaled anesthetics at reduced FGF and thus help him or her to comfortably use inhaled agents and carrier gases with FGF well below 1 l/min. Models are used to develop low-flow administration schedules, in particular to minimize the duration of the high FGF period at the beginning of anesthetic administration that increases anesthetic waste and thus cost and pollution. Models are used to build open loop control systems (Kennedy et al., see Sect. 5) and provide dosage guidelines for the rare CCA enthusiast and for a new liquid agent injection device, the AnaConDa® (Sedana Medical, Sundyberg, Sweden) (Enlund et al. 2006; Enlund et al. 2002). To examine how uptake models can help us better understand the kinetics of inhaled agents in a circle system during low-flow anesthesia, we will first have to expand our interpretation of the F_A/F_I curve.

3 Expanding the Interpretation of the F_A/F_I Curve

F_A/F_I curves that describe how F_A approaches F_I over time (Fig. 4) are widely used to describe the kinetics of inhaled agents in the clinical setting, and have been proven to be of great didactic value to introduce the novice to "uptake and distribution" of inhaled anesthetics (Eger 2000). To correctly interpret the F_A/F_I curve, it is important to understand that these curves do not present actual uptake by the patient. Also, it is important to realize that high FGF and fixed F_I are used (high FGF with constant F_I technique). At a time when no end-expired gas analysis existed and when the introduction of the plenum vaporizer for the first time allowed reasonable control of F_D, a high FGF with constant F_I technique was extremely useful

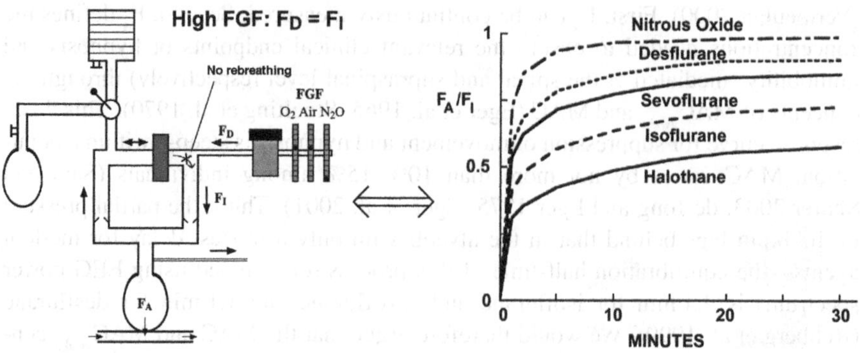

Fig. 4 The interpretation of the F_A/F_I curve when using a circle system requires the understanding that a fixed F_I and a total FGF larger than alveolar ventilation are used (high FGF with constant F_I technique). Under these circumstances, $F_D = F_I$

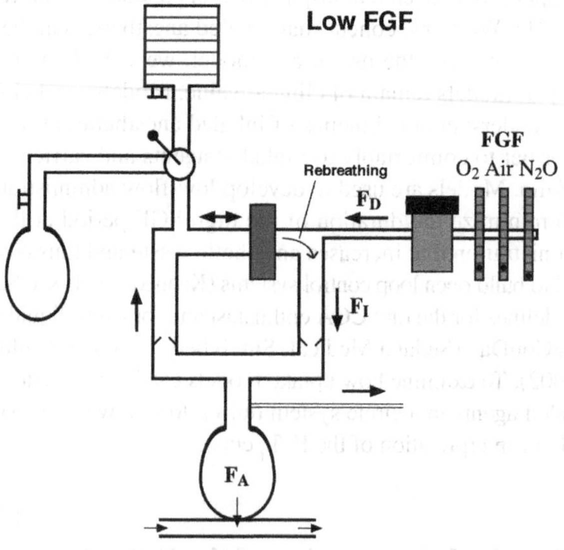

Fig. 5 The circle system and low-flow anesthesia. When FGF is lower than minute ventilation, there will be rebreathing. The lower FGF, the more rebreathing there is, and the larger the discrepancy between F_I and F_D will be

and safe because it ensured F_I matched F_D (F_D=F_I) by avoiding rebreathing. What really is implied when the term "high" FGF is used, is that FGF is higher than alveolar minute ventilation. Let us consider what happens when an inhaled agent is administered to a patient via a circle breathing system of an anesthesia machine with standing bellows when FGF is lower than minute ventilation (Fig. 5). Let us assume ventilation is mechanically controlled. Whenever FGF becomes lower than minute ventilation, FGF alone does not suffice to provide the tidal volume: the ventilator bellows will fill with a mixture of fresh gas and exhaled gas. With the next delivered tidal volume, some of the exhaled gas will thus be inhaled: this is called "rebreathing." The lower FGF, the more rebreathing there is. The rebreathing process is complex, and its effect on the kinetics of vapors depends, on a number of factors, e.g., on the type of carrier gas, the relative percentage of dead space and alveolar ventilation, the configuration of the different parts of the anesthesia circuit, and the location of any leaks. For our purposes, we will only consider the effect of the composition of gas mixture contained in the expired tidal volume. The gas contained in the exhaled tidal volume is not a homogeneous mixture. The first part of tidal volume (about one-third) contains gas that has not participated in gas exchange (dead space ventilation), and will not alter the composition of the inspired mixture to any significant degree when rebreathed because its vapor concentration equals F_I. Next comes alveolar gas, the vapor content of which has been altered by uptake (and all other factors involved in gas exchange across the alveolar–capillary membrane). Overall, the lower the FGF the larger the contribution that the alveolar gas with the lower vapor concentration (F_A) will make to the inspired mixture, leading to a decrease in F_I. To maintain F_I and thus F_A, F_D will have to be increased: a discrepancy has developed between F_D (controlled by the anesthesiologist) and F_I. This discrepancy that has developed between F_D and F_I may be perceived as "lack of control." For this very good reason, anesthesiologists have tended to deliver a fixed inspired partial pressure with a high FGF and watched F_A approach F_I over time. F_A/F_I graphs, discussed extensively by Eger, do graphically explain this process, as well as the effect of ventilation, cardiac output, shunting, and blood/gas partition coefficients (Fig. 6a). The amount of uptake and uptake models themselves are not directly reflected in those graphs—uptake is actually better approximated by the area *above* the F_A/F_I curve, $1\text{-}F_A/F_I$ (Fig. 7; Lin 1994). Still, $1\text{-}F_A/F_I$ is only an approximation of uptake—uptake is the difference between the amount entering and leaving the lungs, and thus has to take inspired and expired volumes into account.

The absence of end-expired gas analysis until the 1980s in most operating rooms did not prevent a few enthusiasts from using FGF well below minute ventilation, down to CCA, where the amount of agent and carrier gases added to the circuit matches the amount taken up by the patient (and lost via leaks) (Lowe and Ernst 1981). The extreme of low FGF, CCA, best illustrates why modeling of uptake became of real interest from a clinical point of view at a time when end-expired gas analysis was not routinely available: knowing the uptake at a certain F_A allowed the anesthesiologist to have a reasonable estimate of the amount of vapor that had to be added to the circuit to maintain the desired (unmeasured) F_A during CCA, because if the amount of vapor added to the circuit equals that removed from it, the concentration of the vapor in the system will remain constant (Lowe and Ernst 1981). The analogy between CCA and intravenous anesthesia is clear: in both cases, models are used to help quantitate the administration of the amount of drug in such a way that the resulting concentration falls within a desired range of concentrations. For inhaled agents, the mass balance also has to take into account the effect of gas sampling, circuit leaks, and circuit absorption. To make the link to a more quantitative

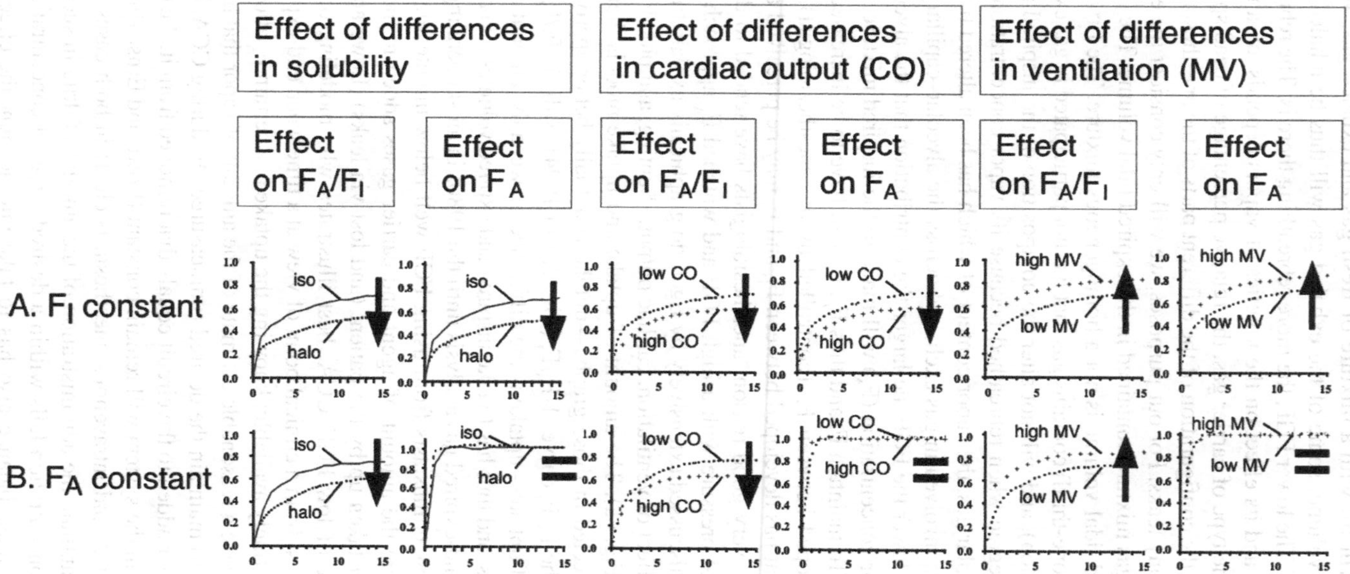

Fig. 6a, b GasMan simulations of how the mode of administration of a potent inhaled agent alters the interpretation of the isoflurane F_A/F_I curve. The qualitative effects on the F_A/F_I curve of an increase in blood/gas solubility (isoflurane vs halothane), cardiac output, and ventilation are the same regardless of whether F_I (**a**) or F_A (**b**) is the controlled variable that is kept constant. However, when F_A is kept constant, differences in solubility, cardiac output, and ventilation will not affect F_A because F_I is adjusted to maintain F_A at the desired concentration approach to the kinetics of inhaled agents, a slightly different approach than the use of the F_A/F_I curve imposes itself: instead of dialing a constant F_D with high FGF and studying the resulting F_A/F_I curve, the anesthesiologist wonders how a certain desired F_A can be attained and maintained in the individual patient by adjusting F_D, and how this is affected by the FGF selected by the anesthesiologist. We will answer these questions by a clinical example (Hendrickx et al. 1998b; Hendrickx 2004): How does the sevoflurane vaporizer setting have to be adjusted to rapidly attain and maintain the F_A at 1.3% sevoflurane with seven different FGF (8, 4, 2, 1, 0.5, 0.3, and 0.2 l/min, all in O_2/N_2O except the 0.2 l/min group in which O_2 was the carrier gas), starting with the maximum vaporizer setting of 8%? Two important points need to be made before analyzing the example. First, we focus on differences between F_D, F_I, and F_A here (F_D-F_A, F_D-F_I, F_I-F_A) rather than their ratios (F_D/F_A, F_D/F_I, F_I/F_A) because this better explains the existing gradients, and because anesthesiologists administer and measure absolute concentrations rather than ratios. Second, F_A and F_I are not presented because they (predictably) will be the same in all FGF groups by design. At the same (constant) F_A, average patient uptake in the different FGF groups logically will be very similar. Uptake can be approximated by the difference between the amount entering (inspired *alveolar* volume×F_I) and leaving the lung (expired *alveolar* volume×F_A; Fig. 7). Ignoring small differences between inspired and expired alveolar minute ventilation, it thus follows that F_I-F_A equals uptake/alveolar minute ventilation. Because F_A, uptake, and alveolar minute ventilation are the same in all FGF groups, it follows that F_I has to be very similar in all FGF groups at the same point in time. Also note that when uptake (and thus F_I-F_A) is constant, at any point in time a constant F_D-F_I implies that F_D-F_A is also constant.

Figure 8 displays the required vaporizer settings for the above example (Hendrickx et al. 1998b; Hendrickx 2004). Each line represents the mean of settings in 8 patients.

Several important findings on the F_D graph deserve mention.

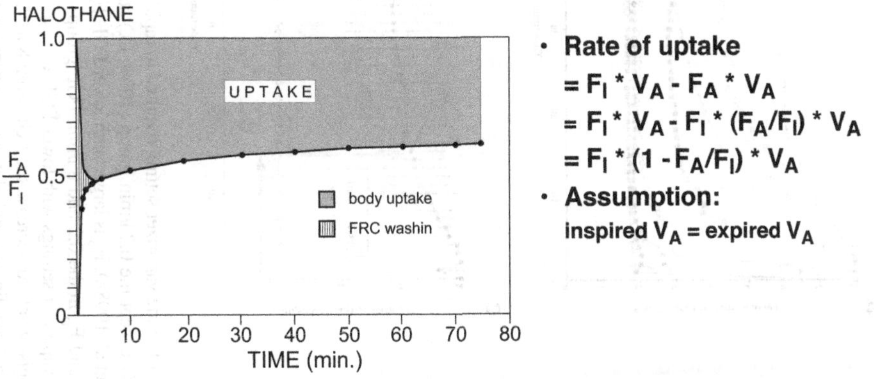

Fig. 7 Uptake is not represented by F_A/F_I itself, but rather by the area above the F_A/F_I curve, called "fraction of uptake" or $1-F_A/F_I$. Rate of uptake=$(1-F_A/F_I)$* alveolar minute ventilation, assuming that inspired and expired alveolar minute ventilation are the same

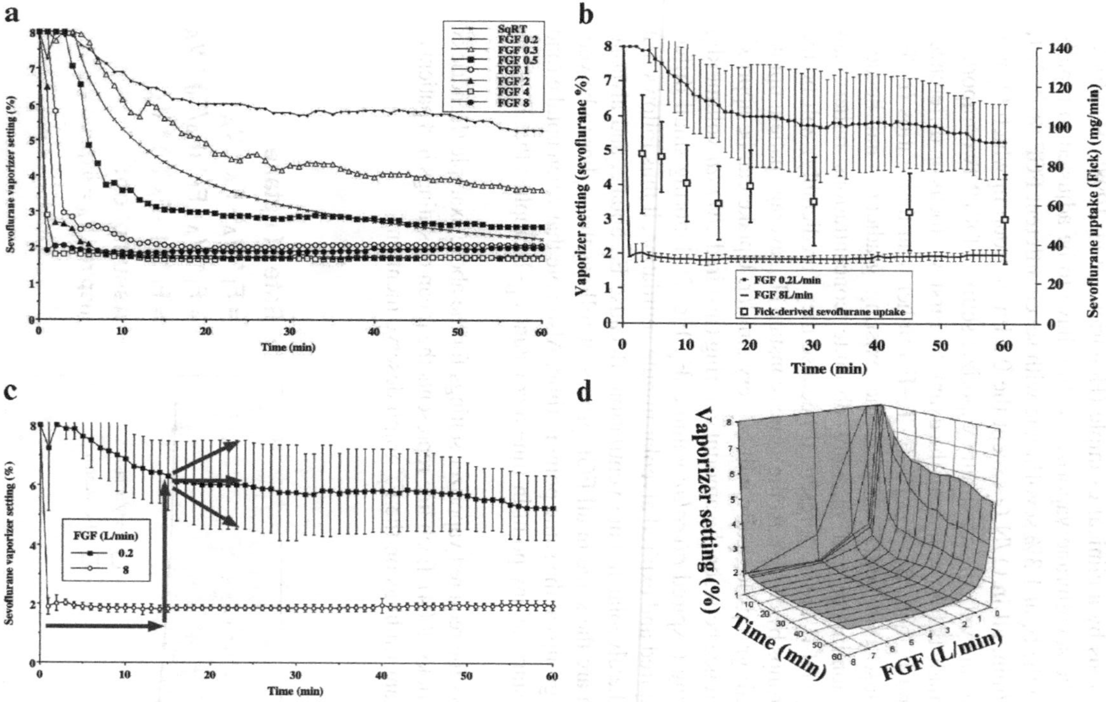

Fig. 8 a Sevoflurane vaporizer setting required to rapidly attain and maintain the F_A at 1.3% sevoflurane with seven different FGF (8, 4, 2, 1, 0.5. 0.3, and 0.2 l/min^{-1}, all in O_2/N_2O except the 0.2 l/min group (100% O_2) starting with the maximum vaporizer setting of 8%. Values in each FGF group represent mean of 8 patients (Hendrickx et al. 1998b). F_D is larger with lower FGF. F_D predicted by the SqRT model (CCA) is added. **b** Overlay of Fick-derived sevoflurane uptake data (Frietman et al. 2001) and F_D in the 0.2 and 8 l/min FGF groups; *error bars* represent standard deviation. The Fick-derived sevoflurane uptake pattern seems to be reflected better in the vaporizer settings with lower FGF. **c** F_D variability increases with lower FGF because of interpatient variability in uptake of up to 50%. As a result, if the anesthesiologist wants to decrease the FGF from 8 to 0.2 l/min, F_D will range from 4% to 8% (*gray arrows*). **d** The information presented in the 2D graph (**a**) can be displayed in a three-dimensional plot, a visual representation of the so-called "general anesthetic equation" or "anesthetic continuum" of sevoflurane

First, a similar vaporizer setting pattern emerges for each FGF (Fig. 8a). After an initial period (30 s to a few minutes) during which the maximum F_D is used to rapidly wash-in the system, F_D can be rapidly decreased, and a phase follows with a more progressive decline over the next 10–15 min (rapidly saturating tissues). After approximately 15 min, no or only a limited number of further F_D changes are needed during the ensuing 45 min (more slowly saturating tissue groups). For example, at an FGF of 1 l/min, the vaporizer setting to maintain the F_A at 1.3% is not different at 60 min than at 15 min (1.9±0.3% at 15 min and 2.0±0.3 at 60 min).

Second, the lower the FGF, the higher the F_D has to be. Said differently, the difference between F_D and F_I increases when FGF is reduced (Fig. 8a). This is caused by rebreathing.

Third, the uptake pattern of sevoflurane seems to be more reflected in the vaporizer settings with lower FGF. At one extreme of FGF, 0.2 l/min, the F_D course can be seen to match the sevoflurane uptake pattern (Fig. 8b). At the other extreme, 8 l/min FGF (FGF > minute ventilation), the uptake pattern is hardly recognizable in the vaporizer settings; the vaporizer setting is high only during the first few minutes because of wash-in of the system combined with high uptake (that is, the first few minutes of the anesthetic). However, if we were to use a very sensitive gas analyzer and an extremely precise vaporizer, the same decreasing F_D pattern observed in the CCA group could be observed in the high FGF groups. Because the difference between F_D and F_I increases with lower FGF (see previous paragraph), the uptake pattern *seems* to be more reflected in lower FGF groups. Nevertheless, the *clinical* implication is that the anesthesiologist has to make barely any F_D changes with high FGF, while with a very low FGF, F_D has to be adjusted in a pattern that follows the decreasing uptake pattern in the body, especially at the beginning of anesthesia when the anesthesiologist may be occupied with a host of other tasks. The reflection of the uptake pattern in the course of F_I (not shown for reasons mentioned above) will be the same in all FGF groups. The difference between F_I and F_A is caused by patient uptake—this is the same for all FGF groups; the difference between F_D and F_I is caused by rebreathing, and thus differs between FGF groups. When FGF is high, there is no rebreathing, and then F_D=F_I.

Fourth, when the F_D predictions by the SqRT model for CCA are compared to those in 0.2 l/min group, it can be appreciated that the SqRT model will initially overestimate and later underestimate F_D (Fig. 8a). This finding is to be expected because the SqRT model initially overestimates and later underestimates uptake of inhaled agents (Fig. 2; Hendrickx et al. 1997, 1998a, 2003; Frietman et al. 2003a, b): the uptake pattern determines the manner in which the anesthesiologist has to adjust F_D. Findings for the 4C models are analogous (Hendrickx 2004).

Fifth, F_D variability increases with lower FGF (Fig. 8b). The lower the FGF, the more uptake by the patient will influence the composition of the inspiratory mixture and therefore the vaporizer setting. Because uptake differs up to 50% between patients (Hendrickx et al. 1997; Frietman et al. 2001), F_D variability increases accordingly with lower FGF (Table 2; Hendrickx 2004; Hendrickx et al. 1999a). The clinical implications of this finding are important. If the anesthesiologist wants to decrease the FGF from 8 to, e.g., 0.2 or 0.3 l/min (Fig. 8c), the F_D for the individual

Table 2 Coefficient of variation of F_D (100×standard deviation/mean) for modern inhaled agents after maintaining 0.65 MAC for 40 min with a range of FGF (Hendrickx 2004; Hendrickx et al. 1999a)

		FGF (l/min)					
Time	Agent	0.3	0.5	1	2	4	8
40 min	Isoflurane	24	12	21	13	10	13
	Sevoflurane	30	19	15	10	3	13
	Desflurane	17	16	6	5	5	6

patient has to be increased to a number that can be anywhere from 4% to 8%, quite a large range. Because patient demographic parameters (e.g., weight) could not be withheld as covariates in most closed-circuit anesthesia studies (Hendrickx et al. 1997, 1998a, 2003; Vermeulen et al. 1997; Westenskow et al. 1983; Lockwood et al. 1993), these covariates cannot be used to help decide which F_D to use in the individual patient, underscoring the need to always use end-expired gas analysis. Even with the application of simple administration schedules (see Sect. 5), clinicians may still find the increased discrepancy between F_D and F_I, coupled with the unpredictability caused by the higher F_D variability at the lower FGF, cumbersome to deal with in a busy operating room. Anesthesia machines that use CCA end-expired feedback control provide a practical solution to these issues—they "black box" these issues (see Chapter 21).

Carrier gas composition also affects F_I–F_A and F_D–F_I. When N_2O is used as the carrier gas instead of O_2 or O_2/air, F_A rises faster and higher because of the second gas effect (Hendrickx et al. 2006b; Slock et al. 2003). Because N_2O increases F_A, to maintain the same F_A, the F_D is slightly lower than when O_2 or O_2/air is used. The use of N_2O also has an effect on the mass balances in the circle system: when N_2O is used, the loss from the circle system will be smaller by the amount of N_2O taken up by the patient (Hendrickx et al. 2002). While the effect of this is small at high FGF because the amount of potent inhaled anesthetic lost via the pop-valve is large relative to uptake by the patient, this effect lowers the required F_D at the lower FGF, such as 500 ml/min: at this low FGF, the amount of gas lost via the pop-off valve with a O_2/N_2O mixture is 100–250 ml/min lower than with 100% O_2. To compensate for these higher losses with O_2 at these low FGF, F_D has to be increased (Hendrickx et al. 2002).

4 The General Anesthetic Equation Concept

The information presented in the 2D graph of the pervious section can be displayed in a three-dimensional plot (Fig. 8d). This 3D figure is a visual representation of the so-called "general anesthetic equation" (GAEq) or "anesthetic continuum" of sevoflurane. "General" and "continuum" refer to the fact that an infinite number of combinations of FGF and F_D can be used to attain and maintain the same F_A (Lowe and Ernst 1981). While the graph only presents the F_D for one particular F_A (1.3% sevoflurane), we nevertheless will further refer to it as the "general" anesthetic equation.

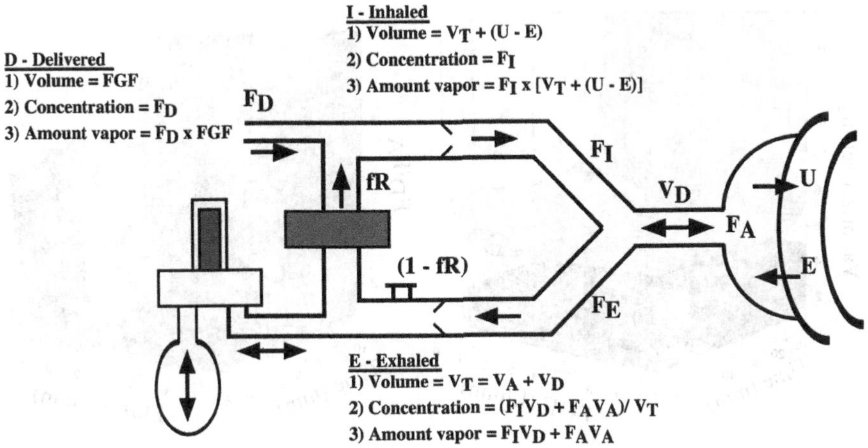

$$F_D = \frac{Qan\,[V_T + (U - E) - V_D \times fR] + (1 - fR)\,F_A \times V_A\,[V_T + (U - E)]}{V_A + (U - E)\,FGF}$$

Fig. 9 Amounts of gases (concentration *x* volume) delivered to the circle system and inhaled and exhaled by the patient. By rearranging these factors Lowe and Ernst derived the general anesthetic equation. F_E, mixed-expired concentration; V_T, V_D, and V_A, minute, dead space, and alveolar minute ventilation, respectively; *U*, uptake of O_2 (VO_2), N_2O (QN_2O), and anesthetic vapor (*Qan*); *E*, elimination of CO_2 (VCO_2) and water vapor (VH_2O); *fR*, fraction rebreathed; *1-fR*, fraction of exhaled vapor exhausted from the system

The word "equation" refers to an actual equation that Lowe and Ernst derived by considering mass balances in the anesthesia system (Fig. 9; Lowe and Ernst 1981). In an extensive treatise, Lowe and Ernst (1981) deduced how the F_D required to attain and maintain a constant F_A in a circle system can be predicted for any FGF if the following are known: (1) uptake of potent inhaled anesthetic, O_2, and N_2O; (2) CO_2 and H_2O production; and (3) alveolar and dead space ventilation. Figure 9 displays those mass balances. The amounts of gases delivered, inhaled, and exhaled can mathematically be quantified. By rearranging the components of these equations, an equation can be derived that mathematically expresses the vaporizer settings over time required to attain and maintain a constant end-expired concentration with a range of FGF: the GAEq (Fig. 9). The equation says that **(1)** F_D is proportional to 1/FGF (F_D–F_I discrepancy increases with lower FGF), **(2)** F_D is proportional to Qan (=uptake; more uptake implies need for higher F_D to maintain F_A), **(3)** and when the factor time is added, ΔF_D is proportional to ΔQan (the uptake pattern or course is reflected in F_D setting over time). Even though many more factors are involved, and a more complex description can be used [incorporating factors such as nitrogen wash-out, physiologic vs anatomical dead-space ventilation, generalization

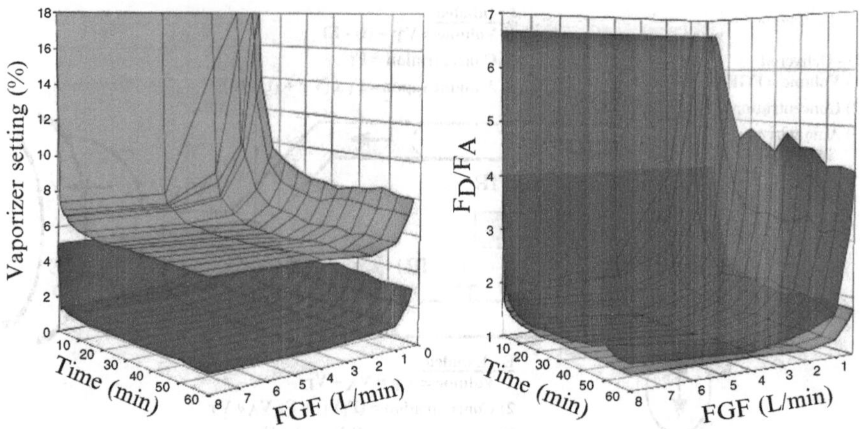

Fig. 10 The 3D representation of the GAEq of 0.65 MAC isoflurane (*purple*) and desflurane (*blue*), with F_D (*left*) and F_D/F_A (*right*) in the Y-axis. While F_D is higher for desflurane because of its higher MAC, the discrepancy between F_D and F_A (or F_D/F_A) is lower for desflurane because of its lower solubility

to STPD (standard temperature and pressure, and dry) conditions, etc.], this concept has didactic value and will help gain insight in how different authors have approached the same "anesthetic plane" from different perspectives.

A 3D plot can be constructed for any F_A with any agent and agent/carrier gas combination (Hendrickx et al. 1998b, c, 1999b; Hendrickx 2004). Figure 10 compares the F_D for isoflurane and desflurane settings to attain and maintain the same MAC (0.65 MAC). The GAEq patterns differ between agents: the agent with the lower blood/gas solubilities (desflurane) has higher absolute F_D because its MAC is higher, but its vaporizer/end-expired ratios (F_D/F_A) are lower than those for isoflurane. The plane for sevoflurane (Fig. 8d) lies between that of isoflurane and desflurane. It has been suggested that the agents with a lower blood/gas partition coefficient would be more "user-friendly" because (1) their F_A/F_I (Fig. 4) is higher (F_A is closer to F_I) and F_D/F_A (Fig. 10) and F_D/F_I are lower—there is less of a discrepancy between the F_D, F_I, and F_A; (2) the more horizontal-shaped plane for desflurane indicates that FGF can be lowered without having to change F_D to a great extent; and (3) vaporizer setting variability is lower with less soluble agents, especially with lower FGF (Table 2; Hendrickx 2004; Hendrickx et al. 1999a).

The plot is also useful to point out how different authors have been studying different parts of the same concept (Fig. 11). From CCA to high FGF one can appreciate the work by Lowe and Ernst (1981; SqRT model, CCA), Virtue (1974; 500 ml/min FGF or minimal flow anesthesia), Foldes et al. (1952; 1 l/min FGF or low-flow anesthesia), and Eger (2000; intermediate- and high-flow regions). Various authors have explored smaller parts of the GAEq, but unfortunately most often using a constant F_D (Johansson et al. 2001, 2002; Park et al. 2005). Nevertheless, the studies by Johansson et al. (2001, 2002) nicely illustrate for both desflurane and sevoflurane

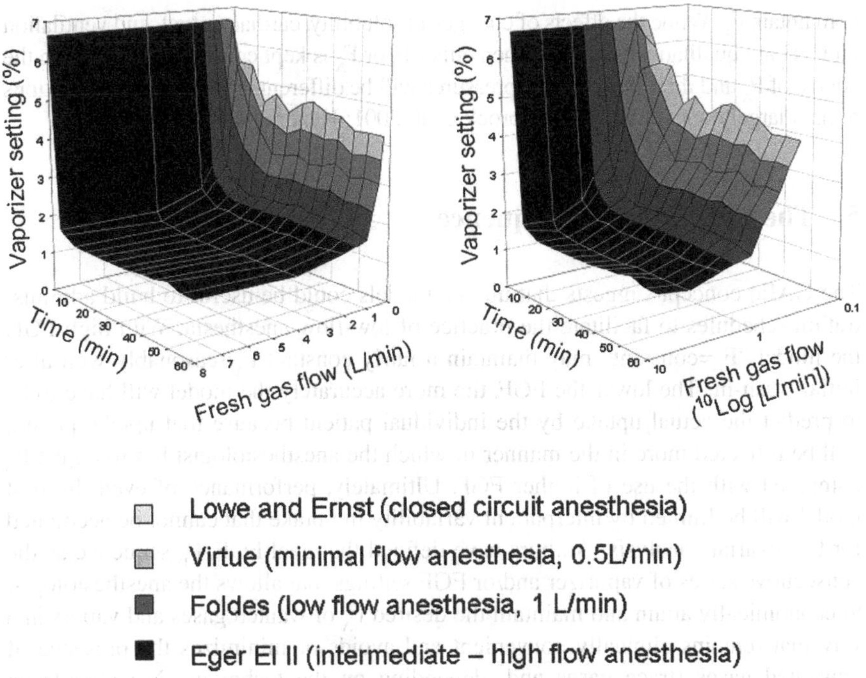

Fig. 11 The 3D plot of the GAEq illustrates how different authors have been studying different parts of the same concept

Table 3 F_A/F_I, F_D/F_I, and F_D/F_I of desflurane and sevoflurane at a FGF of 1 and 2 l/min after 120 min with constant F_D technique (Johansson et al. 2001, 2002)

		Ratios after 120 min of anesthesia with constant F_D		
Agent and carrier gas	FGF (l/min)	F_A/F_I	F_D/F_I	F_D/F_A
Desflurane in O_2/N_2O	1	0.96	1.10	1.14
	2	0.96	1.05	1.09
Sevoflurane in O_2/N_2O	1	0.88	1.38	1.56
	2	0.89	1.22	1.37

how F_A/F_I at 120 min are identical at 1 and 2 l/min FGF, but F_D/F_I and F_D/F_I are higher with the lower FGF (Table 3).

The focus on how to manipulate F_D to attain and maintain a certain F_A when FGF is reduced has implications on how to interpret the effect of cardiac output, ventilation, and solubility on the F_A/F_I curve (Fig. 6). When F_A is kept constant (Fig. 6b), by definition, cardiac output, ventilation, and the use of agents with a different blood/gas partition coefficient will not affect F_A because F_D and thus F_I will be adjusted to maintain F_A. While the effects of changes in solubility, cardiac output, and ventilation on F_A/F_I are qualitatively similar when either F_I or F_A is kept constant, the effect on the course of F_A and thus tissue partial pressures will be different. The clinical implications remain largely unexplored (Neckebroek et al. 2001; Hendrickx et al. 1999c).

5 The Ideal FGF–F_D Sequence

The GAEq concept suggests that uptake models could be useful to build administration schedules to facilitate the practice of low-flow anesthesia. With high FGF, the model "F_D=constant" may maintain a fairly constant F_A reasonably well after initial wash-in. The lower the FGF, the more accurately the model will have to be to predict the actual uptake by the individual patient because that uptake pattern will be reflected more in the manner in which the anesthesiologist has to adjust F_D compared with the use of higher FGF. Ultimately, performance of even the best model will be limited by interpatient variability in uptake that cannot be accounted for by covariate analysis. Authors have defined the ideal FGF–F_D sequence as the consecutive series of vaporizer and/or FGF settings that allows the anesthesiologist to economically attain and maintain the desired F_A of wanted gases and vapors in a way that remains clinically convenient and avoids or minimizes the presence of unwanted gases (trace gases and, depending on the technique, N_2) (Mapleson 1998). This search can be visualized as finding the optimal route of vaporizer and FGF sequence through a 3D representation of the GAEq (Fig. 12a). The number of

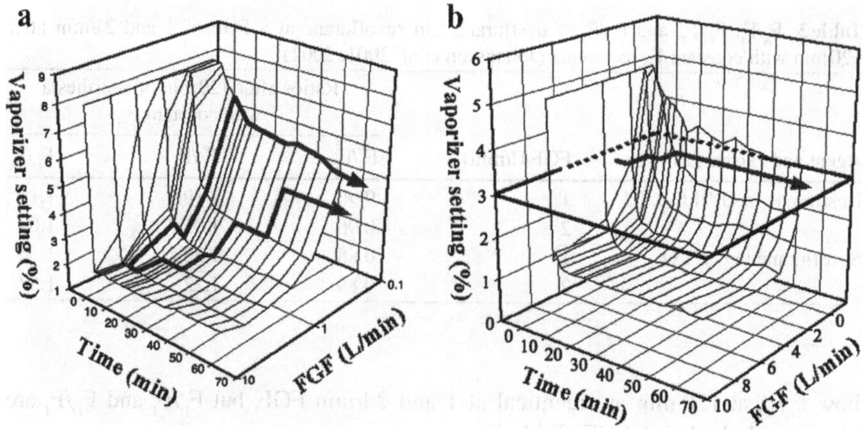

Fig. 12 **a** The search for the ideal FGF–F_D sequence can be visualized as **a** finding the optimal route of vaporizer and FGF sequence through a 3D representation of the GAEq (sevoflurane in this example). **b** The development of a simple low-flow administration schedule for isoflurane in O_2/N_2O with a constant isoflurane F_D by Lerou et al. (Lerou and Booij 2001a, b, 2002; Lerou et al. 2002) can be visualized as the intersection between the plane describing the GAEq for 0.8%–1.1% end-expired isoflurane and the horizontal plane describing a constant vaporizer setting

routes is infinite. Several authors have developed administration schedules but do not explicitly mention the GAEq, yet conceptually they try to approach a certain "path" through this "anesthetic continuum." The attractiveness of the GAEq, and the "planes" or "surfaces" is that they make it clear that in order to keep F_A constant, either FGF or F_D can be adjusted.

When authors search for a "simple" administration schedule, it means "simple to apply but still close enough to the real uptake pattern." Uptake continually changes over time, but because our techniques are crude relative to the uptake changes that actually occur and because these small concentration changes that occur are clinically irrelevant, it may appear as if it does not change during some intervals. Thus, during certain time periods the changes are so small that we can neglect them: This allows us to use "simple" uptake patterns but still be close enough to the real uptake pattern that there is no real penalty to pay for the introduced simplicity.

While the idea of using the uptake pattern to facilitate the administration of inhaled anesthetics is corroborated by other authors (Rietbrock et al. 2000; Lerou et al. 2002), the number of good studies trying to develop these schedules are few, especially those describing strategies to rapidly achieve and maintain a predetermined F_A under low-flow conditions (Lerou et al. 2002). Some of these are reviewed below.

Lowe and Ernst specifically developed the SqRT model to facilitate CCA, yet while mentioning that the 4C physiologic model lacks sufficient clinical validation at the time (Lowe and Ernst 1981), they did not further explore the GAEq clinically themselves. Because their model tends to overestimate initial uptake and thus vaporizer settings, and underestimates them after approximately 30 min (see Fig. 2), it tends to overestimate initial F_D settings and underestimates F_D settings later (Hendrickx 2004).

Mapleson used a multicompartmental physiologic model of the patient and breathing system to predict the ideal FGF sequence at the start of low-flow anesthesia (up to 20 min of anesthesia) using halothane, enflurane, isoflurane, sevoflurane, and desflurane, in a standard male of 40 years old and 70 kg body weight (Mapleson 1998). The goal was to define the FGF and F_D combination that for each anesthetic would raise F_A to 1 MAC as quickly as practically possible and then keep it within ± 5% of that level for 20 min. N_2O was not used. The resulting theoretical combination of FGF and F_D is presented in Fig. 13 (Mapleson 1998). The model has been tested clinically (Ip-Yam et al. 2001; Sobreira et al. 2001): the desired F_A was reached in less than 2 min, but overall mean F_A was at least 10% higher than predicted, and in some instances up to 40%.

Lerou and colleagues' most recent model consists of a physiologic multicompartment model of the body, a three-compartment lung, and a three-compartment breathing system (Lerou and Booij 2001a; Fig. 14). The model meets three criteria: (1) all gases are included, and their partial pressures always add up to 100%; (2) the FGF can range form CCA to higher than minute ventilation; and (3) the breathing system consists of three parts (inspiratory subsystem, sodalime canister, and expiratory tubing plus standing bellows). The model was used to develop a theoretical "ideal FGF and F_D combination schedule" for isoflurane in N_2O. The authors allude to interpatient variability being an issue with the use of a FGF of 0.5 l/min in their

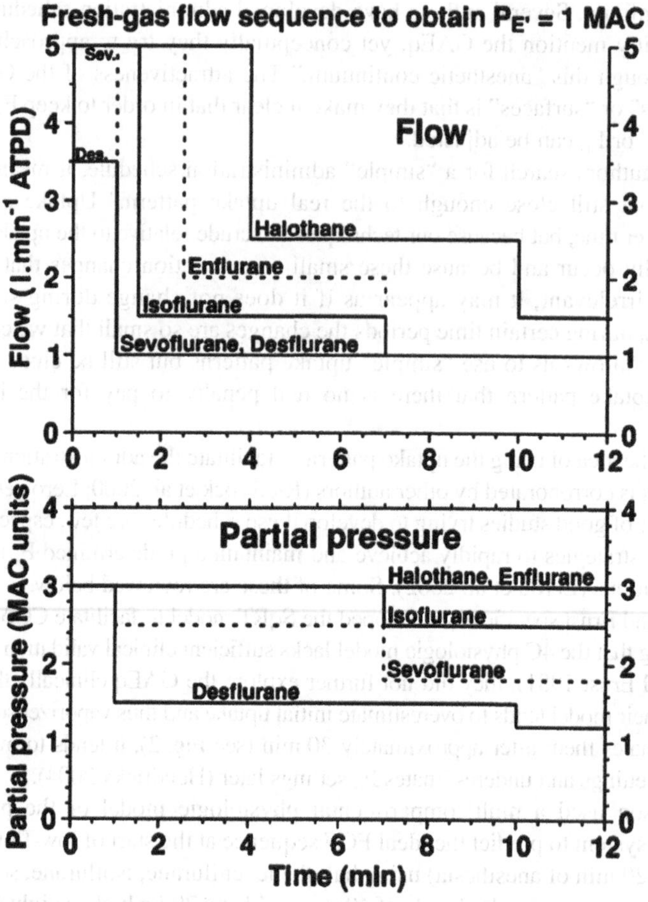

Fig. 13 Theoretical ideal FGF sequence according to Mapleson (1998). Predicted sequence of FGF and partial pressure settings for five anesthetics to achieve and maintain an F_A (labeled $P_{E'}$ here) of 1 MAC using a minimum FGF of 1 l/min

theoretical analysis: the model tends to overshoot for small patients and undershoot in heavier patients (Lerou et al. 2002). The clinically evaluated schedule (Lerou et al. 2002) was started after a 7 to 13 min high O_2/N_2O FGF period without isoflurane, and subsequently consisted of a constant F_D of 3% isoflurane and the following FGF sequence: 2 l/min N_2O+1 l/min O_2 from 0–3 min, 1 l/min N_2O+0.5 l/min from 3–6 min, and 0.2 l/min N_2O+0.3 l/min O_2 after 6 min. Isoflurane F_A reached the desired 0.8%–1.1% range after 2 min (range 1.0–5.67 min), and an average of 72% of individual measurements were within the window from 3–30 min. The approach by Lerou is easy to grasp intuitively if we see their approach in the 3D GAEq graph (Fig. 12b). Lerou describes the intersection between the plane describing the GAEq for 0.8%–1.1% and the plane describing a constant vaporizer setting.

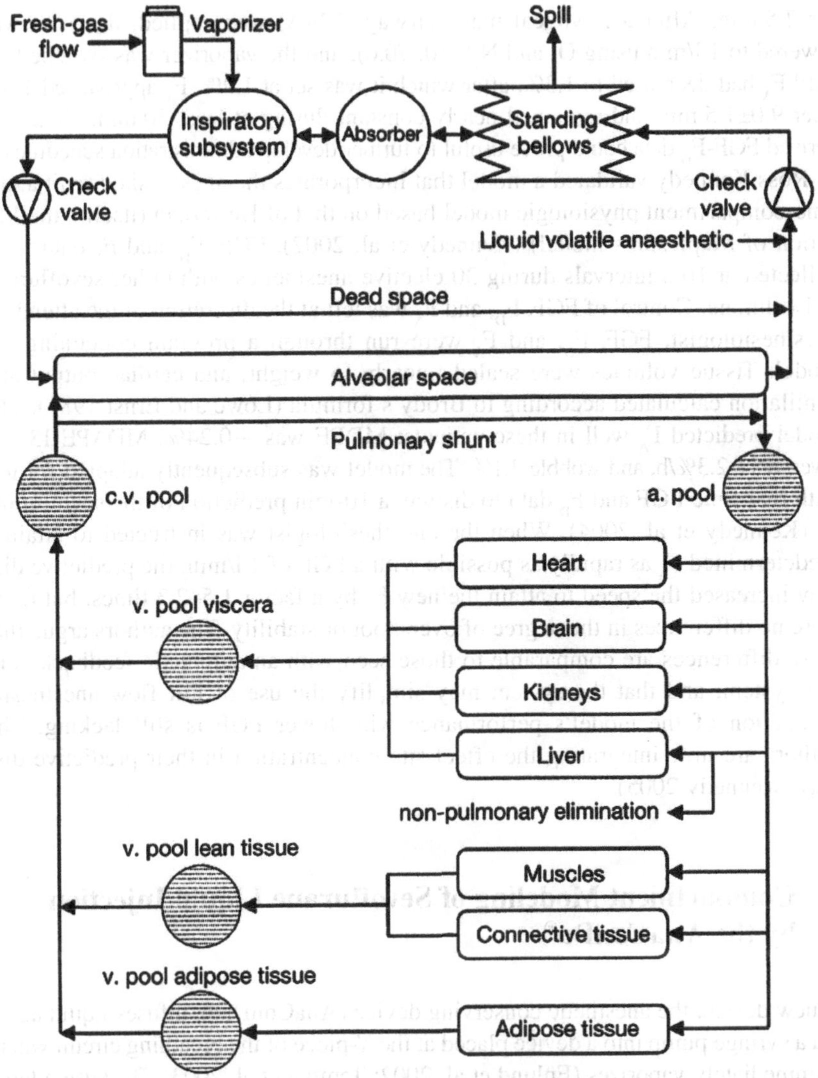

Fig. 14 Diagram of the system model used by Lerou and Booij in their search for a simple low-flow administration schedule for isoflurane in O_2/N_2O (Lerou and Booij 2001a)

Alternative "routes" are obviously possible. We believe administration schedules can be even further optimized and simplified, even with the use of an O_2/N_2O mixture (Carette et al. 2004).

Hendrickx and colleagues did not develop a new model but used the F_D settings from the 1 l/min group in the experiment mentioned section 3 (Hendrickx et al. 1998b; Hendrickx 2004) to develop a simple low-flow anesthesia schedule after overpressure induction (Hendrickx et al. 2000) with sevoflurane (8%) in an 8 l/min O_2/N_2O mixture for 2.5 min. After a laryngeal mask airway (LMA) was applied, the FGF was lowered to 1 l/min using O_2 and N_2O (0.4/0.6), and the vaporizer was switched off until F_A had decreased to 1.3%, after which it was set at 1.9%. F_A approached 1.3% after 9.0±1.5 min and remained nearly constant during at least 30 min. Clinically derived FGF-F_D data could prove useful to further develop administration schedules.

Ross Kennedy validated a model that incorporates the anesthesia circuit and a nine-compartment physiologic model based on that of Heffernan (itself a modification of Mapleson's model) (Kennedy et al. 2002). FGF, F_D, and F_A data were collected at 10-s intervals during 30 elective anesthetics with either sevoflurane or isoflurane. Control of FGF, F_D, and F_A was left at the discretion of the attending anesthesiologist. FGF, F_D, and F_A were run through a program containing the model. Tissue volumes were scaled linearly to weight, and cardiac output and ventilation calculated according to Brody's formula (Lowe and Ernst 1981). The model predicted F_A well in these patients: MDPE was −0.24%, MDAPE 13.7%, divergence 2.3%/h, and wobble 3.1%. The model was subsequently adapted for use with real-time FGF and F_D data to display a 10-min prediction of the sevoflurane F_A (Kennedy et al. 2004). When the anesthesiologist was instructed to attain a predetermined F_A as rapidly as possible with a FGF of 1 l/min, the predictive display increased the speed to attain the new F_A by a factor 1.5–2.3 times, but there were no differences in the degree of overshoot or stability. The authors argue that these differences are comparable to those seen with an automatic feedback control system, and that the system may simplify the use of low-flow anesthesia. Evaluation of the model's performance with lower FGF is still lacking. The authors are now integrating the effect-site concentration in their predictive display (Kennedy 2005).

6 Compartment Modeling of Sevoflurane Liquid Injection by the AnaConDa®

A new device, the anesthetic conserving device (AnaConDa®), infuses liquid agent via a syringe pump into a device placed at the Y-piece of the breathing circuit where it immediately vaporizes (Enlund et al. 2002; Tempia et al. 2003). Because a large part of the agent is retained in the device upon exhalation and reused during the next inhalation, consumption becomes equivalent to that used with a circle system with a FGF of approximately 1.5 l/min. A population pharmacokinetic model analogous to that used for intravenous agents is being developed for sevoflurane administration with the AnaConDa® (Enlund et al. 2006). The sevoflurane concentration-time courses on the patient side of the AnaConDa® were adequately described with a two-compartment model. The model was capable of handling rapid changes in infusion rate, with a precision of the predictions within ±20.4% MDAPE. MDPE was −2.99%. The authors suggest "the possibility of safe open loop administration of sevoflurane even in the absence of end-expired concentration monitoring" because it can be administered with the "predictive performance of [a] model [that] compares favorably with that of pharmacokinetic models used for TCI application of intravenous drugs" (Enlund et al. 2006). Further studies will focus on prospective testing and validation of the model implemented in a TCI device, and will define the place of this device in our clinical armamentarium.

References

Bailey JM (1997) Context-sensitive half-times and other decrement times of inhaled anesthetics. Anesth Analg 85:681–686

Benowitz N, Forsyth FP, Melmon KL, Rowland M (1974) Lidocaine disposition kinetics in monkey and man. I. Prediction by a perfusion model. Clin Pharmacol Ther 16:87–98

Bouillon T, Shafer SL (2000) Hot air or full steam ahead? An empirical pharmacokinetic model of potent inhalational agents. Br J Anaesth 84:429–431

Carette R, Hendrickx J, Deloof T, et al (2004) Bellows volume changes associated with very early O_2/N_2O fresh gas flow (FGF) reductions. Anesthesiology 101:A482

Carpenter RL, Eger EI, Johnson BH, et al (1986) Pharmacokinetics of inhaled anesthetics in humans: measurements during and after the simultaneous administration of enflurane, halothane, isoflurane, methoxyflurane, and nitrous oxide. Anesth Analg 65:575–582

de Jong RH, Eger EI (1975) MAC expanded: AD50 and AD95 values of common inhalation anesthetics in man. Anesthesiology 42:384–389

Doolette DJ, Upton RN, Grant C (1998) Diffusion-limited, but not perfusion-limited, compartmental models describe cerebral nitrous oxide kinetics at high and low cerebral blood flows. J Pharmacokinet Biopharm 26:649–672

Doolette DJ, Upton RN, Zheng D (2001) Diffusion-limited tissue equilibration and arteriovenous diffusion shunt describe skeletal muscle nitrous oxide kinetics at high and low blood flows in sheep. Acta Physiol Scand 172:167–177

Eger EI (1974) Anesthetic uptake and action. Williams & Wilkins, Baltimore

Eger EI (2000) Uptake and distribution. In: Miller R (ed) anesthesia, 5th edn. Churchill Livingstone, New York, pp 74–95

Eger EI, Saidman LJ (2005) Illustrations of inhaled anesthetic uptake, including intertissue diffusion to and from fat. Anesth Analg 100:1020–1033

Eger EI, Shafer SL (2005) Tutorial: context-sensitive decrement times for inhaled anesthetics. Anesth Analg 101:688–696

Eger EI, Sonner JM (2006) Anaesthesia defined (gentlemen, this is no humbug). Best Pract Res Clin Anaesthesiol 20:23–29

Eger EI, Saidman LJ, Brandstater B (1965) Minimum alveolar anesthetic concentration: a standard of anesthetic potency. Anesthesiology 26:756–763

Eger EI, Fisher DM, Dilger JP, et al (2001) Relevant concentrations of inhaled anesthetics for in vitro studies of anesthetic mechanisms. Anesthesiology 94:915–921

Enlund M, Lambert H, Wiklund L (2002) The sevoflurane saving capacity of a new anaesthetic agent conserving device compared with a low flow circle system. Acta Anaesthesiol Scand 46:506–511

Enlund M, Kietzmann D, Bouillon T, et al (2006) Population pharmacokinetics of sevoflurane with the AnaConDa®. Towards volatile-TCI. American Society of Anesthesiologists annual meeting abstracts 105:A1569

Foldes FF, Ceravolo AJ, Carpenter SL (1952) The administration of nitrous oxide-oxygen anesthesia in closed systems. Ann Surg 136:978–981

Frietman P, Hendrickx J, Grouls R, et al (2001) Fick-derived sevoflurane uptake. Anesthesiology 95:A478

Frietman P, Hendrickx J, Grouls R, et al (2003a) The correlation between the sevoflurane uptake pattern and vaporizer dial settings at different fresh gas flows. Eur J Anaesthesiol 30:A451

Frietman P, Hendrickx J, Van Zundert A, et al (2003b) Fick-derived Halothane Uptake: a Comparison with the 4C and SqRT Models and with Closed-Circuit Anesthesia Liquid Injection-derived Halothane Uptake. Eur J Anaesthesiol 30:A511

Fukui Y, Smith NT (1981) Interactions among ventilation, the circulation, and the uptake and distribution of halothane—use of a hybrid computer multiple model. I. The basic model. Anesthesiology 54:107–118

Heffernan PB, Gibbs JM, McKinnon AE (1982) Teaching the uptake and distribution of halothane. A computer simulation program. Anaesthesia 37:9–17

Hendrickx J (2004) The pharmacokinetics of inhaled agents and carrier gases. PhD thesis. Faculty of Medicine and Health Sciences, Department of Anesthesiology. University of Ghent

Hendrickx JF, Soetens M, Van der Donck A, et al (1997) Uptake of desflurane and isoflurane during closed-circuit anesthesia with spontaneous and controlled mechanical ventilation. Anesth Analg 84:413–418

Hendrickx JF, Van Zundert AA, De Wolf AM (1998a) Sevoflurane pharmacokinetics: effect of cardiac output. Br J Anaesth 81:495–501

Hendrickx JF, Van Zundert AAJ, De Wolf AM (1998b) Clinical evaluation of the general anesthetic equation for sevoflurane. Anesthesiology 89:A518

Hendrickx JF, Van Zundert A, De Wolf A (1998c) Clinical evaluation of the general anesthetic equation for isoflurane. Anesth Analg 86:S461

Hendrickx JF, Van Zundert A, De Wolf A (1999a) Vaporizer setting variability increases with lower fresh gas flows. Anesth Analg 88:S344

Hendrickx JF, De Ridder KD, De Geyndt AD, et al (1999b) Clinical evaluation of the general anesthetic equation for desflurane. Anesth Analg 88:S341

Hendrickx JF, Van Zundert A, De Wolf A (1999c) Blood/gas solubility and alveolar rate of rise of potent inhaled anesthetics during open-loop feedback administration using a closed-circuit anesthesia liquid injection technique. Anesth Analg 88:S342

Hendrickx JF, Vandeput DM, De Geyndt AM, et al (2000) Maintaining sevoflurane anesthesia during low-flow anesthesia using a single vaporizer setting change after overpressure induction. J Clin Anesth 12:303–307

Hendrickx JF, Coddens J, Callebaut F, et al (2002) Effect of N_2O on sevoflurane vaporizer settings during minimal- and low-flow anesthesia. Anesthesiology 97:400–404

Hendrickx JF, Dishart MK, De Wolf AM (2003) Isoflurane and desflurane uptake during liver resection and transplantation. Anesth Analg 96:356–362

Hendrickx JF, Lemmens HJ, Shafer SL (2006a) Do distribution volumes and clearances relate to tissue volumes and blood flows? A computer simulation. BMC Anesthesiol 6:7

Hendrickx JF, Carette R, Lemmens HJ, De Wolf AM (2006b) Large volume N_2O uptake alone does not explain the second gas effect of N2O on sevoflurane during constant inspired ventilation. Br J Anaesth 96:391–395

Hull C (1997) Pharmacokinetics for anaesthesia, 1st edn. Heinemann, Oxford

Ip-Yam PC, Goh MH, Chan YH, Kong CF (2001) Clinical evaluation of the Mapleson theoretical ideal fresh gas flow sequence at the start of low-flow anaesthesia with isoflurane, sevoflurane and desflurane. Anaesthesia 56:160–164

Ishibashi T, Hendrickx J, De Wolf A, et al (2006) Isoflurane pharmacokinetics: linking lung uptake to arterial and mixed venous blood concentrations. Anesthesiology 105:A1202

Johansson A, Lundberg D, Luttropp HH (2001) Low-flow anaesthesia with desflurane: kinetics during clinical procedures. Eur J Anaesthesiol 18:499–504

Johansson A, Lundberg D, Luttropp HH (2002) The quotient end-tidal/inspired concentration of sevoflurane in a low-flow system. J Clin Anesth 14:267–270

Kennedy RR (2005) The effect of using different values for the effect-site equilibrium half-time on the prediction of effect-site sevoflurane concentration: a simulation study. Anesth Analg 101:1023–1028

Kennedy RR, French RA, Spencer C (2002) Predictive accuracy of a model of volatile anesthetic uptake. Anesth Analg 95:1616–1621

Kennedy RR, French RA, Gilles S (2004) The effect of a model-based predictive display on the control of end-tidal sevoflurane concentrations during low-flow anesthesia. Anesth Analg 99:1159–1163

Landon MJ, Matson AM, Royston BD, et al (1993) Components of the inspiratory-arterial isoflurane partial pressure difference. Br J Anaesth 70:605–611

Lerou JG, Booij LH (2001a) Model-based administration of inhalation anaesthesia. 1. Developing a system model. Br J Anaesth 86:12–28

Lerou JG, Booij LH (2001b) Model-based administration of inhalation anaesthesia. 2. Exploring the system model. Br J Anaesth 86:29–37

Lerou JG, Booij LH (2002) Model-based administration of inhalation anaesthesia. 3. Validating the system model. Br J Anaesth 88:24–37

Lerou JG, Dirksen R, Beneken Kolmer HH, Booij LH (1991) A system model for closed-circuit inhalation anesthesia. I. Computer study. Anesthesiology 75:345–355

Lerou JG, Verheijen R, Booij LH (2002) Model-based administration of inhalation anaesthesia. 4. Applying the system model. Br J Anaesth 88:175–183

Levitt DG, Schnider TW (2005) Human physiologically based pharmacokinetic model for propofol. BMC Anesthesiol 5:4

Lin CY (1994) Uptake of anaesthetic gases and vapours. Anaesth Intensive Care 22:363–373

Lockhart SH, Cohen Y, Yasuda N, et al (1991) Cerebral uptake and elimination of desflurane, isoflurane, and halothane from rabbit brain: an in vivo NMR study. Anesthesiology 74:575–580

Lockwood GG, Chakrabarti MK, Whitwam JG (1993) The uptake of isoflurane during anaesthesia. Anaesthesia 48:748–752

Lowe J, Ernst E (1981) The quantitative practice of anesthesia—use of a closed circuit. Williams & Wilkins, Baltimore

Mapleson WW (1998) The theoretical ideal fresh-gas flow sequence at the start of low-flow anaesthesia. Anaesthesia 53:264–272

Morris LE (1994) Closed carbon dioxide filtration revisited. Anaesth Intensive Care 22:345–358

Neckebroek M, Hendrickx J, Deloof T, De Wolf A (2001) Effects of ventilation on the isoflurane inspired-expired gradient during low flow anesthesia. Eur J Anaesthesiol 18:A317

NONMEM Project Group (1992) NONMEM user's guide. University of California at San Francisco

Park JY, Kim JH, Kim WY, et al (2005) Effect of fresh gas flow on isoflurane concentrations during low-flow anaesthesia. J Int Med Res 33:513–519

Rehberg B, Bouillon T, Zinserling J, Hoeft A (1999) Comparative pharmacodynamic modeling of the electroencephalography-slowing effect of isoflurane, sevoflurane, and desflurane. Anesthesiology 91:397–405

Rietbrock S, Wissing H, Kuhn I, Fuhr U (2000) Pharmacokinetics of inhaled anaesthetics in a clinical setting: description of a novel method based on routine monitoring data. Br J Anaesth 84:437–442

Sani O, Shafer SL (2003) MAC attack? Anesthesiology 99:1249–1250

Severinghaus JW (1954) The rate of uptake of nitrous oxide in man. J Clin Invest 33:1183–1189

Shafer SL (1998) Principles of pharmacokinetics and pharmacodynamics. In: Longnecker DE, Tinker JH, Morgan GE Jr (eds) Principles and practice of anesthesiology, 2nd edn. Mosby, St. Louis, p 1173

Slock E, Hendrickx J, Van Zundert A, et al (2003) Effect of carrier gases on isoflurane vaporizer dial settings during minimal flow anesthesia. Eur J Anaesthesiol 30:A453

Sobreira DP, Jreige MM, Saraiva R (2001) The fresh-gas flow sequence at the start of low-flow anaesthesia. Anaesthesia 56:379–380

Stoelting RK, Longnecker DE, Eger EI (1970) Minimum alveolar concentrations in man on awakening from methoxyflurane, halothane, ether and fluroxene anesthesia: MAC awake. Anesthesiology 33:5–9

Tempia A, Olivei MC, Calza E, et al (2003) The anesthetic conserving device compared with conventional circle system used under different flow conditions for inhaled anesthesia. Anesth Analg 96:1056–1061

Varvel JR, Donoho DL, Shafer SL (1992) Measuring the predictive performance of computer-controlled infusion pumps. J Pharmacokinet Biopharm 20:63–94

Vermeulen P (2000) Tuning a physiological model for closed-circuit anaesthesia. PhD thesis. University of Utrecht, pp 41–67

Vermeulen PM, Lerou JG, Dirksen R, et al (1995) A system model for halothane closed-circuit anesthesia. Structure considerations and performance evaluation. Anesthesiology 83:515–527

Vermeulen PM, Lerou JG, Dirksen R, et al (1997) Repeated enflurane anaesthetics and model predictions: a study of the variability in the predictive performance measures. Br J Anaesth 79:488–496

Virtue RW (1974) Minimal-flow nitrous oxide anesthesia. Anesthesiology 40:196–198

Westenskow DR, Jordan WS, Hayes JK (1983) Uptake of enflurane: a study of the variability between patients. Br J Anaesth 55:595–601

Wissing H, Kuhn I, Rietbrock S, Fuhr U (2000) Pharmacokinetics of inhaled anaesthetics in a clinical setting: comparison of desflurane, isoflurane and sevoflurane. Br J Anaesth 84:443–449

Yasuda N, Targ AG, Eger EI (1989) Solubility of I-653, sevoflurane, isoflurane, and halothane in human tissues. Anesth Analg 69:370–373

Yasuda N, Lockhart SH, Eger EI, et al (1991a) Kinetics of desflurane, isoflurane, and halothane in humans. Anesthesiology 74:489–498

Yasuda N, Lockhart SH, Eger EI, et al (1991b) Comparison of kinetics of sevoflurane and isoflurane in humans. Anesth Analg 72:316–324

Inhalational Anaesthetics and Cardioprotection

N.C. Weber(✉) and W. Schlack

Abstract The heart has a strong endogenous cardioprotection mechanism that can be triggered by short periods of ischaemia (like during angina) and protects the myocardium during a subsequent ischaemic event (like during a myocardial infarction). This important mechanism, called ischaemic pre-conditioning, has been extensively investigated, but the practical relevance of an intervention by inducing ischaemia is mainly limited to experimental situations. Research that is more recent has shown that many volatile anaesthetics can induce a similar cardioprotection mechanism, which would be clinically more relevant than inducing cardioprotection by ischaemia. In the last few decades, several laboratory investigations have shown that exposure to inhalational anaesthetics leads to a variety of changes in the protein structure of the myocardium. By a functional blockade of these modified (i.e. activated) target enzymes, it was demonstrated that some of these changes in protein structure and distribution can mediate cardioprotection by anaesthetic pre-conditioning. This chapter gives an overview of our current understanding of the signal transduction of this phenomenon. In addition to an intervention before

N.C. Weber
Department of Anaesthesiology, University of Amsterdam (AMC), Meibergdreef 9, 1100 DD Amsterdam, The Netherlands
N.C.hauck@amc.uva.nl

J. Schüttler and H. Schwilden (eds.) *Modern Anesthetics.*
Handbook of Experimental Pharmacology 182.

ischaemia (i.e. pre-conditioning), there are two more time windows when a substance may interact with the ischaemia–reperfusion process and might modify the extent of injury: (1) during ischaemia or (2) after ischaemia (i.e. during reperfusion) (post-conditioning). In animal experiments, the volatile anaesthetics also interact with these mechanisms (especially immediately after ischaemia), i.e. by post-conditioning. Since ischaemia–reperfusion of the heart routinely occurs in a variety of clinical situations such as during transplant surgery, coronary artery bypass grafting, valve repair or vascular surgery, anaesthetic-induced cardioprotection might be a promising option to protect the myocardium in clinical situations. Initial studies now confirm an effect on surrogate outcome parameters such as length of ICU or in-hospital stay or post-ischaemic troponin release. In this chapter, we will summarize our current understanding of the three mechanisms of anaesthetic cardioprotection exerted by inhalational anaesthetics.

1 Effects of Anaesthetics During Ischaemia

The first investigations in 1969 revealed a beneficial role of volatile anaesthetics during myocardial ischaemia (Spieckermann et al. 1969). During halothane anaesthesia, a prolonged tolerance to global ischaemia and enhanced preservation of high-energy compounds in dog hearts was found. Several studies demonstrated that volatile anaesthetics reduced myocardial oxygen demand during ischaemia, resulting in a reduced ischaemic damage (Buljubasic et al. 1992, 1993; Davis et al. 1983). In patients with coronary heart disease, isoflurane improved the tolerance to pacing-induced myocardial ischaemia (Tarnow et al. 1986). Additionally, sevoflurane and desflurane showed anti-ischaemic properties (Oguchi et al. 1995; Pagel et al. 1995; Takahata et al. 1995). As mechanisms behind this protection, the negative inotropic and negative chronotropic action of the anaesthetics is suggested. Moreover, volatile anaesthetics maintain myocardial energy stores and might increase collateral blood flow towards the ischaemic area, thereby reducing the severity of ischaemia. However, one has to take into account that the overall direct anti-ischaemic effect of the anaesthetics is relatively small in comparison to their pre-ischaemic (pre-conditioning, see Sect. 3) effects or their effects against reperfusion injury (post-conditioning). Therefore, the transfer to the clinical setting from the direct anti-ischaemic action of anaesthetics appears to be very limited.

2 Effects of Anaesthetics During Reperfusion (Post-conditioning)

2.1 *Reperfusion Injury*

Subjection of a tissue to ischaemia results in a variety of chemical events that may finally lead to cellular dysfunction and necrosis. If ischaemia is stopped by the restoration of blood flow, a second series of harmful events produces additional injury.

This means whenever there is a transient decrease or even an interruption of blood flow the injury results from two components—the direct injury occurring during the ischaemic period and the indirect or reperfusion injury which follows. The "reperfusion injury" is defined as "metabolic, functional and structural changes after restoration of coronary perfusion, which can be reduced or prohibited by modification of the reperfusion conditions" (Rosenkranz and Buckberg 1983). The reperfusion injury can be divided into a non-lethal, reversible cellular damage and a lethal, irreversible damage. During long-term ischaemia, the ischaemic damage resulting from hypoxia alone is the predominant mechanism. For shorter durations of ischaemia, the reperfusion-mediated damage becomes increasingly more important.

Non-lethal reperfusion injury includes myocardial arrhythmias and the post-ischaemic reduction of myocardial function. The reversible, but delayed recovery of myocardial function after complete restoration of coronary blood flow is called "myocardial stunning" (Braunwald and Kloner 1982). Lethal reperfusion injury is characterized by irreversible cell death (myocardial necrosis) and can be divided into an early (immediately at the beginning of reperfusion) and a late phase of myocardial damage. The different characteristics of the reperfusion injury are caused by distinct pathomechanisms, which can be modified by therapeutic interventions. For detailed description of the pathomechanisms and how anaesthetics can interact see the review by Preckel and Schlack (2002).

2.2 *Interaction of Anaesthetics with Reperfusion Injury*

Already in 1996, a specific protection against myocardial reperfusion injury by halothane was described (Schlack et al. 1996). This study clearly showed for the first time that modification of the reperfusion conditions by administration of a common volatile anaesthetic specifically reduced reperfusion damage. This cardioprotective effect could be confirmed for enflurane, isoflurane, sevoflurane and desflurane and the noble gas xenon under a variety of experimental conditions in vitro and in vivo; cardioprotection against reperfusion damage by anaesthetics was also maintained when the heart was already protected against ischaemic damage by cardioplegic solutions (for review see Preckel and Schlack 2002). The cardioprotection in all these studies was very pronounced, leading to an infarct size reduction of about 50%. In the following years, several specific mechanisms were identified: a direct action at the myocardial cell against immediate damage by an interaction with the ryanodine receptor of the sarcoplasmic reticulum (Siegmund et al. 1997) and indirect effects by modulating neutrophil-mediated damage (Kowalski et al. 1997). A study from Chiari and co-workers identified the phosphatidylinositol-3-kinase (PI_3) as a mediator enzyme when 1MAC (minimum alveolar concentration) isoflurane was administered during reperfusion (Chiari et al. 2005). Recent data from Pagel et al. showed that isoflurane-induced post-conditioning involves extracellular signal-regulated kinase (ERK) 1/2, eNOS and p70s6K (70-kDa ribosomal protein S6 kinase) (Krolikowski et al. 2006). Regarding isoflurane post-conditioning, mitochondrial K_{ATP} channels were also identified as mediators by Tosaka et al. (2005). In patients undergoing coronary bypass grafting, 1.7 vol% of isoflurane given for the first 15 min after the release of the aortic cross clamp led to a substantial reduction in the need for inotropic support and protected against myocardial damage assessed by post-operative troponin release (Buhre 2001). However, in a recent study by De Hert and co-workers the reduction of troponin I release by the volatile anaesthetic did only reach statistical significance when the substance was given throughout the procedure (De Hert et al. 2004a).

In contrast to inhalational anaesthetics, with intravenous anaesthetics there is little evidence of cardioprotection during ischaemia–reperfusion situations. Propofol, for example, is known as a free oxygen radical scavenger and inhibits calcium influx across plasma membranes, but does not improve post-ischaemic myocardial function (Ross et al. 1998). Given only during the reperfusion period, propofol itself provided no protective effect against cellular damage in isolated rat hearts (Ebel et al. 1999).

3 Effects of Anaesthetics Before Ischaemia (Pre-conditioning)

3.1 Background: Ischaemic Pre-conditioning

As the strongest endogenous protective mechanism of the heart against the consequences of ischaemia "ischaemic pre-conditioning" was first described by Murry et al. (1986). First, only the early phase of protection (classic or early pre-conditioning) beginning shortly after the pre-conditioning stimulus and lasting for 2–3 h (Kloner and Jennings 2001a b) was described. However, later studies demonstrated the existence of a second episode of myocardial protection (late pre-conditioning), which begins 12–24 h after the pre-conditioning stimulus and lasts for 48–72 h (Baxter et al. 1994; Marber et al. 1993).

During the phases of pre-conditioning there exist triggers, i.e. mechanisms at the beginning of the signal transduction cascade, and mediators, which finally mediate cardioprotection during the long infarct-inducing (index) ischaemia (Fig. 1). For ischaemic pre-conditioning, the activation of adenosine (Kitakaze et al. 1994), α-adrenergic (Tsuchida et al. 1994), muscarinic (Yao and Gross 1993), opioid (Schultz et al. 1996) or bradykinin (Hartman et al. 1993) receptors during the pre-conditioning ischaemia is known to trigger subsequent steps of the signal transduction pathway (Fig. 1). The activation of these receptors by different drugs (e.g. by anaesthetics) mimics ischaemic pre-conditioning and this results in the activation of inhibitory G proteins (Kirsch et al. 1990) and protein kinase C (PKC) (Light et al. 1996; Speechly-Dick et al. 1995). This activation of PKC affects other signalling pathways such as Raf-MEK1-MAP kinases and the PI3-kinase-Akt cascade (Kuboki et al. 2000; Takahashi et al. 1999). Moreover, the release of free radicals activates different kinases including PKC (mainly its ε-isoform) (Gopalakrishna and Anderson 1989; Yang et al. 1997), tyrosine kinases (Baines et al. 1998; Fryer et al. 1998) and mitogen-activated protein kinases (MAPK) (Weinbrenner et al. 1997; for

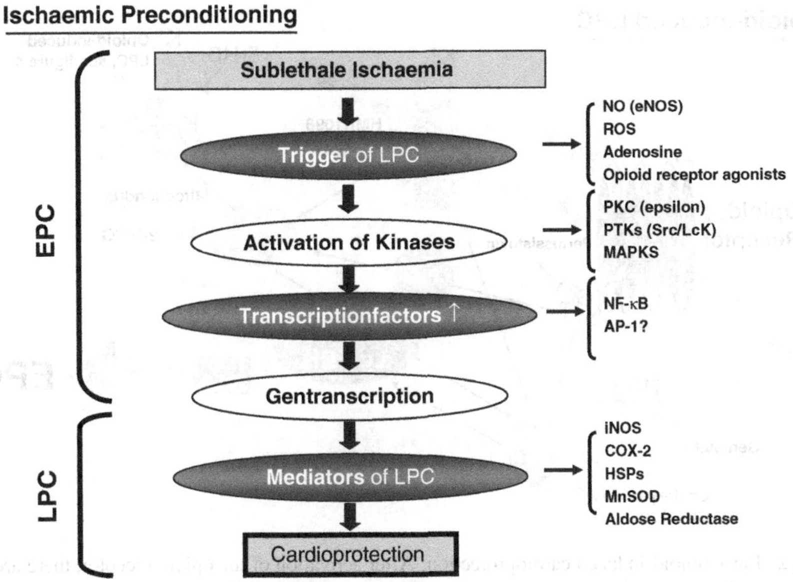

Fig. 1 Overview of the general mechanisms involved in ischaemic pre-conditioning that are activated in early (EPC, day 1) or late (LPC, day 2–3) pre-conditioning. Several of these molecular targets can also be affected by anaesthetics (see Fig. 2). First, during early pre-conditioning, triggers of pre-conditioning like ROS (reactive oxygen species), NO (nitric oxide) derived from endothelial nitrous oxide synthase and adenosine are activated or released in the myocardial cell. Upon their release, they initiate the phosphorylation and/or translocation of different kinases such as PKC (protein kinase C), tyrosine kinases and mitogen-activated protein kinases (MAPK). These activated kinases can up-regulate the activity of different transcription factors such as nuclear factor κ B (NF-κB) and activator protein 1 (AP-1). The up-regulation of transcription factors results in an increased gene transcription of different mediators of pre-conditioning such as inducible nitrous oxide synthase (iNOS), cyclooxygenase 2 (COX-2), aldose reductase, manganese super oxide dismutase (MnSOD), 12-lipoxygenase (12-LO) and heat shock proteins (HSPs)

review see Das et al. 1999) which act as triggers and/or mediators of the resulting cardioprotection (Fryer et al. 1998, 1999; Hattori et al. 2001; Maulik et al. 1998). As this chapter focusses on anaesthetic-induced cardioprotection, ischaemic preconditioning will not be discussed in detail. For an extended review see Kloner and Jennings (2001a, b).

3.2 *Anaesthetic-Induced Pre-conditioning*

Ischaemic pre-conditioning can be mimicked by different inhalational anaesthetics (see Fig. 2). For many years, ischaemic and anaesthetic-induced pre-conditioning were suggested to share a common pathway, but there exists recent evidence from a microarray study by Zaugg and colleagues that anaesthetic-induced pre-conditioning in comparison to ischaemic pre-conditioning has a more homogeneous and predictable

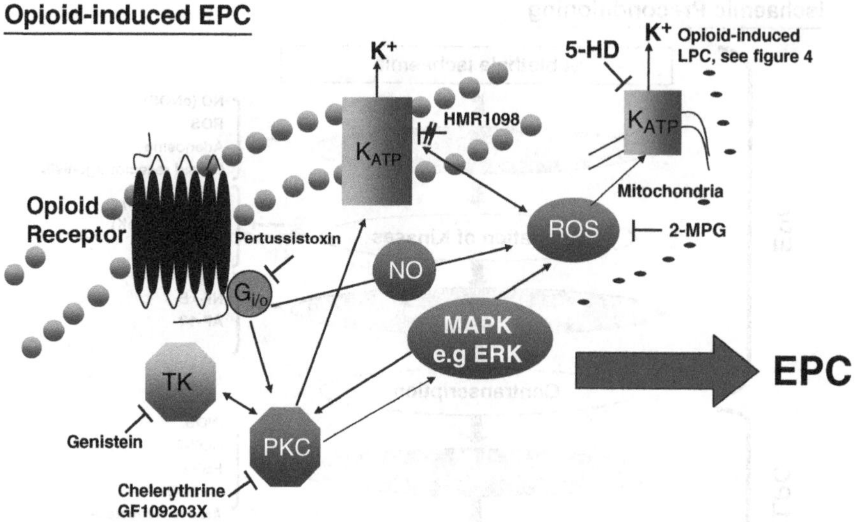

Fig. 2 Early opioid-induced cardioprotection. After activation of the opioid receptor, there are at least two different pathways activated via Gi/o-proteins. 1. Reactive oxygen specimen (ROS), generated from intracellular NO, lead to opening of sarcolemmal ATP sensitive potassium channels (sarcK_{ATP}). K_{ATP}-opening generates additional ROS. 2. Proteinkinase C (PKC) is activated; mainly its isoform ε. At the mitochondrial membrane, PKC-ε phosphorylates mitochondrial K_{ATP} channels (mito K_{ATP}). Blocking mito K_{ATP} channels with the specific antagonist 5-Hydroxydecanoate (5-HD) abolishes acute opioid-induced cardioprotection, while blocking sarcK_{ATP} channels with HMR 1098 did not. Blocking tyrosine kinases (TK) with the unspecific blocking agent genistein, abolishes the cardioprotective effect and prevents the activation of extracellular regulated kinases 1 and 2 (ERK 1/2). Whether TK is downstream or parallel of PKC is currently not clear. If ROS are blocked via 2-mercaptopropionyl glycine (2-MPG), cardioprotection is also abolished, demonstrating the central importance of ROS in acute opioid-induced cardioprotection

cardioprotective phenotype at the transcriptional level (Luchinetti et al. 2004), making anaesthetic-induced pre-conditioning more reliable and safer in clinical applications.

Anaesthetic pre-conditioning by inhalational anaesthetics has been demonstrated in vitro and in vivo in different animal species and in humans. This pre-conditioning effect seems to be a relatively specific action of volatile anaesthetics and the inhalational gas xenon (Weber et al. 2005a). Interestingly, the anaesthetic supplement nitrous oxide did not show pre-conditioning effects on the heart (Weber et al. 2005).

In contrast, the intravenous anaesthetics that have been studied so far, ketamine and propofol, had either no effect (Ebel et al. 1999) or even blocked the cardioprotection induced by pre-conditioning (Mullenheim et al. 2001). However, a very recent study from Zeng and co-workers showed that propofol can pre-condition the isolated heart from renal hypertensive rats and that this effect involves phosphorylation of ERK 1/2 (Cao et al. 2005). With regard to propofol, it is important to mention a recent study by Kehl et al. that demonstrates that this intravenous anaesthetic is able to block desflurane but not ischaemic-induced pre-conditioning in the rabbit (Smul et al. 2005). A similar phenomenon was described for the co-administration of desflurane and metoprolol. Kehl's group showed that metoprolol blocks the pre-conditioning and cardioprotective effects of the volatile anaesthetic desflurane in the rabbit heart in vivo (Lange et al. 2005a). In this context it is interesting that the underlying mechanisms of propofol-induced cardiac effects have been the subject of extensive research in the last few years. Wickley and co-workers showed that propofol in fact induces translocation of different PKC isoforms to distinct subcellular targets in rat ventricular myocytes (Wickley et al. 2006). The same group identified increased NO production as a potential mediator of the negative inotropic actions of propofol in diabetic rat ventricular myocytes (Wickley et al. 2006) and showed that propofol attenuates β_1-adrenoreceptor-mediated cardiac inotropy (Damron et al. 2004). For both effects, PKC activation is suggested as the mediator (Damron et al. 2004; Wickley et al. 2006). However, one has to take into account that these studies are designed as "treatment" studies rather than pre-conditioning studies, since the anaesthetic agent is not eliminated from the myocytes. Nevertheless, these data clearly show that the activation of different cellular targets (e.g. PKC) is not necessarily associated with a cardioprotective effect of anaesthetic agents.

There exists evidence from laboratory investigations that exogenous opioids such as morphine can induce early and late pre-conditioning of the heart. Already in 1996 it was first described that morphine reduces infarct size in rats from 54% to 12% (Schultz et al. 1996). In the rat heart it was shown that δ-opioid receptors mediate ischaemic pre-conditioning (Tsuchida et al. 1998). Interestingly, only δ- and κ-opioid receptors are expressed in the rat heart, but not the μ-receptors to which morphine and fentanyl bind preferentially. G_i protein inhibitors, PKC inhibitors and 5-HD, a selective mitochondrial K_{ATP} channel blocker, can block opioid-induced pre-conditioning. Several additional intracellular mediators similar to those of ischaemic pre-conditioning are involved in opioid-induced pre-conditioning (for extended reviews see Gross 2003; Kato and Foex 2002).

Figure 2 gives an overview over the cellular mediators involved in early pre-conditioning by opioids which are still under investigation.

A recent study showed that also the μ-specific opioid remifentanil when given transiently before ischaemia can modestly reduce infarct size in the rabbit (Kuzume et al. 2004). Surprisingly, the continuous infusion of remifentanil had no infarct size-limiting effect, but even increased the threshold for ischaemic pre-conditioning (Kuzume et al. 2004).

3.3 Animal Experiments, In Vitro

In isolated rat, guinea-pig or rabbit hearts in a Langendorff preparation, 2–10 min administration of 0.5–2.0 MAC of either halothane, enflurane, isoflurane or sevoflurane induced myocardial pre-conditioning (Coetzee et al. 2000; Cope et al. 1997; Novalija et al. 1999). In these experiments, pharmacological-induced pre-conditioning by volatile anaesthetics did not only reduce infarct size (Cope et al. 1997) but it also reduced post-ischaemic myocardial contractile dysfunction ("myocardial stunning") (Coetzee et al. 2000; Novalija et al. 1999) and endothelial dysfunction (Novalija et al. 1999). Extensive research revealed that opening of K_{ATP} channels is an important step in the signal transduction cascade of anaesthetic-induced pre-conditioning: The administration of the unspecific K_{ATP} channel-blocker glibenclamide prior to the administration of the volatile anaesthetics completely abolishes cardioprotection (Coetzee et al. 2000; Novalija et al. 1999). Recent results in cardiac myocytes suggested that anaesthetic-induced pre-conditioning is mediated via sarcolemmal K_{ATP} channels (Marinovic et al. 2006) and also mitochondrial K_{ATP} channels (Mullenheim et al. 2001). In addition, activation of adenosine receptors seems to be involved since pre-conditioning by halothane was blocked by administration of the adenosine receptor blocker 8-(*p*-sulfophenyl)-theophylline during the index-ischaemia (Cope et al. 1997). So far there exists only one study that has investigated the role of PKC during halothane-induced pre-conditioning in isolated rabbit hearts. The study demonstrated that the administration of the PKC blocker chelerythrine during the index-ischaemia blocked halothane-induced cardioprotection (Cope et al. 1997).

The implication of sarcolemmal and mitochondrial K_{ATP} channels in the mechanisms of anaesthetic-induced pre-conditioning in isolated cardiomyocytes was the subject of several studies. Han and co-workers not only demonstrated that isoflurane reduces the inhibitory effect of ATP on K_{ATP} channel opening (Han et al. 1996), but also that the isoflurane metabolite trifluoroacetic acid directly activates K_{ATP} channels. This (in vitro) effect of isoflurane was not prevented by the PKC-blockers polymyxine B and staurosporine, the tyrosine kinase blocker lavendustine A, nor the MAPK blocker SB 203580. In contrast, the group of Bosnjak showed that isoflurane induces prolonged sensitization of sarcolemmal K_{ATP} channels in vitro and in vivo and that this effect was in fact mediated by PKC, since the use of chelerythrine abolished the effect (Marinovic et al. 2005). They could also show that isoflurane pre-conditioning can inhibit the neutrophil-induced apoptotic effect in adult rat cardiomyocytes (Jamnicki-Abegg et al. 2005). Additionally, isoflurane seems to modulate the adenine nucleotide sensitivity of the rat cardiac sarcolemmal K_{ATP} channels differentially (Stadnicka and Bosnjak 2006).

Kohro and co-workers demonstrated in isolated guinea-pig cardiomyocytes that administration of isoflurane or sevoflurane increased the opening probability of mitochondrial K_{ATP} channels in a dose-dependent manner (Kohro et al. 2001). In contrast to these results, a study from Zaugg and co-workers found in isolated rat cardiomyocytes that the administration of isoflurane or sevoflurane did not increase the open-state probability of mitochondrial K_{ATP} channels directly, but that this effect depended on activation of PKC (Zaugg et al. 2002). In the latter study the cardioprotection induced by both volatile anaesthetics did not depend on opening of sarcolemmal K_{ATP} channels (Zaugg et al. 2002). In another study, it has been demonstrated that the administration of isoflurane facilitated opening of sarcolemmal K_{ATP} channels (Fujimoto et al. 2002; Kwok et al. 2002); activation of PKC was crucial for this effect. It has been shown in rabbit vascular smooth muscle cells that isoflurane activates MAPK by translocation of PKCε from the cell membrane to the cytosol (Zhong and Su 2002). This study indicates ERK 1/2 rather than p38 MAPK as a downstream target of PKC after isoflurane administration (Zhong and Su 2002). Using immunohistochemical techniques, Uecker and co-workers confirmed that isoflurane induces cardioprotection by PKC activation. They observed that isoflurane-induced pre-conditioning leads to translocation of PKCδ and PKCε to nuclei (PKCδ and PKCε), to mitochondria (PKCδ) and to the sarcolemma and intercalated disks (PKCε) (Uecker et al. 2003). Only phosphorylation of PKCδ on serine 643 was increased after isoflurane administration but not that of PKCε. The PKC blockers chelerythrine and rottlerin blocked PKC activation and anaesthetic-induced cardioprotection (Uecker et al. 2003). In context with this study one has to take into account that the observed cardioprotection was measured in terms of improved post-ischaemic functional recovery instead of infarct size reduction as the classical endpoint of pre-conditioning studies. Moreover, only one pre-conditioning protocol was used (15 min of isoflurane administration in a concentration of 1.5 MAC) and myocardial tissue samples were collected at only one time point (after the administration of the pre-conditioning stimulus). Another recent study demonstrated a different involvement of MAPK in anaesthetic pre-conditioning (induced by 1.5 MAC isoflurane) and ischaemic pre-conditioning in the isolated rat heart (Da Silva et al. 2004). These in vitro results are in contrast to results of our laboratory using an in vivo model (see the following section) pointing to the fact that the use of different pre-conditioning protocols and experimental conditions may influence the pre-conditioning signal transduction pathways.

Figure 3 gives an overview of the cellular mediators involved in early anaesthetic-induced pre-conditioning which are still under investigation.

3.4 *Animal Experiments, In Vivo*

Pharmacologically induced early pre-conditioning by desflurane, isoflurane or sevoflurane reduced infarct size to the same extent as ischaemic pre-conditioning by a 5-min coronary artery occlusion in rats (Obal et al. 2005; Toma et al. 2004; Weber et al. 2005a), rabbits and dogs (Cason et al. 1997; Ismaeil et al. 1999a, b; Kersten et al. 1997; Piriou et al. 2000; Toller et al. 1999, 2000). The volatile anaesthetics were administered for 5–75 min 15–30 min before the infarct-inducing ischaemia in concentrations corresponding to 0.5–1.0 MAC or in a multiple cycle pre-conditioning protocol (Toma et al. 2004; Weber et al. 2005a).

In contrast to early pre-conditioning, the phenomenon of late pre-conditioning was for a long time thought not to be mediated by volatile anaesthetics (Kehl et al. 2002). Interestingly, there exists increasing evidence from different in vivo models that isoflurane and sevoflurane can produce a second window of cardioprotection (Lutz and Liu 2004; Takahashi et al. 2004; Tsutsumi et al. 2006), in case of sevoflurane up to 72 h after the pre-conditioning insult (Hong 2005). The mechanisms by which volatile anaesthetics may mediate this delayed cardioprotection are currently under investigation and first results revealed that isoflurane-induced late pre-conditioning is mediated by nitrous oxide synthase in the rat heart (Takahashi et al. 2005).

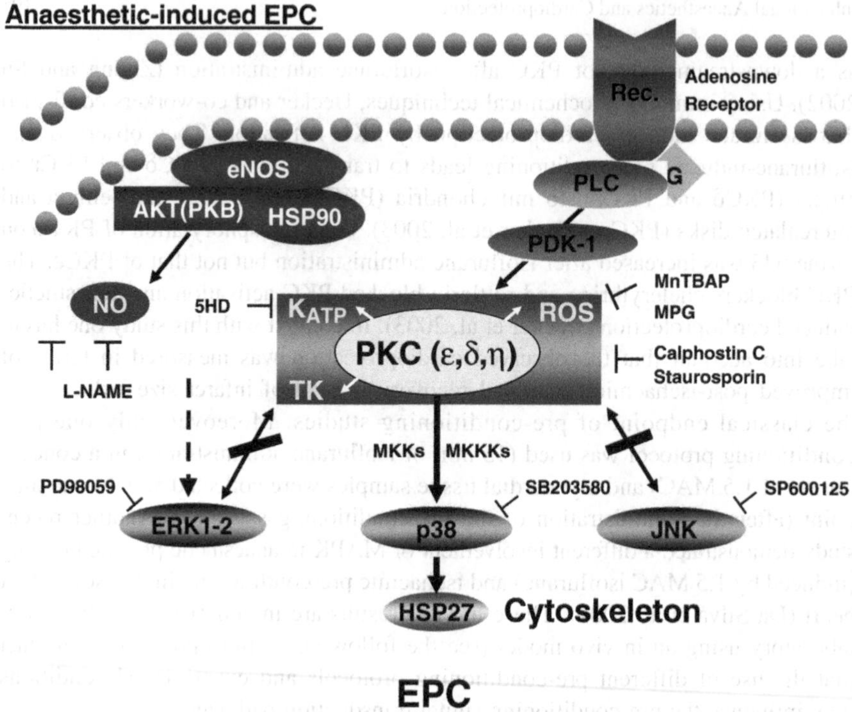

Fig. 3 Overview of the mechanisms of early pre-conditioning. Pre-conditioning by volatile anaesthetics involves the activation of PKC. The effect was shown by the use of specific PKC inhibitors: staurosporine and calphostin C. Also tyrosine kinases (TK) are discussed as mediators of cardioprotection by volatile anaesthetics, but their relationship to PKC is yet not defined. In addition, the family of MAPK: p38, JNK and ERK seems to be involved since the blockade by the specific inhibitors PD 98059 (ERK 1/2) and SB 203580 (p38 MAPK) completely abolished the cardioprotection elicited by volatile anaesthetics. Whether the upstream kinases of MAPK, the mitogen-activated protein kinase kinases (MAPKKs) and mitogen-activated protein kinase kinase kinases (MAPKKKs) are involved is poorly investigated and remains to be determined. Downstream of p38 MAPK, the phosphorylation of a member of the heat shock protein family, HSP27, is upregulated, resulting in cytoskeleton changes of the myocytes. The upstream signalling of PKC is not yet clearly defined. If the activation occurs via the phospholipase C (PLC)/3-phosphoinositide-dependent kinase 1 (PDK-1) pathway involving activation of G protein-linked receptors or via opening of mitochondrial K_{ATP} (mitoK_{ATP}) channels and release of reactive oxygen species (ROS), or in parallel has to be determined in detail. The role of mitoK_{ATP} channels has been extensively studied by the use of 5-hydroxydecanoate (5-HD), a specific blocker of the mitoK_{ATP} channels. Alternatively, it is suggested that the activation of endothelial nitric oxide synthase (eNOS), Akt, HSP90 complex may lead to NO release and that this in turn activates KATP channels. A role for both, NO and ROS, in anaesthetic-induced pre-conditioning has been shown by the use of NG-nitro-l-arginine methyl ester (l-NAME), a specific NOS blocker, and *N*-(2-mercaptopropionyl)gly cine (MPG), a free radical scavenger. The final steps to the still unknown end-effector mediating the protection by ischaemic and anaesthetic-induced pre-conditioning are still under investigation. *AKT (PKB)*, protein kinase B; *eNOS*, endothelial nitric oxide synthase; *ERK 1/2*, extracellular signalling regulated kinase 1 and 2; *mKATP*, mitochondrial ATP-sensitive potassium channel; *HSP27*, heat shock protein 27; *HSP90*, heat shock protein 90; *JNK*, c-jun NH2-terminal kinase; *MKKs*, mitogen activated protein kinase kinases; *MKKKs*, mitogen-activated protein kinase kinase kinases; *p38*, mitogen-activated protein kinase p38; *PDK*, phosphatidylinositol trisphosphate-dependent kinase; *PLC*, protein lipase C. Calphostin C and staurosporine block protein kinase C; l-NAME blocks nitric oxide synthesis; SP 600125 blocks JNK; PD 98059 blocks ERK 1/2; 5HD blocks mitochondrial ATP-sensitive potassium channels

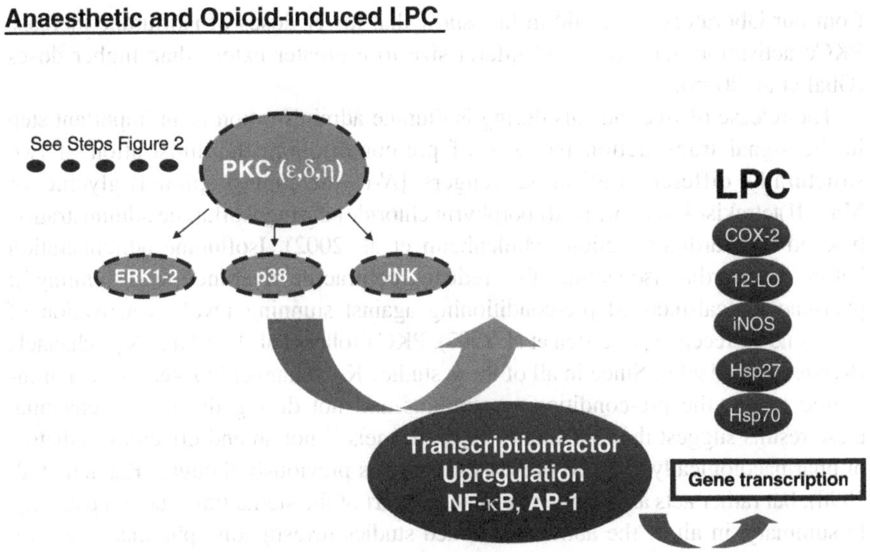

Fig. 4 Delayed anaesthetic and opioid-induced cardioprotection. Following the steps of early pre-conditioning in Fig. 2, PKC and its downstream targets such as extracellular signalling regulated kinase (ERK 1/2) are activated during early pre-conditioning. In the next step the activation of NF-κB is initiated (late pre-conditioning). This activation is thought to mediate the de novo synthesis of at least three mediators of delayed opioid-induced cardioprotection: the inducible isoform of NO-synthetase (iNOS); the COX-2 and 12-LO. How these mediators promote cardioprotection remains unclear

Opioids can also stimulate late pre-conditioning in vivo, and the mechanism is under investigation. A recent study of our laboratory showed that the transcription factor NF-κB is involved in morphine induced pre-conditioning (Fraessdorf et al. 2005). Figure 4 gives an overview of our current concept of the intracellular signalling of anaesthetic and opioid-induced late cardioprotection.

For early pre-conditioning the in vivo experiments confirmed the results of previous in vitro studies that opening of mitochondrial and/or sarcolemmal K_{ATP} channels is a key mechanism of the signal transduction cascade of pharmacologically induced pre-conditioning by volatile anaesthetics (Ismaeil et al. 1999a; Piriou et al. 2000). Activation of adenosine receptors and inhibitory G proteins (Toller et al. 2000) triggers the cardioprotection conferred by isoflurane-induced pre-conditioning. Opening of stretch activated channels is also involved: administration of gadolinium, a blocker of these channels prior to isoflurane administration, also blocked the pre-conditioning effect (Piriou et al. 2000). So far only two studies have investigated whether or not isoflurane-induced early pre-conditioning is dose related. The data from the investigations by Kehl and co-workers provided evidence that the threshold for induction of pre-conditioning by a 30-min period of isoflurane inhalation is 0.25 MAC in dogs. Protection was only dose-dependent in the presence of a low coronary collateral blood flow (Kehl et al. 2002b). In contrast in a recent study from our laboratory we could in fact show that lower doses of isoflurane increase PKCε activation and decreased infarct size to a greater extent than higher doses (Obal et al. 2005).

The release of free radicals during isoflurane administration is an important step in the signal transduction pathway of pre-conditioning: administration of two structurally different radical scavengers [*N*-(2-mercaptopropionyl)-glycine or Mn-(III)tetrakis(4-benzoic acid) porphyrin chloride] during isoflurane administration blocked the cardioprotection (Mullenheim et al. 2002). Isoflurane administration before myocardial ischaemia also reduces contractile dysfunction ("stunning"): pharmacological-induced pre-conditioning against stunning involves activation of adenosine-A_1 receptors (Kersten et al. 1997), PKC (Toller et al. 1999) and K_{ATP} channels (Kersten et al. 1999). Since in all of these studies K_{ATP} channel blockers were administered before the pre-conditioning stimulus and not during the index-ischaemia, these results suggest that opening of K_{ATP} channels is not an end-effector (mediator) of pharmacologically induced pre-conditioning as previously thought (Kersten et al. 1998), but rather acts as a trigger, i.e. an early part of the signal transduction pathway. In summary, in all of the above-mentioned studies investigating pharmacologically induced pre-conditioning by isoflurane, the isoflurane administration was followed by a 15-min washout period, suggesting that isoflurane might trigger other unknown mechanisms of a signal transduction cascade. This hypothesis of the involvement of further downstream targets is also supported by the finding that an intact cytoskeleton is a prerequisite for pharmacologically induced pre-conditioning by isoflurane: administration of colchicine, which disrupts the cytoskeleton, prevents the pre-conditioning effect of isoflurane (Ismaeil et al. 1999b).

In this context, we could detect the activation of small heat shock protein 27 (HSP27) (Weber et al. 2005b) and co-localization of HSP27 with the actin cytoskeleton after both xenon and isoflurane administration in a pre-conditioning manner.

Regarding parallel mechanisms of anaesthetic and ischaemic pre-conditioning, recent laboratory investigations showed that desflurane-induced pre-conditioning is mediated by β-adrenergic receptors in the rabbit heart in vivo (Lange et al. 2005b). In several recent investigations in our laboratory we could confirm the molecular mechanisms found in vitro for in vivo systems. In contrast to the study of Uecker and co-workers, who did not find an increased phosphorylation of PKCε after 15 min of isoflurane (1.5 MAC) administration in the isolated rat heart (Uecker et al. 2003), we could show that isoflurane (0.4 MAC) as well as the inhalative gas xenon administered for 3×5 min before ischaemia reperfusion in an in vivo rat model significantly reduced the infarct size and that this cardioprotection was in fact mediated via an increased phosphorylation and translocation of PKCε (Weber et al. 2005a). Moreover, we could identify the p38 MAPK as a downstream target of PKCε in isoflurane- and xenon-induced pre-conditioning (Weber et al. 2005a). In contrast to our results, Roissant's group could not find a cardioprotective effect of the noble gas xenon (1 MAC) in pigs using a one cycle pre-conditioning model (Baumert et al. 2004) and no influence for xenon on post-ischaemia recovery of left ventricular (LV) function in pigs when given throughout the whole experiment (Hein et al. 2004). Regarding the implication of p38 MAPK in pre-conditioning there exists a current study performed in isolated perfused hearts of guinea-pigs that is in contrast to our findings. This study did not find an involvement of p38 MAPK in the signal transduction of sevoflurane-induced cardioprotection (Sugioka et al. 2004).

The activation of different proteins may follow a certain time course with a rapid return towards normal activity levels for some steps of the signal transduction cascade. Desflurane was shown to activate PKCε and ERK 1/2 in a time-dependent manner (Toma et al. 2004). Moreover, xenon-induced pre-conditioning differentially regulated MAPK. We found that ERK 1/2 is involved in xenon pre-conditioning, but that the functional blockade of c-Jun N-terminal kinase (JNK) did not abolish the cardioprotective effect of xenon (Weber et al. 2006). Most importantly, different concentrations of the anaesthetic may have different effects on the proteins involved in signal transduction: For isoflurane, low but not high concentrations of this anaesthetic protect the heart by pre-conditioning and this effect is mediated via increased phosphorylation and translocation of PKCε (Obal et al. 2005).

It is obvious that the above-mentioned results from in vivo studies are often in contrast to the results obtained from in vitro studies. This divergent data may be explained by distinct discrepancies between in vivo and in vitro situations. This points to the fact that further in vivo studies are needed to expand our knowledge of the underlying molecular mechanisms of anaesthetic-induced cardioprotection in order to allow a limited transfer to the clinical situation.

3.5 *Human Myocardium, In Vitro*

To date there exist few data on studies of isolated human atrial tissue. However, most of the studies could confirm the results from animal studies. In human atrial tissue it was shown that adenosine A_1 receptor activation and K_{ATP} channel opening is essential for pharmacologically induced pre-conditioning by isoflurane (Roscoe et al. 2000). However, for halothane no protective effect was found. In the same study, patch clamp measurements did not demonstrate a direct effect of both volatile anaesthetics on K_{ATP} channel-opening probabilities. Desflurane pre-conditions human atrial myocardium by activation of adenosine A_1 receptors, α- and β-adrenoceptors and mitochondrial K_{ATP} channels (Hanouz et al. 2002). Additionally, for sevoflurane it was demonstrated that pre-conditioning induced by 10 min administration of 2 MAC sevoflurane preserves myocardial and renal function in patients undergoing coronary artery bypass graft surgery under cardioplegic arrest and that PKCδ and -ε are activated and translocated in response to sevoflurane in the human myocardium (Julier et al. 2003).

4 Clinical Implications of Anaesthetic Pre-conditioning?

Concerning the transfer of anaesthetic pre-conditioning to the clinical situation, i.e. administration of the volatile anaesthetic before aortic cross clamping, several studies have shown a pre-conditioning effect for isoflurane (Belhomme et al. 1999;

Haroun-Bizri et al. 2001; Tomai et al. 1999), enflurane (Penta de Peppo et al. 1999) and sevoflurane (Julier et al. 2003). All studies used relatively small groups of patients (*n*=20–72) and consequently, had to focus on surrogate outcome markers such as post-ischaemic dysfunction and release of markers of cellular damage such as troponins. Most of the mentioned studies found a better myocardial function (or less dysfunction) (Haroun-Bizri et al. 2001; Julier et al. 2003; Penta de Peppo et al. 1999), a decrease in myocardial injury markers, or both (Tomai et al. 1999; only a tendency: Belhomme et al. 1999). Two of the studies also demonstrated an increase of biochemical markers indicating crucial signal transduction steps of pre-conditioning in biopsies of human myocardium (Belhomme et al. 1999; Julier et al. 2003).

The first more "clinical" approach that combines the different protective mechanisms was used by De Hert and co-workers in 2002. They gave the volatile anaesthetic sevoflurane throughout the procedure (coronary bypass surgery) and compared the volatile anaesthetic-based anaesthesia with total intravenous anaesthesia by propofol (De Hert et al. 2002). Although only 20 patients with good pre-operative LV function were enrolled, the study could show a clear difference. There was better ventricular function after coming off bypass in the sevoflurane group and less myocardial damage measured by a markedly reduced troponin release in the following 26 h. Interestingly, the results of the latter study could be confirmed in elderly patients with poor ventricular function (De Hert et al. 2003).

A larger trial from July 2004 revealed that desflurane and sevoflurane decreased troponin I release when compared with midazolam and propofol anaesthesia (De Hert et al. 2004b). Moreover, a recent study from De Hert's group investigated different administration modalities of sevoflurane before (pre-conditioning), during and after (i.e. post-conditioning) cardiopulmonary bypass (De Hert et al. 2004a). Interestingly, only the administration of sevoflurane throughout the whole operation procedure had a significant effect on troponin I release and duration of in-hospital stay (De Hert et al. 2004a). In a recent study in our laboratory we observed that the intermitted administration of 1 MAC sevoflurane for two times 5 min before coronary artery bypass grafting (CABG) results in significantly reduced troponin I release, while the administration of only one 5-min pre-conditioning period had no cardioprotective effect (Fraessdorf et al. 2005). These data clearly indicate that the phenomenon of pre-conditioning can be elicited in humans, but that the timing and protocol of the anaesthetic administration seems to be critically important.

Taken together, the optimal dosing and timing for application of the volatile anaesthetic in the clinical setting cannot yet be concluded from the results of the present studies. So far it seems that the application thorough the whole procedure might be the method of choice. However, larger randomized clinical studies need to be conducted in order to understand what mechanisms (i.e. pre- and/or post-conditioning) are responsible for clinical cardioprotection by anaesthetics and how the phenomenon of anaesthetic-induced cardioprotection can be most effectively transferred to the clinical situation.

5 Potential Harmful Mechanisms: Blockade of Cardioprotection by Anaesthetics and Oral Anti-diabetics

Opening of the (mitochondrial) K_{ATP}-channel is a central mechanism in the signal transduction of pre-conditioning (Fig. 2). Both barbiturates and ketamine can block K_{ATP}-channels in isolated cells. While thiopental appeared to be safe and did not block experimental pre-conditioning at clinical doses (Mullenheim et al. 2001), several studies found that ketamine completely blocked the cardioprotection of ischaemic pre-conditioning both in vitro and in vivo (for example: Mullenheim et al. 2001); the effect was stereospecific for the R(−)-isomer. In experimental models, the substances propofol, etomidate, midazolam, dexmedetomidine and mivazerol had no effects on K_{ATP} channel activity (for review see Zaugg et al. 2003). A recent study from our laboratory showed that lidocaine blocks ischaemic pre-conditioning only when used at supratherapeutic concentrations (Barthel et al. 2004). Moreover, it was shown by Kehl and co-workers that propofol might block desflurane-induced pre-conditioning but not ischaemic pre-conditioning (Smul et al. 2005).

While the clinical importance of these findings remains unknown, it seems to be safer to avoid racemic ketamine in clinical settings where ischaemia-reperfusion is likely to occur. Sulphonylurea oral anti-diabetics such as glibenclamide can block the K_{ATP}-channel and prevent cardioprotection by pre-conditioning. Recent evidence suggests that a patient with type II diabetes and coronary artery disease may profit from changing the treatment to insulin (by having less ischaemia-induced myocardial dysfunction) (Scognamiglio et al. 2002). Moreover, hyperglycaemia blocks desflurane-induced early pre-conditioning in the rat in vivo (Ebel et al. 2005) and also the late phase of pre-conditioning induced by isoflurane (Kehl et al. 2002a).

From the data discussed above it is obvious that there exists increasing evidence for a strong cardioprotective mechanisms being exerted by anaesthetic agents and especially inhalational anaesthetics. Anaesthetics may induce myocardial protection and, in some cases, they may block protective mechanisms. The recent results from all the above-discussed studies indicate that the phenomenon of anaesthetic-induced cardioprotection can be transferred in part to the clinical situation. Further progress in elucidating the underlying mechanisms of anaesthetic-induced cardioprotection does not only reflect an important increase in scientific knowledge, but may also offer the new possibility of using different anaesthetics for targeted intraoperative myocardial protection.

References

Baines CP, Wang L, Cohen MV, Downey JM (1998) Protein tyrosine kinase is downstream of protein kinase C for ischemic preconditioning's anti-infarct effect in the rabbit heart. J Mol Cell Cardiol 30:383–392

Barthel H, Ebel D, Mullenheim J, Obal D, Preckel B, Schlack W (2004) Effect of lidocaine on ischaemic preconditioning in isolated rat heart. Br J Anaesth 93:698–704

Baumert JH, Hein M, Roissant R (2004) Effects of Xenon on myocardial infarct size. Anesthesiology 101:A635

Baxter GF, Marber MS, Patel VC, Yellon DM (1994) Adenosine receptor involvement in a delayed phase of myocardial protection 24 hours after ischemic preconditioning. Circulation 90:2993–3000

Belhomme D, Peynet J, Louzy M, Launay JM, Kitakaze M, Menasche P (1999) Evidence for preconditioning by isoflurane in coronary artery bypass graft surgery. Circulation 100: II340–II344

Braunwald E, Kloner RA (1982) The stunned myocardium: prolonged, postischemic ventricular dysfunction. Circulation 66:1146–1149

Buhre W (2001) Cardioprotective and anti-inflammatory action of isoflurane during coronary artery bypass surgery. Thesis/dissertation

Buljubasic N, Marijic J, Stowe DF, Kampine JP, Bosnjak ZJ (1992) Halothane reduces dysrhythmias and improves contractile function after global hypoperfusion in isolated hearts. Anesth Analg 74:384–394

Buljubasic N, Stowe DF, Marijic J, Roerig DL, Kampine JP, Bosnjak ZJ (1993) Halothane reduces release of adenosine, inosine, and lactate with ischemia and reperfusion in isolated hearts. Anesth Analg 76:54–62

Cao H, Gui B, Li J, Lian Q, Zeng Y (2005) p-ERK 1/2 involved in propofol preconditioning on ischemic/reperfused injury in isolated renal hypertension rat hearts. Anesthesiology 103:A546

Cason BA, Gamperl AK, Slocum RE, Hickey RF (1997) Anesthetic-induced preconditioning: previous administration of isoflurane decreases myocardial infarct size in rabbits. Anesthesiology 87:1182–1190

Chiari PC, Bienengraeber MW, Pagel PS, Krolikowski JG, Kersten JR, Warltier DC (2005) Isoflurane protects against myocardial infarction during early reperfusion by activation of phosphatidylinositol-3-kinase signal transduction: evidence for anesthetic-induced postconditioning in rabbits. Anesthesiology 102:102–109

Coetzee JF, le Roux PJ, Genade S, Lochner A (2000) Reduction of postischemic contractile dysfunction of the isolated rat heart by sevoflurane: comparison with halothane. Anesth Analg 90:1089–1097

Cope DK, Impastato WK, Cohen MV, Downey JM (1997) Volatile anesthetics protect the ischemic rabbit myocardium from infarction. Anesthesiology 86:699–709

Da Silva R, Grampp T, Pasch T, Schaub MC, Zaugg M (2004) Differential activation of mitogen-activated protein kinases in ischemic and anesthetic preconditioning. Anesthesiology 100:59–69

Damron DS, Chung KH, Murray PA (2004) Propofol attenuates β1-adrenoreceptor-mediated cardiac inotropy via activation of PKC in diabetic rat cardiomyocytes. Anesthesiology 101: A728

Das DK, Engelman RM, Maulik N (1999) Oxygen free radical signaling in ischemic preconditioning. Ann N Y Acad Sci 874:49–65

Davis RF, DeBoer LW, Rude RE, Lowenstein E, Maroko PR (1983) The effect of halothane anesthesia on myocardial necrosis, hemodynamic performance, and regional myocardial blood flow in dogs following coronary artery occlusion. Anesthesiology 59:402–411

De Hert SG, ten Broecke PW, Mertens E, Van Sommeren EW, De Blier IG, Stockman BA, Rodrigus IE (2002) Sevoflurane but not propofol preserves myocardial function in coronary surgery patients. Anesthesiology 97:42–49

De Hert SG, Cromheecke S, ten Broecke PW, Mertens E, De Blier IG, Stockman BA, Rodrigus IE, Van der Linden PJ (2003) Effects of propofol, desflurane, and sevoflurane on recovery of myocardial function after coronary surgery in elderly high-risk patients. Anesthesiology 99:314–323

De Hert SG, Van der Linden PJ, Cromheecke S, Meeus R, Nelis A, Van Reeth V, ten Broecke PW, De Blier IG, Stockman BA, Rodrigus IE (2004a) Cardioprotective properties of sevoflurane in patients undergoing coronary surgery with cardiopulmonary bypass are related to the modalities of its administration. Anesthesiology 101:299–310

De Hert SG, Van der Linden PJ, Cromheecke S, Meeus R, ten Broecke PW, De Blier IG, Stockman BA, Rodrigus IE (2004b) Choice of primary anesthetic regimen can influence intensive care unit length of stay after coronary surgery with cardiopulmonary bypass. Anesthesiology 101:9–20

Ebel D, Schlack W, Comfere T, Preckel B, Thamer V (1999) Effect of propofol on reperfusion injury after regional ischaemia in the isolated rat heart. Br J Anaesth 83:903–908

Ebel D, Toma O, Weber NC, Huhn R, Preckel B, Schlack W (2005) Hyperglycaemia blocks anaesthetic-induced preconditioning by desflurane during the mediator phase. Eur J Anaesthesiol 22 [Supp34]:A165

Fraessdorf J, Weber NC, Obal D, Toma O, Mullenheim J, Kojda G, Preckel B, Schlack W (2005) Morphine induces late cardioprotection in rat hearts in vivo. Involvement of opioid receptors and NF-κB. Anesth Analg 101:934–941

Fraessdorf J, Weber NC, Feindt P, Borowski A, Schlack W (2005) Sevoflurane-induced preconditioning: evaluation of two different protocols in humans undergoing coronary artery bypass grafting (CABG). Anesthesiology 103:A338

Fryer RM, Schultz JE, Hsu AK, Gross GJ (1998) Pretreatment with tyrosine kinase inhibitors partially attenuates ischemic preconditioning in rat hearts. Am J Physiol 275:H2009–H2015

Fryer RM, Schultz JE, Hsu AK, Gross GJ (1999) Importance of PKC and tyrosine kinase in single or multiple cycles of preconditioning in rat hearts. Am J Physiol 276:H1229–H1235

Fujimoto K, Bosnjak ZJ, Kwok WM (2002) Isoflurane-induced facilitation of the cardiac sarcolemmal K(ATP) channel. Anesthesiology 97:57–65

Gopalakrishna R, Anderson WB (1989) Ca^{2+}- and phospholipid-independent activation of protein kinase C by selective oxidative modification of the regulatory domain. Proc Natl Acad Sci USA 86:6758–6762

Gross GJ (2003) Role of opioids in acute and delayed preconditioning. J Mol Cell Cardiol 35:709–718

Han J, Kim E, Ho WK, Earm YE (1996) Effects of volatile anesthetic isoflurane on ATP-sensitive K+ channels in rabbit ventricular myocytes. Biochem Biophys Res Commun 229:852–856

Hanouz JL, Yvon A, Massetti M, Lepage O, Babatasi G, Khayat A, Bricard H, Gerard JL (2002) Mechanisms of desflurane-induced preconditioning in isolated human right atria in vitro. Anesthesiology 97:33–41

Haroun-Bizri S, Khoury SS, Chehab IR, Kassas CM, Baraka A (2001) Does isoflurane optimize myocardial protection during cardiopulmonary bypass? J Cardiothorac Anesth 15:418–421

Hartman JC, Wall TM, Hullinger TG, Shebuski RJ (1993) Reduction of myocardial infarct size in rabbits by ramiprilat: reversal by the bradykinin antagonist HOE 140. J Cardiovasc Pharmacol 21:996–1003

Hattori R, Otani H, Uchiyama T, Imamura H, Cui J, Maulik N, Cordis GA, Zhu L, Das DK (2001) Src tyrosine kinase is the trigger but not the mediator of ischemic preconditioning. Am J Physiol Heart Circ Physiol 281:H1066–H1074

Hein H, Hecker KE, Horn NA, Roissant R (2004) Xenon anesthesia has no influence on post-ischemia recovery of LV function. Anesthesiology 101:A705

Hong L (2005) Volatile anesthetic preconditioning with sevoflurane provides delayed window of myocardial protection in 72 hours. Anesthesiology 103:A558

Ismaeil MS, Tkachenko I, Gamperl AK, Hickey RF, Cason BA (1999a) Mechanisms of isoflurane-induced myocardial preconditioning in rabbits. Anesthesiology 90:812–821

Ismaeil MS, Tkachenko I, Hickey RF, Cason BA (1999b) Colchicine inhibits isoflurane-induced preconditioning. Anesthesiology 91:1816–1822

Jamnicki-Abegg M, Weihrauch D, Pagel PS, Kersten JR, Bosnjak ZJ, Waltier DC, Bienengraeber M (2005) Isoflurane inhibits cardiac myocyte apoptosis during oxidative and inflammatory stress by activating Akt and enhancing Bcl-2 expression. Anesthesiology 103:1006–1014

Julier K, Da Silva R, Garcia C, Bestmann L, Frascarolo P, Zollinger A, Chassot PG, Schmid ER, Turina MI, von Segesser LK, Pasch T, Spahn DR, Zaugg M (2003) Preconditioning by sevoflurane decreases biochemical markers for myocardial and renal dysfunction in coronary artery bypass graft surgery: a double-blinded, placebo-controlled, multicenter study. Anesthesiology 98:1315–1327

Kato R, Foex P (2002) Myocardial protection by anesthetic agents against ischemia-reperfusion injury: an update for anesthesiologists. Can J Anaesth 49:777–791
Kehl F, Pagel PS, Krolikowski JG, Gu W, Toller W, Warltier DC, Kersten JR (2002) Isoflurane does not produce a second window of preconditioning against myocardial infarction in vivo. Anesth Analg 95:1162–1168
Kehl F, Krolikowski JG, Marinovic B, Pagel PS, Warltier DC, Kersten JR (2002a) Hyperglycemia prevents isoflurane-induced preconditioning against myocardial infarction. Anesthesiology 96:183–188
Kehl F, Krolikowski JG, Mraovic B, Pagel PS, Warltier DC, Kersten JR (2002b) Is isoflurane-induced preconditioning dose related? Anesthesiology 96:675–680
Kersten JR, Orth KG, Pagel PS, Mei DA, Gross GJ, Warltier DC (1997) Role of adenosine in isoflurane-induced cardioprotection. Anesthesiology 86:1128–1139
Kersten JR, Gross GJ, Pagel PS, Warltier DC (1998) Activation of adenosine triphosphate-regulated potassium channels: mediation of cellular and organ protection. Anesthesiology 88:495–513
Kersten JR, Schmeling T, Tessmer J, Hettrick DA, Pagel PS, Warltier DC (1999) Sevoflurane selectively increases coronary collateral blood flow independent of KATP channels in vivo. Anesthesiology 90:246–256
Kirsch GE, Codina J, Birnbaumer L, Brown AM (1990) Coupling of ATP-sensitive K+ channels to A1 receptors by G proteins in rat ventricular myocytes. Am J Physiol 259:H820–H826
Kitakaze M, Hori M, Morioka T, Minamino T, Takashima S, Sato H, Shinozaki Y, Chujo M, Mori H, Inoue M (1994) Infarct size-limiting effect of ischemic preconditioning is blunted by inhibition of 5'-nucleotidase activity and attenuation of adenosine release. Circulation 89:1237–1246
Kloner RA, Jennings RB (2001a) Consequences of brief ischemia: stunning, preconditioning, and their clinical implications: part 2. Circulation 104:3158–3167
Kloner RA, Jennings RB (2001b) Consequences of brief ischemia: stunning, preconditioning, and their clinical implications: part 1. Circulation 104:2981–2989
Kohro S, Hogan QH, Nakae Y, Yamakage M, Bosnjak ZJ (2001) Anesthetic effects on mitochondrial ATP-sensitive K channel. Anesthesiology 95:1335–1340
Kowalski C, Zahler S, Becker BF, Flaucher A, Conzen PF, Gerlach E, Peter K (1997) Halothane, isoflurane, and sevoflurane reduce postischemic adhesion of neutrophils in the coronary system. Anesthesiology 86:188–195
Krolikowski JG, Weihrauch DVM, Bienengraeber MW, Kersten JR, Warltier DC, Pagel PS (2006) Role of Erk1/2, p70s6 K, and eNOS in isoflurane-induced cardioprotection during early reperfusion in vivo. Can J Anaesth 53:174–182
Kuboki K, Jiang ZY, Takahara N, Ha SW, Igarashi M, Yamauchi T, Feener EP, Herbert TP, Rhodes CJ, King GL (2000) Regulation of endothelial constitutive nitric oxide synthase gene expression in endothelial cells and in vivo: a specific vascular action of insulin. Circulation 101:676–681
Kuzume K, Kuzume K, Wolff RA, Chien GL, Van Winkle DM (2004) Remifentanil limits infarct size but attenuates preconditioning-induced infarct limitation. Coron Artery Dis 15:449–455
Kwok WM, Martinelli AT, Fujimoto K, Suzuki A, Stadnicka A, Bosnjak ZJ (2002) Differential modulation of the cardiac adenosine triphosphate-sensitive potassium channel by isoflurane and halothane. Anesthesiology 97:50–56
Lange M, Smul T, Redel A, Roewer N, Kehl F (2005a) Coadministration of desflurane and metoprolol blocks anesthetic-induced preconditioning and cardioprotective effects of beta adrenergic blockade in the rabbit heart in vivo. Anesthesiology 103:A469
Lange M, Smul T, Redel A, Roewer N, Kehl F (2005b) Desflurane-induced anesthetic and ischemic preconditioning are mediated by beta adrenergic receptors. Anesthesiology 103:A550
Light PE, Sabir AA, Allen BG, Walsh MP, French RJ (1996) Protein kinase C induced changes in the stoichiometry of ATP binding activate cardiac ATP-sensitive K+ channels: a possible mechanistic link to ischemic preconditioning. Circ Res 79:399–406

Luchinetti E, Da Silva R, Schaub M, Pasch T, Zaugg M (2004) Ischemic but not pharmacological preconditioning elicits a gene expression profile similar to unprotected myocardium. Physiol Genomics 20:117–130

Lutz MR, Liu H (2004) Sevoflurane produces a delayed window of protection in young rat myocardium and fails to in aged rat myocardium. Anesthesiology 101:A732

Marber MS, Latchman DS, Walker JM, Yellon DM (1993) Cardiac stress protein elevation 24 hours after brief ischemia or heat stress is associated with resistance to myocardial infarction. Circulation 88:1264–1272

Marinovic J, Bosnjak ZJ, Stadnika A (2005) Preconditioning by isoflurane induces lasting sensitization of the cardiac sarcolemmal adenosine triphosphate-sensitive potassium channel by a protein kinase C-delta-mediated mechanism. Anesthesiology 103:540–547

Marinovic J, Bosnjak ZJ, Stadnicka A (2006) Distinct roles for sarcolemmal and mitochondrial adenosine triphosphate-sensitive potassium channels in isoflurane-induced protection against oxidative stress. Anesthesiology 105:98–104

Maulik N, Yoshida T, Zu YL, Sato M, Banerjee A, Das DK (1998) Ischemic preconditioning triggers tyrosine kinase signaling: a potential role for MAPKAP kinase 2. Am J Physiol 275: H1857–H1864

Mullenheim J, Frassdorf J, Preckel B, Thamer V, Schlack W (2001) Ketamine, but not S(+)-ketamine, blocks ischemic preconditioning in rabbit hearts in vivo. Anesthesiology 94:630–636

Mullenheim J, Molojavyi A, Preckel B, Thamer V, Schlack W (2001) Thiopentone does not block ischemic preconditioning in the isolated rat heart. Can J Anaesth 48:784–789

Mullenheim J, Schlack W, Frassdorf J, Heinen A, Preckel B, Thamer V (2001) Additive protective effects of late and early ischaemic preconditioning are mediated by the opening of KATP channels in vivo. Pflugers Arch 442:178–187

Mullenheim J, Ebel D, Frassdorf J, Preckel B, Thamer V, Schlack W (2002) Isoflurane preconditions myocardium against infarction via release of free radicals. Anesthesiology 96:934–940

Murry CE, Jennings RB, Reimer KA (1986) Preconditioning with ischemia: a delay of lethal cell injury in ischemic myocardium. Circulation 74:1124–1136

Novalija E, Fujita S, Kampine JP, Stowe DF (1999) Sevoflurane mimics ischemic preconditioning effects on coronary flow and nitric oxide release in isolated hearts. Anesthesiology 91:701–712

Obal D, Weber NC, Zacharowski K, Toma O, Dettwiller S, Wolter JI, Kratz M, Müllenheim J, Preckel B, Schlack W (2005) Role of protein kinase C-ε (PKC-ε) in isoflurane induced cardioprotection. Low, but not high concentrations of isoflurane activate PKC-ε. Br J Anaesth 94:166–173

Oguchi T, Kashimoto S, Yamaguchi T, Nakamura T, Kumazawa T (1995) Comparative effects of halothane, enflurane, isoflurane and sevoflurane on function and metabolism in the ischaemic rat heart. Br J Anaesth 74:569–575

Pagel PS, Hettrick DA, Lowe D, Tessmer JP, Warltier DC (1995) Desflurane and isoflurane exert modest beneficial actions on left ventricular diastolic function during myocardial ischemia in dogs. Anesthesiology 83:1021–1035

Penta de Peppo A, Polisca P, Tomai F, De Paulis R, Turani F, Zupancich E, Sommariva L, Pasqualetti P, Chiariello L (1999) Recovery of LV contractility in man is enhanced by preischemic administration of enflurane. Ann Thorac Surg 68:112–118

Piriou V, Chiari P, Knezynski S, Bastien O, Loufoua J, Lehot JJ, Foex P, Annat G, Ovize M (2000) Prevention of isoflurane-induced preconditioning by 5-hydroxydecanoate and gadolinium: possible involvement of mitochondrial adenosine triphosphate-sensitive potassium and stretch-activated channels. Anesthesiology 93:756–764

Preckel B, Schlack W (2002) Effect of anesthetics on ischemia-reperfusion injruy of the heart. In: Vincent JL (ed) Springer, Berlin Heidelberg New York, pp 165–176

Roscoe AK, Christensen JD, Lynch C III (2000) Isoflurane, but not halothane, induces protection of human myocardium via adenosine A1 receptors and adenosine triphosphate-sensitive potassium channels. Anesthesiology 92:1692–1701

Rosenkranz ER, Buckberg GD (1983) Myocardial protection during surgical coronary reperfusion. J Am Coll Cardiol 1:1235–1246

Ross S, Munoz H, Piriou V, Ryder WA, Foex P (1998) A comparison of the effects of fentanyl and propofol on left ventricular contractility during myocardial stunning. Acta Anaesthesiol Scand 42:23–31

Schlack W, Hollmann M, Stunneck J, Thamer V (1996) Effect of halothane on myocardial reoxygenation injury in the isolated rat heart. Br J Anaesth 76:860–867

Schultz JE, Hsu AK, Gross GJ (1996) Morphine mimics the cardioprotective effect of ischemic preconditioning via a glibenclamide-sensitive mechanism in the rat heart. Circ Res 78:1100–1104

Scognamiglio R, Avogaro A, Vigili de KS, Negut C, Palisi M, Bagolin E, Tiengo A (2002) Effects of treatment with sulfonylurea drugs or insulin on ischemia-induced myocardial dysfunction in type 2 diabetes. Diabetes 51:808–812

Siegmund B, Schlack W, Ladilov YV, Balser C, Piper HM (1997) Halothane protects cardiomyocytes against reoxygenation-induced hypercontracture. Circulation 96:4372–4379

Smul T, Lange M, Redel A, Roewer N, Kehl M (2005) Propofol blocks desflurane-induced preconditioning, but not ischemic preconditioning. Anesthesiology 103:A462

Speechly-Dick ME, Grover GJ, Yellon DM (1995) Does ischemic preconditioning in the human involve protein kinase C and the ATP-dependent K+ channel? Studies of contractile function after simulated ischemia in an atrial in vitro model. Circ Res 77:1030–1035

Spieckermann PG, Bruckner J, Kubler W, Lohr B, Bretschneider HJ (1969) Preischemic stress and resuscitation time of the heart [in German]. Verh Dtsch Ges Kreislaufforsch 35:358–364

Stadnicka A, Bosnjak ZJ (2006) Impact of in vivo preconditioning by isoflurane on adenosine triphosphate-sensitive potassium channels in the rat heart: lasting modulation of nucleotide sensitivity during early memory period. Anesthesiology 104:503–510

Sugioka S, Miyamae M, Domae N, Figueredo VM, Kotani J (2004) Blockade of p38 mitogene activated protein kinase before and during ischaemia does not abolish sevoflurane-induced cardiac preconditioning in guinea pigs. Anesthesiology 101:A708

Takahashi M, Otani H, Nakao S, Imamura H, Shingu K (2005) Isoflurane induces second window of preconditioning through upregulation of inducible nitric oxide synthase in rat heart. Am J Physiol Heart Circ Physiol 289:H2585–H2591

Takahashi MW, Otani H, Nakao S, Imamura H, Shingu K (2004) The optimal dose, the time window, and the mechanism of delayed cardioprotection by isoflurane. Anesthesiology 101:A632

Takahashi T, Ueno H, Shibuya M (1999) VEGF activates protein kinase C-dependent, but Ras-independent Raf-MEK-MAP kinase pathway for DNA synthesis in primary endothelial cells. Oncogene 18:2221–2230

Takahata O, Ichihara K, Ogawa H (1995) Effects of sevoflurane on ischaemic myocardium in dogs. Acta Anaesthesiol Scand 39:449–456

Tarnow J, Markschies-Hornung A, Schulte-Sasse U (1986) Isoflurane improves the tolerance to pacing-induced myocardial ischemia. Anesthesiology 64:147–156

Toller WG, Montgomery MW, Pagel PS, Hettrick DA, Warltier DC, Kersten JR (1999) Isoflurane-enhanced recovery of canine stunned myocardium: role for protein kinase C? Anesthesiology 91:713–722

Toller WG, Kersten JR, Gross ER, Pagel PS, Warltier DC (2000) Isoflurane preconditions myocardium against infarction via activation of inhibitory guanine nucleotide binding proteins. Anesthesiology 92:1400–1407

Toma O, Weber NC, Wolter JI, Obal D, Preckel B, Schlack W (2004) Desflurane preconditioning induces time-dependent activation of protein kinase C epsilon and extracellular signal-regulated kinase 1 and 2 in the rat heart in vivo. Anesthesiology 101:1372–1380

Tomai F, De Paulis R, Penta de Peppo A, Colagrande L, Caprara E, Polisca P, De Matteis G, Ghini AS, Forlani S, Colella D, Chiariello L (1999) Beneficial impact of isoflurane during coronary bypass surgery on troponin I release. G Ital Cardiol 29:1007–1014

Tosaka S, Cho S, Hara T, Tomiyasu S (2005) Isoflurane administered during early reperfusion protects against myocardial infarction by activating mitochondrial ATP-sensitive K channel in rats. Anesthesiology 103:A470

Tsuchida A, Liu Y, Liu GS, Cohen MV, Downey JM (1994) α1-Adrenergic agonists precondition rabbit ischemic myocardium independent of adenosine by direct activation of protein kinase C. Circ Res 75:576–585

Tsuchida A, Miura T, Tanno M, Nozawa Y, Kita H, Shimamoto K (1998) Time window for the contribution of the delta-opioid receptor to cardioprotection by ischemic preconditioning in the rat heart. Cardiovasc Drugs Ther 12:365–373

Tsutsumi Y, Patel H, Lai C, Takahashi T, Head BP, Roth DM (2006) Isoflurane produces sustained cardiac protection after ischemia-reperfusion injury in mice. Anesthesiology 104:495–502

Uecker M, Da Silva R, Grampp T, Pasch T, Schaub MC, Zaugg M (2003) Translocation of protein kinase C isoforms to subcellular targets in ischemic and anesthetic preconditioning. Anesthesiology 99:138–147

Weber NC, Toma O, Awab S, Fräβdorf J, Preckel B, Schlack W (2005) Effects of nitrous oxide on the rat heart in vivo: another inhalational anesthetic that preconditions the heart? Anesthesiology 103:1174–1182

Weber NC, Toma O, Wolter JI, Obal D, Müllenheim J, Preckel B, Schlack W (2005a) The noble gas xenon induces pharmacological preconditioning in the rat heart in vivo via induction of PKC-epsilon and p38 MAPK. Br J Pharmacol 144:123–132

Weber NC, Toma O, Wolter JI, Wirthle NM, Schlack W, Preckel B (2005b) Mechanisms of xenon and isoflurane induced preconditioning—a potential link to the cytoskeleton via the MAPKAPK-2 HSP27 pathway. Br J Pharmacol 146:445–455

Weber NC, Stursberg J, Wirthle NM, Toma O, Schlack W, Preckel B (2006) Xenon preconditioning differently regulates p44/42 MAPK (ERK 1/2) and p46/54 MAPK (JNK 1/2 and 3) in vivo. Br J Anaesth 97:298–306

Weinbrenner C, Liu GS, Cohen MV, Downey JM (1997) Phosphorylation of tyrosine 182 of p38 mitogen-activated protein kinase correlates with the protection of preconditioning in the rabbit heart. J Mol Cell Cardiol 29:2383–2391

Wickley PJ, Ding X, Murray PA, Damron DS (2006) Propofol-induced activation of protein kinase C isoforms in adult rat ventricular myocytes. Anesthesiology 104:970–977

Wickley PJ, Shiga T, Murray PA, Damron DS (2006) Propofol decreases myofilament Ca^{2+} sensitivity via a protein kinase C-, nitric oxide synthase-dependent pathway in diabetic cardiomyocytes. Anesthesiology 104:978–987

Yang XM, Sato H, Downey JM, Cohen MV (1997) Protection of ischemic preconditioning is dependent upon a critical timing sequence of protein kinase C activation. J Mol Cell Cardiol 29:991–999

Yao Z, Gross GJ (1993) Acetylcholine mimics ischemic preconditioning via a glibenclamide-sensitive mechanism in dogs. Am J Physiol 264:H2221–H2225

Zaugg M, Lucchinetti E, Spahn DR, Pasch T, Schaub MC (2002) Volatile anesthetics mimic cardiac preconditioning by priming the activation of mitochondrial K(ATP) channels via multiple signaling pathways. Anesthesiology 97:4–14

Zaugg M, Lucchinetti E, Garcia C, Pasch T, Spahn DR, Schaub MC (2003) Anaesthetics and cardiac preconditioning. Part II. Clinical implications. Br J Anaesth 91:566–576

Zhong L, Su JY (2002) Isoflurane activates PKC and Ca(2+)-calmodulin-dependent protein kinase II via MAP kinase signaling in cultured vascular smooth muscle cells. Anesthesiology 96:148–154

Non-Immobilizing Inhalational Anesthetic-Like Compounds

M. Perouansky

Abstract Nonimmobilizing, inhalational anesthetic-like compounds are experimental agents developed as a tool to investigate the mechanism of action of general anesthetics. Clinically used for more than 150 years, general anesthesia has until now defied all attempts to formulate a theory of its mechanisms that would link, in an uninterrupted logical chain, observations on the molecular level—via effects on the cellular and network levels—to the in vivo phenomenon. Nonimmobilizers, initially termed nonanesthetics, are substances that disobey the Meyer-Overton rule. Theoretically, in appropriately designed experiments, nonanesthetics can serve as a type of Ockham's razor to separate important from irrelevant observations: processes that, at comparable concentrations, are affected to a similar degree by inhalational anesthetics and by nonanesthetics, do not contribute to anesthesia (the nonanesthetic algorithm). In practice, however, this appealing algorithm has been rather difficult to apply. On one hand, nonanesthetics are not inert on the behavioral level: they cause, *inter alia*, amnesia. This discovery required not only the introduction of the more precise term "nonimmobilizers," but also excluded one important component of anesthesia, i.e., amnesia, from application of the algorithm. On the

M. Perouansky
Department of Anesthesiology, University of Wisconsin School of Medicine,
B6/319 Clinical Science Center, 600 Highland Ave., Madison, WI 53792-3272, USA
mperouansky@wisc.edu

J. Schüttler and H. Schwilden (eds.) *Modern Anesthetics.*
Handbook of Experimental Pharmacology 182.

other hand, compared to inhalational anesthetics, nonimmobilizers interact with relatively few molecular targets, also limiting the usefulness of the nonimmobilizer algorithm. Nevertheless, nonimmobilizers have not only yielded useful results but can, by virtue of those very properties that make them less than ideal for anesthesia research, be used as experimental tools in the neurosciences far beyond anesthetic mechanisms.

1 Introduction

1.1 What Are 'Anesthetic Nondrugs'?

The ability to define "anesthetic nondrugs" rests on two premises: the first is the ability to predict, fairly accurately, anesthetic potencies from their physicochemical properties; the second is the ability to accurately measure anesthetic depth. The Meyer-Overton rule postulates that the anesthetic potency of a substance can be predicted from its lipid solubility, thereby fulfilling the first requirement. The second premise was provided by the development of the MAC concept (minimal alveolar concentration, the concentration that prevents movement in response to a painful stimulus) as a standard index of anesthetic depth (Eger 2002). The availability of a practically useful standardized measure allowed comparisons between drugs and across vertebrate species, a quantum leap for research into anesthetic mechanisms. Since its definition, MAC has been adopted as the standard measure worldwide to define the potency of anesthetic drugs as well as the depth of anesthesia. MAC was unknown to Meyer and Overton (they used nonstandardized descriptions of behavior, e.g., "deeply narcotized," and experimented mostly on tadpoles), but all graphic representations of the "Meyer-Overton correlation" that plot solubility in a lipid phase against MAC illustrate the linear correlation between lipid solubility and anesthetic potency.

Nonanesthetics are in essence substances that disobey the Meyer-Overton rule (Fig. 1). The lack of anesthetic potency was initially determined for perfluoroalkanes (Liu et al. 1994) and later extended to include also other polyhalogenated, perhalogenated or perfluorinated volatile compounds that physicochemically resemble inhalational anesthetics (Koblin et al. 1994). Because all these substances are lipid-soluble, an oil/gas partition coefficient (λ) can be experimentally determined. Using the empirical formula $MAC \times \lambda = 1.82$ atm (the value of the constant is species-specific, 1.82 is the value for rodents) a MAC value can be predicted for these drugs (MAC_{pred}). The distinguishing characteristic of nonanesthetics in vivo is that at MAC_{pred}, and even above, these compounds fail to induce anesthesia as defined by MAC, i.e., they do not immobilize. This, in itself, is remarkable as λ accurately predicts anesthetic potency for hundreds of compounds spanning five orders of magnitude. Therefore, the discovery of compounds that disobey the Meyer-Overton rule has implications for hypotheses about the nature of the anesthetic target site itself. On the biophysical level, the lack of immobilizing potency

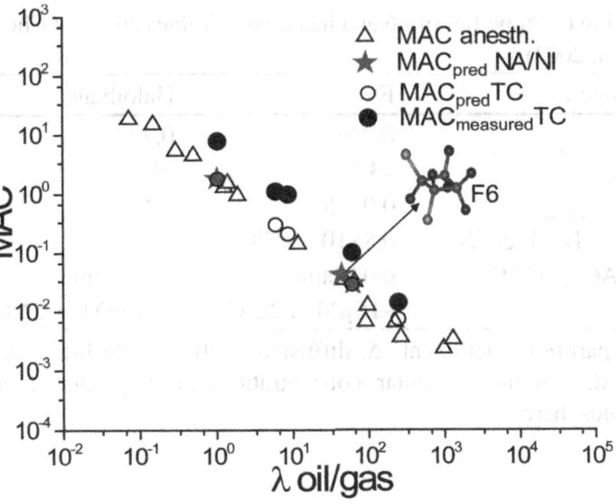

Fig. 1 Anesthetic potency increases with lipid solubility. Lipid solubility correlates well with MAC for anesthetics (*open triangles*) but underestimates experimentally determined MAC for transitional compounds (*TC, open circles*); see TC $MAC_{predicted}$ vs TC $MAC_{measured}$ (*closed circles*). For nonanesthetics/nonimmobilizers (NA/NI, *filled stars*), MAC cannot be determined experimentally as they do not immobilize at testable concentrations. *Insert*: the spoke-and-ball model of 1,2-dichlorohexafluorocyclobutane (*F6*) is courtesy of Dr. J. Trudell. Values *TC* and *NA/NI* are from Koblin et al. (1994)

is typically ascribed to the lack of polarity of these substances that impedes their activity at water–lipid interfaces (Chipot et al. 1997), e.g., their ability to access water-filled cavities in proteins (Eckenhoff 2001). It has also led to the suggestion that, in order to act as an anesthetic, a compound must not only be lipophilic (as postulated by the Meyer-Overton rule) but must also have either a permanent or an inducible dipole moment (North and Cafiso 1997). Primarily, however, nonanesthetics have been used as pharmacological tools to identify sites and mechanisms of anesthetic actions (Raines and Miller 1994).

With respect to anesthetic properties, the 14 nonanesthetics described were classified into transitional compounds (TCs, 9 out of 14) and nonanesthetics proper (Koblin et al. 1994). TCs have the ability to induce anesthesia but at concentrations that are higher than those predicted by the Meyer-Overton correlation. The product of MAC×λ was 2- to 13-fold higher for them than the 1.82 atm for conventional anesthetics. The remaining five drugs had no anesthetic properties (but are not inert, *vide infra*). Over the last decade, some of the originally described drugs have emerged as preferred tools in anesthetic research. The best-characterized and most widely studied compound is 1,2-dichlorohexafluorocyclobutane (F6 or 2N; see Table 1 for a comparison with the anesthetic halothane). Other commonly used experimental compounds are di-(2,2,2,-trifluoroethyl)ether (fluorothyl), and 2,3-dichlorooctafluorobutane (F8).

Table 1 Properties of F6 and halothane. (Values are from Chesney et al. 2003)

Property	F6	Halothane
$\lambda_{saline/gas}$	0.026	0.72
$\lambda_{oil/gas}$	43.5	214
$\lambda_{saline/tissue}$	0.0135	0.125
Δ 0.1×10^{-6} cm²/s	0.8×10^{-6} cm²/s	
MAC_{pred}/MAC	0.042 atm	0.008 atm
	~16 μM at 22°C	~240 μM at 22°C

λ, partition coefficient; Δ, diffusion coefficient in brain tissue; MAC, minimal alveolar concentration; pred, predicted; atm, atmosphere

1.2 Why We Need Them

Since the last edition of this handbook, our model of the mechanism of action of general anesthetics has undergone dramatic changes. I will briefly summarize them here insofar as it is helpful to provide a context for the "raison d'être" of nonimmobilizers. The unitary theory of anesthetic mechanism, commonly accepted in 1972, has been largely replaced by the "multiple sites of anesthetic action" hypothesis. This fundamental change was brought about by:

1. Accumulating inconsistencies and contradictions between experimental results and predictions made from the lipid-based unitary theory.
2. The discovery by Nick Franks and the late Bill Lieb that lipid-free protein systems could interact with anesthetics without violating the Meyer-Overton correlation (Franks and Lieb 1984).
3. Experimental data published in the 1990s also indicated that multiple molecular target sites were matched by multiple (as opposed to a single incremental) behavioral phenotypes of general anesthesia (Rampil et al. 1993; Antognini and Schwartz 1993).

Formerly, the "anesthetic state" was understood as a single, homogeneous condition. Its different elements (amnesia, hypnosis, immobility) were thought to be incremental expressions of the same underlying mechanism, part of a continuum mediated by a unitary, central effector mechanism, sequentially attained by "deepening" anesthesia. Today, by contrast, the majority of researchers active in the field consider the anesthetic state as consisting of multiple substates, each achieved via specific (possibly overlapping) effector mechanisms on the molecular, the network, and the anatomical levels (Eger et al. 1997).

Despite these conceptual changes, the adoption of advanced investigative techniques and the accumulation of large amounts of experimental data, a comprehensive "theory of anesthesia" bridging the molecular and the behavioral levels has not emerged. At least two critical predicaments have thus far prevented an understanding of anesthetic mechanisms profound enough to formulate an inclusive hypothesis. The first one is the lack of a model of the anesthetic state (or of any of its behavioral substates) that is accessible to mechanistic analysis. The other is an "embarrassment of riches" on the molecular level: a multitude of targets and processes are affected to some degree or other by general anesthetics, especially of the inhalational type. Even after excluding "minimal" effects [after all, how little of an effect on a single element in a complex biological cascade is little enough to be considered negligible (Eckenhoff and Johansson 1999)?] at "supra-clinical" concentrations (higher than two to three times MAC) (Sonner 2002), too many molecular targets remain. On this background, the synthesis of nonanesthetics that could be used in a placebo-like manner appeared to offer a chance to escape this experimental impasse.

1.3 The Nonanesthetic Algorithm

The experimental use of nonanesthetics revolves around the following algorithm: If a process on the molecular, cellular, or network level is affected in a similar way by both an anesthetic and a nonanesthetic drug, then this process is unlikely to be relevant for the mechanism of action of anesthetics. One can think of it as an "inverse" placebo—as the compound does not produce the phenotype of interest, whatever effects on the microscopic levels, it can be considered irrelevant. The expectation was that nonanesthetics, used appropriately, would modulate and therefore eliminate many of the proteins that were affected by anesthetics, thereby leaving us with a small pool of anesthesia-relevant targets. This algorithm, of course, had to be modified to exclude amnesia, after the discovery that some nonanesthetics, notably 1,2-dichlorohexafluorocyclobutane (F6, 2N), suppressed learning at similar relative concentrations as the classic inhalational anesthetics (Kandel et al. 1996).

2 Experimental Data

2.1 In Vivo

2.1.1 Pro-convulsant Activity

Nonimmobilizers are defined by their lack of anesthetic action in vivo. It is important, however, to emphasize that they are not inert compounds. It was noted in the initial studies that nonanesthetics had excitatory effects. Indeed, this was considered as evidence that they were able to reach the central nervous system (Koblin et al. 1994). Excitatory effects included tremors, jerking, and convulsant activity (although these were neither defined nor quantitated). F6 above 0.25 MAC_{pred} but below seizure threshold caused a dose-dependent increase in exploratory activity in rats (Perouansky et al. 2005). With certain compounds, excitation progressed to generalized seizures and occasional lethal outcomes. As some clinically used anesthetics also have the potential to induce seizure activity, this property of nonanesthetics has been investigated in some detail. It was found that rat strain (inbred and outbred) had little influence on the convulsant properties, indicating that it was not due to genetic predisposition (Gong et al. 1998). In the case of F6, however, convulsant potency was isomer-dependent, the *cis*- form being almost twice as potent as the *trans*-form (Eger et al. 2001). This pointed to a specific interaction with proteins. Furthermore, the finding of nonadditivity between some convulsant gas combinations (e.g., slight antagonism between F6 and flurothyl when applied together) indicated that nonanesthetics induced seizures via different pathways (Fang et al. 1997). More extensive analysis of 45 nonimmobilizers and transitional compounds revealed that for 36 of them the convulsant ED_{50} correlated closely with lipophilicity ($r^2=0.99$) while for the remaining it did not. This resulted in the hypothesis that this group of compounds produced convulsions via two mechanisms: one that correlated with nonpolarity and the other that did not and that might reflect mixed effects (blocking and enhancing) at γ-aminobutyric acid $(GABA)_A$ receptors (Eger et al. 1999).

2.1.2 Learning and Memory

Three years after the introduction of nonanesthetics as experimental tools, Kandel et al. reported that the nonanesthetics F6 and perfluoropentane suppressed learning at concentrations that, adjusted for lipophilicity, were similar to those of conventional inhalational anesthetics (Kandel et al. 1996). This was an important discovery for a number of reasons. It prompted a name change: nonanesthetics were hence termed nonimmobilizers (Fig. 2), as their defining characteristic was the inability to suppress movement. It also became evident that immobility may not be representative of other components of anesthesia, e.g., amnesia, and that separate mechanisms may underlie these (and other?) anesthetic endpoints (Eger et al. 1997). Moreover, the "nonimmobilizer algorithm" for separating relevant from irrelevant molecular targets had to be amended to account for amnesia. More in-depth analysis of the memory-suppressing effect of nonimmobilizers, particularly F6, revealed additional similarities with conventional anesthetics (exemplified by isoflurane as the best-studied inhalational drug at that time). Fear conditioning is a widely used experimental paradigm for learning and memory in animal models. In its generic form, the experimental animal learns to associate a neutral stimulus (the conditioned stimulus) with a noxious experience (the unconditioned stimulus). Modification of the experimental paradigm can target the learning task toward different, albeit overlapping, neural substrates: fear conditioning to tone depends on the amygdala but not the hippocampus while fear conditioning to context requires processing by the amygdala and the hippocampus. The hippocampus-dependent learning paradigm is significantly more sensitive to interference by isoflurane (ISO), with an EC_{50} of 0.13 MAC (0.19% atm) and is essentially abolished at

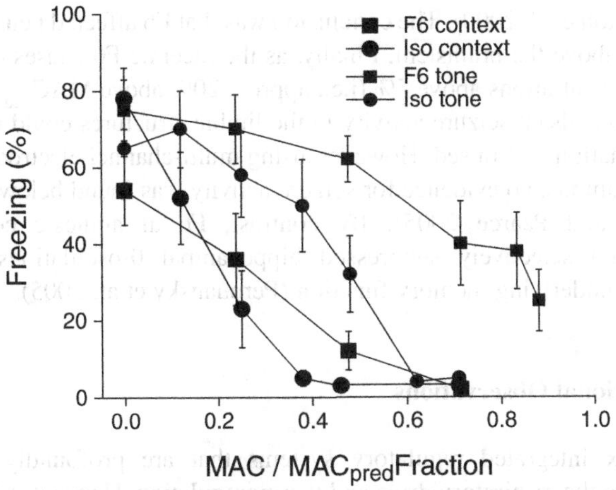

Fig. 2 Nonimmobilizers suppress learning and memory at similar, lipid solubility-corrected concentrations as anesthetics. Freezing is a measure of learning. Learning and memory in the hippocampus-involving paradigm (fear conditioning to context, *closed symbols*) is inhibited by both F6 and isoflurane at similar MAC fractions that are lower than those required to inhibit hippocampus-independent learning (fear conditioning to tone, *open symbols*). F6 and isoflurane data are adapted from published material of Dutton et al. (2002) and Dutton et al. (2001), respectively

0.3–0.4 × MAC ISO, while fear conditioning to tone requires approximately twice the concentration of ISO to achieve a similar degree of inhibition (Dutton et al. 2001). Intriguingly, in MAC equivalents, F6 has a similar differential potency to prevent learning and memory in these two paradigms (Dutton et al. 2002). This similarity was interpreted as an indication of a common amnesic mechanism between nonimmobilizers and anesthetics. However, more recent findings cast doubt on a common mechanism, as coapplication of ISO-antagonized F6 and flurothyl-induced amnesia (Eger et al. 2003).

Suppression of learning in experiments involving noxious stimuli could have been caused by reduced pain perception instead of direct interference with memory formation. In order to exclude this possibility, the amnestic properties of the anesthetic desflurane and F6 were evaluated using unconditioned (i.e., painful) stimuli that were normalized to achieve the same level of response in drug-exposed as in control animals (Sonner et al. 1998). The researchers came to the conclusion that the amnesia induced by both drugs was independent of analgesic effects. Analogously, in experiments using fear conditioning to tone, interference with auditory perception could influence the ability to form associations between conditioned and unconditioned stimuli. Therefore the effect of F6 on middle latency auditory evoked responses was evaluated using epidural electrodes to detect drug-induced depression of sequential loci in the auditory processing pathway. In contrast to isoflurane, desflurane, and nitrous oxide, all of which affected the responses at concentrations at or above 0.2 MAC, F6 had no effect even at 0.8

MAC_{pred} (Dutton et al. 2000). The conclusion was that F6 affected neural processing in structures above the brainstem. Finally, as the racemic F6 causes overt seizures at inhaled concentrations above 5% (i.e., approx. 20% above MAC_{pred}) the possibility that nonconvulsant seizure activity in the limbic structures could interfere with memory formation was raised. However, using multi-channel electrodes implanted in the hippocampus, no evidence for seizure activity was found below one MAC_{pred} (Perouansky and Pearce 2005). By contrast, F6 at amnesic concentrations effectively and selectively suppressed hippocampal θ-oscillations, a network phenomenon underlying memory function (Perouansky et al. 2005).

2.1.3 Additional Observations

Two complex integrated regulatory systems that are profoundly affected by anesthetics are the respiratory drive and thermoregulation. Hence it is interesting to know whether nonimmobilizers modulate them. In anesthetized swine, F6 had no depressant effect on the respiratory drive. In fact, it tended to increase the responsiveness of the respiratory system to imposed increases in CO_2. Qualitatively similar effects were seen with other nonimmobilizers, but toxicity imposed limitations on the experimenters (Steffey et al. 1998). Also, unlike inhaled anesthetics, F6 also had only minimal effects on thermoregulation in rats (Maurer et al. 2000).

Malignant hyperthermia (MH) is an autosomal dominant disorder of skeletal muscle. In genetically predisposed individuals, volatile anesthetics can trigger a potentially life-threatening hypermetabolic state characterized by excessive release of calcium from the sarcoplasmic reticulum. The release is triggered by an interaction with a mutated skeletal muscle sarcoplasmic reticulum calcium release channel, also named the ryanodine receptor type 1 (RY1). Approximately half of all known MH families show linkage to this *RY1* gene (McCarthy et al. 1990), and numerous mutations have been described (McCarthy et al. 2000).

The most sensitive test for diagnosing MH is a bioassay that quantifies the force of contracture of muscle fiber bundles induced by known triggering agents. In tissue obtained from MH-susceptible patients, halothane-induced contractions were on average 15 times stronger than those in response to F6 (Kindler et al. 2002). While the researchers stayed away from the conclusion that F6 could not trigger MH, the results of their experiments indicate that F6 has very limited ability to interact with the ryanodine receptor.

2.2 *In Vitro*

2.2.1 Technical Issues

The delivery of volatile agents to animals by inhalation is technically straightforward. By contrast, delivering volatile drugs via an aqueous carrier to biological preparations in vitro can be problematic. The low aqueous solubility of F6 paired with its moderate lipid solubility has required special attention during in vitro experiments. F6 has a small saline/gas partition coefficient and is therefore quickly lost from the experimental solution unless special precautions are taken. In addition, F6 has no or almost no discernible effect on many proteins. Therefore failure to observe an effect is easily attributed to lack of activity instead of loss of the drug. These pitfalls were relevant enough to be highlighted in an editorial that also urged all researchers to measure the actually delivered F6 concentrations in all experiments (Borghese and Harris 2002). This problem is compounded if F6 is delivered to a preparation (e.g., a brain slice) that, due to its lipid content, has the capacity to take it up in significant quantities. The amount of F6 that can be delivered is limited by the low solubility in water and its diffusion coefficient is low (Table 1), resulting in equilibration time constants that are relatively long compared to the lifetime of biological preparations. Chesney et al. directly addressed this problem (Chesney et al. 2003). This group measured the actual uptake of F6 into brain slices and, using computational modeling, calculated its diffusion coefficient (eight times slower than halothane, Table 1) and modeled concentration depth–time profiles in an acute slice preparation. The study demonstrated the slow equilibration of F6 between the carrier and the slice and suggested that pharmacokinetic modeling is necessary to estimate actual F6 concentrations in brain slices.

2.2.2 Expressed Receptors

Neuronal metabotropic receptors are important modulators of cell excitability, synaptic transmission, network activity, and integrative processes such as learning and memory. Glutamate activates a family of eight metabotropic receptors (mGluR) that are classified into three classes (I–III). Using an amphibian expression system (*Xenopus laevis* oocytes), Harris's laboratory examined the susceptibility of two class I mGluRs (mGluR1 and mGluR5, 60% sequence identity) and of the muscarinic m1 receptor to modulation by a range of anesthetics and nonimmobilizers. The anesthetics ethanol, halothane, and F3 had a similar profile of action, but F6 and F8 differed. At 1 MAC_{pred}, F6 was the only drug that significantly inhibited mGluR1 (~50% block). By contrast, mGluR5 was inhibited by all tested drugs (~40% block) except F8 (Minami et al. 1998). In contrast to the anesthetics, inhibition by F6 was insensitive to manipulations of protein kinase C (PKC), pointing to a separate mechanism of inhibition, similar to its interaction with 5-HT_{2A} receptors (Minami et al. 1997). The muscarinic m1 receptor is coupled via G proteins to inositol triphosphate and diacylglycerol production. The three anesthetics and, to a lesser degree F6 but not F8, inhibited m1-mediated responses (Minami et al. 1997). Similar to the findings with mGluRs, inhibition of PKC abolished anesthetic- but not F6-induced suppression of m1 (Minami et al. 1997). Ionotropic counterparts of these metabotropic receptors in the cholinergic and glutamatergic neurotransmitter systems have also been tested. From the perspective of the nonimmobilizer algorithm, the experiments on neuronal nicotinic acetylcholine (nnAChRs) receptors yielded the clearest results. The predominant nnAChRs type is believed to be composed of α_4 and β_2 subunits (Flores 1992). Nonimmobilizers potently inhibited expressed rat and human $\alpha_4\beta_2$ receptors (Raines et al. 2002). The IC_{50}s for F6, F8, and the anesthetics isoflurane, cyclopropane, and butane all correlated with their lipid solubilities and were below their MAC_{pred} and MAC, respectively. This is the example when application of the nonimmobilizer algorithm yielded a clear conclusion: nicotinic $\alpha_4\beta_2$ do not contribute to anesthetic-induced immobility (Borghese and Harris 2002).

Glutamate activates a large number of ionotropic receptors (GluRs) that belong to four different families. F6 and F8 were found to be inactive on responses mediated by representatives of two families, GluR3 and GluR6, that were modestly inhibited by some volatile anesthetics (Dildy-Mayfield et al. 1996). These results, however, did not yield any conclusions about the involvement of GluRs in anesthetic mechanisms.

There is general agreement that $GABA_A$ receptors contribute importantly to central effects of general anesthetics. Exactly how and to what degree is under debate, especially for the potent inhalational agents. In the CNS, a staggering variety of $GABA_A$ receptors exists (Sieghart and Sperk 2002). Experiments with nonimmobilizers have been carried out only on a few of the existing subunit combinations. $GABA_A$ receptors consisting of $\alpha_1\beta_2\gamma_{2s}$ subunits are widely distributed in synapses throughout the CNS and are enhanced by most general anesthetics (notable exceptions being the gaseous anesthetics N_2O, Xe, and cyclopropane, as well as the injectable anesthetic ketamine). Expressed $\alpha_1\beta_2\gamma_{2s}$ receptors have been found to be resistant to modulation by F6 and F8 (Mihic et al. 1994), implying that (in contrast to $\alpha_4\beta_2$ nnAChRs) nonimmobilizers could not exclude this subunit combination as mediators of any of the anesthetic substates. Recently, it was found that $\alpha_1\beta_2$ receptors were inhibited by F6 and that the γ_{2s} subunit conferred resistance raising the possibility that F6-sensitive $GABA_A$ receptors may be found in the CNS (Zarnowska et al. 2005). The functional consequences of such a selective block are unclear, however.

Background potassium channels have been discussed as targets of anesthetics for some time already (Franks and Lieb 1999). Recently, however, work with genetically manipulated animals produced strong evidence for a role of TREK a widely expressed member of the extensive two-pore domain background potassium channel family (K2P) in some anesthetic substates (Heurteaux et al. 2004). TREK knockout mice were significantly less sensitive to halogenated inhalational anesthetics than the wildtype. TRESK, a recently discovered member of the K2P family that is expressed only in the spinal cord and shares little sequence similarity with the other K2P channels, was also strongly enhanced by volatile anesthetics. As it is not affected by F6, TRESK is a candidate molecular mediator of anesthetic-induced immobility (Liu et al. 2004).

2.2.3 Native Receptors, Channels, Systems

Less data are available on the interaction of nonimmobilizers with native than with expressed receptors. While closer to the in vivo situation, native receptors are typically studied under conditions where the contribution of the protein of interest has to be dissected out of the response of a whole biological system (e.g., the nerve terminal).

Moreover, the exact subunit composition of heteromeric receptors is frequently unknown. Data on the effect of nonimmobilizers is available from three preparations: cortical synaptosomes, dorsal root ganglion (DRG) neurons, and hippocampal slices.

Transmitter Release: Synaptosome

Synaptosomes are "pinched off" nerve terminals that can be obtained from the brain or parts of it and then subjected to various interventions that can simulate, with variable degrees of verisimilitude, certain aspects of physiological transmitter release from synapses. The anesthetic F3 depressed veratridine and 4-amino pyridine-evoked release of the excitatory transmitter glutamate (IC_{50} 0.4 and 0.8 MAC, respectively) and also the veratridine-induced increase in intrasynaptosomal Ca^{2+}, a pharmacological simulation of the release-triggering Ca^{2+}. By contrast, F6 had no effect on either of these parameters at up to $2\times MAC_{pred}$ (Ratnakumari et al. 2000). The conclusion was that anesthetics and nonimmobilizers had different effects on glutamate release. Applying the nonimmobilizer algorithm, these results are consistent with a role for the depression of excitatory transmitter release for some anesthetic endpoints, such as immobility or respiratory depression, but not for amnesia.

Na^+ Channels

In search for a mechanism for the depression of transmitter release, Ratnakumari et al. investigated the effect of F3 and F6 on voltage-gated Na^+ channels in dorsal root ganglion cells. The results were consistent with the findings in synaptosomes: F3 inhibited Na^+ channels much more potently than F6 (70% block at 0.6 MAC vs 18% at 1 MAC_{pred}) (Ratnakumari et al. 2000).

Population Responses in the Hippocampal Slice

Two studies evaluated the effect of nonimmobilizers on evoked extracellular field potentials, a measure of cell excitability and signal propagation. F6 and perfluoropentane had no systematic effect on either the amplitude or the latency of the population spike, nor did they affect excitatory postsynaptic field potentials. This was in contrast to halothane that had depressant effects on these measures of evoked synaptic responses (Taylor et al. 1999). These findings were later confirmed independently for F6 (Chesney et al. 2003).

Synaptic Inhibition

In the hippocampal slice, drug effects on an integrated system can be studied, as both the presynaptic and the postsynaptic elements are present and functional.

Halogenated anesthetics characteristically have a dual effect on $GABA_A$ receptor-mediated inhibitory postsynaptic currents (IPSCs): enhancement at low to moderate concentrations and block at higher agent concentrations (Banks and Pearce 1999). There was no evidence for either presynaptic (GABA release from interneurons) or postsynaptic ($GABA_A$ receptors on pyramidal cells) actions of F6 in the hippocampus (Perouansky and Pearce 2004). In addition, F6 had no effect on currents mediated by $GABA_A$ receptors located at somatic extrasynaptic sites (Perouansky et al. 2005). Taken together, the results of these experiments are consistent with the following interpretations: the amnestic and the convulsant effects of F6 are not due to interactions with $GABA_A$ receptors on the somata of pyramidal neurons, consistent with its classification as a "nonpolar" convulsants (Eger et al. 1999). On the other hand, if viewed through the nonimmobilizer algorithm, these results do not preclude the possibility that isoflurane-induced sedation and hypnosis could be mediated by interaction with $GABA_A$ receptors.

3 Summary and Conclusions

3.1 Implications for Anesthetic Mechanisms

Nonimmobilizers are unusual drugs in that their primary raison d'être is to serve as tools for anesthetic research as inactive controls. More than a decade after their introduction, this book provides an opportunity to summarize their contribution to insights into anesthetic mechanisms. It is probably fair to say that they have not brought about the breakthroughs that optimists expected (Raines and Miller 1994). As with many novel techniques, drugs or approaches (the most recent one being the genetically engineered mouse), the initial enthusiasm gives way to a more sober assessment, as the limitations of the new modality become apparent. In addition, in parallel with the introduction of ever more sophisticated experimental techniques, the sheer complexity of the multimodal "anesthetic state" is becoming apparent, a complexity that was not anticipated a decade ago.

Probably the main reason why the application of the nonimmobilizer algorithm failed to significantly narrow down the number of relevant molecular targets is that, compared to volatile anesthetics, these drugs turned out to be highly selective, not because the algorithm was flawed. The cholinergic ionotropic receptor that was blocked by F6 and F8, the $\alpha_4\beta_2$ nnAChR, could be excluded from a role in anesthetic-induced immobility and, even though not explicitly mentioned by the authors, from sedation and hypnosis. The cholinergic metabotropic muscarinic m2 receptor was also inhibited by F6. However, since F6 does cause amnesia, and as muscarinic receptor block could be a mechanism, the algorithm is not applicable. It is possible, however, that F6s selective suppression of θ-oscillations (Perouansky et al. 2005) is mediated via inhibition of m2.

3.2 *Potential Future Applications*

The other reason for nonimmobilizers' limited success is that they are not inactive, which limits the scope of experiments in vivo and constrains the interpretation of experiments in vitro. Nonimmobilizers have at least three behavioral effects: excitation, amnesia, and seizures, while others may await identification. These limitations in their usefulness as anesthetic "placebos" can be seen as opportunities: these interesting drugs need not necessarily be limited to anesthesia research. The ability to impair memory without causing sedation is a fairly uncommon property and may help separate the involved pathways. The difference between the F6 and isoflurane effect on hippocampal θ- and γ-oscillations may provide a window to understanding the role of network synchronization in memory and consciousness.

Acknowledgements I would like to thank Dr. R.A. Pearce for illuminating discussions, excellent suggestions, and careful reading of the manuscript.

References

Antognini JF, Schwartz K (1993) Exaggerated anesthetic requirements in the preferentially anesthetized brain. Anesthesiology 79:1244–1249

Banks MI, Pearce RA (1999) Dual actions of volatile anesthetics on GABA(A) IPSCs: dissociation of blocking and prolonging effects. Anesthesiology 90:120–134

Borghese CM, Harris RA (2002) Anesthetic-induced immobility: neuronal nicotinic acetylcholine receptors are no longer in the picture. Anesth Analg 95:509–511

Chesney MA, Perouansky M, Pearce RA (2003) Differential uptake of volatile agents into brain tissue in vitro. Measurement and application of a diffusion model to determine concentration profiles in brain slices. Anesthesiology 99:122–130

Chipot C, Wilson MA, Pohorille A (1997) Interactions of anesthetics with the water-hexane interface. A molecular dynamics study. J Phys Chem B 101:782–791

Dildy-Mayfield JE, Eger EI2, Harris RA (1996) Anesthetics produce subunit-selective actions on glutamate receptors. J Pharmacol Exp Ther 276:1058–1065

Dutton RC, Rampil IJ, Eger EI2 (2000) Inhaled nonimmobilizers do not alter the middle latency auditory-evoked response of rats. Anesth Analg 90:213–217

Dutton RC, Maurer AJ, Sonner JM, Fanselow MS, Laster MJ, Eger EI2 (2001) The concentration of isoflurane required to suppress learning depends on the type of learning. Anesthesiology 94:514–519

Dutton RC, Maurer AJ, Sonner JM, Fanselow MS, Laster MJ, Eger EI (2002) Short-term memory resists the depressant effect of the nonimmobilizer 1–2-dichlorohexafluorocyclobutane (2N) more than long-term memory. Anesth Analg 94:631–639

Eckenhoff RG (2001) Promiscuous ligands and attractive cavities: how do the inhaled anesthetics work? Mol Interv 1:258–268

Eckenhoff RG, Johansson JS (1999) On the relevance of "clinically relevant concentrations" of inhaled anesthetics in in vitro experiments. Anesthesiology 91:856–860

Eger EI (2002) A brief history of the origin of minimum alveolar concentration (MAC). Anesthesiology 96:238–239

Eger EI, Koblin DD, Harris RA, Kendig JJ, Pohorille A, Halsey MJ, Trudell JR (1997) Hypothesis: inhaled anesthetics produce immobility and amnesia by different mechanisms at different sites. Anesth Analg 84:915–918

Eger EI, Koblin DD, Sonner J, Gong D, Laster MJ, Ionescu P, Halsey MJ, Hudlicky T (1999) Nonimmobilizers and transitional compounds may produce convulsions by two mechanisms. Anesth Analg 88:884–892

Eger EI, Halsey MJ, Koblin DD, Laster MJ, Ionescu P, Konigsberger K, Fan R, Nguyen BV, Hudlicky T (2001) The convulsant and anesthetic properties of cis-trans isomers of 1, 2-dichlorohexafluorocyclobutane and 1, 2-dichloroethylene. Anesth Analg 93:922–927

Eger EI, Xing Y, Pearce R, Shafer S, Laster MJ, Zhang Y, Fanselow MS, Sonner JM (2003) Isoflurane antagonizes the capacity of flurothyl or 1,2-dichlorohexafluorocyclobutane to impair fear conditioning to context and tone. Anesth Analg 96:1010–1018

Flores CM, Rogers SW, Pabreza LA, Wolfe BB, Kellar KJ (1992) A subtype of nicotinic cholinergic receptor in rat brain is composed of alpha4 and beta2 subunits and is up-regulated by chronic nicotine treatment. Mol Pharmacol 41:31–37

Fang Z, Laster MJ, Gong D, Ionescu P, Koblin DD, Sonner J, Eger EI2, Halsey MJ (1997) Convulsant activity of nonanesthetic gas combinations. Anesth Analg 84:634–640

Franks NP, Lieb WR (1984) Do general anaesthetics act by competitive binding to specific receptors? Nature 310:599–601

Franks NP, Lieb WR (1999) Background K+ channels: an important target for volatile anesthetics? Nat Neurosci 2:395–396

Gong D, Fang Z, Ionescu P, Laster MJ, Terrell RC, Eger EI (1998) Rat strain minimally influences anesthetic and convulsant requirements of inhaled compounds in rats. Anesth Analg 87:963–966

Heurteaux C, Guy N, Laigle C, Blondeau N, Duprat F, Mazzuca M, Lang-Lazdunski L, Widmann C, Zanzouri M, Romey G, Lazdunski M (2004) TREK-1, a K(+) channel involved in neuroprotection and general anesthesia. EMBO J 23:2684–2695

Kandel L, Chortkoff BS, Sonner J, Laster MJ, Eger EI2 (1996) Nonanesthetics can suppress learning. Anesth Analg 82:321–326

Kindler CH, Girard T, Gong D, Urwyler A (2002) The differential effect of halothane and 1,2-dichlorohexafluorocyclobutane on in vitro muscle contractures of patients susceptible to malignant hyperthermia. Anesth Analg 94:1028–1033

Koblin DD, Chortkoff BS, Laster MJ, Eger EI2, Halsey MJ, Ionescu P (1994) Polyhalogenated and perfluorinated compounds that disobey the meyer-overton hypothesis. Anesth Analg 79:1043–1048

Liu C, Au JD, Zou HL, Cotten JF, Yost CS (2004) Potent activation of the human tandem pore domain K channel TRESK with clinical concentrations of volatile anesthetics. Anesth Analg 99:1715–1722

Liu J, Laster MJ, Koblin DD, Eger EI2, Halsey MJ, Taheri S, Chortkoff B (1994) A cutoff in potency exists in the perfluoroalkanes. Anesth Analg 79:238–244

Maurer AJ, Sessler DI, Eger EI2, Sonner JM (2000) The nonimmobilizer 1, 2-dichlorohexafluorocyclobutane does not affect thermoregulation in the rat. Anesth Analg 91:1013–1016

McCarthy TV, Healy JM, Heffron JJ, Lehane M, Deufel T, Lehmann-Horn F, Farrall M, Johnson K (1990) Localization of the malignant hyperthermia susceptibility locus to human chromosome 19q12–13.2. Nature 343:562–564

McCarthy TV, Quane KA, Lynch PJ (2000) Ryanodine receptor mutations in malignant hyperthermia and central core disease. Hum Mutat 15:410–417

Mihic SJ, McQuilkin SJ, Eger EI2, Ionescu P, Harris RA (1994) Potentiation of gamma-aminobutyric acid type a receptor-mediated chloride currents by novel halogenated compounds correlates with their abilities to induce general anesthesia. Mol Pharmacol 46:851–857

Minami K, Minami M, Harris RA (1997) Inhibition of 5-hydroxytryptamine type 2A receptor-induced currents by n-alcohols and anesthetics. J Pharmacol Exp Ther 281:1136–1143

Minami K, Vanderah TW, Minami M, Harris RA (1997) Inhibitory effects of anesthetics and ethanol on muscarinic receptors expressed in Xenopus oocytes. Eur J Pharmacol 339:237–244

Minami K, Gereau RW, Minami M, Heinemann SF, Harris RA (1998) Effects of ethanol and anesthetics on type 1 and 5 metabotropic glutamate receptors expressed in Xenopus laevis oocytes. Mol Pharmacol 53:148–156

North C, Cafiso DS (1997) Contrasting membrane localization and behavior of halogenated cyclobutanes that follow or violate the Meyer-Overton hypothesis of general anesthetic potency. Biophys J 72:1754–1761

Perouansky M, Pearce RA (2004) Effects on synaptic inhibition in the hippocampus do not underlie the amnestic and convulsive properties of the nonimmobilizer 1, 2-dichlorohexafluorocyclobutane (F6). Anesthesiology 101:66–74

Perouansky M, Pearce RA (2005) Non-immobilizers put to the test: F6 and the GABAA receptor. In: Mashimo T, Ogli K, Uchida I (eds) International Congress Series 1283. Elsevier, Amsterdam, pp 73–78

Perouansky M, Banks MI, Pearce RA (2005) Differential effects of the non-immobilizer 1, 2 dichlorohexafluorocyclobutane (F6, 2 N) and isoflurane on extrasynaptic GABAA receptor. Anesth Analg 100:1667–1673

Perouansky M, Hentschke H, Pearce R (2005) The non-immobilizer F6 preferentially suppresses theta vs gamma oscillations at amnestic concentrations. Society for Neuroscience Program No. 886:17

Raines DE, Miller KW (1994) On the importance of volatile agents devoid of anesthetic action. Anesth Analg 79:1031–1033

Raines DE, Claycomb RJ, Forman SA (2002) Nonhalogenated anesthetic alkanes and perhalogenated nonimmobilizing alkanes inhibit alpha (4) beta (2) neuronal nicotinic acetylcholine receptors. [Erratum appears in Anesth Analg 2002 Oct;95(4):869]. Anesth Analg 95:573–577

Rampil IJ, Mason P, Singh H (1993) Anesthetic potency (MAC) is independent of forebrain structures in the rat. Anesthesiology 78:707–712

Ratnakumari L, Vysotskaya TN, Duch DS, Hemmings HC Jr (2000) Differential effects of anesthetic and nonanesthetic cyclobutanes on neuronal voltage-gated sodium channels. Anesthesiology 92:529–541

Sieghart W, Sperk G (2002) Subunit composition, distribution and function of GABA(A) receptor subtypes. Curr Top Med Chem 2:795–816

Sonner JM (2002) Issues in the design and interpretation of minimum alveolar anesthetic concentration (MAC) studies. Anesth Analg 95:609–614

Sonner JM, Li JA, Eger EI (1998) Desflurane and the nonimmobilizer 1, 2-dichlorohexafluorocyclobutane suppress learning by a mechanism independent of the level of unconditioned stimulation. Anesth Analg 87:200–205

Steffey EP, Laster MJ, Ionescu P, Eger EI, Emerson N (1998) Ventilatory effects of the nonimmobilizer 1, 2-dichlorohexafluorocyclobutane (2 N) in swine. Anesth Analg 86:173–178

Taylor DM, Eger EI2, Bickler PE (1999) Halothane, but not the nonimmobilizers perfluoropentane and 1, 2-dichlorohexafluorocyclobutane, depresses synaptic transmission in hippocampal CA1 neurons in rats. Anesth Analg 89:1040–1045

Zarnowska ED, Saad AA, Pearce RA, Perouansky M (2005) The γ-subunit governs the susceptibility of recombinant GABAA receptors to block by the non-immobilizer 1, 2-di2005. The-γ-subunit. The-γ-subunitchlorohexafluorocyclobutane (F6, 2N). Anesth Analg 101:401–406

Part III
Modern Intravenous Anesthetics

Section Editor: F. Camu

Propofol

C. Vanlersberghe(✉) and F. Camu

Abstract The hypnotic agent propofol has pharmacokinetic characteristics that allow for rapid onset and offset of drug effect and fast elimination from the body. Elderly patients show a greater sensitivity to the hypnotic effect of propofol. The drug is extensively metabolized in the liver through the cytochrome P450 system and glucuronidation, with potential for drug interaction. Propofol does not cause significant inotropic depression at clinically relevant concentrations. But in vitro, propofol impairs isotonic relaxation of the heart and decreases free cytosolic Ca^{2+} concentrations in myocardial cells. In animal models, the cardioprotective effects of propofol derive in part from its antioxidant and free radical scavenging properties. Propofol decreases cerebral blood flow and cerebral metabolic rate dose-dependently. The neuroprotective effect of propofol in animal models is attributed to its antioxidant property, the potentiation of γ-aminobutyric acid type A ($GABA_A$)-mediated

C. Vanlersberghe
Department of Anesthesiology, University of Brussels, V.U.B. Medical Center, Laarbeeklaan 101, 1090 Brussels, Belgium
anesvec@uzbrussel.be

J. Schüttler and H. Schwilden (eds.) *Modern Anesthetics.*
Handbook of Experimental Pharmacology 182.

inhibition of synaptic transmission, and the inhibition of glutamate release. Subhypnotic doses of propofol induce sedative, amnestic, and anxiolytic effects in a dose-dependent fashion. Propofol impairs ventilation with a considerable effect on the control of ventilation and central chemoreceptor sensitivity. Propofol reduces the ventilatory response to hypercapnia and the ventilatory adaptation to hypoxia, even at subanesthetic doses. The drug potentiates hypoxic pulmonary vasoconstriction, an effect caused by inhibition of K^{+}_{ATP}-mediated pulmonary vasodilatation. Most of the pharmacological actions of propofol result from interaction with the $GABA_A$ receptor or with calcium channels. Propofol prolongs inhibitory postsynaptic currents mediated by $GABA_A$ receptors, indicating that its effects are associated with enhanced inhibitory synaptic transmission, but propofol also influences presynaptic mechanisms of GABAergic transmission. Propofol modulates various aspects of the host's inflammatory response. It decreases secretion of proinflammatory cytokines, alters the expression of nitric oxide, impairs monocyte and neutrophil functions, and has potent, dose-dependent radical scavenging activity similar to the endogenous antioxidant vitamin E.

1 Pharmacokinetics

Propofol, 2,6-diisopropylphenol (MW 178) is formulated as an emulsion in 10% soybean oil, 2.25% glycerol, 1.2% egg phosphatide, and disodium edetate (EDTA). The formulation is isotonic, has a neutral pH, and the drug has a pK_a in water of 11. The drug is extensively bound to plasma proteins (95%–98%). Propofol does not trigger histamine release and has no inhibitory effect on adrenocortical function or porphyrinogenic activity.

Upon intravenous administration, the pharmacokinetics of propofol is characterized by an initial distribution half-life of 2–8 min, with the slow distribution half-life ranging from 30 to 70 min and the terminal elimination half-life from 4 to 24 h depending on the study conditions using bolus or infusion dosing in healthy (Gepts et al. 1987; Gepts et al. 1988; Campbell et al. 1988; Shafer et al. 1988; Schnider et al. 1998), elderly (Kirkpatrick et al. 1988), and pediatric patients (Kataria et al. 1994). The central volume of distribution (V_1) has been calculated as 20–40 l and the volume of distribution at steady state (V_{dss}) as 150–700 l. Children require significantly larger doses of propofol for induction and maintenance of loss of consciousness than adults. Neither obesity nor hepatic and renal dysfunctions altered the disposition pharmacokinetics of propofol.

More recently, population pharmacokinetic models of propofol including the covariates age, body weight, and gender were published (Schnider et al. 1998; Schüttler and Ihmsen 2000). Weight and age were significant covariates for elimination and intercompartmental distribution clearances and the volumes of distribution (V_1, V_2, and V_3). The estimates for adults were: clearance 1.44 l/min, V_1 9.3 l, and V_{dss} 319.5 l. In children, all parameters were increased when normalized to body weight. In the elderly, V_1 was smaller and clearance decreased.

Moreover, elderly female patients exhibited a larger metabolic clearance of propofol, but a slower distributional clearance when compared with elderly males (Vuyk et al. 2000).

Despite the long terminal half-life, recovery from its clinical effects is rapid, even after prolonged administration. The predicted time for blood propofol concentrations to decrease below 70% of its therapeutic concentration is less than 30 min and is only moderately affected by the duration of drug infusion (Shafer and Varvel 1991; Hughes et al. 1992).

1.1 Hypnotic Potency

Various blood–brain equilibration half-times for propofol have been reported (Wakeling et al. 1999). They range from 1.5 min (k_{e0}=0.456 min^{-1}) to 2.9 min (k_{e0}=0.239 min^{-1}) depending on the effect measured (Schüttler et al. 1986; Schnider et al. 1999). This affects the time to and recovery from loss of consciousness in clinical situations. The median predicted time to peak EEG effect after bolus injection is 1.96 min. The EC_{50} (effect site concentration) for EEG effect was 1.38 µg/ml and for loss of consciousness 1.68 µg/ml (Schnider et al. 1999). The latter was linearly dependent on age. Elderly patients showed increased sensitivity to propofol with EC_{50} values for loss of consciousness decreasing from 2.35 to 1.25 µg/ml for patients aged 25 and 75 years, respectively.

The propofol EC_{50} to prevent movement was 16 µg/ml when used as the sole anesthetic agent, and this concentration decreased by 50% in the presence of 0.6 ng/ml fentanyl plasma concentration (Smith et al. 1994a). Steady state concentrations of propofol during surgery ranged from 2.5 to 6 µg/ml. Awakening from hypnotic effect occurred at blood concentrations averaging 1.6 µg/ml and full orientation at 1.2 µg/ml (Schüttler et al. 1986; Shafer et al. 1988).

In mice the potency of propofol was 1.8 times that of thiopental with similar therapeutic ratio (LD_{50}/ED_{50} ratio of propofol 3.4 compared to 3.9 for thiopental).

1.2 Metabolism

Propofol exhibits a high systemic clearance that exceeds hepatic blood flow (1.5–2.2 l/min). Extrahepatic clearance was demonstrated during the anhepatic phase of liver transplantation (Veroli et al. 1992). Propofol is rapidly and extensively metabolized, with less than 1% excreted unchanged. Metabolic clearance of propofol by the kidneys is extensive with a high renal extraction ratio and accounts for almost one-third of the total body clearance (Hiraoka et al. 2005). Elimination of propofol in lungs and brain does not contribute to total body clearance of propofol.

Approximately 50%–70% of the dose is excreted as propofol glucuronide. Propofol undergoes 4-hydroxylation to 2,6-diisopropyl-1-4-quinol and is excreted as

1-glucuronide, 4-glucuronide, and 4-sulfate conjugates (Guitton et al. 1998). Human liver microsomal propofol oxidation is catalyzed by numerous cytochrome P450 isoforms including CYP 2C9, 1A2, 2A6, 2C8, 2C18, and 2C19 (but not 2E1 or 3A4). Propofol glucuronidation is catalyzed predominantly by uridine diphosphate glucuronosyltransferase I (UGT) family enzymes. Identities of the P450 and UGT enzymes responsible for human propofol metabolism in vivo are not available.

Therapeutically relevant propofol concentrations (up to 50 μM) caused modest inhibition of CYP 2B activity in rat liver microsomes (Baker et al. 1993) and 5%–20% inhibition of CYP 1A, 2B, and 2E1 activities in hamster liver microsomes (Chen et al. 1995). Human liver microsomal metabolism of the CYP 3A substrates alfentanil and sufentanil was inhibited 50% by 50–60 μM propofol (Janicki et al. 1992), whereas that of midazolam was unaffected (Leung et al. 1997). Human liver microsomal propofol glucuronidation was inhibited in vitro by riluzole, enalapril, acetylsalicylic acid, chloramphenicol, ketoprofen, oxazepam, and fentanyl (Le Guellec et al. 1995; Sanderink et al. 1997).

From the anesthetic point of view, the most clinically relevant drug interaction in humans relates to opioids. Propofol infusions at blood concentrations of 0.4–3 μg/ml increased plasma concentrations of alfentanil (Gepts et al. 1988). But fentanyl (5 μg/kg) had no effect on blood propofol concentrations (Dixon et al. 1990). The clinical significance of propofol-opioids pharmacokinetic drug interactions appears modest in comparison with the more prominent pharmacodynamic interactions.

2 Pharmacological Organ Effects

2.1 *The Cardiovascular System*

Propofol administration induces some cardiovascular depression, manifested mainly by a decrease of arterial blood pressure. At clinical concentrations, propofol did not impair myocardial contractility measured from human atrial tissue, in contrast to thiopental and ketamine that showed negative inotropic properties (Gelissen et al. 1996). Mather et al. (2004) studied the direct cardiac effects of propofol in awake, instrumented sheep with infusions of the drug directly into the left coronary arteries. At concentrations in the coronary sinus blood that were at least tenfold higher than in arterial blood, propofol caused rapid dose-related myocardial depression with decreases in dP/dt_{max} and stroke volume, but left coronary blood flow and heart rate increased, thus maintaining cardiac output. The mechanism underlying the negative inotropic effects involves the availability of calcium in myocardial cells. Although in vitro propofol induced no inotropic effect, it impaired isotonic relaxation of the heart (Riou et al. 1992). Propofol decreased free cytosolic Ca^{2+} concentrations in myocardial cells (Li et al. 1997) and altered mitochondrial calcium exchange in myocytes (Sztark et al. 1995), although these effects appeared only at supraclinical concentrations (Kanaya et al. 2001).

The reduced uptake of Ca^{2+} into the sarcoplasmatic reticulum was accompanied by a simultaneous increase in sensitivity of the myofilaments to Ca^{2+} as demonstrated by the leftward shift of the Ca^{2+}-activated actomyosin ATPase activity. This compensated in part the effect of propofol on myocardial contractility (Sprung et al. 2001). The increase in myofilament Ca^{2+} sensitivity involved the protein kinase C (PKC) pathway and an increase in Na^+-H^+ exchange activity (Kanaya et al. 2001; Gable et al. 2005).

Many studies have demonstrated that propofol at clinically relevant concentrations does not cause significant inotropic depression in most species, including humans. The direct negative inotropic effect of propofol in nonfailing and failing human myocardium occurred only at concentrations exceeding typical clinical concentrations (Sprung et al. 2001). Also in rabbits with compensated cardiomyopathy, propofol showed negative inotropic effects only at supraclinical concentrations. The myocardial and coronary effects of propofol were not significantly modified in cardiac hypertrophy (Ouattara et al. 2001). In contrast, a pig model with pacing-induced congestive heart failure suggested that the myocardial depressive effects of propofol might be greater in the presence of left ventricular (LV) dysfunction than in healthy hearts (Hebbar et al. 1997).

Current evidence suggests that cardiovascular depression results from a decreased sympathetic tone with reduction of vascular resistance. In healthy volunteers, cardiac and sympathetic baroslopes were significantly reduced with propofol, especially in response to hypotension, suggesting that propofol-induced hypotension may be mediated by an inhibition of the sympathetic nervous system and impairment of the baroreflex regulatory mechanisms (Ebert 2005). Loss of vascular tone in arteries as a result of a reduced Ca^{2+} influx may also contribute to hypotension following induction with propofol.

Propofol has been suggested to protect the heart from ischemia–reperfusion injury during myocardial surgery. From the metabolic point of view, propofol attenuated the changes in myocardial tissue levels of adenine nucleotides, lactate, and amino acids during myocardial ischemia and reduced cardiac troponin I release on reperfusion. In animal models propofol improved dysfunction of the myocardium, but not of the coronary endothelium, during reperfusion after 15 min of occlusion of the left anterior descending coronary artery (LAD). The protection may be related, at least in part, to its ability to reduce lipid peroxidation, but other mechanisms, such as ion channel modifications, may be involved (Kokita et al. 1998; Yoo et al. 1999; Xia et al. 2003; Lim et al. 2005). Sodium ion-hydrogen ion (Na^+-H^+) exchange inhibitors are effective cardioprotective agents. The Na^+-H^+ exchange inhibitor HOE 642 (cariporide) and propofol provided cardioprotection via different mechanisms, which may explain the additive protection observed with the combination of these drugs. Activation of adenosine triphosphate-sensitive potassium (K_{ATP}) channels produces cardioprotective effects during ischemia (Marthur et al. 1999). Propofol did not affect sarcolemmal K_{ATP} channels at clinically relevant (<2 μm) concentrations (Kawano et al. 2002) although it did inhibit specific subunits of the channel at concentrations 5 to 15 times higher than those encountered during clinical anesthesia.

Free oxygen radicals and reactive oxygen species (ROS) are critical mediators of myocardial injury during ischemia and reperfusion They contribute to myocardial stunning, infarction, and apoptosis, and possibly to the genesis of arrhythmias (Kevin et al. 2005). Propofol has a chemical structure similar to that of phenol-based free-radical scavengers such as endogenous antioxidant vitamin E. It scavenges free oxygen radicals, reduces disulfide bonds in proteins, and inhibits lipid peroxidation induced by oxidative stress in isolated organelles (Eriksson et al. 1992; Murphy et al. 1992). The Intralipid (Fresenius Kabi, Badhomburg, Germany) solvent for propofol also exhibits scavenging activity, but this is negligible at clinical concentrations. The cardioprotective effects of propofol derive at least in part from these antioxidant and free radical scavenging properties (Xia et al. 2004). Propofol attenuated lipid peroxidation induced by hydrogen peroxide and preserved myocardial ATP content (Kokita and Hara 1996).

Another mechanism by which propofol could provide myocardial protection is by inhibiting the mitochondrial permeability transition pore (MPTP) (Javadov et al. 2000). The MPTP involves the opening of nonspecific pores in the inner mitochondrial membrane under conditions of increased oxidative stress, high intracellular Ca^{2+} concentrations, low levels of ATP, and other conditions associated with ischemia–reperfusion and is one of the major causes of reperfusion injury (Halestrap et al. 2004). Opening of the mitochondrial permeability transition pore uncouples mitochondria and interferes with the synthesis of ATP and other mitochondrial functions.

2.2 *The Brain*

In baboons and humans, propofol exerted cerebral vascular and metabolic effects similar to those of barbiturates, decreasing cerebral blood flow (CBF) and reducing the cerebral metabolic rate dose-dependently (Van Hemelrijck et al. 1990; De Cosmo et al. 2005). Despite a reduction in intracranial pressure (ICP) induced by the administration of anesthetic doses of propofol, the decrease in mean arterial pressure usually led to decreased cerebral perfusion pressure (CPP). However, the autoregulatory capacity of the cerebral circulation remained intact during propofol anesthesia, with preservation of the response of the cerebrovascular system to changes in carbon dioxide tension and increases in mean arterial pressure (Fitch et al. 1989; Strebel et al. 1995). In humans, the uptake of propofol by the brain was slow ($t_{1/2}$ k_{e0} of 6.5 min) and accompanied by decreased CBF velocity and EEG slowing. But cerebral oxygen extraction did not change, suggesting parallel changes in cerebral metabolism (Ludbrook et al. 2002).

In the setting of brain injury or tumors, propofol decreased regional CBF, CPP, and ICP without changes in cerebrovascular resistance and cerebral arteriovenous oxygen content difference (Van Hemelrijck et al. 1989; Pinaud et al. 1990).

2.2.1 Proconvulsant Activity

Neuroexcitatory activity is a recognized side effect of propofol anesthesia. These excitatory events (e.g., myoclonus, tremor, dystonic posturing) may be the result from preferential depression of subcortical areas. In mice, pretreatment with propofol increased the convulsive potency of kainic acid and quisqualic acid, which enhance excitatory neurotransmission, and strychnine, a specific glycine antagonist (Bansinath et al. 1995). Propofol induces dose-related changes in EEG, from increased β-activity with sedation to increased δ activity with unconsciousness and burst suppression at higher doses. Propofol depresses somatosensory and motor-evoked potentials but does not appear to affect brainstem auditory evoked potentials (Reddy et al. 1993).

2.2.2 Anticonvulsant Properties

Systematic studies in both humans and animals strongly suggest that propofol possesses antiepileptic properties. In vitro, propofol markedly reduced epileptiform activity in rat hippocampal slices produced by picrotoxin, bicuculline, pilocarpine, and K^+ (Rasmussen et al. 1996), although high propofol concentrations were required for a significant effect against the γ-aminobutyric acid type A ($GABA_A$) receptor antagonists. In animal studies, propofol suppressed seizure activity caused by overdosage of lidocaine (Lee et al. 1998). In rabbits, high-dose propofol suppressed electroencephalographic and pharmacological seizures in pentylenetetrazole-induced generalized epileptic status (De Riu et al. 1992).

Status epilepticus is believed to result from a mechanistic shift from inadequate $GABA_A$ receptor mediated inhibition to excessive *N*-methyl-d-aspartate (NMDA) receptor mediated excitatory transmission (Chen et al. 2007). Propofol is an ideal candidate for the management of refractory status epilepticus. Indeed, in addition to its $GABA_A$ agonist activity, propofol also inhibited the NMDA subtype of glutamate receptors, modulated Ca^{2+} influx through slow calcium ion channels and had protective effects against kainic acid-induced excitotoxicity (Lee and Cheun 1999).

2.2.3 Neuroprotection

Because of its effects on cerebral physiology, propofol was suggested as ideal anesthetic for neurosurgery. Animal models revealed that propofol might protect the brain against ischemic injury as it attenuated neuronal injury after an acute ischemic insult (Young et al. 1997; Yamasaki et al. 1999; Yamaguchi et al. 2000; Wang et al. 2002; Engelhard et al. 2004). Propofol administration for a period of 4 h after focal ischemia significantly reduced infarct volume compared with that in awake, control rats (Bayona et al. 2004) or in isoflurane-anesthetized animals (Young et al. 1997). Neurological and histological outcomes were similar in pentobarbital- and propofol-treated rats subjected to focal ischemia (Pittman et al. 1997).

The neuroprotective effect of propofol has been attributed to its antioxidant property, the potentiation of $GABA_A$-mediated inhibition of synaptic transmission, and its inhibition of glutamate release (Kawaguchi et al. 2005). Indeed propofol directly scavenged free radicals and decreased lipid peroxidation (Wilson and Gelb 2002). Lipid peroxidation induced by transient forebrain ischemia leading to delayed neuronal death in the hippocampal CA1 subfields in gerbils was attenuated by propofol administration (Yamaguchi et al. 2000). These findings suggest that the neuroprotection offered by propofol might reflect a direct scavenging effect against ROS generated during the ischemia and reperfusion. But as pretreatment with the $GABA_A$ antagonist bicuculline significantly inhibited the neuroprotective effects of propofol in a gerbil model of forebrain ischemia, $GABA_A$ receptors have a role in propofol-induced neuroprotection (Ito et al. 1999). This correlates with the finding that cerebral glutamate concentrations decreased by 60% during propofol anesthesia in rats subjected to forebrain ischemia (Engelhard et al. 2003). Accumulation of extracellular glutamate plays an important role in neuronal death during cerebral ischemia. One potential mechanism could be a dysfunction of glutamate transporter (GLT_1) activity. But the propofol neuroprotective effect was demonstrated in vitro to be independent of the glial GLT_1 transporter (Velly et al. 2003).

Propofol may be neuroprotective over a long postischemic period as shown in a model of hemispheric ischemia combined with hemorrhagic hypotension. Propofol reduced neuronal damage and modulated several apoptosis-regulating proteins for at least 28 days (Engelhard et al. 2004). But in endothelin-induced striatal ischemia, propofol delayed, but did not prevent cerebral infarction (Bayona et al. 2004). These contradictory results suggest that the neuroprotective effect of propofol may not be sustained with moderate to severe insults.

Nevertheless, the above data suggest the usefulness of propofol for the management of patients with closed head injuries and status epilepticus. Additional beneficial properties include the dose-dependent reduction of the cerebral metabolic rate and ICP, the potentiation of $GABA_A$ inhibition, the inhibition of the glutamate NMDA receptor, the modulation of voltage-dependent calcium channels, and the prevention of lipid peroxidation. Propofol decreased ICP in patients with either normal or increased ICP (Ravussin et al. 1988) and is associated with the maintenance or increase in CPP. Cerebral metabolic autoregulation is maintained during pharmacological burst suppression with propofol, as shown during cardiopulmonary bypass, where the reduction in CBF was accompanied by the simultaneous decrease of cerebral oxygen delivery and the cerebral metabolic rate for oxygen (Newman et al. 1995).

2.2.4 Mood-Altering Properties and Anxiolytic Effects

Subhypnotic doses of propofol induce sedative, amnestic, and anxiolytic effects in a dose-dependent fashion (Zacny et al. 1992). The use of propofol infusions was shown to decrease anxiety scores and recall in patients undergoing surgery with regional anesthesia (Smith et al. 1994b).

In animals, propofol produced anxiolytic effects at doses that did not induce sedation, similarly to benzodiazepines (Pain et al. 1999). The effects of propofol on tonic inhibition were characterized in the hippocampus, which is crucially involved in learning and memory processes. Hippocampal neurons generate a robust tonic current via activation of α5 subunit-containing $GABA_A$ receptors (Hemmings et al. 2005). These α5 subunit-containing $GABA_A$ receptors are highly sensitive to low concentrations of propofol that produce amnesia but not unconsciousness.

2.3 Respiratory Effects

2.3.1 Pulmonary Ventilation

Propofol has a considerable effect on the control of ventilation by affecting central chemoreceptor sensitivity, reducing the ventilatory response to hypercapnia, and by depressing metabolic ventilatory control, reducing the ventilatory adaptation to hypoxia, even at subanesthetic doses (Blouin et al. 1993; Nieuwenhuijs et al. 2000, 2001). Sedative concentrations of propofol exerted an important effect on the control of breathing, with reduced central carbon dioxide sensitivity. Using dynamic end-tidal forcing of CO_2 tension to determine whether propofol-induced ventilatory depression was primarily central or peripheral in origin, plasma propofol concentrations of 0.5 and 1.3 μg/ml decreased the slope of the ventilatory response to hypercapnia by 20% and 40%, respectively. This change was exclusively related to the more slowly responding central ventilatory control system (Nieuwenhuijs et al. 2001). In contrast to low-dose inhalation anesthetics, the peripheral chemoreflex loop remained unaffected by propofol when stimulated with carbon dioxide. However, animal data showed that high-dose propofol infusion caused cessation of carotid body chemoreceptor activity (Ponte and Sadler 1989). This was confirmed in humans, in whom moderate sedation with propofol depressed the hypoxic ventilatory drive (Nagyova et al. 1995). At propofol plasma concentrations of 0.52 and 2.1 μg/ml, the acute hypoxic response (AHR) decreased by 22% and 61%, respectively. During conscious sedation with propofol the hypoxic respiratory drive also appeared significantly depressed (by 80%) (Blouin et al. 1993). The ventilatory response returned to normal within 30 min after discontinuation of the propofol infusion. Nieuwenhuijs et al. (2000) determined the effect of low concentrations of propofol (0.6 μg/ml) on the AHR and the slower hypoxic ventilatory decline. Propofol significantly decreased the AHR by 50%–60% and increased the magnitude of the hypoxic ventilatory decline relative to the acute hypoxic response. This suggests that propofol affected both the central (the hypoxic ventilatory decline response) and the peripheral (the AHR response) ventilatory control mechanisms.

$GABA_A$ receptors are thought to be involved in the generation of the hypoxic ventilatory decline (Dahan et al. 1996). At clinical concentrations, propofol enhanced GABA-evoked chloride currents and caused direct activation of the receptor in the absence of GABA (Krasowski et al. 1997; Davies et al. 1998).

The relative increase in hypoxic ventilatory decline could be related to the effect of propofol on the $GABA_A$ receptor complex, with increased GABAergic inhibition of ventilation during sustained hypoxia. But in an isolated carotid body preparation, propofol depressed the chemosensitivity of the carotid body in a concentration-dependent manner and with a magnitude proportional to the PO_2 decrease. This effect was clearly demonstrated to be dependent on cholinergic transmission, as the nicotine-induced chemoreceptor response was highly sensitive to propofol. On the other hand, the $GABA_A$ receptor complex was not involved in this preparation (Jonsson et al. 2005).

At doses providing deep sedation or general anesthesia, propofol rapidly decreased resting ventilation and increased resting end-tidal CO_2 ($ETCO_2$). Minute ventilation was always reduced, especially in the first 4 min after bolus administration, while both temporary increases and decreases in respiratory rate have been reported (Goodman et al. 1987; Allsop et al. 1988). Propofol produced dose-dependent depression of ventilation with apnea occurring in 25%–35% of the patients after induction of anesthesia. Peak depression of the ventilatory response to hypercapnia occurred within 90 s after administration of 2.5 mg/kg propofol and remained depressed for 20 min, appreciably longer than clinically assessed sedation. This suggests that propofol-induced ventilatory depression will persist despite clinical recovery of consciousness.

Like other medications used for deep sedation and general anesthesia, propofol may cause significant airway obstruction. Sedative doses of propofol caused a phase shift between abdominal and ribcage movements in spontaneously breathing patients without airway support, thereby decreasing the contribution of rib cage movements to tidal volume and impairing arterial oxygen tensions. These changes may be due in part to upper airway obstruction (Yamakage et al. 1999).

The effects of propofol at preventing induced bronchoconstriction have been extensively evaluated in vitro in the absence of sensitization or following passive sensitization with asthmatic serum or hypoxia (Pedersen et al. 1993; Ouedraogo et al. 1998, 2003; Hanazaki et al. 2000). The airway smooth muscle relaxant effect of propofol is concentration-dependent. Propofol reversed the bronchoconstrictive response to carbachol, histamine, and potassium chloride, even under conditions of hypoxia. This effect was independent of modifications of the intracellular calcium concentration in tracheal myocytes. The bronchodilating effect of propofol has clinical implications, such as decreasing the incidence of intraoperative wheezing in patients with asthma and reducing peripheral airway reactivity in patients requiring mechanical ventilation.

2.3.2 Pulmonary Circulation

Few studies have addressed the effects of propofol on pulmonary circulation. In the isolated perfused lung, K^+ATP channel activation was the major mechanism in mediating propofol pulmonary vasodilatation at clinically relevant concentrations, whereas prostanoids and nitric oxide did not affect the vasodilator effect of propofol

(Erdemli et al. 1995). In patients receiving propofol hypoxic pulmonary vasoconstriction seemed to remain intact (Van Keer et al. 1989). More recent work however showed that propofol potentiated hypoxic pulmonary vasoconstriction, an effect caused by inhibition of K^+ATP-mediated pulmonary vasodilatation (Nakayama and Murray 1999). Others questioned the role of K^+ATP channel activation (Kaye et al. 1999).

In human studies, propofol produced a transient increase in pulmonary vascular resistance in elderly patients, although this effect was not sustained during the infusion of propofol (Claeys et al. 1988). In contrast, propofol caused marked pulmonary vasoconstriction when vasomotor tone was acutely increased with phenylephrine. This propofol effect was concentration-dependent and endothelium independent. Phenylephrine-induced activation of α-adrenoreceptors stimulates both phospholipase C and phospholipase A_2. Stimulation of these signaling pathways increases the release of arachidonic acid, which is metabolized via the cyclooxygenase pathway to produce prostacyclin, thromboxane A_2, and other prostanoids. Prostacyclin is a potent vasodilator, and propofol markedly reduced the synthesis of prostacyclin in response to α-adrenoreceptor activation (Ogawa et al. 2001). Propofol inhibited endothelium-dependent vascular relaxation induced by acetylcholine (Ach) and sodium nitroprusside by interfering at least partly with nitric oxide function (Miyawaki et al. 1995). However, nitric oxide and prostacyclin did not mediate the vasodilator activity of propofol in the isolated blood-perfused rat lung (Kaye et al. 1999).

Taken together, pulmonary vascular responses to propofol appear to be tone-dependent. Indeed, during sympathetic activation propofol may favor α-adrenoreceptor-mediated vasoconstriction over β-adrenoreceptor-mediated vasodilatation.

2.4 Hepatic and Renal System

A bolus dose of propofol did not affect renal or portal venous blood flow in dogs and rabbits (Wouters et al. 1995; Demeure dit Latte et al. 1995). Animal studies using propofol infusions demonstrated dose-related increases in hepatic arterial blood flow, portal tributary, and total liver blood flow. Total liver oxygen delivery and liver oxygen consumption increased, but liver oxygen extraction remained unaltered and hepatic venous oxygen saturation did not decrease (Carmichael et al. 1993).

Alterations in postoperative renal function are common under clinical conditions. Propofol anesthesia did not impair postoperative proteinuria and glucosuria or the protein/creatinine ratio in comparison with inhalation anesthesia in nondiabetic patients (Ebert and Arain 2000). Propofol may cause green discoloration of the urine and the skin due to the production of a phenol green chromophore. This discoloration does not alter renal function. Urinary uric acid excretion is increased after administration of propofol and may manifest as cloudy urine due to crystallization under conditions of low pH and temperature.

3 Effects on Central Nervous System Receptors

3.1 Neuronal $GABA_A$ Receptors

Like other intravenous general anesthetics, propofol produces its hypnotic effects by a positive modulation of the inhibitory function of the neurotransmitter GABA through $GABA_A$ receptors. $GABA_A$ receptors are ligand-gated ion channels coupled to an integral chloride channel, and receptor activation rapidly increases Cl^- conductance and hyperpolarization of the postsynaptic membrane. $GABA_A$ receptors are ubiquitous in the central nervous system.

Propofol allosterically enhanced the actions of GABA at the $GABA_A$ receptor in electrophysiological assays. Propofol reversibly and in a dose-dependent manner potentiated the amplitude of membrane currents evoked by locally applied GABA to bovine adrenomedullary chromaffin cells, which possess high concentrations of $GABA_A$ receptors (Hales and Lambert 1991). Propofol shifted the dose–response curve of GABA-activated current leftwards without altering the maximum of the GABA response (Orser et al. 1994). Furthermore, it prolonged inhibitory postsynaptic currents mediated by $GABA_A$ receptors, indicating that the effects of propofol were associated with enhanced inhibitory synaptic transmission. At higher concentrations, propofol opened $GABA_A$ receptors in the absence of GABA. Propofol slowed desensitization of $GABA_A$ receptors, an important action during rapid repetitive activation of inhibitory synapses (Bai et al. 1999). Early neurochemical studies showed that propofol markedly enhanced [^{3}H]GABA binding in the rat cerebral cortex (Concas et al. 1990) and inhibited the binding of [^{35}S]*tert*-butylbicyclophosphorothionate ([^{35}S] TBPS), a noncompetitive $GABA_A$ antagonist, in a dose-dependent manner (Peduto et al. 1991; Concas et al. 1991). These findings indicate that barbiturates, steroids, and propofol act at separate sites of the $GABA_A$ receptor. Additionally, the action of propofol on the $GABA_A$ receptor could not be antagonized by a benzodiazepine receptor antagonist, suggesting that propofol interacted at a distinct binding site from that of the benzodiazepines. Similarly, propofol did not displace [^{3}H]GABA from its binding site, indicating that the propofol binding site was different from that of GABA on the $GABA_A$ receptor complex (Peduto et al. 1991).

The effect of propofol on $GABA_A$ receptor function was concentration-dependent, with low concentrations of propofol (1–100 μM) potentiating GABA-activated currents and moderate concentrations of propofol directly activating channel opening. These effects occurred within the range of concentrations measured in human blood during propofol anesthesia. This means that at clinically relevant concentrations propofol increases chloride conductance, while at supratherapeutic concentrations propofol desensitizes the $GABA_A$ receptor with suppression of the inhibitory system. Indeed, at higher concentrations the propofol-induced inward Cl^- current decreased considerably (Hara et al. 1993).

Propofol also influenced presynaptic mechanisms of GABAergic transmission. Data suggest that inhibition of GABA uptake, which results in synaptic GABA accumulation, may contribute to propofol-induced anesthesia. Propofol inhibited in a dose-dependent, noncompetitive, and reversible manner [^{3}H]GABA uptake into purified striatal synaptosomes (IC_{50}=46 μM) (Mantz et al. 1995), but did not alter K^+-stimulated [^{3}H]GABA release from striatal nerve terminals. This inhibition was Ca^{2+}-dependent and the general anesthetic action of propofol may involve a facilitation of GABAergic transmission by both presynaptic and postsynaptic mechanisms. However, others have observed that propofol potentiated both spontaneous and K^+-stimulated [^{3}H]GABA release from rat cerebrocortical synaptosomes (Murugaiah and Hemmings 1998).

$GABA_A$ receptors are composed of a number of phylogenetically related subunits (α1–6, β1–4, γ1–3, δ, ε, ρ1–3) that assemble to form a pentameric structure, which contains a central Cl^- channel. Evidence supports the existence of anesthetic binding sites between the second and third transmembrane segments (TM2 and TM3) of $GABA_A$ receptor subunits. Sanna et al. (1995) observed that the direct action of propofol required a β-subunit. Mutations in the β-subunit, particularly at the TM3 position, alter potentiation by propofol. These crucial TM2 and TM3 residues of $GABA_A$ receptors might contribute to anesthetic binding sites or to the allosteric transduction between anesthetic binding and receptor modulation. In fact, propofol produced a strong Cl^- current activation at β1 homomeric receptors as well as at α1β1, α1β1γ2, and β1γ2 receptors, but not at α1γ2 receptors. However, propofol potentiated GABA-evoked responses at β1 and α1γ2 receptors, indicating that an interaction with a receptor different from that mediating the direct effect could be involved. A specific amino acid residue, Met 286, within the β2/3 unit of the $GABA_A$ receptor was identified as essential for potentiation of $GABA_A$ receptor function by propofol. Indeed, a point mutation of TM3 of the β1 subunit (M286W) abolished potentiation of GABA-evoked responses, but not direct receptor activation by propofol. This confirmed the finding that the receptor structural requirements for the positive modulation are distinct from those for direct action (Krasowski et al. 2001) and was consistent with previous studies suggesting the β-subunit of the $GABA_A$ receptor was likely to contain binding sites for this compound.

In contrast to other anesthetics, propofol appears to have marked subcortical effects that may be involved in some of its atypical actions. Microinjections of propofol directly into the tuberomammillary nucleus of the hypothalamus, a nucleus involved in specific sleep pathways, induced sedation that was reversed by a $GABA_A$ receptor antagonist (Nelson et al. 2002). This finding suggests that the sedative effects of propofol may be quite specific and anatomically localized rather than representing a generalized global depression of synaptic activity.

3.2 *Other Sites of Action*

Like most general anesthetic drugs, propofol interacts with different neurotransmitter receptors. Glycine receptors are ligand-gated Cl^- channels and like $GABA_A$

receptors mediate fast neuronal inhibition. Hales and Lambert (1991) demonstrated sensitivity of glycine receptors to propofol, as propofol dose-dependently potentiated strychnine-sensitive currents evoked by glycine in spinal neurons. Pistis et al. (1997) found similar effects of propofol on recombinant glycine receptors expressed in *Xenopus laevis* oocytes.

The effect of propofol on the release of Ach from different brain areas was studied with intracerebral microdialysis. Tonic innervations by GABAergic input regulate the function of cholinergic neurons within specific pathways. GABA agonists, such as muscimol, exerted an inhibitory action on Ach release from both the frontal cortex and hippocampus (Wood et al. 1979). Similarly, propofol decreased markedly the basal Ach release from the same cerebral areas (Kikuchi et al. 1998), but Ach release from the striatum was almost completely insensitive to propofol. These observations suggest brain region selectivity for this effect of propofol.

Alterations in the central cholinergic neurotransmission may contribute to the mechanism by which general anesthetic drugs produce unconsciousness. Neuronal nicotinic Ach receptors (nAchRs) represent very sensitive target sites for propofol. Two types of nAchRs ($\alpha4\beta2$ and $\alpha7$) were examined in vitro in *Xenopus* oocytes. The IC_{50} for propofol was 19 μM for the $\alpha4\beta2$ receptor whereas the $\alpha7$ receptors were unaffected (Flood et al. 1997). But in another cell line (PC12 pheochromocytoma cells), propofol inhibited nAchRs at larger than clinically relevant concentrations in a noncompetitive fashion and had no effect on adenosine triphosphate-induced currents from P2X purinoreceptors (Furuya et al. 1999). Propofol also interacted with G protein-coupled receptors. Indeed, propofol inhibited muscarinic Ach M1 receptor function by interacting at the receptor site and/or at the site of interaction between the receptor and the associated G protein (Trapani et al. 2000). Physostigmine, a carbamyl tertiary amine anticholinesterase that crosses the blood–brain barrier, reversed the propofol-induced unconsciousness, and this reversal was blocked by pretreatment with scopolamine, a nonselective muscarinic antagonist that also crosses the blood–brain barrier (Meuret et al. 2000). These findings suggest that modulation of nAchRs and interruption of central cholinergic muscarinic neurotransmission mediate at least in part the unconsciousness induced by propofol.

Some excitatory glutamate receptors are also sensitive to propofol. Glutamate receptors selective to kainate appeared to be generally insensitive, as propofol failed to produce a consistent effect on kainate-evoked responses in mouse hippocampal neurons (Orser et al. 1995). It is noteworthy that propofol enhanced the convulsive potency of kainate and quisqualate, while it reduced the incidence of NMDA-induced convulsions (Bansinath et al. 1995). This suggests different sensitivities of the glutamatergic receptors to propofol. Indeed, hippocampal NMDA receptors underwent allosteric modulation of channel gating by propofol, although their sensitivity to propofol was low (IC_{50} 160 μM) and the inhibition incomplete. Propofol did not influence the apparent affinity of the receptor for NMDA nor modify its channel conductance. Propofol caused a noncompetitive inhibition of the NMDA receptor and is thought to modulate the NMDA receptor at a domain other than the agonist recognition sites (Orser et al. 1995).

Aside from kainate and *S*-alpha-amino-3-hydroxy-5-methyl-4-isoxazolepropionic acid (AMPA) ion channels, propofol also inhibited voltage-dependent sodium (Na^+) channels in human brain cortex tissue, leading to a voltage-independent reduction in the fractional channel-open time (Frenkel and Urban 1991).

Propofol did not enhance the function of serotonin 5-HT_3 receptors expressed in *Xenopus* oocytes. Due to the role of 5-HT_3 receptors in the control of emesis, their insensitivity to propofol may explain the clinically low incidence of nausea and vomiting after propofol anesthesia (Machu and Harris 1994).

Nonneuronal cell populations such as astrocytes may be affected by propofol. The drug induced changes in the concentration of intracellular Ca^{2+} and disrupted cellular communication by closing the gap junctions between astrocytes at clinically relevant concentrations (Mantz et al. 1993; Mantz et al. 1994). Propofol also disrupted CNS function by nonspecific changes in the cytoskeletal organization of cultured neurons and glial cells caused by increases in cytosolic free Ca^{2+}, particularly of actin, while tubulin organization remained unaffected (Jensen et al. 1994).

Altogether, these data indicate that the mechanism of action of propofol is rather complex with interactions at distinct neurotransmitter receptors being involved.

4 Effects of Propofol on Inflammation

4.1 Immunomodulating Properties

Propofol has been shown to modulate various aspects of the host's inflammatory response; it decreased secretion of proinflammatory cytokines, altered the expression of nitric oxide, and impaired monocyte and neutrophil functions of the nonspecific immune system, including chemotaxis, oxidative burst, and phagocytosis (Krumholz et al. 1994; Galley and Webster 1997). Propofol impaired neutrophil chemotaxis, phagocytosis, and production of ROS in vitro in a dose-dependent manner, probably through a decrease of intracellular Ca^{2+} (Mikawa et al. 1998).

In animal models, propofol exhibited antiinflammatory effects during endotoxinemia, with marked attenuation of the plasma cytokine response [tumor necrosis factor (TNF)-α, interleukin (IL)-6, IL-10] and of neutrophil infiltration of the lungs, together with a lesser degree of metabolic acidosis (Taniguchi et al. 2000). Furthermore, early treatment of rats with propofol after endotoxin-induced shock drastically decreased their mortality rate and reduced their cytokine responses (Taniguchi et al. 2002). Propofol treatment attenuated the endotoxin-induced increase of bronchoalveolar lavage fluid and the lung tissue levels of nitrite, TNF-α, and inducible nitric oxide synthase (iNOS) mRNA, while reducing pulmonary microvascular permeability (Gao et al. 2004).

The molecular mechanisms of this immunomodulating effect have not been established in detail yet. Propofol did not depress the activation of the nuclear transcription factor κB (NF-κB), or the subsequent expression of the cytokines IL-2, IL-6, and IL-8 in human T lymphocytes in vitro (Loop et al. 2002). But NF-κB activation was reduced in lipopolysaccharide (LPS)-stimulated endothelial cells cultured from human umbilical veins (Gao et al. 2006). In this model, propofol also reduced the LPS-enhanced iNOS mRNA and the LPS-induced increase in endothelial cell permeability. Propofol did not affect the intracellular increase of IL-8 mRNA following LPS stimulation of isolated human polymorphonuclear leukocytes, but the extracellular transport or secretion of IL-8 was suppressed (Galley et al. 1998). More recently, it was suggested that propofol affected neutrophil chemotaxis by inhibiting phosphorylation of the p44/42 mitogen-activated protein kinases (MAPK) involved in signal transduction (Nagata et al. 2001).

In animal model testing for bacterial clearance in vivo, propofol induced a dysfunction of the reticuloendothelial system with increased accumulation of bacteria in lungs and spleen. However, this impaired immune function was attributed to the propofol solvent Intralipid, as the lipid emulsion induced the same effect (Kelbel et al. 1999). Others demonstrated that the lipid solvent activated complement and produced concentrations of C3a similar to propofol (Ohmizo et al. 1999).

Such immunosuppressive effects of propofol were not demonstrated in healthy volunteers under clinical anesthetic conditions. Lymphocyte proliferation and cytokine release in response to concanavalin A or endotoxin were unaffected by propofol in cultured human mononuclear leukocytes (Pirttikangas et al. 1995; Salo et al. 1997; Larsen et al. 1998; Hoff et al. 2001). In these studies, propofol increased TNF-α gene expression and the lipopolysaccharide-stimulated TNF-α response, even at low concentrations of propofol. This suggested a proinflammatory immune response of propofol. LPS stimulation of whole blood cultures obtained from patients under anesthesia with propofol enhanced TNF-α and IL-1β release while the antiinflammatory cytokine IL-10 decreased. Also, the profile of peripheral immune cells changed with a decrease of natural killer cells and increased percentages of the T lymphocyte subpopulation $CD4^+$ cells and B lymphocytes (Brand et al. 2003). Others, however, demonstrated that propofol decreased the production of both the proinflammatory cytokine IL-6 and the antiinflammatory cytokine IL-10 from LPS-stimulated mononuclear cells in healthy volunteers (Takaono et al. 2002).

4.2 Antioxidant Properties

Propofol has potent, dose-dependent radical scavenging activity similar to the endogenous antioxidant vitamin E. Propofol contains a phenol hydroxyl group that confers antioxidant activity by reacting with free radicals to form a phenoxyl radical, a property common to all phenol-based free radical scavengers (Murphy et al. 1992; Green et al. 1994). The lipid emulsion Intralipid was not found to possess significant antioxidant activity. The added preservatives have biological activity: EDTA has antiinflammatory properties, whereas metabisulfite may cause lipid peroxidation. Propofol was efficient in blocking formation of malondialdehyde

(MDA) degradation products generated from lipid hydroperoxides of arachidonic acid. But no radical scavenging activities occurred at concentration ranges of less than 10 μg/ml. This is approximately an order of magnitude higher than therapeutic doses of propofol used in anesthesia, suggesting that its scavenging activity during anesthesia is likely very limited (Green et al. 1994). In animal experiments, however, repeated boluses or an infusion of propofol delayed the onset of lipid peroxidation in rat liver microsomes, suggesting a significantly increased resistance to lipid peroxidation at anesthetic doses (Murphy et al. 1993). The antioxidant potencies of propofol and vitamin E to inhibit lipid peroxidation induced by three free radical systems (hydroxyl, ferryl, and oxo-ferryl radicals) were compared in vitro and found to be similar, with higher efficacy against the hydroxyl than the ferryl and oxo-ferryl radicals (Hans et al. 1996).

Activated polymorphonuclear neutrophils may damage tissues through the release of biochemical mediators. Among them, peroxynitrite ($ONOO^-$) is a potent biological oxidant formed by the near diffusion-limited reaction of nitric oxide with superoxide. $ONOO^-$ is responsible for hydroxylation reactions and nitration of proteins, or is metabolized into nitrate. In addition to having hydroxyl radical-like oxidative reactivity, $ONOO^-$ is capable of nitrating phenol rings, including protein-associated tyrosine residues. Nitric oxide does not directly nitrate tyrosine residues. Therefore, demonstration of tissue nitrotyrosine residues infers the action of $ONOO^-$ or related nitrogen-centered oxidants. Propofol protected endothelial cells against the toxicity of $ONOO^-$. The antioxidant properties of propofol can be partially attributed to its scavenging effect on $ONOO^-$ and was as effective as tyrosine. Propofol reacted with $ONOO^-$ more rapidly than did tyrosine, inhibiting nitrotyrosine formation (Mathy-Hartert et al. 2000). Propofol dose-dependently inhibited nitration of proteins and nitrate production by activated human polymorphonuclear neutrophils in a concentration range from 10^{-3} to 10^{-6} mM, consistent with the scavenging effect of propofol on $ONOO^-$ (Thiry et al. 2004).

The antiinflammatory and antioxidant properties of propofol may have beneficial effects in patients with sepsis and systemic inflammatory response syndrome (SIRS) due to noninfective causes. Acute pulmonary inflammation induces toxicity mediated by nitrogen-derived oxidants in human acute lung injury. The contribution of $ONOO^-$ was demonstrated in lung tissue with specific monoclonal antibodies to nitrotyrosine (Kooy et al. 1995). Similarly, the antiinflammatory and antioxidant properties of propofol may have beneficial effects in patients with ischemia–reperfusion injury. In an isolated rat heart preparation simulating cardiac ischemia and reperfusion, the application of high-concentration propofol during ischemia combined with low-concentration propofol (1.2 μg/ml) administered before ischemia and during reperfusion significantly improved postischemic myocardial functional recovery and reduced heart tissue lipid peroxidation (Xia et al. 2003). Free radical scavenging also occurred in vivo in patients undergoing coronary artery bypass surgery and in tourniquet-induced ischemia-reperfusion. Propofol strongly attenuated lipid peroxides, measured as thiobarbituric acid-reacting substances, in atrial tissue samples obtained before and during cardiopulmonary bypass (Sayin et al. 2002). Also, concentrations of lipid peroxides in both plasma and muscle tissue samples were significantly lower than pre-reperfusion concentrations in the propofol group in patients undergoing peripheral surgery under tourniquet (Kahraman et al. 1997).

The neuroprotective effect of propofol might also be related to the antioxidant potential of the drug's phenol ring structure. Oxidative damage has been implicated in the pathogenesis of cerebral ischemia. The exposure to oxidative stress of cultured astrocytes decreased the rate of Na^+-dependent glutamate uptake, and both propofol and vitamin E attenuated this glutamate transport inhibition. Furthermore, anesthetic concentrations of propofol overcame the inhibition of the Na/H exchanger isoform (NHE1) activation by intracellular protons (Sitar et al. 1999; Daskalopoulos et al. 2001). This suggests that propofol and other lipophilic antioxidants may contribute to neuroprotection by preserving the NHE1 response to cytosolic protons and preventing intracellular acidification. Propofol also inhibited the production of MDA in rat brain synaptosomes treated with lipid peroxidation inducers (Musacchio et al. 1991) and in acute spinal cord contusion injury, although this was not accompanied by an improvement of the ultrastructure of the spinal cord (Kaptanoglu et al. 2002). Increased levels of MDA due to cerebral lipid peroxidation were related to decreased intraparenchymal ascorbic acid levels. Astrocyte clearance of dehydroascorbic acid from the extracellular fluid and increased intracellular ascorbate concentrations modulate glutamate uptake by astrocytes. Oxidative stress decreased intracellular glutathione concentration and impaired accumulation of intracellular ascorbate. Both vitamin E and propofol restored the ability of astrocytes to accumulate intracellular ascorbate from dehydroascorbic acid after oxidative stress induced by a lipophilic radical generator, but did not affect intracellular glutathione concentration (Daskalopoulos et al. 2002). The neuroprotection effect in cerebral ischemia was found to be independent of tissue ascorbate and glutathione concentrations (Bayona et al. 2004)

References

Allsop P, Taylor MB, Grounds RM, Morgan M (1988) Ventilatory effects of propofol infusion using a method to rapidly achieve steady-state equilibrium. Eur J Anaesthesiol 5:293–303

Bai D, Pennefather PS, MacDonald JF, Orser B (1999) The general anesthetic propofol slows deactivation and desensitization of GABA(A) receptors. J Neurosci 19:10635–10646

Baker MT, Chadam MV, Ronnenberg WC (1993) Inhibitory effects of propofol on cytochrome P450 activities in rat hepatic microsomes. Anesth Analg 76:817–821

Bansinath M, Shukla VK, Turndorf H (1995) Propofol modulates the effects of chemoconvulsants acting at GABAergic, glycinergic and glutamate receptor subtypes. Anesthesiology 83:809–815

Bayona NA, Gelb AW, Jiang Z, Wilson JX, Urquhart BL, Cechetto DF (2004) Propofol neuroprotection in cerebral ischemia and its effects on low molecular weight antioxidants and skilled motor tasks. Anesthesiology 100:1151–1159

Blouin RT, Seifert HA, Babenco HD, Conard PF, Gross JB (1993) Propofol depresses the hypoxic ventilatory response during conscious sedation and isohypercapnia. Anesthesiology 79:1177–1182

Brand JM, Frohn C, Luhm I, Kirchner H, Schmucker P (2003) Early alterations in the number of circulating lymphocyte subpopulations and enhanced proinflammatory immune response during opioid-based general anesthesia. Shock 20:213–217

Campbell GA, Morgan DJ, Kumar K, Crankshaw DP (1988) Extended blood collection period required to define distribution and elimination kinetics of propofol. Br J Clin Pharmacol 26:187–190

Carmichael FJ, Crawford MW, Khayyam N, Saldivia V (1993) Effect of propofol infusion on splanchnic hemodynamics and liver oxygen consumption in the rat. A dose-response study. Anesthesiology 79:1051–1060

Chen JW, Naylor DE, Wasterlain CG (2007) Advances in the pathophysiology of status epilepticus. Acta Neurol Scand 115:7–15

Chen TL, Ueng TH, Chen SH, Lee PH, Fan SZ, Liu CC (1995) Human cytochrome P450 monooxygenase system is suppressed by propofol. Br J Anaesth 74:558–562

Claeys MA, Gepts E, Camu F (1988) Haemodynamic changes during anaesthesia induced and maintained with propofol. Br J Anaesth 60:3–9

Concas A, Santoro G, Mascia MP, Serra M, Sanna E, Biggio G (1990) The general anesthetic propofol enhances the function of gamma-aminobutyric acid-coupled chloride channel in the rat cerebral cortex. J Neurochem 55:2135–2138

Concas A, Santoro G, Serra M, Sanna E, Biggio G (1991) Neurochemical action of the general anesthetic propofol on the chloride ion channel coupled with GABAA receptors. Brain Res 542:225–232

Dahan A, Ward D, Van den Elsen M, Temp J, Berkenbosch A (1996) Influence of reduced carotid body drive during sustained hypoxia on hypoxic depression of ventilation in humans. J Appl Physiol 81:565–572

Daskalopoulos R, Korcok J, Farhangkhgoee P, Karmazyn M, Gelb AW, Wilson JX (2001) Propofol protection of sodium-hydrogen exchange activity sustains glutamate uptake during oxidative stress. Anesth Analg 93:1199–1204

Daskalopoulos R, Korcok J, Tao L, Wilson JX (2002) Accumulation of intracellular ascorbate from dehydroascorbic acid by astrocytes is decreased after oxidative stress and restored by propofol. Glia 39:124–132

Davies M, Thuynsma RP, Dunn SM (1998) Effects of propofol and pentobarbital on ligand binding to GABAA receptors suggest a similar mechanism of action. Can J Physiol Pharmacol 76:46–52

De Cosmo G, Cancelli I, Adduci A, Merlino G, Aceta P, Valente M (2005) Changes in the hemodynamics during isoflurane and propofol anesthesia: a comparative study. Neurol Res 27:433–435

De Riu PL, Petruzzi V, Testa C, Mulas M, Melis F, Caria MA, Mameli O (1992) Propofol anticonvulsant activity in experimental epileptic status. Br J Anaesth 69:177–181

Demeure dit Latte D, Bernard JM, Blanloeil Y, Peltier P, Francois T, Chatal JF (1995) Induction of anesthesia by propofol and hepatic blood flow in the rabbit. Clin Physiol 15:515–522

Dixon J, Roberts FL, Tackley RM, Lewis GT, Connell H, Prys-Roberts C (1990) Study of the possible interaction between fentanyl and propofol using a computer controlled infusion of propofol. Br J Anaesth 64:142–147

Ebert TJ (2005) Sympathetic and hemodynamic effects of moderate and deep sedation with propofol in humans. Anesthesiology 103:20–24

Ebert TJ, Arain SR (2000) Renal responses to low-flow desflurane, sevoflurane and propofol in patients. Anesthesiology 93:1401–1406

Engelhard K, Werner C, Hoffman WE, Matthes B, Blobner M, Kochs E (2003) The effect of sevoflurane and propofol on cerebral neurotransmitter concentrations during cerebral ischemia in rats. Anesth Analg 97:1155–1161

Engelhard K, Werner C, Eberspacher E, Pape M, Stegemann U, Kellermann K, Hollweck R, Hutzler P, Kochs E (2004) Influence of propofol on neuronal damage and apoptotic factors after incomplete cerebral ischemia and reperfusion in rats: a long-term observation. Anesthesiology 101:912–917

Erdemli O, Tel BC, Gumusel B, Sahin-Erdemli I (1995) The pulmonary vascular response to propofol in the isolated perfused rat lung. Eur J Anaesthesiol 12:617–623
Eriksson O, Pollesello P, Saris NE (1992) Inhibition of lipid peroxidation in isolated rat liver mitochondria by the general anesthetic propofol. Biochem Pharmacol 44:391–393
Fitch W, Van Hemelrijck J, Mattheussen M, Van Aken H (1989) Responsiveness of the cerebral circulation to acute alterations in mean arterial pressure during the administration of propofol. J Neurosurg Anesthesiol 1:375–376
Flood P, Ramirez-Latorre J, Role L (1997) Alpha 4 beta 2 neuronal nicotinic acetylcholine receptors in the central nervous system are inhibited by isoflurane and propofol, but alpha 7-type nicotinic acetylcholine receptors are unaffected. Anesthesiology 86:859–865
Frenkel C, Urban BW (1991) Human brain sodium channels as one of the molecular target sites for the new intravenous anesthetic propofol (2,6 di-isopropylphenol). Eur J Pharmacol 12:75–79
Furuya R, Oka K, Watanabe I, Kamiya Y, Itoh H, Andoh T (1999) The effects of ketamine and propofol on neuronal nicotinic acetylcholine receptors and P2X purinoceptors in PC12 cells. Anesth Analg 88:174–180
Gable BD, Shiga T, Murray PA, Damron DS (2005) Propofol increases contractility during alpha1a-adrenoreceptor activation in adult rat cardiomyocytes. Anesthesiology 103:335–343
Galley HF, Webster NR (1997) Effects of propofol and thiopentone on the immune response. Anaesthesia 52:921–923
Galley HF, Dubbels AM, Webster NR (1998) The effect of midazolam and propofol on interleukin-8 from human polymorphonuclear leukocytes. Anesth Analg 86:1289–1293
Gao I, Zeng BX, Zhou LJ, Yuan SY (2004) Protective effects of early treatment with propofol on endotoxin-induced acute lung injury in rats. Br J Anaesth 92:277–279
Gao I, Zhao WX, Zhou LI, Zeng BX, Yao SL, Liu D, Chen ZQ (2006) Protective effects of propofol on lipopolysaccharide activated endothelial cell barrier dysfunction. Inflamm Res 55:385–392
Gelissen HP, Epema AH, Henning RH, Krijnen HJ, Hennis PJ, Den Hertog A (1996) Inotropic effects of propofol, thiopental, midazolam, etomidate, and ketamine on isolated human atrial muscle. Anesthesiology 84:397–403
Gepts E, Camu F, Cockshott ID, Douglas EJ (1987) Disposition of propofol administered as constant rate intravenous infusions in humans. Anesth Analg 42:1256–1263
Gepts E, Jonckheer K, Maes V, Sonck W, Camu F (1988) Disposition kinetics of propofol during alfentanil anaesthesia. Anaesthesia 43 [Suppl]:8–13
Goodman NW, Black AM, Carter JA (1987) Some ventilatory effects of propofol as sole anaesthetic agent. Br J Anaesth 59:1497–1503
Green TR, Bennett SR, Nelson VM (1994) Specificity and properties of propofol as an antioxidant free radical scavenger. Toxicol Appl Pharmacol 129:163–169
Guitton J, Buronfosse T, Desage M, Flinois JP, Perdrix JP, Brazier JL, Beaune P (1998) Possible involvement of multiple human cytochrome P450 isoforms in the liver metabolism of propofol. Br J Anaesth 80:788–795
Hales TG, Lambert JJ (1991) The actions of propofol on inhibitory amino acid receptors of bovine adrenomedullary chromaffin cells and rodent central neurones. Br J Pharmacol 104:619–628
Halestrap AP, Clarke SJ, Javadov SA (2004) Mitochondrial permeability transition pore opening during myocardial reperfusion—a target for cardioprotection. Cardiovasc Res 61:372–385
Hanazaki M, Jones KA, Warner DO (2000) Effects of intravenous anesthetics on Ca^{2+} sensitivity in canine tracheal smooth muscle. Anesthesiology 92:133–139
Hans P, Deby C, Deby-Dupont G, Vrijens B, Albert A, Lamy M (1996) Effect of propofol on in vitro lipid peroxidation induced by different free radical generating systems: a comparison with vitamin E. J Neurosurg Anesthesiol 8:154–158
Hara M, Kai Y, Ikemoto Y (1993) Propofol activates GABAA receptor-chloride ionophore complex in dissociated hippocampal pyramidal neurons of the rat. Anesthesiology 79:781–788

Hebbar L, Dorman BH, Clair MJ, Roy RC, Spinale FG (1997) Negative and selective effects of propofol on isolated swine myocyte contractile function in pacing-induced congestive heart failure. Anesthesiology 86:649–659

Hemmings HC, Akabas MH, Goldstein PA, Trudell JR, Orser BA, Harrison NL (2005) Emerging molecular mechanisms of general anesthetic action. Trends Pharmacol Sci 26:503–510

Hiraoka H, Yamamoto K, Miyoshi S, Morita T, Nakamura K, Kadoi Y, Kunimoto F, Horiuchi R (2005) Kidneys contribute to the extrahepatic clearance of propofol in humans, but not lungs and brain. Br J Clin Pharmacol 60:176–182

Hoff G, Bauer I, Larsen B, Bauer M (2001) Modulation of endotoxin-stimulated TNF alpha gene expression by ketamine and propofol in cultured human whole blood. Anaesthesist 50:494–499

Hughes MA, Glass PSA, Jacobs JR (1992) Context-sensitive half-time in multicompartment pharmacokinetic models for intravenous anesthetic drugs. Anesthesiology 76:334–341

Ito H, Watanabe Y, Isshiki A, Uchino H (1999) Neuroprotective properties of propofol and midazolam, but not pentobarbital, on neuronal damage induced by forebrain ischemia, based on the GABAA receptors. Acta Anaesthesiol Scand 43:153–162

Janicki PK, James MF, Erskine WA (1992) Propofol inhibits enzymatic degradation of alfentanil and sufentanil by isolated liver microsomes in vitro. Br J Anaesth 68:311–312

Javadov SA, Lim KH, Kerr PM, Suleiman MS, Angelini GD, Halestrap AP (2000) Protection of hearts from reperfusion injury by propofol is associated with inhibition of the mitochondrial permeability transition. Cardiovasc Res 45:360–369

Jensen AG, Lindroth M, Sjolander A, Eintrei C (1994) Propofol induced changes in the cytosolic free calcium concentration and the cytoskeletal organization of cultured human glial cells and primary embryonic rat brain cells. Anesthesiology 81:1220–1229

Jonsson MM, Lindahl SG, Eriksson LI (2005) Effect of propofol on carotid body chemosensitivity and cholinergic chemotransduction. Anesthesiology 102:110–116

Kahraman S, Kilinc K, Dal D, Erdem K (1997) Propofol attenuates formation of lipid peroxides in tourniquet-induced ischaemia-reperfusion injury. Br J Anaesth 78:279–281

Kanaya N, Murray PA, Damron DS (1998) Propofol and ketamine only inhibit intracellular Ca^{2+} transients and contraction in rat ventricular myocytes at supraclinical concentrations. Anesthesiology 88:781–791

Kanaya N, Murray PA, Damron DS (2001) Propofol increases myofilament Ca^{2+} sensitivity and intracellular pH via activation of Na+-H+ exchange in rat ventricular myocytes. Anesthesiology 94:1096–1104

Kaptanoglu E, Sen S, Beskonakli E, Surucu HS, Tuncel M, Kilinc K, Taskin Y (2002) Antioxidant actions and early ultrastructural findings of thiopental and propofol in experimental spinal cord injury. J Neurosurg Anesthesiol 14:114–122

Kataria BK, Ved SA, Nicodemus F, Hoy Gr, Lea D, Dubois MY, Mandema JW, Shafer SL (1994) The pharmacokinetics of propofol in children using three different data analysis approaches. Anesthesiology 80:104–122

Kawaguchi M, Furuya H, Patel PM (2005) Neuroprotective effects of anesthetic agents. J Anesth 19:150–156

Kawano T, Oshita S, Tsutsumi Y, Tomiyama Y, Kitahata H, Kuroda Y, Takahashi A, Nakaya Y (2002) Clinically relevant concentrations of propofol have no effect on adenosine triphosphate-sensitive potassium channels in rat ventricular myocytes. Anesthesiology 96:1472–1477

Kaye A, Anwar M, Bansiter R, Feng C, Turner K, Kadowitz P, Nossaman B (1999) Responses to propofol in the pulmonary vascular bed of the rat. Acta Anaesthesiol Scand 43:431–437

Kelbel I, Koch T, Weber A, Schiefer HG, Van Ackern K, Neuhof H (1999) Alterations of bacterial clearance induced by propofol. Acta Anaesthesiol Scand 43:71–76

Kevin LG, Novalija E, Stowe DF (2005) Reactive oxygen species as mediators of cardiac injury and protection: the relevance to anesthesia practice. Anesth Analg 101:1275–1287

Kikuchi T, Wang Y, Sato K, Okumura F (1998) In vivo effects of propofol on acetylcholine release from the frontal cortex, hippocampus and striatum studied by intracerebral microdialysis in freely moving rats. Br J Anaesth 80:644–648

Kirkpatrick T, Cockshott ID, Douglas EJ, Nimmo WS (1988) Pharmacokinetics of propofol (Diprivan) in elderly patients. Br J Anaesth 60:146–150

Kokita N, Hara A (1996) Propofol attenuates hydrogen peroxide-induced mechanical and metabolic derangements in the isolated rat heart. Anesthesiology 84:117–127

Kokita N, Hara A, Abiko Y, Arakawa J, Hashizume H, Namiki A (1998) Propofol improves functional and metabolic recovery in ischemic reperfused isolated rat hearts. Anesth Analg 86:252–258

Kooy NW, Royall JA, Ye YZ, Kelly DR, Beckman JS (1995) Evidence for in vivo peroxynitrite production in human acute lung injury. Am J Respir Crit Care Med 151:1250–1254

Krasowski MD, O'Shea SM, Rick CE, Whiting PJ, Hadingham KL, Czajkowski C, Harrison NL (1997) Alpha subunit isoform influences GABA(A) receptor modulation by propofol. Neuropharmacology 36:941–949

Krasowski MD, Nishikawa K, Nikolaeva N, Lin A, Harrison NL (2001) Methionine 286 in transmembrane domain 3 of the GABAA receptor beta subunit controls a binding cavity for propofol and other alkylphenol general anesthetics. Neuropharmacology 41:952–964

Krumholz W, Endrass I, Hempelmann G (1994) Propofol inhibits phagocytosis and killing of Staphylococcus aureus and Escherichia Coli by polymorphonuclear leukocytes in vitro. Can J Anaesth 41:446–449

Larsen B, Hoff G, Wilhelm W, Buchinger H, Wanner GA, Bauer M (1998) Effect of intravenous anesthetics on spontaneous and endotoxin-stimulated cytokine response in cultured human whole blood. Anesthesiology 89:1218–1227

Le Guellec C, Lacarelle B, Villard PH, Point H, Catalin J, Durand A (1995) Glucuronidation of propofol in microsomal fractions from various tissues and species including humans: effect of different drugs. Anesth Analg 81:855–861

Lee SR, Cheun JK (1999) Propofol administration reduces hippocampal neuronal damage induced by kainic acid in rats. Neurol Res 21:225–228

Lee VC, Moscicki JC, DiFazio CA (1998) Propofol sedation produces dose-dependent suppression of lidocaine-induced seizures in rats. Anesth Analg 86:652–657

Leung BP, Miller E, Park GR (1997) The effect of propofol on midazolam metabolism in human liver microsome suspension. Anaesthesia 52:945–948

Li YC, Ridefelt P, Wiklund L, Bjerneroth G (1997) Propofol induces a lowering of free cytosolic calcium in myocardial cells. Acta Anaesthesiol Scand 41:633–638

Lim KH, Halestrap AP, Angelini GD, Suleiman MS (2005) Propofol is cardioprotective in a clinically relevant model of normothermic blood cardioplegic arrest and cardiopulmonary bypass. Exp Biol Med 230:413–420

Loop T, Liu Z, Humar M, Hoetzel A, Benzing A, Pahl HL, Geiger KK, I Pannen BH (2002) Thiopental inhibits the activation of nuclear factor kappa B. Anesthesiology 96:1202–1213

Ludbrook GL, Visco E, Lam AM (2002) Propofol: relation between brain concentrations, electroencephalogram, middle cerebral artery blood flow velocity and cerebral oxygen extraction during induction of anesthesia. Anesthesiology 97:1363–1370

Machu TK, Harris RA (1994) Alcohols and anesthetics enhance the function of 5-hydroxytryptamine3 receptors expressed in Xenopus laevis oocytes. J Pharmacol Exp Ther 271:898–905

Mantz J, Cordier J, Giaume C (1993) Effects of general anesthetics on intercellular communications mediated by gap junctions between astrocytes in primary culture. Anesthesiology 78:892–901

Mantz J, Delumeau JC, Cordier J, Petitet F (1994) Differential effects of propofol and ketamine on cytosolic calcium concentrations of astrocytes in primary culture. Br J Anaesth 72:351–353

Mantz J, Lecharny JB, Laudenbach V, Henzel D, Peytavin G, Desmonts JM (1995) Anesthetics affect the uptake but not the depolarisation-evoked release of GABA in rat striatal synaptosomes. Anesthesiology 82:502–511

Marthur S, Farhangkhgoee P, Karmazyn M (1999) Cardioprotective effects of propofol and sevoflurane in ischemic and reperfused rat hearts: role of K(ATP) channels and interaction with the sodium-hydrogen exchange inhibitor HOE 642 (cariporide). Anesthesiology 91:1349–1360

Mather LE, Duke CC, Ladd LA, Copeland SE, Gallagher G, Chang DH (2004) Direct cardiac effects of coronary site-directed thiopental and its enantiomers: a comparison to propofol in conscious sheep. Anesthesiology 101:354–364

Mathy-Hartert M, Mouithys-Mickalad A, Kohnen S, Deby-Dupont G, Lamy M, Hans P (2000) Effects of propofol on endothelial cells subjected to a peroxynitrite donor (SIN-1). Anaesthesia 55:1066–1071

Meuret P, Backman SB, Bonhomme V, Plourde G, Fiset P (2000) Physostigmine reverses propofol-induced unconsciousness and attenuation of the auditory steady state response and Bispectral Index in human volunteers. Anesthesiology 93:708–717

Mikawa K, Akamatsu H, Nishina K, Shiga M, Maekawa N, Obara H, Niwa Y (1998) Propofol inhibits human neutrophil functions. Anesth Analg 87:695–700

Miyawaki I, Nakamura K, Terasako K, Toda H, Kakuyama M, Mori K (1995) Modification of endothelium-dependent relaxation by propofol, ketamine and midazolam. Anesth Analg 81:474–479

Murphy PG, Myers DS, Davies MJ, Webster NR, Jones JG (1992) The antioxidant potential of propofol (2,6-diisopropylphenol). Br J Anaesth 68:613–618

Murphy PG, Bennett JR, Myers DS, Davies MJ, Jones JG (1993) The effect of propofol anaesthesia on free radical-induced lipid peroxidation in rat liver microsomes. Eur J Anaesthesiol 10:261–266

Murugaiah KD, Hemmings HC (1998) Effects of intravenous general anesthetics on (3H)GABA release from rat cortical synaptosomes. Anesthesiology 89:919–928

Musacchio E, Rizzoli V, Bianchi M, Bindoli A, Galzigna L (1991) Antioxidant action of propofol on liver microsomes, mitochondria and brain synaptosomes in the rat. Pharmacol Toxicol 69:75–77

Nagata T, Kansha M, Irita K, Takahashi S (2001) Propofol inhibits FMLP-stimulated phosphorylation of p42 mitogen-activated protein kinase and chemotaxis in human neutrophils. Br J Anaesth 86:853–858

Nagyova B, Dorrington KL, Gill EW, Robbins PA (1995) Comparison of the effects of subhypnotic concentrations of propofol and halothane on the acute ventilatory response to hypoxia. Br J Anaesth 75:713–718

Nakayama M, Murray PA (1999) Ketamine preserves and propofol potentiates hypoxic pulmonary vasoconstriction compared with the conscious state in chronically instrumented dogs. Anesthesiology 91:760–771

Nelson LE, Guo TZ, Lu J, Saper CB, Franks NP, Maze M (2002) The sedative component of anesthesia is mediated by GABAA receptors in an endogenous sleep pathway. Nat Neurosci 5:979–984

Newman MF, Murkin JM, Roach G, Croughwell ND, White WD, Clements FM, Reves JG (1995) Cerebral physiologic effects of burst suppression doses of propofol during nonpulsatile cardiopulmonary bypass. CNS subgroup of McSPI. Anesth Analg 81:452–457

Nieuwenhuijs D, Sarton E, Teppema LJ, Dahan A (2000) Propofol for monitored anesthesia care: implications on hypoxic control of cardiorespiratory responses. Anesthesiology 92:46–54

Nieuwenhuijs D, Sarton E, Teppema LJ, Kruyt E, Olievier I, Van Kleef J, Dahan A (2001) Respiratory sites of action of propofol: absence of depression of peripheral chemoreflex loop by low-dose propofol. Anesthesiology 95:889–895

Ogawa K, Tanaka S, Murray PA (2001) Propofol potentiates phenylephrine-induced contraction via cyclooxygenase inhibition in pulmonary artery smooth muscle. Anesthesiology 94:833–839

Ohmizo H, Iwama H, Sugita T (1999) Complement activation by propofol and its effect during propofol anesthesia. Anaesth Intensive Care 27:623–627

Orser BA, Wang LY, Pennefather PS, MacDonald JF (1994) Propofol modulates activation and desensitization of GABAA receptors in cultured murine hippocampal neurons. J Neurosci 14:7747–7760

Orser BA, Bertlik M, Wang LY, MacDonald JF (1995) Inhibition by propofol (2,6 di-isopropylphenol) of the N-methyl-D-aspartate subtype of glutamate receptor in cultured hippocampal neurones. Br J Pharmacol 116:1761–1768

Ouattara A, Langeron O, Souktani R, Mouren S, Coriat P, Riou B (2001) Myocardial and coronary effects of propofol in rabbits with compensated cardiac hypertrophy. Anesthesiology 95:699–707

Ouedraogo N, Roux E, Forestier F, Rossetti M, Savineau JP, Marthan R (1998) Effects of intravenous anesthetics on normal and passively sensitized human isolated airway smooth muscle. Anesthesiology 88:317–326

Ouedraogo N, Marthan R, Roux E (2003) The effects of propofol and etomidate on airway contractility in chronically hypoxic rats. Anesth Analg 96:1035–1041

Pain L, Oberling P, Launoy A, Di Scala G (1999) Effect of nonsedative doses of propofol on an innate anxiogenic situation in rats. Anesthesiology 90:191–196

Pedersen CM, Thirstrup S, Nielsen-Kudsk JE (1993) Smooth muscle relaxant effects of propofol and ketamine in isolated guinea-pig trachea. Eur J Pharmacol 238:75–80

Peduto VA, Concas A, Santoro G, Biggio G, Gessa GL (1991) Biochemical and electrophysiological evidence that propofol enhances GABAergic transmission in the rat brain. Anesthesiology 75:1000–1009

Pinaud M, Lelausque JN, Chetanneau A, Fauchoux N, Menegalli D, Souron R (1990) Effects of propofol on cerebral hemodynamics and metabolism in patients with brain trauma. Anesthesiology 73:404–409

Pirttikangas CO, Salo M, Riutta A, Perttila J, Pletola O, Kirvela O (1995) Effects of propofol and Intralipid on immune response and prostaglandin E2 production. Anaesthesia 50:317–321

Pistis M, Belelli D, Peters JA, Lambert JJ (1997) The interaction of general anesthetics with recombinant GABAA and glycine receptors expressed in Xenopus laevis oocytes: a comparative study. Br J Pharmacol 122:1707–1717

Pittman JE, Sheng H, Pearlstein R, Brinkhous A, Dexter F, Warner DS (1997) Comparison of the effects of propofol and pentobarbital on neurologic outcome and cerebral infarct size after temporary focal ischemia in the rat. Anesthesiology 87:1139–1144

Ponte J, Sadler CL (1989) Effect of thiopentone, etomidate and propofol on carotid body chemoreceptor activity in the rabbit and the cat. Br J Anaesth 62:41–45

Rasmussen PA, Yang Y, Rutecki PA (1996) Propofol inhibits epileptiform activity in rat hippocampal slices. Epilepsy Res 25:169–175

Ravussin P, Guinard JP, Ralley F, Thorin D (1988) Effect of propofol on cerebrospinal fluid pressure and cerebral perfusion pressure in patients undergoing craniotomy. Anaesthesia 43 [Suppl]:37–41

Reddy RV, Moorthy SS, Dierdorf SE, Deitch RD, Link L (1993) Excitatory effects and electroencephalographic correlation of etomidate, thiopental, methohexital and propofol. Anesth Analg 77:1008–1011

Riou B, Besse S, Lecarpentier Y, Viars P (1992) In vitro effects of propofol on rat myocardium. Anesthesiology 76:609–616

Salo M, Pirttikangas CO, Pulkki K (1997) Effects of propofol emulsion and thiopentone on T-helper cell type-1/type-2 balance in vitro. Anaesthesia 52:341–344

Sanderink GJ, Bournique B, Stevens J, Petry M, Martinet M (1997) Involvement of human CYP1A isoenzymes in the metabolism and drug interactions of riluzole in vitro. J Pharmacol Exp Ther 282:1465–1472

Sanna E, Mascia MP, Klein RL, Whiting PJ, Biggio G, Harris RA (1995) Actions of the general anesthetic propofol on recombinant human $GABA_A$ receptors: influence of receptor subunits. J Pharmacol Exp Ther 274:353–360

Sayin MM, Ozatamer O, Tasoz R, Kilinc K, Unal N (2002) Propofol attenuates myocardial lipid peroxidation during coronary artery bypass grafting surgery. Br J Anaesth 89:242–246

Schnider TW, Minto CF, Gambus PL, Andresen C, Goodale DB, Shafer SL, Youngs EJ (1998) The influence of method of administration and covariates on the pharmacokinetics of propofol in adult volunteers. Anesthesiology 88:1170–1182

Schnider TW, Minto CF, Shafer SL, Gambus PL, Andresen C, Goodale DB, Youngs EJ (1999) The influence of age on propofol pharmacodynamics. Anesthesiology 90:1502–1516

Schüttler J, Ihmsen H (2000) Population pharmacokinetics of propofol: a multicenter study. Anesthesiology 92:727–738

Schüttler J, Schwilden H, Stoeckel H (1986) Pharmacokinetic modeling of diprivan. Anesthesiology 65:A549

Shafer A, Doze VA, Shafer SL, White PF (1988) Pharmacokinetics and pharmacodynamics of propofol infusions during general anesthesia. Anesthesiology 69:348–356

Shafer SL, Varvel JR (1991) Pharmacokinetics, pharmacodynamics and rational opioid selection. Anesthesiology 74:53–63

Sitar SM, Hanifi-Moghaddam P, Gelb A, Cechetto DF, Siushansian R, Wilson JX (1999) Propofol prevents peroxide-induced inhibition of glutamate transport in cultured astrocytes. Anesthesiology 90:1446–1453

Smith C, McEwan AI, Jhaveri R, Wilkinson M, Goodman D, Smith LR, Canada AT, Glass PS (1994a) The interaction of fentanyl on the Cp50 of propofol for loss of consciousness and skin incision. Anesthesiology 81:820–828

Smith I, Monk TG, White PF, Ding Y (1994b) Propofol infusion during regional anesthesia: sedative, amnestic and anxiolytic properties. Anesth Analg 79:313–319

Sprung J, Ogletree-Hughes ML, McConnell BK, Zakhary DR, Smolsky SM, Moravec CS (2001) The effects of propofol on the contractility of failing and nonfailing human heart muscles. Anesth Analg 93:550–559

Strebel S, Lam AM, Matta B, Mayberg TS, Aaslid R, Newell DW (1995) Dynamic and static cerebral autoregulation during isoflurane, desflurane and propofol anesthesia. Anesthesiology 83:66–76

Sztark F, Ichas F, Ouhabi R, Dabadie P, Mazat JP (1995) Effects of the anesthetic propofol on the calcium-induced permeability transition of rat heart mitochondria: direct pore inhibition and shift of the gating potential. FEBS Lett 368:101–104

Takaono M, Yogosawa T, Okawa-Takatsuji M, Aotsuka S (2002) Effects of intravenous anesthetics on interleukin (IL)-6 and IL-10 production by lipopolysaccharide-stimulated mononuclear cells from healthy volunteers. Acta Anaesthesiol Scand 46:176–179

Taniguchi T, Yamamoto K, Ohmoto N, Ohta K, Kobayashi T (2000) Effects of propofol on hemodynamic and inflammatory responses to endotoxinemia in rats. Crit Care Med 28:1101–1106

Taniguchi T, Kanakura H, Yamamoto K (2002) Effects of posttreatment with propofol on mortality and cytokine responses to endotoxin-induced shock in rats. Crit Care Med 30:904–907

Thiry JC, Hans P, Deby-Dupont G, Mouythis-Mickalad A, Bonhomme V, Lamy M (2004) Propofol scavenges reactive oxygen species and inhibits the protein nitration induced by activated polymorphonuclear neutrophils. Eur J Pharmacol 499:29–33

Trapani G, Altomare C, Liso G, Sanna E, Biggio G (2000) Propofol in anesthesia. Mechanism of action, structure-activity relationships and drug delivery. Curr Med Chem 7:249–271

Van Hemelrijck J, Van Aken H, Plets C, Goffin J, Vermaut G (1989) The effects of propofol on intracranial pressure and cerebral perfusion pressure in patients with brain tumors. Acta Anaesthesiol Belg 40:95–100

Van Hemelrijck J, Fitch W, Mattheussen M, Van Aken H, Plets C, Lauwers T (1990) Effect of propofol on cerebral circulation and autoregulation in the baboon. Anesth Analg 71:49–54

Van Keer L, Van Aken H, Vandermeersch E, Vermaut G, Lerut T (1989) Propofol does not inhibit hypoxic pulmonary vasoconstriction in humans. J Clin Anesth 1:284–288

Velly LJ, Guillet BA, Masmejean FM, Nieoullon AL, Bruder NJ, Gouin FM, Pisano PM (2003) Neuroprotective effects of propofol in a model of ischemic cortical cell cultures: role of glutamate and its transporters. Anesthesiology 99:368–375

Veroli P, O'Kelly B, Bertrand F, Trouvin JH, Farinotti R, Ecoffey C (1992) Extrahepatic metabolism of propofol in man during the anhepatic phase of orthotopic liver transplantation. Br J Anaesth 68:183–186

Vuyk J, Oostwouder CJ, Vletter AA, Burm AG, Bovill JG (2000) Gender differences in the pharmacokinetics of propofol in elderly patients during and after continuous infusion. Br J Anaesth 86:183–188

Wakeling HG, Zimmerman JB, Howell S, Glass PS (1999) Targeting effect compartment or central compartment concentration of propofol: what predicts loss of consciousness? Anesthesiology 90:92–97

Wang J, Yang X, Camporesi CV, Yang Z, Bosco G, Chen C, Camporesi EM (2002) Propofol reduces infarct size and striatal dopamine accumulation following transient middle cerebral artery occlusion: a microdialysis study. Eur J Pharmacol 452:303–308

Wilson JX, Gelb AW (2002) Free radicals, antioxidants and neurologic injury: possible relationship to cerebral protection by anesthetics. J Neurosurg Anesthesiol 14:66–79

Wood PL, Cheney DL, Costa E (1979) An investigation of whether septal gamma-aminobutyrate-containing interneurons are involved in the reduction in the turnover rate of acetylcholine elicited by substance P and beta-endorphin in the hippocampus. Neuroscience 4:1479–1484

Wouters PF, Van de Velde MA, Marcus MA, Deruyter HA, Van Aken H (1995) Hemodynamic changes during induction of anesthesia with eltanolone and propofol in dogs. Anesth Analg 81:125–131

Xia Z, Godin DV, Ansley DM (2003) Propofol enhances ischemic tolerance of middle-aged rat hearts: effects on 15-F(2t)-isoprostane formation and tissue antioxidant capacity. Cardiovasc Res 59:113–121

Xia Z, Godin DV, Ansley DM (2004) Application of high-dose propofol during ischemia improves postischemic function of rat hearts: effects on tissue antioxidant capacity. Can J Physiol Pharmacol 82:919–926

Yamaguchi S, Hamagushi S, Mishio M, Okuda Y, Kitajima T (2000) Propofol prevents lipid peroxidation following transient forebrain ischemia in gerbils. Can J Anaesth 47:1025–1030

Yamakage M, Kamada Y, Toriyabe M, Honma Y, Namiki A (1999) Changes in respiratory pattern and arterial blood gases during sedation with propofol or midazolam in spinal anesthesia. J Clin Anesth 11:375–379

Yamasaki T, Nakakimura K, Matsumoto M, Xiong L, Ishikawa T, Sakabe T (1999) Effects of graded suppression of the EEG with propofol on the neurological outcome following incomplete cerebral ischaemia in rats. Eur J Anaesthesiol 16:320–329

Yoo KY, Yang SY, Lee J, Im WM, Jeong CY, Chung SS, Kwak SH (1999) Intracoronary propofol attenuates myocardial but not coronary endothelial dysfunction after brief ischemia and reperfusion in dogs. Br J Anaesth 82:90–96

Young Y, Menon DK, Tisavipat N, Matta BF, Jones JG (1997) Propofol neuroprotection in a rat model of ischaemia reperfusion injury. Eur J Anaesthesiol 14:320–326

Zacny JP, Lichtor JL, Coalson DW, Finn RS, Uitvlugt AM, Glosten B, Flemming DC, Apfelbaum JL (1992) Subjective and psychomotor effects of subanesthetic doses of propofol in healthy volunteers. Anesthesiology 76:696–702

Pharmacokinetics and Pharmacodynamics of GPI 15715 or Fospropofol (Aquavan Injection) – A Water-Soluble Propofol Prodrug

J. Fechner(✉), H. Schwilden, and J. Schüttler

Abstract Propofol (2,6-diisopropylphenol) is inadequably soluble in water and is therefore formulated as a lipid emulsion. This may have disadvantages when propofol is used to provide total intravenous anaesthesia or especially during long-term sedation. There has been considerable interest in the development of new propofol formulations or propofol prodrugs. GPI 15715 or fospropofol (Aquavan injection; Guilford Pharmaceutical, Baltimore, MD) is the first water-soluble prodrug that has been thoroughly studied in human volunteers and patients. GPI 15751 or fospropofol is cleaved by alkaline phosphatase to phosphate, formaldehyde and propofol. Formaldehyde is rapidly metabolised to formate. Although a formate accumulation is the principal pathomechanism responsible for the toxicity of methanol ingestion, so far there has been no report of toxicity due to the administration of fospropofol or other phosphate ester prodrugs, such as fosphenytoin. Fosphenytoin has been successfully introduced into the market for the treatment of status epilepticus in 1996. The main side-effects were a feeling of paraesthesia after rapid i.v. administration of GPI 15715 or fospropofol, which has also been described for fosphenytoin. The pharmacokinetics of GPI 15715 or fospropofol could be described by a combined pharmacokinetic model with a submodel of two compartments for GPI 15715 and of three compartments for propofol$_G$. The liberated propofol$_G$ compared to lipid-formulated propofol showed unexpected pharmacokinetic and pharmacodynamic differences.

J. Fechner
Klinik für Anästhesiologie, Universität Erlangen-Nürnberg, Krankenhausstrasse. 12, 91054 Erlangen, Germany
joerg.fechner@kfa.imed.uni-erlangen.de

J. Schüttler and H. Schwilden (eds.) *Modern Anesthetics. Handbook of Experimental Pharmacology 182.*

We found a significantly greater V_c, V_{dss}, significantly shorter α- and β-half-life and a longer MRT (mean residence time) for $propofol_G$. The pharmacodynamic potency of $propofol_G$ appears to be higher than propofol when measured by EEG and clinical signs of hypnosis. In summary, GPI 15715 or fospropofol was well suited to provide anaesthesia or conscious sedation.

1 Introduction

Due to its unique pharmacokinetic and pharmacodynamic profile propofol (2,6-diisopropylphenol) is the most often used intravenous anaesthetic to provide total intravenous anaesthesia. It is also often used to provide procedural and long-term sedation. Propofol is an oil at room temperature and is inadequably soluble in aqueous solutions. It is formulated in a 10% (w/v) Intralipid (Baxter Healthcare, Deerfield, IL) solution or other lipid-containing solvents (see chapter by C. Vanlersberghe and F. Camu, this volume). There is considerable concern about the side-effects of these lipid solutions and/or the lipid solvent Intralipid. When anaesthesia is induced with a bolus application of propofol, about 30% of patients (Bachmann-Mennenga et al. 2003) have mild to moderate pain on injection. Although propofol lipid emulsion is bactericidal or bacteriostatic for some micro-organisms such as *Staphylococcus aureus* (Crowther et al. 1996), it does support the growth of other clinically relevant pathogens such as *Escherichia coli* or *Candida albicans* (Graystone et al. 1997; Wachowski et al. 1999). Propofol lipid solutions containing 0.005% (w/v) disodium edetate may have a reduced potency to support bacterial growth, although no clear effect on the rate of bacterial growth after contamination at room temperature could be demonstrated, and Intralipid itself clearly supports bacterial growth (Fukada and Ozaki 2007; Langevin et al. 1999; Vidovich et al. 1999). Prolonged infusion of propofol for sedation may cause hypertriglyceridemia, which is a limitation for the use of propofol for long-term sedation (Lindholm 1992; McKeage and Perry 2003). Therefore during the last several years there has been considerable interest in the development of new propofol formulations or a propofol prodrug. The first reports of propofol in aqueous solutions with the solvent propylene glycol, hydroxy-β-cyclodextrin or 2-hydroxypropyl-γ-cyclodextrin have been published (Egan et al. 2003; Trapani et al. 2004). A propofol micro-emulsion with the solvent Poloxamer 188 (BASF Company, Florham Park, NJ) has been tested in an animal model in dogs (Morey et al. 2006) and a propofol micro-emulsion with the solvent propylene glycol 660 hydroxystearate (Solutol HS 15, BASF Company, Seoul) has been tested in the first study for anaesthesia in man (Kim et al. 2007). Besides the approach of developing a better-suited solvent, it is also possible today to administer propofol as a prodrug. A different propofol formulation does not necessarily change the pharmacokinetics and pharmacodynamics (PK/PD) of the administered propofol, although in studies with a lipid-free propofol solution in rats these PK/PD differences have been reported (Dutta and Ebling 1997a; Dutta and Ebling 1998a, b). Propofol liberated from a prodrug of propofol will definitely show different pharmacokinetics and possibly different pharmacodynamics when compared to lipid-formulated propofol solutions. To date three propofol prodrugs have been synthesised and tested. Propofol sodium hemisuccinate (Sagara et al. 1999; Vansant et al. 2007) has clearly neuroprotective properties even in a rat model of experimental autoimmune encephalitis (EAE). Nothing is known about the anaesthetic effects of propofol sodium hemisuccinate in man, as it was found unsuitable for commercial development because of its instability in aqueous solutions (Banaszczyk et al. 2002). Propofol phosphate liberates inorganic phosphate and propofol. So far it has only been studied in mice, rabbits, rats and pigs. GPI 15715 or fospropofol is the first propofol prodrug that has been studied in volunteers and patients and was administered to provide conscious sedation and total intravenous anaesthesia.

2 GPI 15715 or Fospropofol Disodium (Aquavan Injection)

GPI 15715 or fospropofol disodium is a water-soluble phosphate ester of propofol (2,6-diisopropylphenol). It is chemically described as $C_{13}H_{19}O_5PNa_2$ or 2,6-diisopropylphenol methoxyphosphonic acid. The structural formula is given in Fig. 1. The molecular weight of fospropofol is 332.24 and the molecular weight ratio of fospropofol to propofol is 1.86:1. Fospropofol, as compared to propofol, has attached a methyl phosphate side-chain to the C_1 atom of the phenol ring. The polarity of the attached phosphate group makes the new fospropofol molecule water-soluble. Fospropofol is not the first phosphate ester prodrug that has been studied in man. In 1984 in a comparable approach, fosphenytoin was synthesised; it contains the identical methyl phosphate side-chain as fospropofol. Fosphenytoin ((2,5-dioxo-4,4-diphenyl-imidazolidin-1-yl) methoxyphosphonic acid) (Varia and Stella 1984a, b) is a water-soluble prodrug of phenytoin, a classical anti-epileptic drug, and was successfully licensed for the treatment of status epilepticus in 1996. Phenytoin is also inadequately soluble in water and the solvents ethanol 10% and propylene glycol 40% are added to the commercially available solution. Comparably to propofol, many patients have severe pain when phenytoin is injected into a peripheral vein and often a peripheral phlebitis develops (Jamerson et al. 1990).

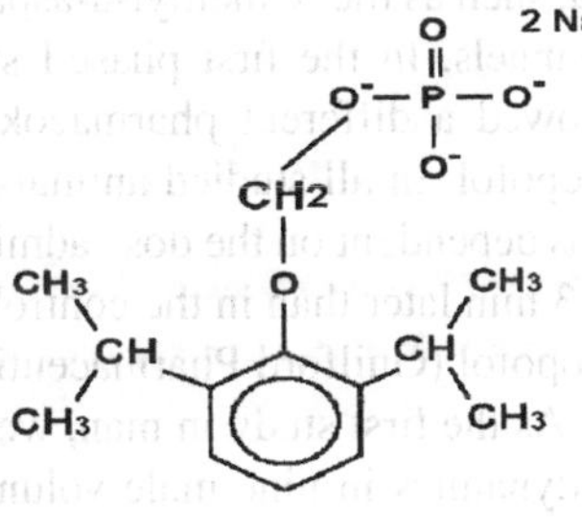

Fig. 1 Chemical structure of GPI 15715 or fospropofol disodium

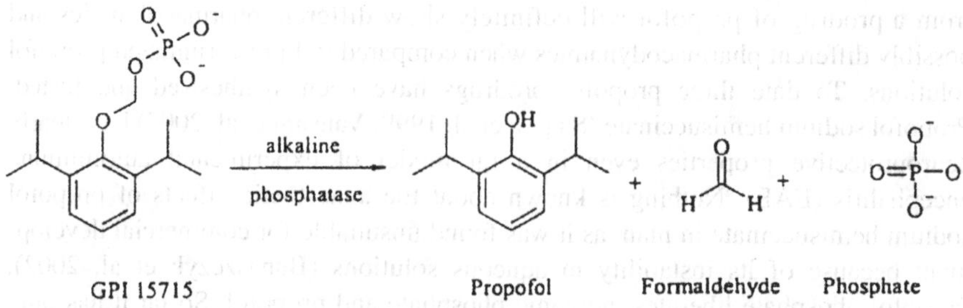

Fig. 2 Degradation of GPI 15715 to propofol, formaldehyde and phosphate by alkaline phosphatase

Fospropofol disodium is hydrolysed by alkaline phosphatases to release propofol, formaldehyde and phosphate (Fig. 2). Formaldehyde is rapidly converted by the enzyme aldehyde dehydrogenase to formic acid or formate, and levels of formaldehyde are only transiently found and difficult to measure. Formate is a naturally occurring substance in the metabolism of mammalian organisms and in humans, and is further metabolised to CO_2 and H_2O in the presence of tetrahydrofolic acid as coenzyme. Although formate is principally responsible for the methanol toxicity and is capable of inhibiting the cytochrome oxidase chain, increasing lactate production which can lead to metabolic acidosis, this is the case only when the amount of formate produced is extremely high or there is an acquired severe deficiency of tetrahydrofolic acid. Also fosphenytoin does produce the same metabolites as fospropofol, as mentioned before, and to date there has been no report of formate toxicity caused by the administration of fosphenytoin. The physiologically occurring formate concentrations in man are in the range of 13 ± 7 μg ml^{-1} (d'Alessandro et al. 1994), and so far all measured formate concentrations during the administration of fospropofol have been no higher than this physiological range.

GPI 15715 is formulated as 2% solution in 0.4% normal saline (w/v, aqua ad injectabilis). The glass ampoules contain N_2O, and the pH of the intravenously injectable solution is 8.4 ± 0.4. It can be reasonably assumed that the pharmacologically active anaesthetic agent of fospropofol is the liberated propofol, which interacts with the $GABA_A$ receptors of the CNS. In receptor studies GPI 15715 showed no direct binding to the $GABA_A$ receptor up to a concentration of 10 mM, which is equivalent to 3,322.4 μg ml^{-1}. As far as can be ascertained, there was also no binding or effect of GPI 15715 at other known relevant receptor systems for anaesthesia, such as the *N*-methyl-d-aspartate (NMDA) receptor or potassium or sodium ion channels. In the first phase I studies in mice, rats, rabbits and dogs, GPI 15715 showed a different pharmacokinetic profile when compared to lipid-formulated propofol. In all studied animals GPI 15715 showed a hypnotic/sedative effect that was dependent on the dose administered. The hypnotic/sedative effect was achieved 2–3 min later than in the control group of animals, which received lipid-formulated propofol (Guilford Pharmaceutical Industries, now MGI Pharma, data on file).

As the first study in man, we studied the pharmacokinetics and clinical pharmacodynamics in nine male volunteers who received 290, 580 and 1,160 mg of GPI as a constant rate infusion over 10 min (Fechner et al. 2003). In a second study, based on the pharmacokinetic results of the first, 9 male volunteers initially received a target-controlled infusion (TCI infusion of GPI 15715, and after a wash-out period of 14 days a TCI infusion of lipid-formulated propofol (Diprivan, AstraZeneca, London) with the same propofol target concentrations as before (crossover design). At the start of infusion there was a linear increase of the TCI target up to 5 μg ml^{-1} over 20 min, then the TCI target was reduced to 3 μg ml^{-1} for the next 20 min and then further reduced to 1.5 μg ml^{-1} for the last 20 min. After 60 min the infusion was stopped (Fechner et al. 2004). The following sections present some of the PK/PD results of these two studies. To make the difference between lipid-formulated propofol and propofol liberated from GPI 15715 more clear, the lipid-formulated propofol will be called $propofol_L$ and the propofol liberated from the prodrug GPI 15715 $propofol_G$.

2.1 Comparative Pharmacokinetics of $Propofol_G$ Liberated from GPI 15715 and Lipid-Formulated Propofol

Using a population pharmacokinetic analysis (NONMEM, GloboMax, Hanover, MD), the pharmacokinetics of GPI 15715 and the liberated $propofol_G$ could be reasonably well modelled. The pharmacokinetics of GPI 15715 could be described with a two-compartment model. GPI 15715 showed a relatively small central volume of distribution of 0.072±0.011 L kg^{-1} and a V_{dss} of 0.1±0.17 L kg^{-1}. The distribution half-life of GPI 15715 was 6.5±1.1 min and the elimination half-life of GPI 15715 was 46±11 min. There was a markedly fast conversion of GPI 15715 to propofol. The half-life for the hydrolysis of GPI 15715 was estimated from the first study as 7.1±1.1 and in the second study, 7.9±1.5 min. The value is well in agreement with the data published for fosphenytoin. For fosphenytoin a half-life for the hydrolysis to phenytoin of 8.1±1.5 min has been published (Gerber et al. 1988).

The liberated propofol could be adequately described with a three-compartment model. At the conclusion of both studies we found a combined pharmacokinetic model with two compartments for GPI 15715 and three compartments for $propofol_G$. This model is shown in Fig. 3. The mean pharmacokinetic data of GPI 1515 as well as $propofol_G$ compared to $propofol_L$ are given in Table 1. As a measure for goodness of fit of this population pharmacokinetic model, Figs. 4 and 5 show the prediction error over time of the model-predicted and measured $propofol_G$ and $propofol_L$ concentrations. In contrast to the phenytoin liberated from fosphenytoin, which behaved pharmacokinetically similar to normal administered phenytoin, we found unexpected pharmacokinetic differences when $propofol_G$ was compared with $propofol_L$. $Propofol_G$ showed a significantly greater central volume of distribution and a significantly greater volume at steady state as well as significantly shorter α- and β-distribution half-lives. These values are also given in Table 1. In Fig. 3 the term $Fk_{10}{}^G$ denotes the amount of $propofol_G$ mass input into the central compartment of $propofol_G$ after liberation of $propofol_G$ from GPI 15715 in the central compartment of GPI. The second arrow illustrates the possibility

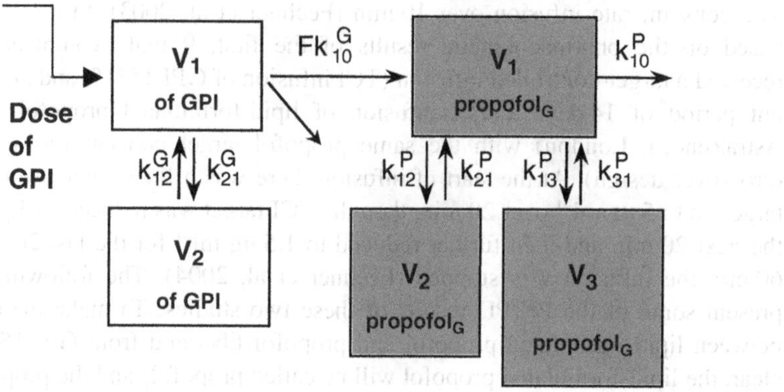

Fig. 3 Pharmacokinetic model of GPI 15715 and liberated propofol$_G$

Table 1 PK parameter of propofol$_L$ and propofol$_G$ estimated in the crossover study by Fechner et al. (2004). The asterisk stands for statistically significant differences. MRT (mean residence time) was estimated as the model-independent PK parameter. V_c, V_{ss} and CL of propofol$_G$ are given for a metabolism factor F=0.54

Parameter	Propofol$_L$	Propofol$_G$	GPI 15715
k_{12} (min^{-1})	0.017±0.005	0.16±0.09*	0.012±0.006
k_{21} (min^{-1})	0.014±0.007	0.078±0.032*	0.022±0.004
k_{13} (min^{-1})	0.025±0.010	0.048±0.025*	–
k_{31} (min^{-1})	0.0029±0.004	0.0023±0.0005	–
k_{10} (min^{-1})	0.11±0.02	0.07±0.02*	0.090±0.017
CL (ml kg^{-1} min^{-1})	23.7±2.9	37.8±9.4*	6.7±1.0
V_c (l kg^{-1})	0.23±0.03	0.55±0.14*	0.08±0.01
V_{dss} (l kg^{-1})	4.5±2.1	12.4±4.6*	0.11±0.01
$t_{1/2}\alpha$ (min)	4.7±0.8	2.5±1.2*	6.9±1.3
$t_{1/2}\beta$ (min)	58.2±17.9	26.3±9.3*	37.7±4.6
$t_{1/2}\gamma$ (min)	651±194	543±223	–
MRT (min)	185±99	348±265*	17.1±2.5

k_{12}, k_{21}, k_{13}, k_{31}: transfer rate constants between the central and the peripheral compartments; k_{10}, elimination rate constant; CL, elimination clearance; V_c, central volume of distribution; V_{ss}, volume of distribution at steady state; $t_{1/2}\alpha$, fast half-life; $t_{1/2}\beta$, intermediate half-life; $t_{1/2}\gamma$, terminal half-life

*p<0.05 propofol$_G$ vs propofol$_L$

that not all liberated propofol$_G$ is transferred to the central propofol$_G$ compartment. F is the conversion factor, and theoretically—based on the molecular weight ratio GPI to propofol of 1,86:1—F should be 0.54 if all GPI 15715 is converted to propofol and all liberated propofol$_G$ is transferred to the central propofol$_G$ compartment. Also based on the measured concentrations and dose administered, F can be calculated as

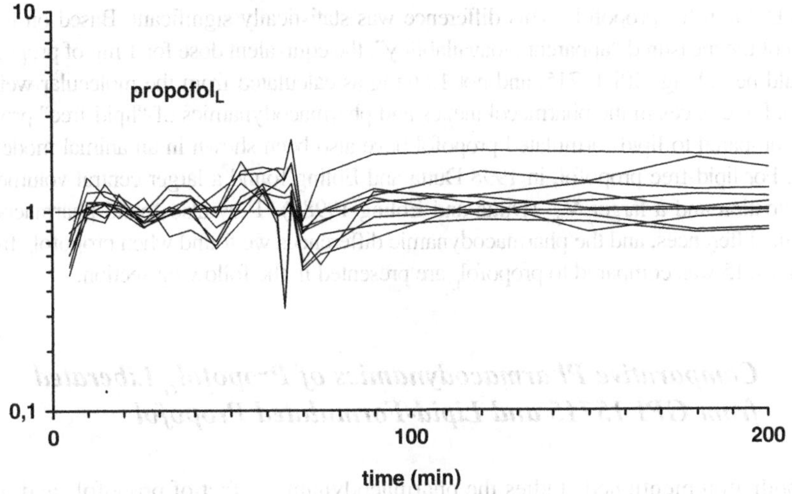

Fig. 4 Prediction error of the estimated PK model for propofol$_L$

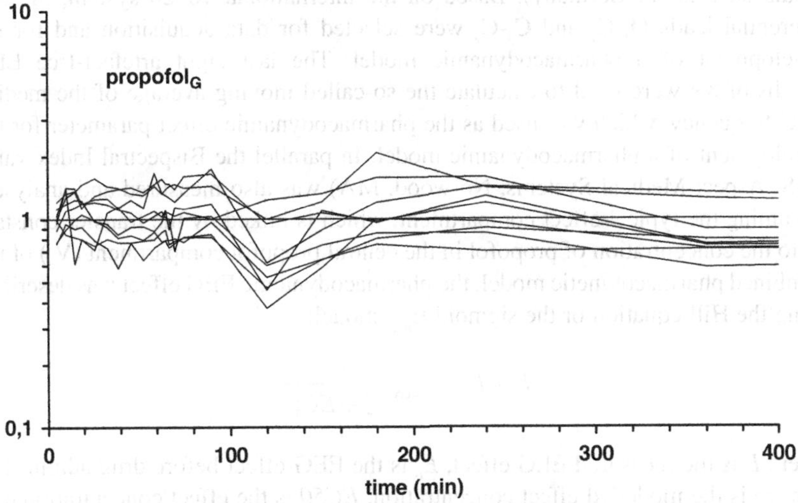

Fig. 5 Prediction error of the estimated PK model for propofol$_G$

$$F = \frac{AUC_{\mathrm{Propofol}_G} D_{\mathrm{Propofol}_L}}{AUC_{\mathrm{Propofol}_L} D_{GPI}}$$

For F in the crossover study we found a value of 0.35±0.09, which is equivalent to an "apparent bioavailability" of 65%. In contrast for fosphenytoin, a 100% apparent bioavailability of was measured (Browne et al. 1989). Additionally, the model-independent mean residence time (MRT) was calculated as 348±265 min for propofol$_G$ and as

185±99 min for $propofol_L$. This difference was statistically significant. Based on these data of the measured "apparent bioavailability", the equivalent dose for 1 mg of $propofol_L$ would be 2.9 mg GPI 15715, and not 1.86 mg as calculated from the molecular weight ratio. Differences in the pharmacokinetics and pharmacodynamics of "lipid-free" propofol compared to lipid-formulated propofol have also been shown in an animal model in rats. For lipid-free propofol, in 1998 Dutta and Ebling found a larger central volume of distribution and a larger V_{dss} (Dutta and Ebling 1998b). They also found pharmacodynamic differences, and the pharmacodynamic differences we found when $propofol_G$ from GPI 15715 was compared to $propofol_L$ are presented in the following section.

2.2 *Comparative Pharmacodynamics of $Propofol_G$ Liberated from GPI 15715 and Lipid-Formulated Propofol*

In both aforementioned studies the pharmacodynamic effect of $propofol_G$ and $propofol_L$ was quantified using EEG. EEG data were stored and analysed with the CATEEM Monitoring system (Computer Aided Topographical Encephalometry, Medisyst, Linden, Germany). Based on the international 10–20 system, the two referential leads O_1-C_z and C_3-C_z were selected for data acquisition and for the development of a pharmacodynamic model. The last eight artefact-free EEG epochs of 8 s were used to calculate the so-called moving average of the median EEG frequency, which was used as the pharmacodynamic effect parameter for the development of a pharmacodynamic model. In parallel the Bispectral Index value (BIS; Aspect Medical Systems, Norwood, MA) was also measured and analysed. Assuming the typical effect compartment, which is linked by the transfer constant k_{eo} to the concentration of propofol in the central propofol compartment (V_c) of the combined pharmacokinetic model, the pharmacodynamic EEG effect was described using the Hill equation or the sigmoid E_{max} model:

$$E = E_0 - E_{\max} \frac{c_e^\gamma}{c_e^\gamma + EC_{50}^\gamma},$$

where E is the measured EEG effect, E_0 is the EEG-effect before drug administration, *ce* is the modelled effect concentration, *EC50* is the effect concentration corresponding to the observed half-maximal EEG effect and E_{max} is the maximal observed EEG effect, γ is the Hill coefficient. Especially in the volunteers receiving lipid-formulated propofol, we observed increasing β-band activity during induction of anaesthesia/sedation and during recovery. Therefore for modelling purposes the Hill equation was modified to:

$$E = E_0 - \left(E_{\max} + E_\beta\right)\frac{c_e^\gamma}{c_e^\gamma + EC_{50}^\gamma} + E_\beta \frac{c_e^\kappa}{c_e^\kappa + EC_\beta^\kappa}$$

The comparative pharmacodynamics of GPI 15715 and lipid-formulated propofol could be described analysing the data of the crossover study (see Sect. 2 above), where each volunteer received first a TCI infusion of GPI 15715 with three propofol target concentrations and, after a 14-day washout period, a TCI of lipid-formulated propofol with identical propofol target concentrations, so that the pharmacodynamic effect could be directly compared. As clinical measures of the sedative/hypnotic effect, a modified Observer's Assessment of Alertness/Sedation Scale (OAA/S) score (Chernik et al. 1990)—loss and recovery of consciousness (tested as reaction or no reaction to loud verbal command), and loss and recovery of lid reflex and loss and recovery of corneal reflex—was used. Finally hysteresis loops were calculated and the area minimised to determine the hysteresis of both propofol_G and propofol_L.

Figure 6 shows the observed EEG effect of propofol_G and propofol during the TCI infusions with a linear increasing target concentration of 5 µg ml^{-1} over 20 min, TCI target concentration of 3 µg ml^{-1} from 20 to 40 min and TCI target concentration of 1.5 µg ml^{-1} from 40 to 60 min. After 60 min the infusion was stopped. The pharmacodynamic analyses from the crossover study as described above again showed unexpected results. Propofol_G liberated from GPI 15715 behaved differently from propofol_L. During the start of infusion of GPI 15715 and after administration there was less β-activity in the EEG. Although propofol_G had to be liberated from GPI 15715 before a pharmacodynamic effect could occur and although the half-life for hydrolysis was about 7.9 ± 1.5 min in this investigation with a linear increase of a TCI target concentration over 20 min, the clinical as well as the EEG effects were observed earlier and at a lower effect concentration of propofol_G than of propofol_L. In addition, the measured hysteresis loop was counter-clockwise for propofol_L, as expected, but clockwise for propofol_G (see Fig. 7). Although the k_{eo} as a measure of hysteresis could be estimated for propofol_L using the approach of minimising the area of the hysteresis loop, there was only a very small area of the hysteresis loop for pro-

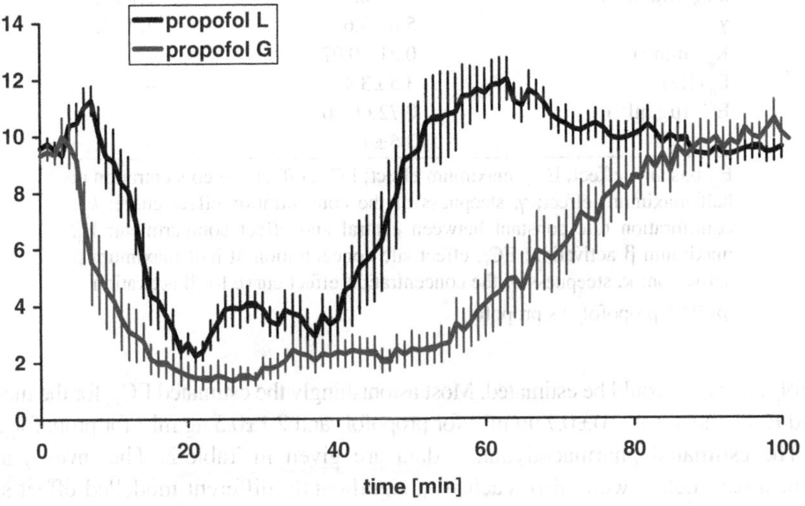

Fig. 6 Median EEG frequency (mean ± SEM) during TCI infusion of propofol_G (GPI 15715) and propofol_L (crossover study)

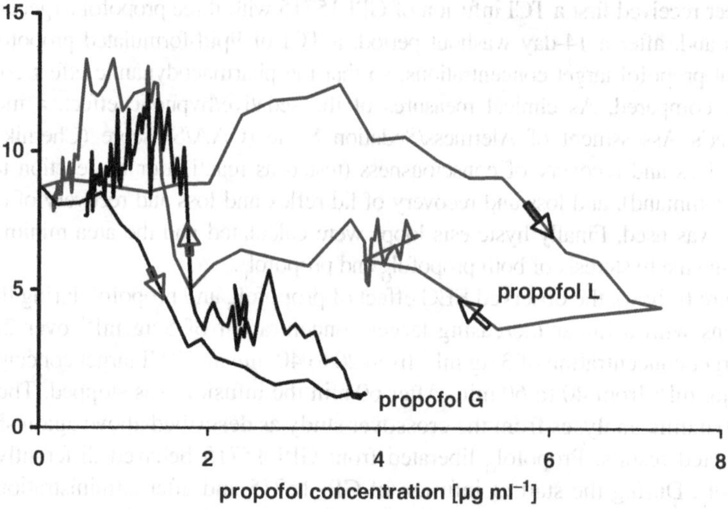

Fig. 7 Hysteresis loops (measured propofol concentration and measured EEG median frequency) of propofol$_L$ and propofol$_G$. *Arrows* indicate direction of the hysteresis loop

Table 2 Estimated pharmacodynamic parameters for propofol$_L$ and propofol$_G$ using the EEG median frequency as pharmacodynamic parameter (Fechner et al. 2004). Values are given as mean plus/minus standard deviation

Estimated parameter	Propofol$_L$	Propofol$_G$
E_0 (Hz)	9.1±0.8	9.7±1.1
E_{max} (Hz)	7.8±1.0	8.4±0.8
EC_{50} (µg ml^{-1})	3.0±0.7	2.1±0.5*
γ	5.6±3.6	7.2±3.6
K_{e0} (min^{-1})	0.21±0.07	–
E_β (Hz)	3.5±3.4	–
EC_β (µg ml^{-1})	0.72±0.20	–
κ	3.6±1.4	–

E_0, baseline effect; E_{max}, maximum effect; EC_{50}, effect site concentration at half-maximum effect; γ, steepness of the concentration-effect curve; k_{e0}, equilibration rate constant between central and effect compartment; E_β, maximum β activation; EC_β, effect site concentration at half-maximum β activation; κ, steepness of the concentration-effect curve for β activation

*$p<0.05$ propofol$_G$ vs propofol$_L$

pofol$_G$ and no k_{eo} could be estimated. Most astonishingly the estimated EC_{50} for the measured EEG effect was 3.0±0.7 µg ml^{-1} for propofol$_L$ and 2.1±0.5 µg ml^{-1} for propofol$_G$.

The estimated pharmacodynamic data are given in Table 2. The investigated clinical parameters were also reached at significantly different modelled effect site concentrations of propofol$_G$ and propofol$_L$. For example, loss of response to loud verbal command was achieved with a propofol$_G$ effect site concentration of 1.9±0.5 µg ml^{-1} and a propofol$_L$ effect site concentration of 3.2±1.0 µg ml^{-1} (see Table 3).

Table 3 Compared clinical pharmacodynamic parameters of propofol$_L$ and propofol$_G$ (Fechner et al. 2004). Time since start of TCI infusion with linear increasing propofol plasma concentration of up to 5 μg ml^{-1} at 20 min, corresponding plasma concentrations (C_{plasma}), modeled effect site concentrations (C_{effect}) and observed EEG median frequencies for the investigated clinical endpoints

	Propofol$_L$				Propofol$_{GPI}$			
	Time since start of infusion (min)	C_{plasma} (μg ml^{-1})	C_{effect} (μg ml^{-1})	EEG median frequency (Hz)	Time since start of infusion (min)	C_{plasma} (μg ml^{-1})	C_{effect} (μg ml^{-1})	EEG median frequency (Hz)
LOC	13±2	4.6±0.8	3.2±1.0	5.6±3.9	9±2	1.9±0.5	1.9±0.5*	4.6±4.1
LOCR	19±6	6.1±1.2	4.7±1.2	2.4±1.2	16±5	3.5±1.4	3.5±1.4*	2.0±1.3
ROCR	32±10	4.7±1.3	4.8±0.8	3.3±1.3	46±15	3.4±3.3	3.4±3.3*	2.1±1.3
ROC	47±10	2.0±0.8	2.8±0.8	6.3±5.3	73±13	1.8±0.4	1.8±0.4*	6.6±3.4
OAA/S=5	82±26	0.50±0.39	0.61±0.44	9.8±1.0	128±17	0.67±0.16	0.67±0.16	9.6±1.3

LOC, loss of response to verbal command; ROC, recurrence of response to verbal command. LOCR, loss of corneal reflex; ROCR, recurrence of corneal reflex. OAA/S=5, alert

*$p<0.005$ propofol$_{GPI}$ vs propofol$_D$

In summary, this investigation of propofol$_G$ compared to propofol$_L$ showed significant pharmacodynamic differences. Based on the modelled effect site concentration, propofol$_G$ has a higher pharmacodynamic potency and we could not model a hysteresis or k_{eo} of propofol$_G$ after it was liberated from GPI 15715. In part, similar results have been described by Dutta and Ebling (1997). They also found a higher steady state pharmacodynamic potency of lipid-free propofol compared to lipid-formulated propofol in rats. However, they did see the opposite with regard to hysteresis, with a longer time to effect for lipid-free propofol.

3 Summary of Published Study Result of GPI 15715 or Fospropofol

Besides the studies presented above, which were the first two investigating possible PK/PD differences after infusion and TCI-infusion of GPI 15715 or fospropofol in volunteers (Fechner et al. 2004; Fechner et al. 2003), two other combined studies presenting the PK/PD results after bolus dosing of GPI 15715 or fospropofol compared to lipid-formulated propofol in human volunteers have been published (Gibiansky et al. 2005; Struys et al. 2005). They found a combined pharmacokinetic model with three compartments for GPI 15715 and three compartments for propofol$_G$ best described their data. By non-compartmental analysis they also describe higher volumes of distribution and higher clearance values for propofol$_G$. In contrast to the initial studies, this group describes many non-linearities of the fitted compartment model. For example, the rate of GPI 15715 metabolism to propofol increased linearly with the GPI 15715 plasma concentration. They also describe an EC_{50} value of around 2 μg ml^{-1} for propofol$_G$ and the BIS as the effect parameter, which is well in agreement with our data. The effect on the EEG of GPI 15715 has also been studied in rats (Schywalsky et al. 2003). In this investigation very similar results to the above-presented investigations of Dutta et al. ¯(Dutta and Ebling 1997; Dutta and Ebling 1998a, b) with lipid-free propofol in rats were found. Schywalsky et al. also describe a different pharmacokinetic behaviour of propofol$_G$, with an increased volume of distribution, a longer half-life and an increased pharmacodynamic potency. Additionally, an investigation from our group of the pharmacodynamics of GPI 15715 when given as TCI infusion for sedation in male and female volunteers has been published (Fechner et al. 2005). In this study sedation in male and female volunteers over 2 h was achieved with a TCI infusion of GPI 15715 and was rated with the modified OAAS (Chernik et al. 1990). OAAS scale values of 3 could be achieved with propofol$_G$ concentrations of 1.72 ± 0.15 μg ml^{-1}. Unfortunately, in this study propofol$_G$ was not directly compared with propofol$_L$. In summary, GPI 15715 or fospropofol has been extensively studied in human volunteers. The pharmacokinetic differences for propofol$_G$ we found are in agreement with the results of other study groups (Gibiansky et al. 2005; Struys et al. 2005), but the higher pharmacodynamic potency of propofol$_G$ compared to propofol$_L$ that we found has not been proved in other investigations.

References

Bachmann-Mennenga B, Ohlmer A, Heesen M (2003) Incidence of pain after intravenous injection of a medium-/long-chain triglyceride emulsion of propofol. An observational study in 1375 patients. Arzneimittelforschung 53:621–626

Banaszczyk MG, Carlo AT, Millan V, Lindsey A, Moss R, Carlo DJ, Hendler SS (2002) Propofol phosphate, a water-soluble propofol prodrug: in vivo evaluation. Anesth Analg 95:1285–1292

Browne TR, Davoudi H, Donn KH, Dougherty CL, Dukes GE, Evans B, Evans JE, Jamerson B, Kres J, McEntegart CM, et al (1989) Bioavailability of ACC-9653 (phenytoin prodrug). Epilepsia 30[Suppl 2]:S27–S32

Chernik DA, Gillings D, Laine H, Hendler J, Silver JM, Davidson AB, Schwam EM, Siegel JL (1990) Validity and reliability of the Observer's Assessment of Alertness/Sedation Scale: study with intravenous midazolam. J Clin Psychopharmacol 10:244–251

Crowther J, Hrazdil J, Jolly DT, Galbraith JC, Greacen M, Grace M (1996) Growth of microorganisms in propofol, thiopental, and a 1:1 mixture of propofol and thiopental. Anesth Analg 82:475–478

d'Alessandro A, Osterloh JD, Chuwers P, Quinlan PJ, Kelly TJ, Becker CE (1994) Formate in serum and urine after controlled methanol exposure at the threshold limit value. Environ Health Perspect 102:178–181

Dutta S, Ebling WF (1997) Emulsion formulation reduces propofol's dose requirements and enhances safety. Anesthesiology 87:1394–1405

Dutta S, Ebling WF (1998a) Formulation-dependent brain and lung distribution kinetics of propofol in rats. Anesthesiology 89:678–685

Dutta S, Ebling WF (1998b) Formulation-dependent pharmacokinetics and pharmacodynamics of propofol in rats. J Pharm Pharmacol 50:37–42

Egan TD, Kern SE, Johnson KB, Pace NL (2003) The pharmacokinetics and pharmacodynamics of propofol in a modified cyclodextrin formulation (Captisol) versus propofol in a lipid formulation (Diprivan): an electroencephalographic and hemodynamic study in a porcine model. Anesth Analg 97:72–79

Fechner J, Ihmsen H, Hatterscheid D, Schiessl C, Vornov JJ, Burak E, Schwilden H, Schuttler J (2003) Pharmacokinetics and clinical pharmacodynamics of the new propofol prodrug GPI 15715 in volunteers. Anesthesiology 99:303–313

Fechner J, Ihmsen H, Hatterscheid D, Jeleazcov C, Schiessl C, Vornov JJ, Schwilden H, Schuttler J (2004) Comparative pharmacokinetics and pharmacodynamics of the new propofol prodrug GPI 15715 and propofol emulsion. Anesthesiology 101:626–639

Fechner J, Ihmsen H, Schiessl C, Jeleazcov C, Vornov JJ, Schwilden H, Schuttler J (2005) Sedation with GPI 15715, a water-soluble prodrug of propofol, using target-controlled infusion in volunteers. Anesth Analg 100:701–706

Fukada T, Ozaki M (2007) Microbial growth in propofol formulations with disodium edetate and the influence of venous access system dead space. Anaesthesia 62:575–580

Gerber N, Mays DC, Donn KH, Laddu A, Guthrie RM, Turlapaty P, Quon CY, Rivenburg WK (1988) Safety, tolerance and pharmacokinetics of intravenous doses of the phosphate ester of 3-hydroxymethyl-5,5-diphenylhydantoin: a new prodrug of phenytoin. J Clin Pharmacol 28:1023–1032

Gibiansky E, Struys MM, Gibiansky L, Vanluchene AL, Vornov J, Mortier EP, Burak E, Van Bortel L (2005) AQUAVAN injection, a water-soluble prodrug of propofol, as a bolus injection: a phase I dose-escalation comparison with DIPRIVAN (part 1): pharmacokinetics. Anesthesiology 103:718–729

Graystone S, Wells MF, Farrell DJ (1997) Do intensive care drug infusions support microbial growth? Anaesth Intensive Care 25:640–642

Jamerson BD, Donn KH, Dukes GE, Messenheimer JA, Brouwer KL, Powell JR (1990) Absolute bioavailability of phenytoin after 3-phosphoryloxymethyl phenytoin disodium (ACC-9653) administration to humans. Epilepsia 31:592–597

Kim KM, Choi BM, Park SW, Lee SH, Christensen LV, Zhou J, Yoo BH, Shin HW, Bae KS, Kern SE, Kang SH, Noh GJ (2007) Pharmacokinetics and pharmacodynamics of propofol microemulsion and lipid emulsion after an intravenous bolus and variable rate infusion. Anesthesiology 106:924–934

Langevin PB, Gravenstein N, Doyle TJ, Roberts SA, Skinner S, Langevin SO, Gulig PA (1999) Growth of Staphylococcus aureus in Diprivan and Intralipid: implications on the pathogenesis of infections. Anesthesiology 91:1394–1400

Lindholm M (1992) Critically ill patients and fat emulsions. Minerva Anestesiol 58:875–879

McKeage K, Perry CM (2003) Propofol: a review of its use in intensive care sedation of adults. CNS Drugs 17:235–272

Morey TE, Modell JH, Shekhawat D, Shah DO, Klatt B, Thomas GP, Kero FA, Booth MM, Dennis DM (2006) Anesthetic properties of a propofol microemulsion in dogs. Anesth Analg 103:882–887

Sagara Y, Hendler S, Khoh-Reiter S, Gillenwater G, Carlo D, Schubert D, Chang J (1999) Propofol hemisuccinate protects neuronal cells from oxidative injury. J Neurochem 73:2524–2530

Schywalsky M, Ihmsen H, Tzabazis A, Fechner J, Burak E, Vornov J, Schwilden H (2003) Pharmacokinetics and pharmacodynamics of the new propofol prodrug GPI 15715 in rats. Eur J Anaesthesiol 20:182–190

Struys MM, Vanluchene AL, Gibiansky E, Gibiansky L, Vornov J, Mortier EP, Van Bortel L (2005) AQUAVAN injection, a water-soluble prodrug of propofol, as a bolus injection: a phase I dose-escalation comparison with DIPRIVAN (part 2): pharmacodynamics and safety. Anesthesiology 103:730–743

Trapani A, Laquintana V, Lopedota A, Franco M, Latrofa A, Talani G, Sanna E, Trapani G, Liso G (2004) Evaluation of new propofol aqueous solutions for intravenous anesthesia. Int J Pharm 278:91–98

Vansant G, Trauger RJ, Cameron A, Vendemelio M, Kreitschitz S, Carlo AT, Banaszczyk MG, Carlo DJ, Hendler S, Ill CR (2007) Propofol hemisuccinate suppression of experimental autoimmune encephalomyelitis. Autoimmunity 40:180–186

Varia SA, Stella VJ (1984a) Phenytoin prodrugs V: in vivo evaluation of some water-soluble phenytoin prodrugs in dogs. J Pharm Sci 73:1080–1087

Varia SA, Stella VJ (1984b) Phenytoin prodrugs VI: in vivo evaluation of a phosphate ester prodrug of phenytoin after parenteral administration to rats. J Pharm Sci 73:1087–1090

Vidovich MI, Peterson LR, Wong HY (1999) The effect of lidocaine on bacterial growth in propofol. Anesth Analg 88:936–938

Wachowski I, Jolly DT, Hrazdil J, Galbraith JC, Greacen M, Clanachan AS (1999) The growth of microorganisms in propofol and mixtures of propofol and lidocaine. Anesth Analg 88:209–212

Etomidate and Other Non-Barbiturates

C. Vanlersberghe(✉) and F. Camu

Abstract It is today generally accepted that anesthetics act by binding directly to sensitive target proteins. For certain intravenous anesthetics, such as propofol, barbiturates, and etomidate, the major target for anesthetic effect has been identified as the γ-aminobutyric acid type A ($GABA_A$) receptor, with particular subunits playing a crucial role. Etomidate, an intravenous imidazole general anesthetic, is thought to produce anesthesia by modulating or activating ionotropic Cl^--permeable $GABA_A$ receptors. For the less potent steroid anesthetic agents the picture is less clear, although a relatively small number of targets have been identified as being the most likely candidates. In this review, we summarize the most relevant clinical and experimental pharmacological properties of these intravenous anesthetics, the molecular targets mediating other endpoints of the anesthetic state in vivo, and the work that led to the identification of the $GABA_A$ receptor as the key target for etomidate and aminosteroids.

C. Vanlersberghe
Department of Anesthesiology, University of Brussels V.U.B. Medical Center, Laarbeeklaan 101, 1090 Brussels, Belgium
anesvec@uzbrussel.be

J. Schüttler and H. Schwilden (eds.) *Modern Anesthetics.*
Handbook of Experimental Pharmacology 182.

1 Etomidate

Etomidate [R(+)-ethyl-1-(α-methyl-benzyl)-1H-imidazole-5-carboxylate, MW 342.4] is a short-acting anesthetic agent, unstable in water, and is currently marketed as a preparation containing 2 mg/ml solubilized in either propylene glycol (pH solution 5.1, 4,965 mOsmol/kg) or a lipid emulsion (pH solution 7.6, 400 mOsmol/kg). Etomidate has a very high therapeutic index in animals (26.4 compared to 9.5 for methohexital). The drug is optically active and exists in two mirror-image enantiomeric forms. Only the dextro isomer is active as a hypnotic. The salt is water soluble, but the base is soluble in ethanol, propylene glycol, and chloroform. The pK_a of etomidate is 4.24. The imidazole ring renders etomidate water soluble at acidic pH and lipid soluble at physiological pH, with almost 99% of the drug unionized in the blood (Fig. 1).

The drug is used as hypnotic component for the induction of anesthesia. It is considered by many to be the ideal agent for induction of anesthesia in cardiac-compromised or hypovolemic patients. The recommended dose in humans is 0.3 mg/kg, which produces an equal duration of sleep to methohexital 1.5 mg/kg (Kay 1976). The duration of sleep is dose-dependent and there is little evidence of accumulation of the drug even with repeated dosing. The speed of onset and short duration of action is the result of rapid uptake and elimination by the brain and a fast redistribution of the drug from the plasma to other tissues. Minor side effects (pain on injection, thrombophlebitis, involuntary muscle movements, coughing, and hiccups) may accompany the injection of etomidate. The occurrence of thrombophlebitis has been attributed to the solvent propylene glycol. Both the emulsion formulation and the use of 2-hydroxypropyl-β-cyclodextrin as solvent significantly reduce the incidence of pain on injection, thrombophlebitis, and red cell hemolysis without affecting the pharmacokinetics and -dynamics of etomidate (Doenicke et al. 1994).

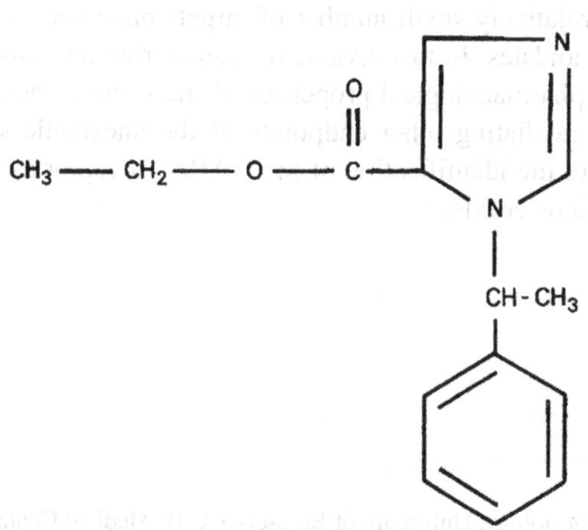

Fig. 1 Chemical structure of etomidate

1.1 Pharmacokinetics

In initial studies by Heykants et al. (1973) in man, the plasma concentration of etomidate after intravenous injection decayed in a biphasic manner with elimination half-life of 75 min. The plasma concentration of the metabolites increased over the first 30 min after administration, and then decreased with a slower half-life of 160 min. The distribution of both stereoisomers of etomidate (R(+) and S(−)) does not differ substantially in blood, brain, or liver. However, the S(−) form has considerably less hypnotic effect, suggesting stereospecificity of the receptor area in the brain.

Later kinetic studies in humans under general anesthesia showed wide variations in the clearance of etomidate after single doses and continuous infusions. In the investigations of Van Hamme et al. (1978), the plasma concentrations of etomidate following a single dose were consistent with a three-compartment distribution model, with individual plasma half-lives of 2.6 min, 28.7 min, and 275.4 min, respectively. The apparent volume of distribution (V_{dss}) was 4.51 l/kg and the systemic or plasma clearance rate 11.7 ml/kg per minute. Data from infusion studies were best fitted to a two-compartment model with mean elimination half-lives ranging from 1.13 to 2.9 h, mean apparent volumes of distribution of 154 to 310 l, and mean systemic clearance varying between 1,175 and 2,550 ml/min (Schüttler et al. 1980; De Ruiter et al. 1981; Hebron et al. 1983; Schüttler et al. 1985). In the presence of a steady-state concentration of fentanyl (10 ng/ml) the clearance of etomidate was reduced from about 1,600 to 400 ml/min, with little alteration of the elimination half-life. However, the initial volume of distribution (V_c) decreased from 21 l to 5 l and V_{dss} from 160 l to about 40 l. The exact nature of this kinetic drug interaction is not known, but may possibly involve saturation of the enzymes responsible for the metabolism of etomidate (Schüttler et al. 1983).

The relationship between concentration and drug effect is well established. Etomidate penetrates the brain rapidly. Anesthesia was associated with concentrations between 300 and 500 ng/ml, with burst suppression of the electroencephalogram (EEG) found at concentrations greater than 1.0 µg/ml. The mean half-time for blood/brain equilibration ($t_{1/2}$ k_{e0}), which represents the speed of equilibration between concentrations in plasma and effect compartment or biophase, was 1.6 min. Brain sensitivity expressed as the magnitude of the maximal slowing of the EEG spectral edge (E_{max}) was 7.2 Hz and the mean plasma drug concentration that caused 50% of the maximal EEG slowing (IC_{50}) was 0.39 µg/ml (Arden et al. 1986). Studies in volunteers using EEG median frequency as surrogate for hypnotic effect and pharmacokinetic/-dynamic modeling established a mean IC_{50} value (which is the plasma concentration of etomidate necessary to cause half of the possible EEG depressant effect) of 0.32 µg/ml. Of the greatest possible EEG-depressant effect, 90% was achieved at mean plasma concentration of 0.56 µg/ml (Schwilden et al. 1985). Based on the concentration response curves from these studies and the IC_{50} values, the relative potency ratio for pure hypnotic effect of etomidate versus thiopental was 50:1.

Etomidate is metabolized by enzymes present in plasma, but mainly in the liver by ether hydrolysis to pharmacologically inactive metabolites. The main metabolite in man is the corresponding carboxylic acid of etomidate. In man, approximately 75% of the dose administered is excreted in the urine during the first 24 h after administration, mainly as inert metabolites, with only 2% of the etomidate excreted unchanged (Heykants et al. 1975).

In vitro protein binding of etomidate has been studied by equilibrium dialysis using radiolabeled etomidate. Human serum albumin was found to bind 78.5% etomidate, while human γ-globulin bound not more than 3% etomidate. Total plasma protein binding of etomidate was 76.5% in man, with distribution percentages for blood cells, plasma proteins, and plasma water being 37.7%, 47.6%, and 14.7%, respectively.

1.2 Pharmacological Organ Effects

Etomidate induces a hypnotic effect within one arm–brain circulation time, with no detectable histamine release, minimal cardiovascular and respiratory depressive effects, and a reduction in cerebral metabolism, cerebral blood flow (CBF), and intracranial pressure, and with a rapid recovery of consciousness and orientation to time, space, and person.

1.2.1 The Cardiovascular System

Animal Data

In animals, therapeutic doses had no depressant effect on atrial muscle function or conduction, while high doses (1.25–2.5 mg/kg) induced a slight decrease of arterial pressure. Etomidate had little effect on myocardial contractility of isolated normal and cardiomyopathic rat papillary muscle, presumably by maintaining the availability of intracellular Ca^{2+} for contractile activation in vitro (Komai et al. 1985; Riou et al. 1993; Gelissen et al. 1996). Etomidate also caused little or no myocardial depression in dogs, as evaluated with isovolumetric and ejection-phase indexes of contractility (Kissin et al. 1983; De Hert et al. 1990). However, the actions of etomidate on load-independent measures of contractile state and on diastolic function have not been specifically addressed.

The effects of etomidate on vascular smooth muscle cells have been widely investigated. In rat aortic vascular smooth muscle cells, etomidate (5×10^{-5} M–5×10^{-4} M) moderately inhibited the angiotensin II-induced calcium influx. Etomidate also produced a significant rightward shift in the dose–response curves of acetylcholine (receptor-mediated endothelium-dependent agonist), phenylephrine, and 5-hydroxytryptamine, and potassium chloride-induced contraction in rat aorta. The underlying mechanism was an inhibitory effect on the calcium influx by blocking the L-type calcium channels. Indeed, these effects of etomidate were absent in aorta rings pretreated with verapamil (Pili-Floury et al. 2004; Shin et al. 2005). These data indicate that etomidate may alter the vascular response to endogenous and exogenous vasoactive agents. However, these effects of etomidate occurred at concentrations exceeding the clinically relevant concentration, and thus the effect of etomidate on blood pressure regulatory systems in clinical conditions is limited.

Etomidate, however, may affect blood pressure in a different way. Bovine adrenal chromaffin cells, which express functional γ-aminobutyric acid type A ($GABA_A$) receptors, were excited by etomidate at clinically relevant concentrations, thereby stimulating catecholamine release. Etomidate directly activated $GABA_A$ receptors found in chromaffin cells and increased intracellular Ca^{2+} concentrations. This depolarized chromaffin cells, thus activating voltage-dependent Ca^{2+} channels and stimulating catecholamine release (Xie et al. 2004). Etomidate also showed agonist effects at α2-adrenoceptors in mice lacking individual α2-adrenoceptor subtypes (α2-KO). In membranes from HEK293 cells transfected with α2-receptors, etomidate inhibited binding of the α2-antagonist [3H]RX821002. In α2B-receptor-expressing HEK293 cells, etomidate rapidly increased phosphorylation of the extracellular signal-related kinases (ERK)1/2. (Paris et al. 2003). Thus, the interaction of etomidate with α2B-adrenoceptors could in vivo primarily increase blood pressure and may contribute to the cardiovascular stability observed in patients after induction of anesthesia with etomidate.

Human Data

Investigations in normal patients (Gooding and Corssen 1977; Patschke et al. 1977; Criado et al. 1980) and those with cardiovascular disease (Colvin et al. 1979; Gooding et al. 1979) have repeatedly demonstrated that etomidate produced little change in hemodynamics.

In humans, etomidate did not affect heart contractility or mean aortic pressure. During infusion of etomidate, coronary blood flow slightly increased and coronary resistance decreased to the same extent, leaving a constant coronary perfusion pressure. Myocardial oxygen consumption was unaltered and cardiac work diminished in proportion to any decrease in mean arterial pressure (MAP) (Kettler et al. 1974). Only at high infusion rates did etomidate decrease cardiac output and liver blood flow, causing greater plasma drug concentrations than might otherwise have been predicted (Van Lambalgan et al. 1982; Thomson et al. 1984).

Patients with severe coronary artery disease showed no major alterations in cardiac function or hemodynamics. Patients with aortic or mitral valve disease responded to etomidate with a 19% fall in MAP, which was associated with decreased systemic vascular resistance and left ventricular stroke work index. Cardiac index and pulmonary artery pressures decreased slightly, and central venous pressure and heart rate remained unchanged (Colvin et al. 1979).

As with other anesthetic agents, etomidate induced modest decreases in MAP, presumably resulting from depressed neural control of the peripheral vasculature by depression of central generation of neural tone, which may contribute to attenuated activity of the central sympathetic nervous system. No direct effect of etomidate has been established concerning receptor organ function or afferent transmission when reflexes are involved, or on the synaptic transmission at the level of the autonomic ganglion or at the vascular smooth muscle neuromuscular junction (Prakash et al. 1981).

1.2.2 The Brain

Etomidate decreased CBF, the cerebral metabolic rate for oxygen ($CMRO_2$), and intracranial pressure in humans, while blood pressure was well maintained (Van Aken and Rolly 1976; Moss et al. 1979). In dogs receiving continuous infusions, etomidate decreased CBF and cerebral metabolic oxygen requirements by 35%–45%, with marked increases in cerebrovascular resistance (Milde et al. 1985). The decrease in CBF was independent of changes in cerebral metabolic rate of oxygen ($CMRO_2$) as $CMRO_2$ decreased more slowly than CBF. At increasing doses of etomidate after suppression of EEG activity, a minimal $CMRO_2$ was established and maintained (2.6 ml/min/100 g). Normal levels of ATP and phosphocreatine and a normal energy charge of the brain tissue indicated, despite small increases in lactate, that energy production remained adequate to supply the energy requirements of the brain.

Because of these properties, etomidate was considered a neuroprotective agent and has often been used to attenuate the effects of cerebral ischemia in neurovascular surgical procedures that require temporary cerebral arterial occlusion. The neuroprotective effects of etomidate have been investigated in several animal models of cerebral ischemia, neurodegenerative diseases, and spinal cord trauma. Ates et al. (2006) investigated the effects of high-dose etomidate (2 mg/kg) on oxidative stress in streptozotocin-induced (STZ-induced) hyperglycemia in the rat brain and spinal cord. Malondialdehyde (MDA), total nitrite, and xanthine oxidase activity were used as markers. Etomidate treatment partly prevented the elevation of MDA, xanthine oxidase, and nitrite levels in the hippocampus, cortex, cerebellum, brain stem, and spinal cord of the rats. These data suggested a neuroprotective effect on the neuronal tissue against diabetic oxidative damage. A similar neuroprotective effect was demonstrated in experimental spinal cord injury in rats with etomidate (2 mg/kg), methylprednisolone, and the combination of both drugs. When administered immediately after spinal cord injury etomidate offered similar neuroprotection to methylprednisolone. However, the combined treatment with methylprednisolone and etomidate did not provide better protection than that obtained with each drug given separately (Cayli et al. 2006).

In models of cerebral mitochondrial dysfunction after temporary middle cerebral artery occlusion in rats, however, etomidate showed an adverse effect on ischemic injury. Prior inhibition of nitric oxide synthase (NOS) with l-NAME did not influence the volume of cerebral injury. Administration of a large dose of l-arginine, a NO donor, prevented the adverse effect of etomidate. These data suggest that etomidate impaired mitochondrial function by inhibition of NOS early in the setting of temporary focal cerebral ischemia (Drummond et al. 2005).

In humans, the effects of etomidate and temporary cerebral arterial occlusion on brain tissue oxygen pressure (PO_2), carbon dioxide pressure (PCO_2), and pH were evaluated during intracranial aneurysm surgery. Etomidate was administered to produce EEG burst suppression before temporary cerebral arterial occlusion. This resulted in cerebral deoxygenation as brain tissue PO_2 decreased 30% compared with before etomidate administration. Overall, supplemental oxygen therapy returned brain oxygen tensions to pre-etomidate baseline values, but subsequent temporary cerebral artery occlusion decreased tissue PO_2 again (32% below preclip values), while tissue PCO_2 increased (23%) and acidosis set in (pH decrease 0.1-unit). Thus, brain tissue PO_2 decreased during cerebral aneurysm surgery despite etomidate administration (Edelman et al. 1997). In patients who had middle cerebral artery occlusion for 30 min after craniotomy, tissue PO_2 decreased with etomidate with significant tissue acidosis (7.09 to 6.63) (Hoffman et al. 1998). These results suggest that tissue hypoxia and acidosis were often observed during etomidate treatment in the setting of cerebral ischemia and that etomidate enhanced hypoxic risk during middle cerebral artery occlusion.

Etomidate may activate seizure foci manifesting as fast activity on the EEG and has been observed to augment the amplitude of somatosensory evoked potentials. Myoclonus is frequently observed and may resemble seizures, but it is not associated with epileptiform discharges on the EEG. Etomidate-induced myoclonus could be related to disinhibition of subcortical structures that normally suppress extrapyramidal motor activity (Laughlin and Newberg 1985).

1.2.3 The Respiratory System

Etomidate depressed the medullar centers that modify the ventilatory drive in response to changing CO_2 tensions, but this effect was less marked than that of the barbiturates (Choi et al. 1985). Induced reductions in tidal volume were offset by compensatory increases in breathing frequency, and these effects on ventilation were transient, lasting only a few minutes.

The ability of etomidate to prevent airway constriction or bronchospasm under normal and pathological conditions was explored in vitro. General anesthetics modify airway responsiveness via, at least partially, a direct inhibitory effect on calcium signaling in airway smooth muscle cells. Contraction experiments were done in human airway rings that were either normal or passively sensitized with asthmatic serum. The lowest effective concentration of etomidate that altered the intracellular Ca^{2+} response was 10^{-4} M. Etomidate reduced histamine-induced contraction in human isolated airway smooth muscles that were either not sensitized or passively sensitized with asthmatic serum. In rat isolated tracheal myocytes, etomidate (10^{-4} M) altered the intracellular Ca^{2+} signal in response to the depolarizing agent potassium chloride and acetylcholine (Ouedraogo et al. 1998). Another model evaluated the ability of etomidate to relax and prevent agonist-induced contraction in tracheal rings isolated from chronically hypoxic rats and precontracted with the muscarinic agonist carbachol (CCh) and the depolarizing agent KCl. Etomidate (10^{-4} M) inhibited chronic hypoxic tracheal ring contraction in response to cumulative concentrations of CCh and KCl (Ouedraogo et al. 2003).

1.3 Effects on Adrenal and Gonadal Steroidogenesis

Etomidate inhibits stress- and drug-induced corticosteroid production in the adrenal gland, as well as the adrenocorticotropic hormone (ACTH)-induced stress response, in a dose-related and reversible fashion. Studies in vivo and with rat adrenal mitochondrial fractions and isolated rat adrenal cells indicated that there are four different sites of enzyme inhibition with apparent dose dependence: 11β hydroxylase, 17α hydroxylase, 18 hydroxylase, and probably the cholesterol side chain cleavage enzyme (20, 22 lyase) (de Jong et al. 1984; Fry and Griffiths 1984; Wagner et al. 1984; de Coster et al. 1985; Moore et al. 1985; Allolio et al. 1985). The main hormonal effects of etomidate are therefore to decrease cortisol and aldosterone synthesis and secretion, and increase the plasma concentrations of their precursors, 11-deoxycortisol and 18-deoxycorticosterone. The effect of etomidate on 11β hydroxylation is concentration-related. Crozier et al. (1988) found a sigmoid relationship between the relative inhibition of cortisol in response to ACTH stimulation and the log of the plasma etomidate concentration. The ED_{50} etomidate concentration was 110 nM, with suppression negligible at concentrations below 40 nM. On the basis of these data and the known kinetics of the drug, the expected duration of inhibition in humans will be about 4–8 h after administration.

Etomidate had no significant effect on microsomal enzymes in the glucocorticoid pathway (Wagner et al. 1984).

1.4 Effects on Other Microsomal Enzymes

Studies using antipyrine indicated that etomidate inhibited hepatic cytochrome oxidase P450-dependent drug metabolism in a concentration-dependent manner with IC_{50} concentrations in the order of 10 μM (Horai et al. 1985; Atiba et al. 1988). The minimal degree of in vivo inhibition of hepatic metabolism may delay elimination of low clearance drugs (diazepam, propranolol, carbamazepine, phenytoin), but is unlikely to affect drugs with high hepatic clearance, such as opioids and ketamine.

1.5 Effects on Central Nervous System Receptors

Central nervous system depression may reflect a $GABA_A$-like effect of etomidate. Indeed, etomidate is a selective modulator of this receptor and has, at clinically relevant concentrations, no effect on other ligand-gated ion channels. Etomidate acts by binding to and enhancing the function of $GABA_A$ receptors, which mediate inhibitory neurotransmission in the brain. The EC_{50} concentrations for general anesthesia in animals for the R(+) and S(−) isomers were 3.4 μM and 57 μM, respectively. The R(+) isomer was also much more effective than the S(−) isomer at potentiating GABA-induced currents (Tomlin et al. 1998). Etomidate is more potent than barbiturates in activating $GABA_A$ receptor channels, with potency comparable to that of GABA (Robertson 1989). In cortical homogenates, etomidate, like alphaxalone and pentobarbital, enhanced GABA or muscimol binding, apparently by increasing the number of binding sites (Thyagarajan et al. 1983). Etomidate also potentiated benzodiazepine binding by increasing the affinity of the benzodiazepine-binding site, an effect shown to be dose dependent, stereospecific, and antagonized by bicuculline or picrotoxin. It is noteworthy that in the presence of more than one anesthetic agent (e.g., pentobarbital plus etomidate) the enhancement in GABA and muscimol binding was additive. These results suggest that binding sites for different classes of intravenous anesthetic agents are distinct from each other as well as from benzodiazepine binding sites.

The site of action of etomidate is at the β_3 subunit of the receptor, where amino acid residues have been identified that are essential for activation of the $GABA_A$ receptor function by etomidate. Within the ion channel pore, the amino acid Asp265 located in the membrane-spanning region TM2 of the β_3 subunits conferred anesthetic activity for etomidate, but not for pentobarbital, propofol, or steroid anesthetics (Tomlin et al. 1998; Belelli et al. 1997). However, recent studies using a photoreactive etomidate analog ([(3)H]azietomidate) yielded different results. R(+)azietomidate, a diazirine derivative of etomidate, retained the anesthetic potency of etomidate in vivo. Both agents equally enhanced $GABA_A$ receptor function in vitro. The enantioselectivity was comparable to etomidate's, with an approximate potency ratio of the enantiomers being R:S 1:10 (Husain et al. 2003). [(3)H]Azietomidate established photolabeling of two residues: one within the αTM1 transmembrane helix at α1Met-236 (and/or the homologous methionines in α2,3,5), not previously implicated in etomidate function, and one within the βTM3 transmembrane helix at β3Met-286 (and/or the homologous methionines in β1,2), an etomidate sensitivity determinant. The pharmacological specificity of labeling indicates that these methionines contribute to a single binding pocket for etomidate located in the transmembrane domain at the interface between β- and α-subunits, rather than in the β-subunit (Li et al. 2006).

These binding data have functional significance: under voltage-clamp conditions, etomidate potentiated GABA-induced chloride currents, which causes membrane hyperpolarization and a reduction in neuronal excitability (Proctor et al. 1986). But direct activation of chloride currents in the absence of GABA has also been observed with etomidate at concentrations slightly higher than those needed for potentiation of GABA-evoked currents (Evans and Hill 1978). Etomidate thus differs from the benzodiazepines, which are unable to activate $GABA_A$ receptors.

Other studies indicate that there is distinct subunit dependence for different pharmacological actions of etomidate on the $GABA_A$ receptor. These studies used knockout mice or mice carrying point mutations in neurotransmitter receptor subunits to assess the contribution of the respective receptor subtype to the pharmacological actions of etomidate. It was recently shown, using β2 knockout mice to completely remove any contribution of the β2 subunit to the effects of etomidate, that the β2 subunit contributed to the sedative properties of etomidate (O'Meara et al. 2004). Etomidate was equally anesthetic in wildtype and knockout mice, indicating that the β3 subunit was responsible for its anesthetic properties.

Another study addressed the involvement of the β3 subunit in the respiratory, cardiovascular, hypothermic, and sedative actions of etomidate, using β3 knockin mice carrying etomidate-insensitive β3-containing $GABA_A$ receptors. The respiratory depressant action of etomidate, determined by blood gas analysis, was almost absent in β3 mice, but the cardiac depressant and hypothermic effects, and the sedative effect were still present. Thus, respiratory depression was mediated by β3-containing $GABA_A$ receptors, while the hypothermic, cardiac depressant, and sedative actions were largely independent of β3-containing $GABA_A$ receptors (Zeller et al. 2005).

Studies with hippocampus pyramidal neurons showed that deletion of the α5 subunit of the $GABA_A$ receptor reduced the amnestic but not the sedative-hypnotic properties of etomidate. Etomidate markedly increased the tonic inhibitory conductance generated by $GABA_A$ receptors and reduced long-term potentiation (LTP) of field excitatory postsynaptic potentials (EPSPs) in wildtype but not α5 null mutant ($\alpha5^{-/-}$) mice. The sedative-hypnotic effects were similar in wildtype and $\alpha5^{-/-}$ mice (Cheng et al. 2006).

1.6 Contraindications

The use of etomidate is contraindicated in patients with acute porphyria and with depressed adrenocortical activity, at least in the absence of any substitution therapy. Although allergic reactions to etomidate are very rare, caution is warranted in patients with history of atopy.

2 5β-Pregnanolone (Eltanolone)

This steroid with a 5β pregnane structure (5β-pregnan-3α-ol-20-one) has anesthetic properties with a high therapeutic index (<40). The drug is water insoluble and formulated in a 10% Intralipid (Fresenius Kabi, Badhomburg, Germany) emulsion. There is rapid hepatic metabolism to inactive glucuronide and sulfate conjugates, with excretion via the kidneys and the biliary tract.

Clinical investigations in humans indicated that the blood concentration needed to achieve hypnotic effect was 0.46 μg/ml. The drug is, therefore, as potent as etomidate (concentration for hypnotic effect 0.32 μg/ml) and five times more potent than propofol (concentration for hypnotic effect 2.3 μg/ml). Loss of consciousness is usually obtained with doses of 0.4–0.6 mg/kg eltanolone.

Investigations in volunteers have addressed the infusion pharmacokinetics of eltanolone and used EEG effect data for full pharmacodynamic modeling of a power spectral parameter of the EEG (median frequency) to the serum concentration using a sigmoid E_{max} model, including an effect compartment to minimize possible hysteresis. Population pharmacokinetics was analyzed using a three-compartment mammillary model with central elimination. Eltanolone showed a high total clearance (1.75±0.22 l/min), small volumes of distribution (V_c=7.65±3.40 l; V_{dss}=91.6±22 l), and relatively short half-lives ($t_{1/2}\alpha$=1.5±0.6 min; $t_{1/2}\beta$=27±5 min; $t_{1/2}\gamma$=184±32 min). With regard to the pharmacodynamic model parameters, eltanolone proved to be a potent hypnotic agent (Cp_{50}=0.46±0.09 μg/ml). The equilibration half-time blood/brain is long (between 6 and 8 min, k_{e0}=0.087±0.013 min^{-1}) compared with barbiturates or propofol (Hering et al. 1996a).

Such a long equilibration time between blood and the biophase makes eltanolone difficult to be administered by titration of dose to hypnotic effect. It also affects the context-sensitive times following infusions of eltanolone. Context-sensitive time is the time required for the plasma drug concentration to decline by 20%, 50%, or 80% after terminating the infusion, where context refers to infusion duration. Context-sensitive times were estimated for a 50% and 80% drop in the concentration of eltanolone after different infusion times. A 50% drop in concentration was estimated to occur after 8 min following a 3-h infusion and after 10 min for a 10-h infusion. Following a 1-h infusion, an 80% drop in concentration was estimated to occur after 55 min and this delay increased to 70–80 min following an infusion of 10 h (Parivar et al. 1996). During recovery, the corneal reflex reappeared on average 9.4 min after stopping infusion, with the first reactions to loud verbal commands being recorded after 24 min; full orientation was regained after an average of 35 min (Hering et al. 1996b). Concentration–effect relationships during recovery from a bolus dose and constant rate intravenous infusion in healthy male volunteers established Cp_{50} values for "eye opening" at 0.38 μg/ml after a bolus dose and 0.51 μg/ml after eltanolone infusions. Median time to eye opening was 16 min after a bolus dose and up to 49 min after eltanolone infusion (Wessen et al. 1996). Thus, the long time between the administration of the drug in the blood and the equilibration with the biophase implicates the potential disadvantage of drug accumulation, with prolonged recovery foreseen if larger-than-necessary doses are used to induce and maintain anesthesia.

The clinical effects on organ functions after i.v. administrations of eltanolone were generally mild. There was slight respiratory depression and a maximum reduction in arterial blood pressure of 31% compared to the resting level after a bolus dose of eltanolone. Diastolic arterial blood pressure decreased about 10%, while heart rate increased 24% (Hering et al. 1996b). In patients scheduled for coronary artery bypass grafting, systemic vascular resistance decreased significantly 2 min after induction with eltanolone at all doses (0.5–1 mg/kg). Mean arterial pressure reduction induced by eltanolone was most likely the result of the combination of a decrease in cardiac contractility and peripheral vasodilatation (Tassani et al. 1996).

After a single dose of 0.6 mg/kg eltanolone, CBF decreased by 34%, with a comparable fall in cerebral oxygen consumption, thereby maintaining a coupling between metabolism and blood flow (Wolff et al. 1994).

Eltanolone administration may produce side effects such as skin rash, urticaria, short-lasting excitation, minor involuntary movements, and convulsions. Considering the lack of clinical advantages over existing anesthetic drugs, the drug has been withdrawn from clinical use.

The molecular targets for eltanolone are also the $GABA_A$ receptor and the glycine receptor. Of the anesthetic isomers, 5α-pregnan-3α-ol-20-one and 5β-pregnan-3α-ol-20-one (eltanolone), only the latter has anesthetic effects. Both isomers enhanced $GABA_A$ receptor-mediated currents with similar potency and efficacy, but only 5α-pregnan-3α-ol-20-one enhanced glycine currents. On the other hand, eltanolone caused inhibition of the glycine currents (Weir et al. 2004). These data indicate that steroid modulation at the $GABA_A$ and glycine receptors differs.

3 ORG 21465 and ORG 20599

Two other 2-substituted aminosteroids, ORG 21465 and ORG 20599, have been evaluated in animals and humans. These agents are water-soluble. ORG 21465 (2β-3α-5α-3-hydroxy-2-(2,2-dimethylmorpholin-4-yl)-pregnan-11,20-dione) has a high therapeutic index in mice (13.8). The neuroactive aminosteroids differ in potency, but not in intrinsic efficacy at the $GABA_A$ receptor in vivo, as the estimates for the maximum activation of the receptor are similar (Visser et al. 2002).

In humans, ORG 21465 administration caused no cardiovascular or respiratory depression. Anesthetic effects were observed at doses of at least 1 mg/kg. However, as with other steroids, ORG 21465 produced a high incidence of excitatory side effects that was dose-related, but without accompanying EEG spike activity (Sneyd et al. 1997a).

With regard to pharmacokinetics following an i.v. dose, the decay of plasma concentrations supported a three-compartment model with compartmental volumes V_c, V_2, and V_3 of 4.31, 14.2, and 89.4 l, respectively. Clearance from the central compartment, V_c, was 1.55 l/min (Sneyd et al. 1997a). Using computer-controlled infusions of ORG 21465, a steady-state plasma concentration of 1.18 μg/ml depressed the EEG spectral edge frequency by 50%. The equilibration rate constant of the effect compartment was 0.112/min ($t_{1/2}$ k_{e0} 6.2 min) (Sneyd et al. 1997b).

ORG 20599 [(2β, 3α, 5α)-21-chloro-3-hydroxy-2-(4-morpholinyl)pregnan-20-one methanesulfonate], intravenously administered produced a rapid onset and short duration loss of the righting reflex in mice. The anesthetic potency of ORG 20599 exceeded that of propofol, thiopental, and pentobarbital. ORG 20599 produced a concentration-dependent and reversible potentiation of the peak amplitude of GABA-evoked currents at human recombinant α1, β2, γ2L-subunit-containing $GABA_A$ receptors expressed in *Xenopus laevis* oocytes (EC_{50} = 1.1 μM), and for the $GABA_A$ receptors expressed by bovine adrenal chromaffin cells maintained in culture. At concentrations greater than those required for potentiation of GABA, ORG 20599 exhibited GABA-mimetic effects (Hill-Venning et al. 1996; Weir et al. 2004). The results suggest positive allosteric regulation of $GABA_A$ receptor function to be a plausible molecular mechanism of action for the drug.

The effect of ORG 20599 on strychnine-sensitive glycine receptors (the principal mediators of fast, inhibitory neurotransmission in the brain stem and spinal cord) were investigated at human recombinant α1, β2, γ2L-subunit-containing $GABA_A$ receptors and α1-glycine receptors expressed in *X. laevis* oocytes under voltage-clamp. ORG 20599 enhanced currents mediated by glycine receptors, although with higher EC_{50} values (22.9 μM) than for $GABA_A$ receptors (Weir et al. 2004).

The aminosteroids were also investigated for antinociceptive effects following intrathecal injection in rats. ORG 20599 had no antinociceptive properties as assessed by tail flick and electrical current nociceptive tests (Goodchild et al. 2000). These data suggest that the modulatory effects of the aminosteroids on the cerebral $GABA_A$ receptors cannot be transposed to the $GABA_A$ receptors of the spinal cord.

References

Allolio B, Dorr H, Stuttmann R, Knorr D, Engelhardt D, Winkelmann W (1985) Effect of a single bolus of etomidate upon eight major corticosteroid hormones and plasma ACTH. Clin Endocrinol (Oxf) 22:281–286

Arden JR, Holley FO, Stanski DR (1986) Increased sensitivity to etomidate in the elderly: initial distribution versus altered brain response. Anesthesiology 65:19–27

Ates O, Yucel N, Cayli SR, Altinoz E, Yologlu S, Kocak A, Cakir CO, Turkoz Y (2006) Neuroprotective effect of etomidate in the central nervous system of streptozotocin-induced diabetic rats. Neurochem Res 31:777–783

Atiba JO, Horai Y, White PF, Trevor AJ, Blaschke TF, Sung ML (1988) Effect of etomidate on hepatic drug metabolism in humans. Anesthesiology 68:920–924

Belelli D, Lambert JJ, Peters JA, Wafford K, Whiting PJ (1997) The interaction of the general anesthetic etomidate with the gamma-aminobutyric acid type A receptor is influenced by a single amino acid. Proc Natl Acad Sci USA 94:11031–11036

Cayli SR, Ates O, Karadag N, Altinoz E, Yucel N, Yologlu S, Kocak A, Cakir CO (2006) Neuroprotective effect of etomidate on functional recovery in experimental spinal cord injury. Int J Dev Neurosci 24:233–239

Cheng VY, Martin LJ, Elliott EM, Kim JH, Mount HT, Taverna FA, Roder C, Macdonald JF, Bhambri A, Collinson N, Wafford KA, Orser BA (2006) Alpha5 GABAA receptors mediate the amnestic but not the sedative-hypnotic effects of the general anesthetic etomidate. J Neurosci 26:3713–3720

Choi SD, Spaulding BC, Gross JB, Apfelbaum JL (1985) Comparison of the ventilatory effects of etomidate and methohexital. Anesthesiology 62:442–447

Colvin MP, Savege TM, Newland PE, Weaver EJM, Waters AF, Brookers JM, Innias R (1979) Cardiorespiratory changes following induction of anesthesia with etomidate in patients with cardiac disease. Br J Anaesth 51:551–556

Criado A, Maseda J, Navarro E, Escarpa A, Avello F (1980) Induction of anesthesia with etomidate. Hemodynamic study of 36 patients. Br J Anaesth 52:803–806

Crozier TA, Beck D, Wuttke W, Kettler D (1988) In vivo suppression of steroid synthesis by etomidate is concentration-dependent. Anaesthesist 37:337–339

De Coster R, Helmers JH, Noorduin H (1985) Effect of etomidate on cortisol biosynthesis: site of action after induction of anesthesia. Acta Endocrinol (Copenh) 110:526–531

De Hert SG, Vermeyen KM, Adriaensen HF (1990) Influence of thiopental, etomidate and propofol on regional myocardial function in the normal and acute ischemic heart segment in dogs. Anesth Analg 70:600–607

De Jong FH, Mallios C, Jansen C, Scheck PAE, Lamberts SWJ (1984) Etomidate suppresses adrenocortical function by inhibition of 11β hydroxylation. J Clin Endocrinol Metab 59:1143–1147

De Ruiter G, Popescu DT, De Boer AG, Smekens JB, Breimer DD (1981) Pharmacokinetics of etomidate in surgical patients. Arch Int Pharmacodyn Ther 249:180–188

Doenicke AW, Roizen MF, Nebauer AE, Kugler A, Hoernecke R, Beger-Hintzen H (1994) Comparison of two formulations of etomidate, 2-hydroxypropyl-β-cyclodextrin (HPCD) and propylene glycol. Anesth Analg 79:933–939

Drummond JC, McKay LD, Cole DJ, Patel PM (2005) The role of nitric oxide synthase inhibition in the adverse effects of etomidate in the setting of focal cerebral ischemia in rats. Anesth Analg 100:841–846

Edelman GJ, Hoffman WE, Charbel FT (1997) Cerebral hypoxia after etomidate administration and temporary cerebral artery occlusion. Anesth Analg 85:821–825

Evans RH, Hill RG (1978) GABA-mimetic action of etomidate. Experientia 34:1325–1327

Fry DE, Griffiths H (1984) The inhibition by etomidate of the 11β hydroxylation of cortisol. Clin Endocrinol (Oxf) 20:625–629

Gelissen HP, Epema AH, Henning RH, Krijnen HJ, Hennis PJ, den Hertog A (1996) Inotropic effects of propofol, thiopental, midazolam, etomidate and ketamine on isolated human atrial muscle. Anesthesiology 84:397–403

Goodchild CS, Guo Z, Nadeson R (2000) Antinociceptive properties of neurosteroids. I. Spinally mediated antinociceptive effects of water-soluble aminosteroids. Pain 88:23–29

Gooding JM, Corssen G (1977) Effect of etomidate on the cardiovascular system. Anesth Analg 56:717–719

Gooding JM, Weng JT, Smith RA, Berninger GT, Kirby RR (1979) Cardiovascular and pulmonary responses following etomidate induction of anesthesia in patients with demonstrated cardiac disease. Anesth Analg 58:40–41

Hebron BS, Edbrooke DL, Mather LE, Newby DM (1983) Pharmacokinetics of etomidate associated with a prolonged intravenous infusion. Br J Anaesth 55:281–287

Hering W, Ihmsen H, Uhrlau C, Schüttler J (1996b) Concentration-effect relationship, hemodynamics and respiration after infusion of the steroid anesthetic eltanolone in healthy subjects. Anaesthesist 45:1142–1150

Hering WJ, Ihmsen H, Langer H, Uhrlau C, Dinkel M, Geisslinger G, Schüttler J (1996a) Pharmacokinetic-pharmacodynamic modeling of the new steroid hypnotic eltanolone in healthy volunteers. Anesthesiology 85:1290–1299

Heykants J, Brugmans J, Doenicke A (1973) Pharmacokinetics of etomidate (R26490) in human volunteers: plasma levels, metabolism and excretion. Janssen Research Products Information Service. Clinical Research Report R 26490/1

Heykants J, Meuldermans W, Michiels L, Lewi P, Janssen P (1975) Distribution, metabolism and excretion of etomidate, a short acting hypnotic drug, in the rat. Comparative study of R(+) and S(–) etomidate. Arch Int Pharmacodyn Ther 216:113–129

Hill-Venning C, Peters JA, Callachan H, Lambert JJ, Gemmell DK, Anderson A, Byford A, Hamilton N, Hill DR, Marshall RJ, Campbell AC (1996) The anesthetic action and modulation of GABAA receptor activity by the novel water-soluble aminosteroid ORG 20599. Neuropharmacology 35:1209–1222

Hoffman WE, Charbel FT, Edelman G, Misra M, Ausman JI (1998) Comparison of the effect of etomidate and desflurane on brain tissue gases and pH during prolonged middle cerebral artery occlusion. Anesthesiology 88:1188–1194
Horai Y, White PF, Trevor AJ (1985) The effects of etomidate on rabbit liver microsomal drug metabolism in vitro. Drug Metab Dispos 13:364–367
Husain SS, Ziebell MR, Ruesch D, Hong F, Arevalo E, Kosterlitz JA, Olsen RW, Forman SA, Cohen JB, Miller KW (2003) 2-(3-Methyl-3H-diaziren-3yl)ethyl 1-(1-phenylethyl)-1H-imidazole-5-carboxylate: a derivative of the stereoselective general anesthetic etomidate for photolabeling ligand-gated ion channels. J Med Chem 46:1257–1265
Kay B (1976) A dose-response relationship for etomidate with some observations on cumulation. Br J Anaesth 48:213–216
Kettler D, Sonntag H, Donath U, Regensburger D, Schenk HD (1974) Hemodynamics, myocardial function, oxygen requirement and oxygen supply of the human heart after administration of etomidate. Anaesthesist 23:116–121
Kissin I, Motomura S, Aultman DF, Reves JG (1983) Inotropic and anesthetic potencies of etomidate and thiopental in dogs. Anesth Analg 62:961–965
Komai H, DeWitt DE, Rusy BF (1985) Negative inotropic effects of etomidate in rabbit papillary muscle. Anesth Analg 64:400–404
Laughlin TP, Newberg LA (1985) Prolonged myoclonus after etomidate anesthesia. Anesth Analg 64:80–82
Li GD, Chiara DC, Sawyer GW, Husain SS, Olsen RW, Cohen JB (2006) Identification of a GABAA receptor anesthetic binding site at subunit interfaces by photolabeling with an etomidate analog. J Neurosci 8:11599–11605
Milde LN, Milde JH, Michenfelder JD (1985) Cerebral functional, metabolic and hemodynamic effects of etomidate in dogs. Anesthesiology 63:371–377
Moore RA, Allen MC, Wood PJ, Rees LH, Sear JW (1985) Perioperative endocrine effects of etomidate. Anaesthesia 40:124–130
Moss E, Powell D, Gibson RM, McDowall DG (1979) Effect of etomidate on intracranial pressure and cerebral perfusion pressure. Br J Anaesth 51:347–352
O'Meara GF, Newman RJ, Fradley RL, Dawson GR, Reynolds DS (2004) The GABA-A beta3 subunit mediates anesthesia induced by etomidate. Neuroreport 15:1653–1656
Ouedraogo N, Roux E, Forestier F, Rossetti M, Savineau JP, Marthan R (1998) Effects of intravenous anesthetics on normal and passively sensitized human isolated airway smooth muscle. Anesthesiology 88:317–326
Ouedraogo N, Marthan R, Roux E (2003) The effects of propofol and etomidate on airway contractility in chronically hypoxic rats. Anesth Analg 96:1035–1041
Paris A, Philipp M, Tonner PH, Steinfath M, Lohse M, Scholz J, Hein L (2003) Activation of alpha 2B-adrenoceptors mediates the cardiovascular effects of etomidate. Anesthesiology 99:889–895
Parivar K, Wessen A, Widman M, Nilsson A (1996) Pharmacokinetics of eltanolone following bolus injection and constant rate infusion. J Pharmacokinet Biopharm 24:535–549
Patschke D, Bruckner JB, Eberlein JH, Hess W, Tarnow J, Weymar A (1977) Effects of althesin, etomidate and fentanyl on hemodynamics and myocardial oxygen consumption in man. Can Anaesth Soc J 24:57–69
Pili-Floury S, Samain E, Bouillier H, Rucker-Martin C, Safar M, Dagher G, Marty J, Renaud JF (2004) Etomidate alters calcium mobilization induced by angiotensin II in rat aortic smooth muscle cells. J Cardiovasc Pharmacol 43:485–488
Prakash O, Dhasmana M, Verdouw PD, Saxena PR (1981) Cardiovascular effects of etomidate with emphasis on regional myocardial blood flow and performance. Br J Anaesth 53:591–599
Proctor WR, Mynlieff M, Dunwiddie TV (1986) Facilitatory action of etomidate and pentobarbital on recurrent inhibition in rat hippocampal pyramidal neurons. J Neurosci 6:3161–3168
Riou B, Lecarpentier Y, Viars P (1993) Effects of etomidate on the cardiac papillary muscle of normal hamsters and those with cardiomyopathy. Anesthesiology 78:83–90

Robertson B (1989) Actions of anesthetics and avermectin on GABAA chloride channels in mammalian dorsal root ganglion neurons. Br J Pharmacol 98:167–176

Schüttler J, Wilms M, Lauven P, Stoeckel H, Koenig A (1980) Pharmakokinetische Untersuchungen über Etomidat beim Menschen. Anaesthesist 29:658–661

Schüttler J, Wilms M, Stoeckel H, Schwilden H, Lauven P (1983) Pharmacokinetic interaction of etomidate and fentanyl. Anesthesiology 59:A247

Schüttler J, Schwilden H, Stoeckel H (1985) Infusion strategies to investigate the pharmacokinetics and pharmacodynamics of hypnotic drugs: etomidate as an example. Eur J Anaesthesiol 2:133–142

Schwilden H, Schüttler J, Stoeckel H (1985) Quantitation of the EEG and pharmacodynamic modeling of hypnotic drugs: etomidate as an example. Eur J Anaesthesiol 2:121–131

Shin IW, Sohn JT, Kim HJ, Kim C, Lee HK, Chang KC, Chung YK (2005) Etomidate attenuates phenylephrine-induced contraction in isolated rat aorta. Can J Anaesth 52:927–934

Sneyd JR, Wright PM, Cross M, Thompson P, Voortman G, Weideman MM, Andrews CJ, Daniell CJ (1997a) Administration to humans of ORG 21465, a water soluble steroid i.v. anaesthetic agent. Br J Anaesth 79:427–432

Sneyd JR, Wright PM, Harris D, Taylor PA, Vijn PC, Cross M, Dale H, Voortman G, Boen P (1997b) Computer-controlled infusion of ORG 21465, a water soluble steroid i.v. anaesthetic agent, into human volunteers. Br J Anaesth 79:433–439

Tassani P, Janicke U, Ott E, Conzen P (1996) Hemodynamic effects of three different dosages of the induction hypnotic, eltanolone, in coronary surgery patients. Anaesthesist 45:249–254

Thomson IA, Fitch W, Hughes RI, Campbell D, Watson R (1984) Effects of certain i.v. anaesthetics on liver blood flow and hepatic oxygen consumption in the greyhound. Br J Anaesth 58:69–80

Thyagarajan R, Ramanjaneyulu R, Tick MK (1983) Enhancement of diazepam and gamma-aminobutyric acid binding by (+) etomidate and pentobarbital. J Neurochem 41:578–585

Tomlin SL, Jenkins A, Lieb WR, Franks NP (1998) Stereoselective effects of etomidate optical isomers on gamma-aminobutyric acid type A receptors and animals. Anesthesiology 88:708–717

Van Aken J, Rolly G (1976) Influence of etomidate, a new short-acting anesthetic agent, on cerebral blood flow in man. Acta Anaesthesiol Belg 27:175–180

Van Hamme MJ, Ghoneim MM, Ambre JJ (1978) Pharmacokinetics of etomidate, a new intravenous anesthetic. Anesthesiology 49:274–277

Van Lambalgan AA, Bronsveld W, Van den Bos GC (1982) Cardiovascular and biochemical changes in dogs during etomidate-nitrous oxide anesthesia. Cardiovasc Res 15:599–606

Visser SA, Gladdines WW, van der Graaf PH, Peletier LA, Danhof M (2002) Neuroactive steroids differ in potency but not in intrinsic efficacy at the GABA(A) receptor in vivo. J Pharmacol Exp Ther 303:616–626

Wagner RL, White PF, Kan PB, Rosenthal MH, Feldman D (1984) Inhibition of adrenal steroidogenesis by the anesthetic etomidate. N Engl J Med 310:1415–1421

Weir CJ, Ling AT, Belelli D, Wildsmith JA, Peters JA, Lambert JJ (2004) The interaction of anaesthetic steroids with recombinant glycine and GABAA receptors. Br J Anaesth 92:704–711

Wessen A, Parivar K, Widman M, Nilsson A, Hartvig P (1996) Concentration-effect relationships of eltanolone given as a bolus dose or constant rate intravenous infusion to healthy male volunteers. Anesthesiology 84:1317–1326

Wolff J, Carl P, Bo Hansen P, Hogskilde S, Christensen MS, Sorensen MB (1994) Effects of eltanolone on cerebral blood flow and metabolism in healthy volunteers. Anesthesiology 81:623–627

Xie Z, Currie KP, Fox AP (2004) Etomidate elevates intracellular calcium levels and promotes catecholamine secretion in bovine chromaffin cells. J Physiol 460:677–690

Zeller A, Arras M, Lazaris A, Jurd R, Rudolph U (2005) Distinct molecular targets for the central respiratory and cardiac actions of the general anesthetics etomidate and propofol. FASEB J 19:1677–1679

Remifentanil and Other Opioids

F.S. Servin(✉) and V. Billard

Abstract Most opioids used in anaesthesia are of the anilidopiperidine family, including fentanyl, alfentanil, sufentanil and remifentanil. While all share similar pharmacological properties, remifentanil, the newest one, is probably the most original, which is the reason this review focusses especially on this drug. Remifentanil is a potent μ-agonist that retains all the pharmacodynamic characteristics of its class (regarding analgesia, respiratory depression, muscle rigidity, nausea and vomiting, pruritus, etc.) but with a unique pharmacokinetic profile that combines a short onset and the fastest offset, independent of the infusion duration. Consequently, it offers a unique titratability when its effects need to be quickly achieved or suppressed, but it requires specific drug delivery schemes such as continuous infusion, target-controlled

F.S. Servin
CHU Bichat Claude Bernard, Paris, France, Institut Gustave Roussy, Villejuif, France
fservin@magic.fr

J. Schüttler and H. Schwilden (eds.) *Modern Anesthetics.*
Handbook of Experimental Pharmacology 182.

infusion and anticipated postoperative pain treatment. Kinetic differences between opioids used in anaesthesia and some clinical uses of remifentanil are reviewed in this chapter.

1 Introduction

Historically, anaesthesia was provided as a single agent, first as a volatile (since the nineteen century) and later an intravenous (as thiopentone since World War II) compound. The quality of anaesthesia was obviously far from perfect, and no drug could provide both immobility and stable haemodynamics during the noxious stimulations of surgery, even in unconscious patients. "Balanced" anaesthesia was first proposed by combining hypnotic drugs with local anaesthetics for pain relief around 1926, but a great improvement was made in 1947 by the introduction of an opioid analgesic, meperidine, in the combination (Bovill et al. 1984). Then pure μ-agonists such as fentanyl (1960), sufentanil (1978) and alfentanil (1984) were released and became progressively widely employed because of their high potency, few side-effects and large therapeutic index.

Remifentanil, the newest one, is probably the most original, which is the reason this review is especially focussed on this drug. It is a potent μ-agonist which retains all the pharmacodynamic characteristics of its class (regarding analgesia, respiratory depression, muscle rigidity, nausea and vomiting, pruritus...) but with a unique pharmacokinetic (PK) profile due to a rapid metabolism by non-specific tissue esterases (Egan et al. 1993). Its potency is in the same order of magnitude as that of fentanyl, and it is about 20 times more potent than alfentanil (Egan et al. 1996). Its onset of action is similar to that of alfentanil, which reflects similar equilibration times between blood and effect-site concentrations, but its duration of effect is much shorter (Glass et al. 1999), and its measured context-sensitive half-time averages 3 min after an infusion of 3 h (Kapila et al. 1995). To integrate remifentanil and its interesting pharmacological properties in clinical practice, a major obstacle needs to be overcome: there must be an important "cultural" change in the way opioids are dealt with intra-operatively and in the way postoperative analgesia is planned and carried out.

After about 10 years of release in everyday practice, remifentanil use is still increasing for several reasons:

- Recently released sophisticated drug delivery systems such as target-controlled infusion (TCI) (Egan and Shafer 2003) allow for precise titration and safe administration in patients with very narrow therapeutic margin.
- Some new clinical applications are currently growing, such as remifentanil's use as the sole agent for "sedation" during painful procedures in patients breathing spontaneously, or as the analgesic component in intensive care sedation.
- Simultaneously, remifentanil has permitted important scientific research, both experimental and clinical, in the study of interactions between opioids and glutamatergic systems, leading to a better understanding of postoperative hyperalgesia and acute tolerance to the analgesic action of opioids.

2 Remifentanil: Basic Pharmacological Properties

2.1 Chemical and Physical Properties

Remifentanil is a μ-receptor agonist of the 4-anilidopiperidine series (Burkle et al. 1996; Egan 1995), chemically related to fentanyl, alfentanil and sufentanil (Fig. 1). It is the hydrochloride salt of the 3-(4-methoxycarbonyl-4-[(1-oxopropyl)-phenylamino]-1 piperidine) propionic acid, methyl ester. Its molecular weight is 413 and it is a lipophilic drug with an octanol/water partition coefficient of 17.9 at a pH of 7.4 (Table 1). It does not have a chiral centre, and therefore exists in a single form. The modification of the basic anilidopiperidine structure by the introduction of a methyl ester group onto the *N*-acyl side chain of the piperidine ring confers to the molecule an increased susceptibility to hydrolytic metabolism by non-specific esterases, which leads to a rapid systemic elimination. It is not a substrate for

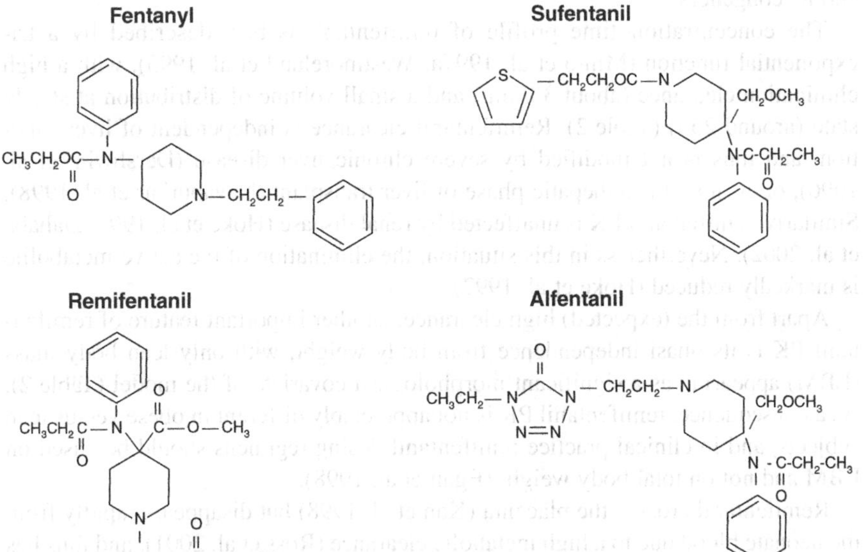

Fig. 1 Chemical structure of opioids used in anaesthesia

Table 1 Physicochemical properties of commonly used opioids (Bailey and Egan 1997)

	Fentanyl	Sufentanil	Alfentanil	Remifentanil
pK_a	8.4	8.0	6.5	7.1
% Unionized at pH 7.4	<10	20	90	67
Octanol/H_2O partition coefficient	813	1 778	129	18
% Bound to plasma proteins	84	93	92	70
Hepatic extraction ratio	0.8–1.0	0.7–0.9	0.3–0.5	-

butyrylcholinesterases and thus its clearance is not affected by cholinesterases deficiency or anti-cholinergic drugs (Manullang and Egan 1999). It is presented as a water-soluble lyophilized powder containing the free base and glycine as a vehicle to buffer the solution (pH 3; pK_a in water 7.07), to be reconstituted in water or 5% dextrose solution for injection. Glycine potentially produces reversible, naloxone-insensitive motor dysfunction after continuous, but not after acute, bolus intrathecal administration in rodents (Buerkle and Yaksh 1996). Hence, the spinal or epidural administration of remifentanil in its current formulation is not recommended in humans.

2.2 Pharmacokinetics

Remifentanil was primarily designed to cover the need for a short-acting fast-eliminating opioid, retaining the desirable pharmacodynamic features of fentanyl and its congeners.

The concentration–time profile of remifentanil is best described by a tri-exponential function (Minto et al. 1997a; Westmoreland et al. 1993), with a high elimination clearance (about 3 l/min) and a small volume of distribution at steady state (around 25 l) (Table 2). Remifentanil clearance is independent of liver function, and thus is not modified by severe chronic liver disease (Dershwitz et al. 1996), or even by the anhepatic phase of liver transplant (Navapurkar et al. 1998). Similarly, remifentanil PK is unaffected by renal disease (Hoke et al. 1997; Dahaba et al. 2002). Nevertheless in this situation, the elimination of the active metabolite is markedly reduced (Hoke et al. 1997).

Apart from the (expected) high clearance, another important feature of remifentanil PK is its quasi independence from body weight, with only lean body mass (LBM) appearing as a significant morphological covariate of the model (Table 2). As a consequence, remifentanil PK is not appreciably different in obese versus lean subjects, and in clinical practice remifentanil dosing regimens should be based on LBM and not on total body weight (Egan et al. 1998).

Remifentanil crosses the placenta (Kan et al. 1998) but disappears rapidly from the neonate blood due to a high metabolic clearance (Ross et al. 2001), and thus has no clinical consequences on the child. Remifentanil PK is very similar in children and in adult patients (Ross et al. 2001). In the elderly remifentanil clearance is reduced (Minto et al. 1997b). This observation, associated with the well-known increase of elderly patients' susceptibility to the pharmacological action of opioids, should lead to markedly decreased dosing recommendations in this population (Kabbaj et al. 2005; Pitsiu et al. 2004; Bouillon et al. 2002).

Propofol decreases the remifentanil central volume of distribution and distributional clearance of remifentanil by 41% as already described with alfentanil (Mertens et al. 2001). Consequently, the bolus dose to achieve a chosen target concentration should be reduced, but the infusion rate to maintain it is unchanged in the presence of propofol compared to remifentanil alone (Bouillon et al. 2002).

Table 2 Comparison of remifentanil pharmacokinetic macro-constants as described by Minto et al. (1997a) to other μ-agonists and values for a 40-year-old, 70-kg, 1.70-m male patient

Estimated parameters	Fentanyl (Scott and Stanski 1987)	Alfentanil (Maitre et al. 1987)	Sufentanil (Gepts et al. 1995)	Remifentanil Full model (Minto et al. 1997a)	Value
Covariates	None	Weight, gender	None	LBM, age, gender	
Volumes (l)					
Central (V_1)	12.7	7.77	14.3	5.1–0.0201 × (age–40) + 0.072 × (LBM– 55)	5.1
Rapid peripheral (V_2)	50	12	63	9.82–0.0811 × (age–40) + 0.108 × (LBM– 55)	9.8
Slow peripheral (V_3)	295	10.48	262	5.42	5.4
Clearances ($l.min^{-1}$)					
Metabolic (Cl_1)	0.62	0.356	0.92	2.6–0.0162 × (age–40) + 0.0191 × (LBM– 55)	2.6
Rapid peripheral (Cl_2)	4.8	0.808	1.55	2.05–0.0301 × (age–40)	2.05
Slow peripheral (Cl_3)	2.3	0.132	0.33	0.076–0.00113 × (age–40)	0.08
$t_{1/2}\ k_{e0}$ (min)	4.7	0.35	6.2 (Scott et al. 1991)	0.69/[0.595–0.007 (age– 40)]	1.16
Time to peak after bolus (min)	3.7	1.4	5.6		1.52

LBM, lean body mass

2.2.1 Effect-Site Concentration

Remifentanil equilibration half-time between plasma and the effect compartment ($t_{1/2}\ k_{e0}$) has been modelled using continuous EEG recording and is brief (1.0–1.5 min) (Glass et al. 1993). As this transfer to CNS competes with distribution processes, $t_{1/2}\ k_{e0}$ is not a directly clinically relevant parameter, and time to peak effect should be considered instead. It is also short for remifentanil (around 1.5 min in young adults, increasing markedly with age) (Gambus et al. 1995). Thus, remifentanil has a short onset after a bolus dose, similar to alfentanil, and it is much shorter than fentanyl or sufentanil (Egan et al. 1996; Shafer and Varvel 1991). Nevertheless, as remifentanil plasma concentration decreases very quickly after a bolus dose, the peak effect-site concentration of remifentanil is proportionally lower than that of alfentanil but higher than others (Fig. 2).

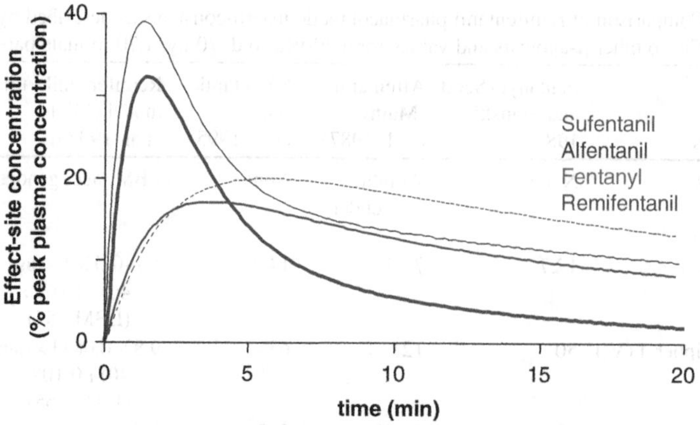

Fig. 2 Effect-site concentration time course after a bolus. Simulation obtained with Stanpump (Steve Shafer, Palo Alto; http://anesthesia.stanford.edu/pkpd/) with the pharmacokinetic parameters from Scott et al. (1991), Gepts et al. (1995), Maitre et al. (1987) and Minto et al. (1997) for fentanyl, sufentanil, alfentanil and remifentanil

2.2.2 Context-Sensitive Half-Time

Remifentanil was introduced at a time when anaesthetists, through the work of Shafer and Varvel (1991) and Hughes et al. (1992), understood the importance of considering the decrease in concentration during the early phases after an infusion as opposed to terminal half-time. If a rapid decrease in concentration is desired after an infusion, simulation studies demonstrated that it was always beneficial to have a small central volume of distribution (V_1) and a large elimination clearance (Cl_1) (Youngs and Shafer 1994).

The time for the effect-site concentration to decrease by 50% after the end of a remifentanil infusion (context-sensitive half-time, CSHT ; Hughes et al. 1992) modelled from early remifentanil PK analyses (Egan et al. 1993; Westmoreland et al. 1993; Glass et al. 1993) was found to average 3 min and to be independent of the duration of infusion conversely to all other μ-agonists (Fig. 3). This result was subsequently confirmed by an actual measurement in 30 volunteers receiving a 3-h infusion of remifentanil or alfentanil (Kapila et al. 1995). Remifentanil CSHT was 3.2 ± 0.9 min, compared to 47.3 ± 12 min for alfentanil (Kapila et al. 1995).

2.2.3 Active Metabolite

Remifentanil is predominantly metabolized by non-specific esterases to an acid metabolite GI-90291 and to a lesser extend by *N*-dealkylation to a second metabolite GI-94219 (Westmoreland et al. 1993). GI-90291 is an analgesic, but its potency (about 0.1% that of remifentanil) renders its clinical impact negligible. It is excreted through the kidney. Even when accumulation occurs in renal failure patients, the concentrations obtained after a few hours of infusion are insufficient to generate pharmacological effects (Hoke et al. 1997; Pitsiu et al. 2004).

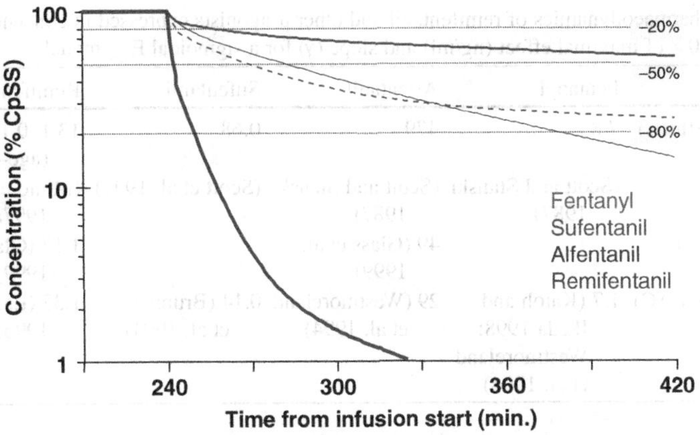

Fig. 3 Concentration decrease of anaesthesia opioids after 4 h infusion. Simulation obtained with Stanpump (Steve Shafer, Palo Alto; http://anesthesia.stanford.edu/pkpd/) with the pharmacokinetic parameters from Scott et al. (1991), Gepts et al. (1995), Maitre et al. (1987) and Minto et al. (1997) for fentanyl, sufentanil, alfentanil and remifentanil

2.3 *Pharmacodynamics*

Remifentanil is a pure μ-agonist analgesic drug whose effects are antagonized by naloxone. The analgesic effect is mediated through coupling of a guanine nucleotide binding protein (G protein) which concomitantly results presynaptically in an inhibition of excitatory neurotransmitter release and postsynaptically in an inhibition of cyclic adenosine monophosphatase, suppression of voltage-sensitive calcium channels, and hyperpolarization of the postsynaptic membrane through increased potassium conductance (Marker et al. 2005).

2.3.1 Potency

Remifentanil is slightly more potent than fentanyl (Lang et al. 1996), and about 20 (Egan et al. 1996) to 40 (Glass et al. 1999; Black et al. 1999) times more potent than alfentanil (Table 3). As a consequence, its range of clinically useful concentrations in anaesthesia is approx. 1–20 ng/ml.

2.3.2 Respiratory Effects

Remifentanil induces a significant depression in hypoxic drive, reversed by naloxone in a dose-related fashion (Amin et al. 1995). As might be expected from the PK of the drug, this depression disappears rapidly at the end of administration (Wuesten et al. 2001). After administration to healthy volunteers of a remifentanil bolus of 0.5 μg/kg, there was a decrease in slope and downward shift of the carbon dioxide ventilatory response curve which reached a nadir approximately 2.5 min

Table 3 Pharmacodynamics of remifentanil and other μ-agonists expressed in concentrations inducing 50% of maximal effect (ng/ml) and slope (γ) for a sigmoidal E_{max} model

	Fentanyl	Alfentanil	Sufentanil	Remifentanil
C_{50} (EEG effects)	7.8	479	0.68	13.1–0.148 (age-40)
	(Scott and Stanski 1987)	(Scott and Stanski 1987)	(Scott et al. 1991)	(Minto et al. 1997a)
C_{50} (50% resp depr)		49 (Glass et al. 1999)		1.17 (Glass et al. 1999)
Ce (50% ↘ MAC)	1.7 (Katoh and Ikeda 1998; Westmoreland et al. 1994)	29 (Westmoreland et al. 1994)	0.14 (Brunner et al. 1994)	1.37 (Lang et al. 1996)[1]

after injection, and completely recovered within 15 min after injection (Babenco et al. 2000). This allowed the estimation of k_{e0} (0.24 min^{-1}) and EC50 (1.12 ng/ml) for respiratory effect. This k_{e0} value corresponds to a longer onset time than that observed by Egan et al. for EEG effects (Egan et al. 1996). This difference may be related in part to the fact that the EEG and ventilatory drive depend on different neural pathways, and that local blood flows may also differ, as well as blood–brain barrier characteristics and neural responsiveness to opioids (Bouillon et al. 2003; Karan et al. 2005; Hsu et al. 2004; Nieuwenhuijs et al. 2003).

2.3.3 Haemodynamic Effects

Remifentanil induces a dose-dependent decrease in heart rate, arterial blood pressure and cardiac output consistent with μ-opioid agonism (James et al. 1992). As fentanyl, remifentanil exerts a central vagotonic action, leading to bradycardia and hypotension, and associated with a marked increase in sympathetic nerve activity mediated by arterial baroreflex (Shinohara et al. 2000). These effects have a rapid onset and a short duration, but they may be marked if remifentanil potency is underestimated, specifically in elderly or β-adrenergic blocker-treated patients (Elliott et al. 2000; Reid and Mirakhur 2000). In those patients, titration to effect and slow administration are advocated. When properly used, remifentanil conveys a haemodynamic stability similar to that of sufentanil, with a more effective blunting of the increase in arterial pressure at intubation even in haemodynamically compromised patients (Mouren et al. 2001). In isolated human right atria fibres, remifentanil has no negative inotropic effect (Hanouz et al. 2001). The haemodynamic effects of remifentanil are not related to histamine release (Sebel et al. 1995).

2.3.4 Central Nervous System

Like other μ-opioid agonists, remifentanil reduces cerebral blood flow in dogs (Hoffman et al. 1993). This effect, which is independent of blood pressure control, is predominant in the forebrain and modest in lower brain regions. A positron emission tomography study in human volunteers further refined those topographic findings (Wagner et al. 2001). Remifentanil induces dose-dependent changes in relative cerebral blood flow in areas involved in pain processing. At the highest infusion rate used (0.15 μg/kg per minute), regional cerebral blood flow was also modified in structures known to participate in modulation of vigilance and alertness. Under remifentanil/N_2O anaesthesia, the global cerebral blood flow is reduced (Ostapkovich et al. 1998). As a consequence, intracranial pressure is reduced and autoregulation is preserved.

Non-invasive assessments of cerebral capacity in awake volunteers showed no influence of low remifentanil infusion rates (0.1 μg/kg per minute) on this parameter (Lorenz et al. 2000). Remifentanil in rabbits did not influence cerebrospinal fluid formation nor resistance to reabsorption (Artru and Momota 2000), and under remifentanil/N_2O anaesthesia, cerebrovascular reactivity to CO_2 remains intact (Baker et al. 1997).

Remifentanil has a powerful spinal opioid action (Buerkle and Yaksh 1996). Nevertheless, supramaximal doses of intrathecal remifentanil sufficient to inhibit initial nociceptive behavioural response still permit sufficient glutamate release to allow spinal facilitation (Buerkle et al. 1998).

It also induces muscle rigidity with an incidence similar to that observed with equipotent doses of alfentanil (Jhaveri et al. 1997). This is probably related to the very rapid onset of effect the drug (Nieuwenhuijs et al. 2003; Habib et al. 2002; Dimitriou et al. 2006; Lecomte et al. 2006; Bilgin et al. 2006; Chanavaz et al. 2005; Locala et al. 2005; Pleym et al. 2004; Ouattara et al. 2004; Godet et al. 2004; Heijmans et al. 2004; Joo et al. 2004; Unlugenc et al. 2003; Jellish et al. 2003; Manyam et al. 2006; Albertin et al. 2006; Mustola et al. 2005; Albertin et al. 2004; Bouillon et al. 2004; Kern et al. 2004; Drover et al. 2004; Mertens et al. 2003; Milne et al. 2003; Fechner et al. 2003; Criado and Gomez e Segura 2003; Bothtner et al. 2002).

At high concentrations, remifentanil induces EEG changes similar to that of other μ-opioids (Gambus et al. 1995), transforming high frequency, low-voltage desynchronized signals to low-frequency, high-voltage synchronized. This feature has been very useful to understand the pharmacology of all opioids, because numeric parameters derived from raw EEG, such as spectral edge, median power frequency, semi-linear canonical correlation or Bispectral Index (Aspect Medical Systems, Norwood, MA, USA) could be calculated and used as a continuous, quantitative measure of EEG effect. These surrogate measures of effect have then been linked to the plasma concentration in order to model the concentration–effect relationship and they have allowed for estimations of the blood-to-CNS equilibration time ($t_{1/2}$ k_{e0}) (Billard and Shafer 1995).

2.3.5 Interactions with Hypnotics

All opioids act similarly in synergism with both volatile (Lang et al. 1996) and intravenous hypnotics (Ropcke et al. 2001) and remifentanil is not an exception to this general rule.

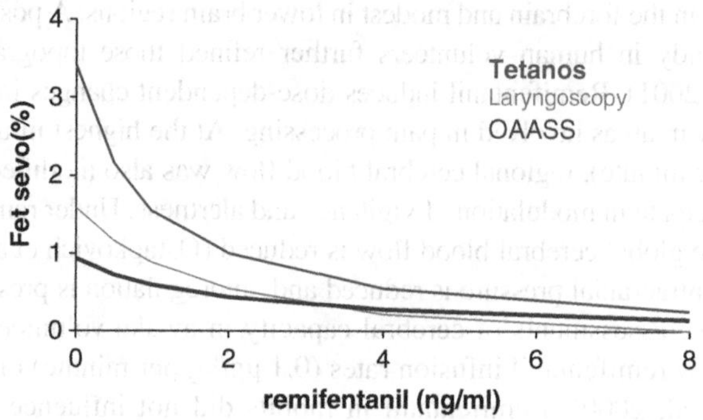

Fig. 4 Influence of remifentanil on sevoflurane C_{50} for various end-points. (From Manyam et al. 2006)

The minimal hypnotic concentration required to control noxious stimuli is markedly reduced (50%–60%) when a low concentration of opioid is added (Fig. 4; Manyam et al. 2006). Intermediate opioid concentrations allow a further reduction in hypnotic requirement by 15%–20%. As remifentanil offset is shorter than the offset of all hypnotics, especially for long-term infusions, the combination which allows the quickest recovery is shifted towards high remifentanil, low hypnotic concentrations [just above the minimum alveolar concentration (MAC)-awake] (Vuyk et al. 1997). Thereafter (i.e. remifentanil concentration above 8 ng/ml for laryngoscopy or incision), the decrease in MAC/Cp50 with increasing opiate concentration tends to flatten until a ceiling effect is observed (Fig. 4; Vuyk et al. 1997) and increasing remifentanil further does not lead to additional reductions in hypnotic requirements.

This synergistic interaction is also observed for the hypnotic effect but is of a lower magnitude. Without opioid, the hypnotic concentration required for loss of consciousness is lower than the one to prevent response to noxious stimulations (around 1/3 MAC). It is moderately reduced by low-dose opioids: for example, propofol concentration for loss of consciousness is reduced by 25% in the presence of remifentanil 6 ng/ml (Nieuwenhuijs et al. 2003; Manyam et al. 2006; Albertin et al. 2006; Mustola et al. 2005; Albertin et al. 2004; Bouillon et al. 2004; Kern et al. 2004; Drover et al. 2004; Mertens et al. 2003; Milne et al. 2003; Fechner et al. 2003; Criado and Gomez e Segura 2003; Bothtner et al. 2002). Consequently, at high opioid concentrations the hypnotic needs for loss of consciousness may be higher than those to prevent response to noxious stimuli, and a patient might show no response to surgery and be completely awake, especially if he cannot move to signal his awareness because of neuromuscular blockade. This situation should be prevented either by staying at an intermediate remifentanil concentration, or by systematically monitoring the depth of anaesthesia when high opioid concentrations are used.

Unfortunately, opioids also enhance the adverse effects of hypnotics: remifentanil is synergistic to propofol on respiratory depression (Peacock et al. 1998), and moderately additive on cardiovascular status (Nieuwenhuijs et al. 2003).

2.3.6 Remifentanil and Acute Tolerance

Opioids, administered to experimental animals, may rapidly induce acute tolerance to their effects (Cox et al. 1968). Remifentanil, administered for 4 h to volunteers, induced an analgesic effect which started to decrease after 60–90 min despite a constant rate infusion (Vinik and Kissin 1998). After 3 h of infusion, the effect was only one-fourth of the peak value. This result was confirmed in the clinical setting, when Guignard et al. demonstrated an increase in morphine requirements associated with higher pain scores after high intraoperative doses of remifentanil (Guignard et al. 2000a). Such an effect is not unheard of, and similar findings have already been published with fentanyl (Chia et al. 1999) and alfentanil (Kissin et al. 1996; Mandema and Wada 1995). Nevertheless, this acute tolerance to remifentanil has not always been demonstrated in the clinical setting (Billard et al. 2004; Cortinez et al. 2001; Schraag et al. 1999). Schraag et al. administered remifentanil as a TCI for postoperative pain and could not demonstrate any increase in effective remifentanil concentrations over time (Cortinez et al. 2001; Schraag et al. 1999). This might nevertheless be compatible with tolerance associated to a reduction in the level of painful stimulus over the first postoperative hours. Cortinez et al. have designed a study very similar to that of Guignard, using sevoflurane instead of desflurane (Cortinez et al. 2001; Schraag et al. 1999). The main difference was that they administered nitrous oxide, which is an *N*-methyl-d-aspartate (NMDA) receptor antagonist (Jevtovic-Todorovic et al. 1998), to their patients. Indeed, acute tolerance to the effect of opioids seems at least in part mediated through the control of μ-opioid receptors by glutaminergic pathways in the central nervous system (Kissin et al. 2000). Several studies have attempted to demonstrate an improvement in postoperative pain control with infra-analgesic doses of ketamine, an NMDA antagonist readily available to anaesthetists (Fu et al. 1997; Jaksch et al. 2002). These studies led to contradictory results which might be due to difficulties in defining the proper ketamine dose/concentration and to wide interindividual variability.

Thus, remifentanil, like other potent opioids, induces acute tolerance which, due the rapid disappearance of its analgesic effect, may lead to difficult postoperative pain control after high doses. The co-administration of an NMDA receptor antagonist (ketamine, nitrous oxide) may help.

3 Remifentanil: Clinical Use as Derived from the Pharmacological Properties

3.1 Administration Modes

The kinetics of remifentanil renders its administration by continuous infusion quasi-mandatory. Even if it is a very forgiving drug, administration diluted through a usual infusion line by gravity (Fragen and Fitzgerald 2000) is not recommended if haemodynamics, drug interactions and even recovery time are to be properly controlled. The three-way stopcock, which is usually used to bring remifentanil into the main infusion line, should be as close as possible to the patient to avoid useless dead space. If a one-way valve is not used, the infusion line should always be carefully purged before recovery and extubation, to avoid delayed boluses leading to apnoea (Bowdle et al. 1996; Fourel et al. 1999). The risks of muscle rigidity at induction of anaesthesia (Schuttler et al. 1997) and/or of haemodynamic instability in risk patients (Elliott et al. 2000) preclude the use of important bolus doses unless administered over at least 30 s. Nevertheless, titration and experience will reduce the incidence of unwanted side-effects (Joshi et al. 2000).

The short remifentanil time-to-peak effect after a bolus allows a deep analgesia to be achieved very rapidly, but its fast elimination requires combining the bolus with a continuous infusion to maintain it more than a few minutes (Fig. 2). The relative doses of bolus and infusions to achieve and maintain a chosen concentration might be tricky to select, especially if the desired concentration changes over time (titration).

A great help has been the launching in clinical practice of TCI devices suitable for opioids (sufentanil or remifentanil), which allow a direct application of the concentration–effect relationship (Egan and Shafer 2003) without risk of administration mistakes (Milne and Kenny 1998). TCI has been used in many pharmacodynamic studies, using software prototypes such as Stanpump (Steve Shafer, Palo Alto; http://anaesthesia.stanford.edu/pkpd) or commercial devices, and allowed the description of drug interactions for various clinical end-points independently of time.

In clinical practice such devices are particularly helpful when remifentanil is used in obese or elderly patients (because of adjusted models) or in cardiac patients because of easier and more precise titration (Olivier et al. 2000). They can improve haemodynamic stability (De Castro et al. 2003). TCI might also represent a safer way to use remifentanil for postoperative pain control, either through doctor or patient controlled administration (Schraag et al. 1998).

With sufentanil, the PK model incorporated in current commercial devices is not weight-adjusted (Gepts et al. 1995) but has been shown to have an acceptable precision in obese patients (Slepchenko et al. 2003). The expected benefits of sufentanil TCI for characterizing drug interactions (Forestier et al. 2003; Hentgen et al. 2002) or titrating to haemodynamic stability are similar to those expected with remifentanil. Additionally, a real time display of sufentanil decrement time by the TCI device might warn the anaesthesia team and suggest a shift to higher hypnotic and lower sufentanil target concentration to optimize recovery delay (Vuyk et al. 1997).

3.2 *Induction and Airway Control*

As remifentanil was initially proposed for anaesthesia in controlled ventilation, inserting a device to control the airway [endotracheal tube or laryngeal mask (LMA)] is usually required.

Tracheal intubation may be performed with or without neuromuscular blocking agents (NMBA) and the dose of remifentanil to recommend will depend on this choice and on the intensity of response tolerated.

Despite serious allergic side-effects, NMBA remain in clinical use to facilitate tracheal intubation and prevent morbidity due to motor response. In the last few years, several anaesthetic protocols combining propofol for its depression of laryngeal reflexes (Sundman et al. 2001) with various doses of opioids have attempted to challenge the quality of intubation provided by muscle relaxants. Nevertheless, laryngoscopy and tracheal intubation create very intense but brief noxious stimuli and therefore call for a very deep level of analgesia to be maintained only for a short duration. The lingering effect of a bolus of fentanyl, sufentanil or alfentanil precludes the use of high opioid concentrations at the time of laryngoscopy for fear of subsequent haemodynamic effects. The PK properties of remifentanil appear ideal for the purpose of blunting the haemodynamic and motor response to tracheal intubation without useless prolonged effect.

In the absence of NMBA and combined with propofol, a remifentanil bolus dose of 4 μg/kg (corresponding in young adults to a predicted peak effect-site concentration around 16 ng/ml) was necessary to ensure good intubation conditions and prevent motor response in adults (Klemola et al. 2000) and in children (Klemola and Hiller 2000). In TCI mode, a concentration above 8–10 ng/ml has been recommended (Troy et al. 2002), but it induced a dose-dependant decrease in blood pressure (BP) and HR (Leone et al. 2004a).

If hypnosis was provided by sevoflurane (Fet 2.5%–3%) and maintained for several minutes with assisted ventilation, remifentanil doses might be reduced to a 1 μg/kg bolus plus a 0.25 μg/kg per minute infusion rate (Cros et al. 2000) or to a 3–4 ng/ml target concentration in TCI (Sztark et al. 2005), thereby creating satisfying intubating conditions.

When a NMBA is used, the only concern is the haemodynamic response to intubation. Target concentrations exceeding 8 ng/ml are necessary to completely blunt the BP and HR response when compared to pre-intubation values (Guignard et al. 2000b), but they result in prolonged reduction in arterial pressure. Target concentrations of 5–7 ng/ml appear as a good compromise to maintain BP and HR response around the pre-induction values (Billard et al. 2004). A single bolus of 1 μg/kg induces only a moderate HR increase (McAtamney et al. 1998).

These doses should be reduced in the elderly (Habib et al. 2002) as well as in hypertensive patients, where a bolus dose of 0.5 μg/kg plus a 0.1-μg/kg per minute infusion rate (i.e. predicted concentration around 3 ng/ml) already induced hypotension in 7/20 hypertensive patients (Maguire et al. 2001).

The remifentanil dose required to insert a laryngeal mask is lower and has been estimated as 0.25–0.3 μg/kg in association with propofol (Grewal and Samsoon 2001; Lee et al. 2001), without the need for NMBA.

3.3 *Control Over Intra-operative Stimuli*

During general anaesthesia, the opioid concentration should permanently be adjusted to the intensity of noxious stimulations to avoid both relative overdose with adverse haemodynamic effects and a dangerous response to surgical stimulation (Glass et al. 1994).

The situations where remifentanil may represent a significant clinical improvement are therefore those where a potent analgesic effect is required with a short onset and a rapid offset, specifically if postoperative pain is easily controlled (i.e. with a regional technique). Clinically, remifentanil titratability translates into a better control over adrenergic stimuli whatever the type of surgery or the patients (Kapila et al. 1995; Mouren et al. 2001; Schuttler et al. 1997; Cartwright et al. 1997; Gemma et al. 2002; Guy et al. 1997; Howie et al. 2001; McGregor et al. 1998; Sneyd et al. 2001; Ahonen et al. 2000; Balakrishnan et al. 2000; Casati et al. 2000; Doyle et al. 2001; Fleisher et al. 2001; Natalini et al. 1999; Twersky et al. 2001; Wee et al. 1999; Wilhelm et al. 2001). For example, intubation is a stronger stimulus than laryngoscopy, which in turn is stronger than skin incision. Intra-abdominal surgery represents a very strong stimulus and requires remifentanil concentrations between 4 and 10 ng/ml (Billard et al. 2004; Dershwitz et al. 1995). Other particular contexts will be described below.

For a given noxious stimulation, however, the opioid concentration to maintain may be influenced by the hypnotic concentration it is combined with, in order to stay above both interaction curves (Fig. 4), namely the curve for response to stimulation and the curve for loss of consciousness.

If the opioid is fentanyl, which accumulates very early and has a long context-sensitive half-time (Fig. 3), low fentanyl high hypnotic doses should be maintained to optimize the recovery delay (Vuyk et al. 1997). For sufentanil or alfentanil, intermediate doses of both hypnotic and opioid, i.e. maximal synergy, provide the shortest recovery. With remifentanil—since any dosage may be used during surgery without undue lengthening of emergence times (Dershwitz et al. 1995)—the hypnotic opioid/balance may be shifted to high opioid to spare some hypnotic and thus save money, limit pollution and shorten recovery time. Such high doses of remifentanil may nevertheless have drawbacks:

- A combination with the "usual" doses of hypnotic may increase the incidence of hypotension and bradycardia (Vuyk et al. 1997; Hogue et al. 1996).
- If the hypnotic is used at lower concentrations than with other opioids to maintain haemodynamic stability, this reduction increases the risk of awareness during anaesthesia, specifically if the patient is paralysed (Hogue et al. 1996).
- A high intraoperative opioid dosage increases postoperative morphine requirements through the development of acute tolerance (Guignard et al. 2000a).
- The incidence of postoperative nausea and vomiting is high in opioid-based anaesthetic techniques, and remifentanil is no exception (Bowdle et al. 1996).

3.3.1 Absence of Residual Opioid Effect: An Advantage or a Drawback?

Micro-laryngoscopy represents a very intense but short adrenergic stimulus, and it is mandatory that the patients, often suffering from chronic obstructive pulmonary disease (COPD) and frequently with some degree of airway obstruction, recover with as little respiratory impairment as possible. In this situation, the absence of residual remifentanil effect is clearly an advantage (Wuesten et al. 2001). In upper intra-abdominal surgery, a degree of postoperative respiratory impairment directly related to surgery is also present, and an effective postoperative analgesia is readily provided by central blockade. In this situation, remifentanil provides shorter time to extubation and fewer effects on postoperative SpO_2 than sufentanil in the first 7 h after surgery (Casati et al. 2000).

On the other hand, remifentanil lack of residual effect may be a major drawback if postoperative pain control is sub-optimal (Davis et al. 2000; Fletcher et al. 2000).

3.4 Postoperative Analgesia

A major concern when using remifentanil during general anaesthesia is postoperative pain control, which must be planned and initiated before the end of the procedure. Local or regional analgesia, when available, are obvious options which brings satisfying results (Casati et al. 2000). The absence of postoperative respiratory depression is an advantage in this situation (Casati et al. 2000).

In moderately painful surgery, adequate analgesia is usually obtained through multimodal analgesia associating various non-opioid analgesics. The major point is to administer the analgesics early enough to account for their onset time, i.e. between 30 and 60 min before stopping remifentanil infusion (Pendeville et al. 2001). In major surgery when regional techniques are not available, an elegant solution is to reduce remifentanil infusion at the end of the procedure to allow spontaneous breathing and extubation while maintaining adequate analgesia (Calderon et al. 2001). After surgical procedures leading to significant postoperative pain, an infusion rate of remifentanil between 0.05 and 0.15 $\mu g.kg^{-1}.min^{-1}$ ensured adequate analgesia in 78% of the patients during the first hour after surgery, but some patients required doses well outside this range (Bowdle et al. 1996). Even in the carefully controlled setting of clinical investigation, 8% of the patients became apnoeic or required the administration of naloxone for severe respiratory depression. These events were usually triggered by the administration of a remifentanil bolus. Another risk is the rapid flush of an infusion line containing remifentanil. This risk can be avoided by reducing as much as possible the dead space between the remifentanil line and the patient's blood. The wide interindividual variability in the dosages required calls for each patient to have control over remifentanil infusion rates. This is best obtained with a remifentanil TCI (Schraag et al. 1998).

If postoperative remifentanil infusion is not considered, adequate analgesia can usually be obtained with morphine 0.15–0.20 mg/kg given intravenously more than 30 min before the end of surgery, then titrated to effect in the post-anaesthesia care unit (PACU) before the institution of a patient-controlled analgesia (PCA) (Kochs et al. 2000; Minkowitz 2000). An intraoperative dose of morphine 0.25 mg/kg would be excessive in some patients (Fletcher et al. 2000). Adjuvant analgesics (acetaminophen, ketamine) may enhance morphine analgesia.

4 Remifentanil: A Few Examples of Specific Clinical Situations

Since its launch, remifentanil has been assessed in numerous clinical situations with rather predictable results when considering its pharmacology. Their descriptions would unduly lengthen this review. Only specific fields which have been under discussion are therefore considered here.

4.1 Remifentanil and Regional Anaesthesia

Due to the glycine contained in the current formulation, remifentanil should not be used in regional blocks, for fear of toxic motor impairment (Buerkle and Yaksh 1996).

It has been proposed that remifentanil alone (Lauwers et al. 1999; Mingus et al. 1998; Servin et al. 2002) or associated with propofol (Holas et al. 1999) be used for intraoperative sedation in patients undergoing surgery under regional anaesthesia. In this situation, remifentanil may offer some advantages in terms of sedation control, but respiratory depression should be monitored closely, and anti-emetic prophylaxis should be used in patients at risk.

4.2 Monitored Anaesthesia Care

The first experiences with remifentanil in spontaneously breathing patients were not entirely persuasive: in the PACU, the use of remifentanil infusions to prevent and treat postoperative severe pain led to some serious respiratory depression when accidental boluses were administered, most of the time through flushes of the infusion line (Bowdle et al. 1996). This technique is now seldom used. Similarly, the use of remifentanil as "sedative" agent in patients undergoing surgery under regional anaesthesia was impaired by the incidence of respiratory depression and post-operative nausea and vomiting (PONV) during surgery (Servin et al. 1999). Then, remifentanil was proposed to ensure analgesia during painful procedures, associated or not with propofol, and remifentanil TCI further increased its titratability. Thus, new indications have appeared and their number is growing. These include extracorporeal shock wave lithotripsy (Cortinez et al. 2005), colonoscopies (Akcaboy et al. 2006), awake endotracheal intubation (Machata et al. 2003), paediatric fibreoptic bronchoscopies (Dilger et al. 2004), outpatient facial laser resurfacing (Ramos-Zabala et al. 2004), third molar extraction (Fong and Kwan 2005), etc. In all those circumstances, remifentanil is used alone (the addition of small doses of propofol or midazolam may lead to dangerous respiratory depression and should be carefully monitored), and titrated to effect, best through TCI. The efficient target concentrations may vary widely from 0.5 ng/ml or less to 5 ng/ml or even more. Another interesting titration technique is patient controlled administration of the drug, which can be combined with TCI (Schraag et al. 1998).

4.3 Intensive Care Sedation

Current intensive care sedation protocols are often unsatisfactory: during sedation, the control over stimulating events is frequently poor and recovery may be delayed leading to prolonged weaning periods and withdrawal syndromes. The titratability of remifentanil appears appealing in this context. Even if controlled trials are still rare, some promising results have demonstrated that remifentanil was at least as effective as comparator opioids such as fentanyl, morphine and sufentanil in providing pain relief and sedation in mechanically ventilated ICU patients (Karabinis et al. 2004; Baillard et al. 2005), plus it allowed faster awakening and extubation, thus shortening ICU stay (Breen et al. 2005; Muellejans et al. 2006). Similarly, an analgesic-based sedation with remifentanil as the main component, when compared to hypnotic-based sedation with either propofol or midazolam, appeared more comfortable for the patients (Park et al. 2007), even providing acceptance of stressful therapies such as non-invasive ventilation (Constantin et al. 2007). On the other hand, further assessments are still required before a sound position can be taken on the problem of acute tolerance or pain-free transition to recovery (Muellejans et al. 2004). Furthermore, dosing schemes are still to be refined for fear no clinical benefit can be demonstrated (Leone et al. 2004b).

4.4 Cardiac Anaesthesia

Administration of high doses of opioids is a very good way to blunt stress response, which explains their wide use in cardiac-compromised patients. Nevertheless, such administration may lead to delayed recovery and extubation if long-acting opioids are used, and other possibly less optimal but cost saving anaesthetic regimens have therefore been advocated to shorten extubation and ICU stay in cardiac surgery (Cheng et al. 1996). Remifentanil might combine the requirements of intraoperative control of stress response and rapid recovery. A first step towards the use of remifentanil in cardiac surgery was to assess whether remifentanil retained its unique PK profile during cardiopulmonary bypass (CPB) and hypothermia. In fact, during hypothermic CPB the volume of distribution of remifentanil increases with the institution of CPB and the elimination clearance decreases with hypothermia (Michelsen et al. 2001). If hypothermia remains mild (around 32°C), the effect of both CPB and hypothermia tend to maintain a fairly stable remifentanil concentration. Conversely, a deeper hypothermia will lead to higher remifentanil concentrations, and the infusion rate should therefore be reduced during CPB.

In open-heart clinical studies, haemodynamic stability in the remifentanil groups usually compares favourably with that in the fentanyl (Howie et al. 2001) or sufentanil (Latham et al. 2000; Lehmann et al. 2000) groups, with a better or an equivalent control over major stimuli (sternal spread) and an equivalent control during the rest of the procedure. Nevertheless several reports of difficult haemodynamic control or of adverse events have been published (Elliott et al. 2000; Mollhoff et al. 2001; Wang et al. 1998). An attentive examination of those reports brings out the difficulties in assessing the potency of the drug and its interactions with other anaesthetic agents, and in most cases a relative overdose in patients taking β-blockers is likely. The initially recommended remifentanil infusion rate of 1 μg/kg per minute generates a stable concentration around 27 ng/ml, whereas a bolus dose of 10 μg/kg fentanyl will allow the fentanyl concentration to peak at 11 ng/ml, when remifentanil is slightly more potent than fentanyl. Anaesthesia with high doses of remifentanil leads to alterations in myocardial perfusion not observed with lower remifentanil doses associated with propofol (Kazmaier et al. 2000). Only a careful titration of both the hypnotic and the analgesic component of the anaesthetic protocol may optimize intraoperative control. It might be helpful in that respect to titrate the hypnotic component through EEG monitoring and administer remifentanil through a TCI device. Apart from still sparse experiences of ultra-fast track and minimally invasive surgery (Ahonen et al. 2000; Djaiani et al. 2001), the time to extubation is usually not different whether remifentanil is used or not (Howie et al. 2001; Cheng et al. 2001; Engoren et al. 2001; Zarate et al. 2000). With the ability to readily obtain spontaneous ventilation, a new perspective today is planned extubation rather than fast-track (Olivier et al. 2000). Postoperative respiratory impairment is less with remifentanil than with sufentanil (Guggenberger et al. 2006).

Of course another issue as to the use of remifentanil in cardiac surgery is postoperative pain control. Several analgesic protocols have demonstrated their efficiency including intrathecal morphine administration (Latham et al. 2000; Zarate et al. 2000) and i.v. morphine (Olivier et al. 2000; Ahonen et al. 2000), and remifentanil (Krishnan et al. 2005) patient-controlled analgesia.

4.5 Neuranaesthesia

During craniotomy, the intensity of painful stimuli varies a lot, and a rapid and predictable emergence is warranted to assess early neurological status after surgery. Remifentanil therefore appears a useful drug in this situation. It allows a better intraoperative haemodynamic control than alfentanil (Sneyd et al. 1998) or fentanyl (Guy et al. 1997), and less intraoperative isoflurane administration (Balakrishnan et al. 2000). The recovery time is shorter with remifentanil (Balakrishnan et al. 2000; Coles et al. 2000) without naloxone administration (Guy et al. 1997).

Remifentanil titratability, usually associated with propofol TCI, allows the necessary control over anaesthesia in minimally invasive neurosurgical procedures. These include awake craniotomies (Berkenstadt et al. 2001; Johnson and Egan

1998; Sarang and Dinsmore 2003; Manninen et al. 2006), stereotaxic neurosurgery (Debailleul et al. 2002), epilepsy surgery (Herrick et al. 2002; Wass et al. 2001) and magnetic resonance-guided neurosurgery (Berkenstadt et al. 2001).

4.6 Obstetrics

The gold standard for labour pain is epidural analgesia. Nevertheless, this technique may be contraindicated in cases of sepsis or coagulation disorders for example. In these situations, remifentanil analgesia might be proposed, considering the fact that newborns are able to metabolize remifentanil and are therefore not at risk of prolonged respiratory depression at birth (Kan et al. 1998). Interest in this technique arose from several case reports describing successful remifentanil analgesia in labour (Jones et al. 1999; Owen et al. 2002; Roelants et al. 2001; Thurlow and Waterhouse 2000). Nevertheless, contradiction was brought by the results of a preliminary investigation of remifentanil as a labour analgesic which was discontinued due to inadequate pain relief and the presence of significant opioid-related side-effects (Olufolabi et al. 2000). This issue was addressed by Saunders in an editorial outlining the fact that not only the pharmacological properties of the drug were important but also the administration mode (Saunders and Glass 2002). It seems that the best way to administer remifentanil in labour is to provide basal analgesia through a small-dose continuous infusion to which small boluses are added by patient-controlled administration. PCA without background infusions usually provides incomplete analgesia (Volikas et al. 2005), though superior to that provided by meperidine (Blair et al. 2005). A patient-controlled remifentanil TCI (Schraag et al. 1998) might be worth studying. Adequate continuous respiratory monitoring is mandatory.

4.7 Bariatric Surgery and Morbidly Obese

Remifentanil has a very small volume of distribution which does not seem to increase much in obese patients (Egan et al. 1998). The absence of lingering effects in the postoperative period may be an advantage specifically in the presence of sleep apnoea syndrome. Thus, remifentanil has the pharmacological characteristics of a drug of choice in morbidly obese patients. Its use in this population first appeared in the literature through case reports (Gaszynski et al. 2003). Its interest was further demonstrated in original investigations (De Baerdemaeker et al. 2006; Gaszynski et al. 2004). TCI seems the most logical choice in this population since the device takes into account the PK of the drug. Nevertheless, a difficulty not yet solved is the estimation of the LBM, which is a significant covariate in remifentanil PK parameters as described by Minto et al. (1997a). The most frequently used formula for LBM estimation is extrapolated over 135 kg and is therefore not suited to these morbidly obese patients. Thus, current TCI devices do not estimate LBM if the BMI of the patient is too high. This problem is currently under investigation.

5 Conclusion

The pharmacodynamic profile of remifentanil in clinical practice corresponds to what was expected from this drug from the start: it is versatile and manageable. When used adequately, it increases the patient's safety by its unique reversibility of both adverse and expected effects.

Nevertheless, clinical studies have also confirmed that an adequate use of remifentanil could not be achieved without major changes in our management of analgesia, both intra- and postoperatively, and in our prescribing habits.

New methods to administer opioids have renewed the interest in those drugs and brought about a shift in the relative position of hypnotics and opioids.

References

Ahonen J, Olkkola KT, Verkkala K, et al (2000) A comparison of remifentanil and alfentanil for use with propofol in patients undergoing minimally invasive coronary artery bypass surgery. Anesth Analg 90:1269–1274

Akcaboy ZN, Akcaboy EY, Albayrak D, et al (2006) Can remifentanil be a better choice than propofol for colonoscopy during monitored anesthesia care? Acta Anaesthesiol Scand 50:736–741

Albertin A, Casati A, Bergonzi P, et al (2004) Effects of two target-controlled concentrations (1 and 3 ng/ml) of remifentanil on MAC(BAR) of sevoflurane. Anesthesiology 100:255–259

Albertin A, Dedola E, Bergonzi PC, et al (2006) The effect of adding two target-controlled concentrations (1–3 ng mL −1) of remifentanil on MAC BAR of desflurane. Eur J Anaesthesiol 23:510–516

Amin HM, Sopchak AM, Esposito BF, et al (1995) Naloxone-induced and spontaneous reversal of depressed ventilatory responses to hypoxia during and after continuous infusion of remifentanil or alfentanil. J Pharmacol Exp Ther 274:34–39

Artru AA, Momota T (2000) Rate of CSF formation and resistance to reabsorption of CSF during sevoflurane or remifentanil in rabbits. J Neurosurg Anesthesiol 12:37–43

Babenco HD, Conard PF, Gross JB (2000) The pharmacodynamic effect of a remifentanil bolus on ventilatory control. Anesthesiology 92:393–398

Bailey JM, Egan TD (1997) Fentanyl and congeners. In: White PF (ed) Text book on intravenous anesthesia. Lippincott Williams & Wilkins, Baltimore, pp 213–245

Baillard C, Cohen Y, Le Toumelin P, et al (2005) Remifentanil-midazolam versus sufentanil-midazolam pour la sedation prolongee en reanimation. Ann Fr Anesth Reanim 24:480–486

Baker KZ, Ostapkovich N, Sisti MB, et al (1997) Intact cerebral blood flow reactivity during remifentanil/nitrous oxide anesthesia. J Neurosurg Anesthesiol 9:134–140

Balakrishnan G, Raudzens P, Samra SK, et al (2000) A comparison of remifentanil and fentanyl in patients undergoing surgery for intracranial mass lesions. Anesth Analg 91:163–169

Berkenstadt H, Perel A, Hadani M, et al (2001) Monitored anesthesia care using remifentanil and propofol for awake craniotomy. J Neurosurg Anesthesiol 13:246–249

Bilgin H, Basagan Mogol E, Bekar A, et al (2006) A comparison of effects of alfentanil, fentanyl, and remifentanil on hemodynamic and respiratory parameters during stereotactic brain biopsy. J Neurosurg Anesthesiol 18:179–184
Billard V, Shafer SL (1995) Does the EEG measure therapeutic opioid drug effect? In: Schwilden H, Stoeckel H (eds) Control and automation in anaesthesia. Springer, Berlin Heidelberg New York, pp 79–95
Billard V, Servin F, Guignard B, et al (2004) Desflurane-remifentanil-nitrous oxide anaesthesia for abdominal surgery: optimal concentrations and recovery features. Acta Anaesthesiol Scand 48:355–364
Black ML, Hill JL, Zacny JP (1999) Behavioral and physiological effects of remifentanil and alfentanil in healthy volunteers. Anesthesiology 90:718–726
Blair JM, Dobson GT, Hill DA, et al (2005) Patient controlled analgesia for labour: a comparison of remifentanil with pethidine. Anaesthesia 60:22–27
Bothtner U, Milne SE, Kenny GN, et al (2002) Bayesian probabilistic network modeling of remifentanil and propofol interaction on wakeup time after closed-loop controlled anesthesia. J Clin Monit Comput 17:31–36
Bouillon T, Bruhn J, Radu-Radulescu L, et al (2002) Non-steady state analysis of the pharmacokinetic interaction between propofol and remifentanil. Anesthesiology 97:1350–1362
Bouillon T, Bruhn J, Radu-Radulescu L, et al (2003) A model of the ventilatory depressant potency of remifentanil in the non-steady state. Anesthesiology 99:779–787
Bouillon TW, Bruhn J, Radulescu L, et al (2004) Pharmacodynamic interaction between propofol and remifentanil regarding hypnosis, tolerance of laryngoscopy, Bispectral Index, and electroencephalographic approximate entropy. Anesthesiology 100:1353–1372
Bovill JG, Sebel PS, Stanley TH (1984) Opioid analgesics in anesthesia: with special reference to their use in cardiovascular anesthesia. Anesthesiology 61:731–755
Bowdle TA, Camporesi EM, Maysick L, et al (1996) A multicenter evaluation of remifentanil for early postoperative analgesia. Anesth Analg 83:1292–1297
Breen D, Karabinis A, Malbrain M, et al (2005) Decreased duration of mechanical ventilation when comparing analgesia-based sedation using remifentanil with standard hypnotic-based sedation for up to 10 days in intensive care unit patients: a randomised trial [ISRCTN47583497]. Crit Care 9:R200–R210
Brunner M, Braithwaite P, Jhaveri R, et al (1994) MAC reduction of isoflurane by sufentanil. Br J Anaesth 72:42–46
Buerkle H, Yaksh TL (1996) Comparison of the spinal actions of the mu-opioid remifentanil with alfentanil and morphine in the rat. Anesthesiology 84:94–102
Buerkle H, Marsala M, Yaksh TL (1998) Effect of continuous spinal remifentanil infusion on behaviour and spinal glutamate release evoked by subcutaneous formalin in the rat. Br J Anaesth 80:348–353
Burkle H, Dunbar S, Van Aken H (1996) Remifentanil: a novel, short-acting, mu-opioid. Anesth Analg 83:646–651
Calderon E, Pernia A, De Antonio P, et al (2001) A comparison of two constant-dose continuous infusions of remifentanil for severe postoperative pain. Anesth Analg 92:715–719
Cartwright DP, Kvalsvik O, Cassuto J, et al (1997) A randomized, blind comparison of remifentanil and alfentanil during anesthesia for outpatient surgery. Anesth Analg 85:1014–1019
Casati A, Albertin A, Fanelli G, et al (2000) A comparison of remifentanil and sufentanil as adjuvants during sevoflurane anesthesia with epidural analgesia for upper abdominal surgery: effects on postoperative recovery and respiratory function. Anesth Analg 91:1269–1273
Chanavaz C, Tirel O, Wodey E, et al (2005) Haemodynamic effects of remifentanil in children with and without intravenous atropine. An echocardiographic study. Br J Anaesth 94:74–79
Cheng DC, Newman MF, Duke P, et al (2001) The efficacy and resource utilization of remifentanil and fentanyl in fast-track coronary artery bypass graft surgery: a prospective randomized, double-blinded controlled, multi-center trial. Anesth Analg 92:1094–1102
Cheng DCH, Karski J, Peniston C, et al (1996) Early tracheal extubation after coronary artery bypass graft srugery reduces costs and improves resource use. Anesthesiology 85:1300–1310

Chia YY, Liu K, Wang JJ, et al (1999) Intraoperative high dose fentanyl induces postoperative fentanyl tolerance. Can J Anaesth 46:872–877

Coles JP, Leary TS, Monteiro JN, et al (2000) Propofol anesthesia for craniotomy: a double-blind comparison of remifentanil, alfentanil, and fentanyl. J Neurosurg Anesthesiol 12:15–20

Constantin JM, Schneider E, Cayot-Constantin S, et al (2007) Remifentanil-based sedation to treat noninvasive ventilation failure: a preliminary study. Intensive Care Med 33:82–87

Cortinez LI, Brandes V, Munoz HR, et al (2001) No clinical evidence of acute opioid tolerance after remifentanil-based anaesthesia. Br J Anaesth 87:866–869

Cortinez LI, Munoz HR, De la Fuente R, et al (2005) Target-controlled infusion of remifentanil or fentanyl during extra-corporeal shock-wave lithotripsy. Eur J Anaesthesiol 22:56–61

Cox BM, Ginsburg M, Osman OH (1968) Acute tolerance to narcotic analgesic drugs in rats. Bri Pharm Chemother 33:245–256

Criado AB, Gomez e Segura IA (2003) Reduction of isoflurane MAC by fentanyl or remifentanil in rats. Vet Anaesth Analg 30:250–256

Cros AM, Lopez C, Kandel T, Sztark F (2000) Determination of sevoflurane alveolar concentration for tracheal intubation with remifentanil, and no muscle relaxant. Anaesthesia 55:965–969

Dahaba AA, Oettl K, von Klobucar F, et al (2002) End-stage renal failure reduces central clearance and prolongs the elimination half life of remifentanil. Can J Anaesth 49:369–374

Davis PJ, Finkel JC, Orr RJ, et al (2000) A randomized, double-blinded study of remifentanil versus fentanyl for tonsillectomy and adenoidectomy surgery in pediatric ambulatory surgical patients. Anesth Analg 90:863–871

De Baerdemaeker LE, Jacobs S, Den Blauwen NM, et al (2006) Postoperative results after desflurane or sevoflurane combined with remifentanil in morbidly obese patients. Obes Surg 16:728–733

De Castro V, Godet G, Mencia G, et al (2003) Target-controlled infusion for remifentanil in vascular patients improves hemodynamics and decreases remifentanil requirement. Anesth Analg 96:33–38

Debailleul AM, Bortlein ML, Touzet G, Krivosic-Horber R (2002) Particularités anesthésiques de la neurochirurgie stéréotaxique. Ann Fr Anesth Reanim 21:170–178

Dershwitz M, Randel GI, Rosow C, et al (1995) Initial clinical experience with remifentanil, a new opioid metabolized by esterases. Anesth Analg 81:619–623

Dershwitz M, Hoke JF, Rosow CE, et al (1996) Pharmacokinetics and pharmacodynamics of remifentanil in volunteer subjects with severe liver disease. Anesthesiology 84:812–820

Dilger JA, Sprung J, Maurer W, Tetzlaff J (2004) Remifentanil provides better analgesia than alfentanil during breast biopsy surgery under monitored anesthesia care. Can J Anaesth 51:20–24

Dimitriou V, Chantzi C, Zogogiannis I, et al (2006) Remifentanil preventing hemodynamic changes during laparoscopic adrenalectomy for pheochromocytoma. Middle East J Anesthesiol 18:947–954

Djaiani GN, Ali M, Heinrich L, et al (2001) Ultra-fast-track anesthetic technique facilitates operating room extubation in patients undergoing off-pump coronary revascularization surgery. J Cardiothorac Vasc Anesth 15:152–157

Doyle PW, Coles JP, Leary TM, et al (2001) A comparison of remifentanil and fentanyl in patients undergoing carotid endarterectomy. Eur J Anaesthesiol 18:13–19

Drover DR, Litalien C, Wellis V, et al (2004) Determination of the pharmacodynamic interaction of propofol and remifentanil during esophagogastroduodenoscopy in children. Anesthesiology 100:1382–1386

Egan TD (1995) Remifentanil pharmacokinetics and pharmacodynamics. A preliminary appraisal. Clin Pharmacokinet 29:80–94

Egan TD, Shafer SL (2003) Target-controlled infusions for intravenous anesthetics: surfing USA not! Anesthesiology 99:1039–1041

Egan TD, Lemmens HJ, Fiset P, et al (1993) The pharmacokinetics of the new short-acting opioid remifentanil (GI87084B) in healthy adult male volunteers. Anesthesiology 79:881–892

Egan TD, Minto CF, Hermann DJ, et al (1996) Remifentanil versus alfentanil: comparative pharmacokinetics and pharmacodynamics in healthy adult male volunteers. Anesthesiology 84:821–833

Egan TD, Huizinga B, Gupta SK, et al (1998) Remifentanil pharmacokinetics in obese versus lean patients. Anesthesiology 89:562–573

Elliott P, O'Hare R, Bill KM, et al (2000) Severe cardiovascular depression with remifentanil. Anesth Analg 91:58–61

Engoren M, Luther G, Fenn-Buderer N (2001) A comparison of fentanyl, sufentanil, and remifentanil for fast-track cardiac anesthesia. Anesth Analg 93:859–864

Fechner J, Hering W, Ihmsen H, et al (2003) Modelling the pharmacodynamic interaction between remifentanil and propofol by EEG-controlled dosing. Eur J Anaesthesiol 20:373–379

Fleisher LA, Hogue S, Colopy M, et al (2001) Does functional ability in the postoperative period differ between remifentanil- and fentanyl-based anesthesia? J Clin Anesth 13:401–406

Fletcher D, Pinaud M, Scherpereel P, et al (2000) The efficacy of intravenous 0.15 versus 0.25 mg/kg intraoperative morphine for immediate postoperative analgesia after remifentanil-based anesthesia for major surgery. Anesth Analg 90:666–671

Fong CC, Kwan A (2005) Patient-controlled sedation using remifentanil for third molar extraction. Anaesth Intensive Care 33:73–77

Forestier F, Hirschi M, Rouget P, et al (2003) Propofol and sufentanil titration with the Bispectral Index to provide anesthesia for coronary artery surgery. Anesthesiology 99:334–346

Fourel D, Almanza L, Aubouin JP, Guiavarch M (1999) [Remifentanil: postoperative respiratory depression after purging of the infusion line]. Ann Fr Anesth Reanim 18:358–359

Fragen RJ, Fitzgerald PC (2000) Is an infusion pump necessary to safely administer remifentanil? Anesth Analg 90:713–716

Fu ES, Miguel R, Scharf JE (1997) Preemptive ketamine decreases postoperative narcotic requirements in patients undergoing abdominal surgery. Anesth Analg 84:1086–1090

Gambus PL, Gregg KM, Shafer SL (1995) Validation of the alfentanil canonical univariate parameter as a measure of opioid effect on the electroencephalogram. Anesthesiology 83:747–756

Gaszynski T, Gaszynski W, Strzelczyk J (2003) General anaesthesia with remifentanil and cisatracurium for a superobese patient. Eur J Anaesthesiol 20:77–78

Gaszynski TM, Strzelczyk JM, Gaszynski WP (2004) Post-anesthesia recovery after infusion of propofol with remifentanil or alfentanil or fentanyl in morbidly obese patients. Obes Surg 14:498–503

Gemma M, Tommasino C, Cozzi S, et al (2002) Remifentanil provides hemodynamic stability and faster awakening time in transsphenoidal surgery. Anesth Analg 94:163–168

Gepts E, Shafer SL, Camu F, et al (1995) Linearity of pharmacokinetics and model estimation of sufentanil. Anesthesiology 83:1194–1204

Glass PS, Hardman D, Kamiyama Y, et al (1993) Preliminary pharmacokinetics and pharmacodynamics of an ultra-short-acting opioid: remifentanil (GI87084B). Anesth Analg 77:1031–1040

Glass PS, Iselin-Chaves IA, Goodman D, et al (1999) Determination of the potency of remifentanil compared with alfentanil using ventilatory depression as the measure of opioid effect. Anesthesiology 90:1556–1563

Glass PSA, Shafer SL, Jacobs JR, Reves JG (1994) Intravenous drug delivery systems. In: Miller RD (ed) Anesthesia. Livingstone, New York, pp 389–416

Godet G, Reina M, Raux M, et al (2004) Anaesthesia for carotid endarterectomy: comparison of hypnotic- and opioid-based techniques. Br J Anaesth 92:329–334

Grewal K, Samsoon G (2001) Facilitation of laryngeal mask airway insertion: effects of remifentanil administered before induction with target-controlled propofol infusion. Anaesthesia 56:897–901

Guggenberger H, Schroeder TH, Vonthein R, et al (2006) Remifentanil or sufentanil for coronary surgery: comparison of postoperative respiratory impairment. Eur J Anaesthesiol 23:832–840

Guignard B, Bossard AE, Coste C, et al (2000a) Acute opioid tolerance: intraoperative remifentanil increases postoperative pain and morphine requirement. Anesthesiology 93:409–417

Guignard B, Menigaux C, Dupont X, et al (2000b) The effect of remifentanil on the Bispectral Index change and hemodynamic responses after orotracheal intubation. Anesth Analg 90:161–167

Guy J, Hindman BJ, Baker KZ, et al (1997) Comparison of remifentanil and fentanyl in patients undergoing craniotomy for supratentorial space-occupying lesions. Anesthesiology 86:514–524

Habib AS, Parker JL, Maguire AM, et al (2002) Effects of remifentanil and alfentanil on the cardiovascular responses to induction of anaesthesia and tracheal intubation in the elderly. Br J Anaesth 88:430–433

Hanouz JL, Yvon A, Guesne G, et al (2001) The in vitro effects of remifentanil, sufentanil, fentanyl, and alfentanil on isolated human right atria. Anesth Analg 93:543–549

Heijmans JH, Maessen JG, Roekaerts PM (2004) Remifentanil provides better protection against noxious stimuli during cardiac surgery than alfentanil. Eur J Anaesthesiol 21:612–618

Hentgen E, Houfani M, Billard V, et al (2002) Propofol-sufentanil anesthesia for thyroid surgery: optimal concentrations for hemodynamic and electroencephalogram stability, and recovery features. Anesth Analg 95:597–605

Herrick IA, Craen RA, Blume WT, et al (2002) Sedative doses of remifentanil have minimal effect on ECoG spike activity during awake epilepsy surgery. J Neurosurg Anesthesiol 14:55–58

Hoffman WE, Cunningham F, James MK, et al (1993) Effects of remifentanil, a new short-acting opioid, on cerebral blood flow, brain electrical activity, and intracranial pressure in dogs anesthetized with isoflurane and nitrous oxide. Anesthesiology 79:107–113

Hogue CW Jr, Bowdle TA, O'Leary C, et al (1996) A multicenter evaluation of total intravenous anesthesia with remifentanil and propofol for elective inpatient surgery. Anesth Analg 83:279–285

Hoke JF, Shlugman D, Dershwitz M, et al (1997) Pharmacokinetics and pharmacodynamics of remifentanil in persons with renal failure compared with healthy volunteers. Anesthesiology 87:533–541

Holas A, Krafft P, Marcovic M, Quehenberger F (1999) Remifentanil, propofol or both for conscious sedation during eye surgery under regional anaesthesia. Eur J Anaesthesiol 16:741–748

Howie MB, Cheng D, Newman MF, et al (2001) A randomized double-blinded multicenter comparison of remifentanil versus fentanyl when combined with isoflurane/propofol for early extubation in coronary artery bypass graft surgery. Anesth Analg 92:1084–1093

Hsu YW, Cortinez LI, Robertson KM, et al (2004) Dexmedetomidine pharmacodynamics: part I: crossover comparison of the respiratory effects of dexmedetomidine and remifentanil in healthy volunteers. Anesthesiology 101:1066–1076

Hughes MA, Glass PS, Jacobs JR (1992) Context-sensitive half-time in multicompartment pharmacokinetic models for intravenous anesthetic drugs. Anesthesiology 76:334–341

Jaksch W, Lang S, Reichhalter R, et al (2002) Perioperative small-dose S(+)-ketamine has no incremental beneficial effects on postoperative pain when standard-practice opioid infusions are used. Anesth Analg 94:981–986

James MK, Vuong A, Grizzle MK, et al (1992) Hemodynamic effects of GI 87084B, an ultra-short acting mu-opioid analgesic, in anesthetized dogs. J Pharmacol Exp Ther 263:84–91

Jellish WS, Sheikh T, Baker WH, et al (2003) Hemodynamic stability, myocardial ischemia, and perioperative outcome after carotid surgery with remifentanil/propofol or isoflurane/fentanyl anesthesia. J Neurosurg Anesthesiol 15:176–184

Jevtovic-Todorovic V, Todorovic SM, Mennerick S, et al (1998) Nitrous oxide (laughing gas) is an NMDA antagonist, neuroprotectant and neurotoxin. Nat Med 4:460–463

Jhaveri R, Joshi P, Batenhorst R, et al (1997) Dose comparison of remifentanil and alfentanil for loss of consciousness. Anesthesiology 87:253–259

Johnson KB, Egan TD (1998) Remifentanil and propofol combination for awake craniotomy: case report with pharmacokinetic simulations. J Neurosurg Anesthesiol 10:25–29

Jones R, Pegrum A, Stacey RG (1999) Patient-controlled analgesia using remifentanil in the parturient with thrombocytopaenia. Anaesthesia 54:461–465

Joo HS, Salasidis GC, Kataoka MT, et al (2004) Comparison of bolus remifentanil versus bolus fentanyl for induction of anesthesia and tracheal intubation in patients with cardiac disease. J Cardiothorac Vasc Anesth 18:263–268
Joshi GP, Jamerson BD, Roizen MF, et al (2000) Is there a learning curve associated with the use of remifentanil? Anesth Analg 91:1049–1055
Kabbaj M, Vachon P, Varin F (2005) Impact of peripheral elimination on the concentration-effect relationship of remifentanil in anaesthetized dogs. Br J Anaesth 94:357–365
Kan RE, Hughes SC, Rosen MA, et al (1998) Intravenous remifentanil: placental transfer, maternal and neonatal effects. Anesthesiology 88:1467–1474
Kapila A, Glass PS, Jacobs JR, et al (1995) Measured context-sensitive half-times of remifentanil and alfentanil. Anesthesiology 83:968–975
Karabinis A, Mandragos K, Stergiopoulos S, et al (2004) Safety and efficacy of analgesia-based sedation with remifentanil versus standard hypnotic-based regimens in intensive care unit patients with brain injuries: a randomised, controlled trial. Crit Care 8:R268–R280
Karan S, Voter W, Palmer L, Ward DS (2005) Effects of pain and audiovisual stimulation on the opioid-induced depression of the hypoxic ventilatory response. Anesthesiology 103:384–390
Katoh T, Ikeda K (1998) The effects of fentanyl on sevoflurane requirements for loss of consciousness and skin incision. Anesthesiology 88:18–24
Kazmaier S, Hanekop GG, Buhre W, et al (2000) Myocardial consequences of remifentanil in patients with coronary artery disease. Br J Anaesth 84:578–583
Kern SE, Xie G, White JL, Egan TD (2004) A response surface analysis of propofol-remifentanil pharmacodynamic interaction in volunteers. Anesthesiology 100:1373–1381
Kissin I, Lee SS, Arthur GR, Bradley EL Jr (1996) Time course characteristics of acute tolerance development to continuously infused alfentanil in rats. Anesth Analg 83:600–605
Kissin I, Bright CA, Bradley EL Jr (2000) Acute tolerance to continuously infused alfentanil: the role of cholecystokinin and N-methyl-D-aspartate-nitric oxide systems. Anesth Analg 91:110–116
Klemola UM, Hiller A (2000) Tracheal intubation after induction of anesthesia in children with propofol-remifentanil or propofol-rocuronium. Can J Anaesth 47:854–859
Klemola UM, Mennander S, Saarnivaara L (2000) Tracheal intubation without the use of muscle relaxants: remifentanil or alfentanil in combination with propofol. Acta Anaesthesiol Scand 44:465–469
Kochs E, Cote D, Deruyck L, et al (2000) Postoperative pain management and recovery after remifentanil-based anaesthesia with isoflurane or propofol for major abdominal surgery. Remifentanil Study Group. Br J Anaesth 84:169–173
Krishnan K, Elliot SC, Berridge JC, Mallick A (2005) Remifentanil patient-controlled analgesia following cardiac surgery. Acta Anaesthesiol Scand 49:876–879
Lang E, Kapila A, Shlugman D, et al (1996) Reduction of isoflurane minimal alveolar concentration by remifentanil. Anesthesiology 85:721–728
Latham P, Zarate E, White PF, et al (2000) Fast-track cardiac anesthesia: a comparison of remifentanil plus intrathecal morphine with sufentanil in a desflurane-based anesthetic. J Cardiothorac Vasc Anesth 14:645–651
Lauwers M, Camu F, Breivik H, et al (1999) The safety and effectiveness of remifentanil as an adjunct sedative for regional anesthesia. Anesth Analg 88:134–140
Lecomte P, Ouattara A, Le Manach Y, et al (2006) The coronary and myocardial effects of remifentanil and sufentanil in the erythrocyte-perfused isolated rabbit heart. Anesth Analg 103:9–14
Lee MP, Kua JS, Chiu WK (2001) The use of remifentanil to facilitate the insertion of the laryngeal mask airway. Anesth Analg 93:359–362
Lehmann A, Zeitler C, Thaler E, et al (2000) Comparison of two different anesthesia regimens in patients undergoing aortocoronary bypass grafting surgery: sufentanil-midazolam versus remifentanil-propofol. J Cardiothorac Vasc Anesth 14:416–420
Leone M, Rousseau S, Avidan M, et al (2004a) Target concentrations of remifentanil with propofol to blunt coughing during intubation, cuff inflation, and tracheal suctioning. Br J Anaesth 93:660–663

Leone M, Albanese J, Viviand X, et al (2004b) The effects of remifentanil on endotracheal suctioning-induced increases in intracranial pressure in head-injured patients. Anesth Analg 99:1193–1198

Locala JA, Irefin SA, Malone D, et al (2005) The comparative hemodynamic effects of methohexital and remifentanil in electroconvulsive therapy. J Ect 21:12–15

Lorenz IH, Kolbitsch C, Hormann C, et al (2000) The effects of remifentanil on cerebral capacity in awake volunteers. Anesth Analg 90:609–613

Machata AM, Gonano C, Holzer A, et al (2003) Awake nasotracheal fiberoptic intubation: patient comfort, intubating conditions, and hemodynamic stability during conscious sedation with remifentanil. Anesth Analg 97:904–908

Maguire AM, Kumar N, Parker JL, et al (2001) Comparison of effects of remifentanil and alfentanil on cardiovascular response to tracheal intubation in hypertensive patients. Br J Anaesth 86:90–93

Maitre PO, Vozeh S, Heykants J, et al (1987) Population pharmacokinetics of alfentanil: average dose-plasma concentraiton relationship and interindividual variability. Anesthesiology 66:3–12

Mandema JW, Wada DR (1995) Pharmacodynamic model for acute tolerance development to the electroencephalographic effects of alfentanil in the rat. J Pharmacol Exp Ther 275:1185–1194

Manninen PH, Balki M, Lukitto K, Bernstein M (2006) Patient satisfaction with awake craniotomy for tumor surgery: a comparison of remifentanil and fentanyl in conjunction with propofol. Anesth Analg 102:237–242

Manullang J, Egan TD (1999) Remifentanil's effect is not prolonged in a patient with pseudocholinesterase deficiency. Anesth Analg 89:529–530

Manyam SC, Gupta DK, Johnson KB, et al (2006) Opioid-volatile anesthetic synergy: a response surface model with remifentanil and sevoflurane as prototypes. Anesthesiology 105:267–278

Marker CL, Lujan R, Loh HH, Wickman K (2005) Spinal G-protein-gated potassium channels contribute in a dose-dependent manner to the analgesic effect of mu- and delta- but not kappa-opioids. J Neurosci 25:3551–3559

McAtamney D, O'Hare R, Hughes D, et al (1998) Evaluation of remifentanil for control of haemodynamic response to tracheal intubation. Anaesthesia 53:1223–1227

McGregor RR, Allan LG, Sharpe RM, et al (1998) Effect of remifentanil on the auditory evoked response and haemodynamic changes after intubation and surgical incision. Br J Anaesth 81:785–786

Mertens MJ, Vuyk J, Olofsen E, et al (2001) Propofol alters the pharmacokinetics of alfentanil in healthy male volunteers. Anesthesiology 94:949–957

Mertens MJ, Olofsen E, Engbers FH, et al (2003) Propofol reduces perioperative remifentanil requirements in a synergistic manner: response surface modeling of perioperative remifentanil-propofol interactions. Anesthesiology 99:347–359

Michelsen LG, Holford NH, Lu W, et al (2001) The pharmacokinetics of remifentanil in patients undergoing coronary artery bypass grafting with cardiopulmonary bypass. Anesth Analg 93:1100–1105

Milne SE, Kenny GN (1998) Future applications for TCI systems. Anaesthesia 53 [Suppl 1]:56–60

Milne SE, Kenny GN, Schraag S (2003) Propofol sparing effect of remifentanil using closed-loop anaesthesia. Br J Anaesth 90:623–629

Mingus ML, Monk TG, Gold MI, et al (1998) Remifentanil versus propofol as adjuncts to regional anesthesia. Remifentanil 3010 Study Group. J Clin Anesth 10:46–53

Minkowitz HS (2000) Postoperative pain management in patients undergoing major surgery after remifentanil vs. fentanyl anesthesia. Multicentre Investigator Group. Can J Anaesth 47:522–528

Minto CF, Schnider TW, Egan TD, et al (1997a) Influence of age and gender on the pharmacokinetics and pharmacodynamics of remifentanil. I. Model development. Anesthesiology 86:10–23

Minto CF, Schnider TW, Shafer SL (1997b) Pharmacokinetics and pharmacodynamics of remifentanil. II Model application. Anesthesiology 86:24–33

Mollhoff T, Herregods L, Moerman A, et al (2001) Comparative efficacy and safety of remifentanil and fentanyl in 'fast track' coronary artery bypass graft surgery: a randomized, double-blind study. Br J Anaesth 87:718–726

Mouren S, De Winter G, Guerrero SP, et al (2001) The continuous recording of blood pressure in patients undergoing carotid surgery under remifentanil versus sufentanil analgesia. Anesth Analg 93:1402–1409

Muellejans B, Lopez A, Cross MH, et al (2004) Remifentanil versus fentanyl for analgesia based sedation to provide patient comfort in the intensive care unit:a randomized, double-blind controlled trial. Crit Care 8:R1–R11

Muellejans B, Matthey T, Scholpp J, Schill M (2006) Sedation in the intensive care unit with remifentanil/propofol versus midazolam/fentanyl: a randomised, open-label, pharmacoeconomic trial. Crit Care 10:R91

Mustola ST, Baer GA, Neuvonen PJ, Toivonen KJ (2005) Requirements of propofol at different end-points without adjuvant and during two different steady infusions of remifentanil. Acta Anaesthesiol Scand 49:215–221

Natalini G, Fassini P, Seramondi V, et al (1999) Remifentanil vs. fentanyl during interventional rigid bronchoscopy under general anaesthesia and spontaneous assisted ventilation. Eur J Anaesthesiol 16:605–609

Navapurkar VU, Archer S, Gupta SK, et al (1998) Metabolism of remifentanil during liver transplantation. Br J Anaesth 81:881–886

Nieuwenhuijs DJ, Olofsen E, Romberg RR, et al (2003) Response surface modeling of remifentanil-propofol interaction on cardiorespiratory control and Bispectral Index. Anesthesiology 98:312–322

Olivier P, Sirieix D, Dassier P, et al (2000) Continuous infusion of remifentanil and target-controlled infusion of propofol for patients undergoing cardiac surgery: a new approach for scheduled early extubation. J Cardiothorac Vasc Anesth 14:29–35

Olufolabi AJ, Booth JV, Wakeling HG, et al (2000) A preliminary investigation of remifentanil as a labor analgesic. Anesth Analg 91:606–608

Ostapkovich ND, Baker KZ, Fogarty-Mack P, et al (1998) Cerebral blood flow and CO2 reactivity is similar during remifentanil/N2O and fentanyl/N2O anesthesia. Anesthesiology 89:358–363

Ouattara A, Boccara G, Kockler U, et al (2004) Remifentanil induces systemic arterial vasodilation in humans with a total artificial heart. Anesthesiology 100:602–607

Owen MD, Poss MJ, Dean LS, Harper MA (2002) Prolonged intravenous remifentanil infusion for labor analgesia. Anesth Analg 94:918–919

Park G, Lane M, Rogers S, Bassett P (2007) A comparison of hypnotic and analgesic based sedation in a general intensive care unit. Br J Anaesth 98:76–82

Peacock JE, Luntley JB, O'Connor B, et al (1998) Remifentanil in combination with propofol for spontaneous ventilation anaesthesia. Br J Anaesth 80:509–511

Pendeville PE, Kabongo F, Veyckemans F (2001) Use of remifentanil in combination with desflurane or propofol for ambulatory oral surgery. Acta Anaesthesiol Belg 52:181–186

Pitsiu M, Wilmer A, Bodenham A, et al (2004) Pharmacokinetics of remifentanil and its major metabolite, remifentanil acid, in ICU patients with renal impairment. Br J Anaesth 92:493–503

Pleym H, Stenseth R, Wiseth R, et al (2004) Supplemental remifentanil during coronary artery bypass grafting is followed by a transient postoperative cardiac depression. Acta Anaesthesiol Scand 48:1155–1162

Ramos-Zabala A, Perez-Mencia MT, Fernandez-Garcia R, Cascales-Nunez MR (2004) Anesthesia technique for outpatient facial laser resurfacing. Lasers Surg Med 34:269–272

Reid JE, Mirakhur RK (2000) Bradycardia after administration of remifentanil. Br J Anaesth 84:422–423

Roelants F, De Franceschi E, Veyckemans F, Lavand'homme P (2001) Patient-controlled intravenous analgesia using remifentanil in the parturient. Can J Anaesth 48:175–178

Ropcke H, Konen-Bergmann M, Cuhls M, et al (2001) Propofol and remifentanil pharmacodynamic interaction during orthopedic surgical procedures as measured by effects on Bispectral Index. J Clin Anesth 13:198–207

Ross AK, Davis PJ, Dear Gd GL, et al (2001) Pharmacokinetics of remifentanil in anesthetized pediatric patients undergoing elective surgery or diagnostic procedures. Anesth Analg 93:1393–1401

Sarang A, Dinsmore J (2003) Anaesthesia for awake craniotomy—evolution of a technique that facilitates awake neurological testing. Br J Anaesth 90:161–165

Saunders TA, Glass PS (2002) A trial of labor for remifentanil. Anesth Analg 94:771–773

Schraag S, Kenny GN, Mohl U, Georgieff M (1998) Patient-maintained remifentanil target-controlled infusion for the transition to early postoperative analgesia. Br J Anaesth 81:365–368

Schraag S, Checketts MR, Kenny GN (1999) Lack of rapid development of opioid tolerance during alfentanil and remifentanil infusions for postoperative pain. Anesth Analg 89:753–757

Schuttler J, Albrecht S, Breivik H, et al (1997) A comparison of remifentanil and alfentanil in patients undergoing major abdominal surgery. Anaesthesia 52:307–317

Scott JC, Stanski DR (1987) Decreased fentanyl and alfentanil dose requirements with age. A simultaneous pharmacokinetic and pharmacodynamic evaluation. J Pharmacol Exp Ther 240:159–166

Scott JC, Cooke JE, Stanski DR (1991) EEG quantitation of opiate effect: comparative pharmacodynamics of fentanyl and sufentanil. Anesthesiology 74:34–42

Sebel PS, Hoke JF, Westmoreland C, et al (1995) Histamine concentrations and hemodynamic responses after remifentanil. Anesth Analg 80:990–993

Servin F, Desmonts JM, Watkins WD (1999) Remifentanil as an analgesic adjunct in local/regional anesthesia and in monitored anesthesia care. Anesth Analg 89:S28–32

Servin FS, Raeder JC, Merle JC, et al (2002) Remifentanil sedation compared with propofol during regional anaesthesia. Acta Anaesthesiol Scand 46:309–315

Shafer SL, Varvel JR (1991) Pharmacokinetics, pharmacodynamics, and rational opioid selection. Anesthesiology 74:53–63

Shinohara K, Aono H, Unruh GK, et al (2000) Suppressive effects of remifentanil on hemodynamics in baro-denervated rabbits. Can J Anaesth 47:361–366

Slepchenko G, Simon N, Goubaux B, et al (2003) Performance of target-controlled sufentanil infusion in obese patients. Anesthesiology 98:65–73

Sneyd JR, Whaley A, Dimpel HL, Andrews CJ (1998) An open, randomized comparison of alfentanil, remifentanil and alfentanil followed by remifentanil in anaesthesia for craniotomy. Br J Anaesth 81:361–364

Sneyd JR, Camu F, Doenicke A, et al (2001) Remifentanil and fentanyl during anaesthesia for major abdominal and gynaecological surgery. An open, comparative study of safety and efficacy. Eur J Anaesthesiol 18:605–614

Sundman E, Witt H, Sandin R, et al (2001) Pharyngeal function and airway protection during subhypnotic concentrations of propofol, isoflurane, and sevoflurane: volunteers examined by pharyngeal videoradiography and simultaneous manometry. Anesthesiology 95:1125–1132

Sztark F, Chopin F, Bonnet A, Cros AM (2005) Concentration of remifentanil needed for tracheal intubation with sevoflurane at 1 MAC in adult patients. Eur J Anaesthesiol 22:919–924

Thurlow JA, Waterhouse P (2000) Patient-controlled analgesia in labour using remifentanil in two parturients with platelet abnormalities. Br J Anaesth 84:411–413

Troy AM, Huthinson RC, Easy WR, Kenney GN (2002) Tracheal intubating conditions using propofol and remifentanil target-controlled infusions. Anaesthesia 57:1204–1207

Twersky RS, Jamerson B, Warner DS, et al (2001) Hemodynamics and emergence profile of remifentanil versus fentanyl prospectively compared in a large population of surgical patients. J Clin Anesth 13:407–416

Unlugenc H, Itegin M, Ocal I, et al (2003) Remifentanil produces vasorelaxation in isolated rat thoracic aorta strips. Acta Anaesthesiol Scand 47:65–69

Vinik HR, Kissin I (1998) Rapid development of tolerance to analgesia during remifentanil infusion in humans. Anesth Analg 86:1307–1311

Volikas I, Butwick A, Wilkinson C, et al (2005) Maternal and neonatal side-effects of remifentanil patient-controlled analgesia in labour. Br J Anaesth 95:504–509

Vuyk J, Mertens MJ, Olofsen E, et al (1997) Propofol anesthesia and rational opioid selection. Anesthesiology 87:1549–1562

Wagner KJ, Willoch F, Kochs EF, et al (2001) Dose-dependent regional cerebral blood flow changes during remifentanil infusion in humans: a positron emission tomography study. Anesthesiology 94:732–739

Wang J, Winship S, Russell G (1998) Induction of anaesthesia with sevoflurane and low-dose remifentanil: asystole following laryngoscopy. Br J Anaesth 81:994–995

Wass CT, Grady RE, Fessler AJ, et al (2001) The effects of remifentanil on epileptiform discharges during intraoperative electrocorticography in patients undergoing epilepsy surgery. Epilepsia 42:1340–1344

Wee LH, Moriarty A, Cranston A, Bagshaw O (1999) Remifentanil infusion for major abdominal surgery in small infants. Paediatr Anaesth 9:415–418

Westmoreland CL, Hoke JF, Sebel PS, et al (1993) Pharmacokinetics of remifentanil (GI87084B) and its major metabolite (GI90291) in patients undergoing elective inpatient surgery. Anesthesiology 79:893–903

Westmoreland CL, Sebel PS, Gropper A (1994) Fentanyl or alfentanil decreases the minimum alveolar anesthetic concentration of isoflurane in surgical patients. Anesth Analg 78:23–28

Wilhelm W, Schlaich N, Harrer J, et al (2001) Recovery and neurological examination after remifentanil-desflurane or fentanyl-desflurane anaesthesia for carotid artery surgery. Br J Anaesth 86:44–49

Wuesten R, Van Aken H, Glass PS, Buerkle H (2001) Assessment of depth of anesthesia and postoperative respiratory recovery after remifentanil- versus alfentanil-based total intravenous anesthesia in patients undergoing ear-nose-throat surgery. Anesthesiology 94:211–217

Youngs EJ, Shafer SL (1994) Pharmacokinetic parameters relevant to recovery from opioids. Anesthesiology 81:833–842

Zarate E, Latham P, White PF, et al (2000) Fast-track cardiac anesthesia: use of remifentanil combined with intrathecal morphine as an alternative to sufentanil during desflurane anesthesia. Anesth Analg 91:283–287

Ketamine

B. Sinner and B.M. Graf(✉)

Abstract There are two optical isomers of the 2-(2-chlorophenyl)-2-(methylamino)-cyclohexanone ketamine: S(+) ketamine and R(−) ketamine. Effects of this drug are mediated by *N*-methyl-d-aspartate (NMDA), opioid, muscarinic and different voltage-gated receptors. Clinically, the anaesthetic potency of the S(+)-isomer is approximately three to four times that of the R(−)-isomer, which is attributable to the higher affinity of the S(+)-isomer to the phencyclidine binding sites on the NMDA receptors. Ketamine is water- and lipid-soluble, allowing it to be administered conveniently via various routes and providing extensive distribution in the body. Ketamine metabolism is mediated by hepatic microsomal enzymes. It causes

B.M. Graf
Zentrum für Anaesthesie, Rettungs- und Intensivmedizin, Georg August Universität Göttingen, Robert-Koch-Str. 40, 37075 Göttingen, Germany
bgraf@ZARI.de

J. Schüttler and H. Schwilden (eds.) *Modern Anesthetics.*
Handbook of Experimental Pharmacology 182.

bronchodilation and stimulation of the sympathetic nervous system and cardiovascular system. In clinics, ketamine and particularly S(+)-ketamine are used for premedication, sedation, and induction and maintenance of general anaesthesia, which is than termed "dissociative anaesthesia". Ketamine and its S(+)-isomer are ideal anaesthetic agents for trauma victims, patients with hypovolemic and septic shock and patients with pulmonary diseases. Even subanaesthetic doses of this drug have analgesic effects, so ketamine is also recommended for post-operative analgesia and sedation. The combination of ketamine with midazolam or propofol can be extremely useful and safe for sedation and pain relief in intensive care patients, especially during sepsis and cardiovascular instability. In the treatment of chronic pain ketamine is effective as a potent analgesic or substitute together with other potent analgesics, whereby it can be added by different methods. There are some important patient side-effects, however, that limit its use, whereby psycho-mimetic side-effects are most common.

1 History

In 1959 the search for a safe but potent sedative agent led pharmacologists to the phencyclidines (PCPs) (CI-395 and CI-400). Although CI-395 and CI-400 produced reliable sedation, the hallucinogenic effects that patients experienced upon reawakening were too severe to warrant widespread use, and therefore the search for related, but less hallucinogenic, compounds began (Johnson 1959). This finally led to the discovery of ketamine (CI-581), which was first synthesized in 1962 by Calvin Stevens at Parke-Davis and Co. Ketamine showed fewer severe adverse effects of the PCPs and was introduced into clinical practice by 1970, in time for use during the Vietnam War. But in the 1970s patients began also to report unwanted visions during ketamine's influence.

2 Pharmacology of Ketamine

Ketamine is frequently described as a "unique drug" because it shows hypnotic (sleep producing), analgesic (pain relieving) and amnesic (short-term memory loss) effects; no other drug used in clinical practice combines these three important features at the same time. Ketamine is chemically (+/–) 2-(2-chlorophenyl)-2-(methylamino)-cyclohexanone (Ketalar, Pfizer, Karlsruhe; Ketaject, Phoenix Pharmaceutical, St. Joseph, MO; Ketaset, Wyeth, Madison, NJ; Vetalar, Fort Dodge Animal Health, Fort Dodge, IA) and most commonly comes as a white crystalline powder, but can also be seen in liquid and tablet form.

Ketamine is characterized by a molecular weight of 274.4 M with the chemical formula: $C_{13}H_{16}ClNO$ (Fig. 1). The melting point of ketamine is found between 258°C and 261°C. Ketamine is water- and lipid-soluble, allowing it to be administered

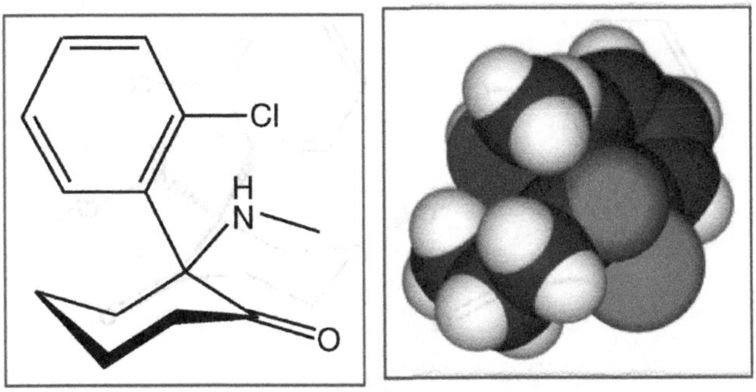

Fig. 1 Chemical structure of ketamine

conveniently via various routes while still rapidly crossing the blood–brain barrier. This agent has been administered by intramuscular injection, intravenous drip and bolus injection, intranasal solution, rectal solution and as an oral elixir.

Ketamine is characterized by a chiral structure consisting of two pure optically isomers. This is the result of an optic active centre in the C2 position of the molecule, which allows the existence of two molecules with the same empirical formula but different spatial structures resulting in an image and its mirror image. Both isomers possess identical chemical and physical properties except that one isomer turns polarized light left (−) and the other turns it right (+). As racemate—containing 50% of each isomer—the polarized light is not turned, since it turns to the left from half of the isomers and then back again from the other half. In order to denominate the assembly of the substitutes at the optic active centre, isomers are named S- and R-ketamine (Fig. 2).

Both enantiomers exhibit different clinical potencies and different affinities to the various receptors, which are also optically active. Different bindings of the enantiomers to receptors are called stereoselective bindings. Clinically, the anaesthetic potency of the S(+)-isomer is approximately three or four times that of the R(−)-isomer (White et al. 1980).

2.1 Pharmacokinetic Properties

Ketamine produces an anaesthetic state, which has been termed "dissociative anaesthesia", characterized by analgesia and changes in vigilance and perception, but it is not a sedative or hypnotic. It appears that ketamine selectively interrupts the thalamocortical system. The patient rapidly goes into a trance-like state, with widely open eyes and nystagmus. He is unconscious, amnesic and deeply analgesic. His airway is remarkably open, with only slightly depressed pharyngeal-laryngeal reflexes preserved while the patient's head in almost any position, far more so than with any other anaesthetic. Dissociative anaesthesia is a result of reduced activation in the thalamocortical structures and increased activity in the limbic system and hippocampus (Domino et al. 1965).

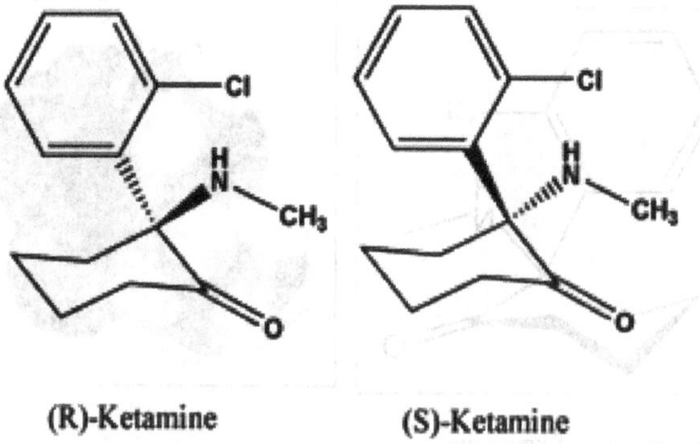

Fig. 2 Optical isomers of ketamine

Bioavailability following an intramuscular dose is 93%, an intranasal dose 25%–50%, an oral dose only 17%. Ketamine is rapidly distributed into the brain and other highly perfused tissues; 12% are protein-bound in the plasma. Therefore oral administration produces lower peak concentrations of ketamine, but increased amounts of the metabolites norketamine and dehydro-norketamine (Larenza et al. 2007). When intravenously administered, the onset of the first effects is seen within seconds, 1–5 min if injected intramuscularly, 5–10 min if snorted and 15–20 min if orally administered. If injected effects generally last 30–45 min, if snorted 45–60 min, and 1–2 h following oral ingestion. There is no direct correlation between ketamine concentrations and behaviour. Drowsiness and perceptual distortions may be dose related in a concentration range of 50–200 ng/ml, and analgesia begins at plasma concentrations of about 100 ng/ml. During anaesthesia, blood ketamine concentrations of 2,000–3,000 ng/ml are used, and patients may begin to awaken from a surgical procedure when concentrations have been gradually reduced to 500–1,000 ng/ml.

Both ketamine isomers are characterized by a short α half-life (2–4 min). The β half-life as determined mainly by redistribution is 8–16 min in adults. Ketamine has a low protein binding of 20%–30%. In vivo, S(+)-ketamine is not inverted to R(−)-ketamine; however, after racemate administration a statistically significant smaller clearance and volume of distribution for R(−)-ketamine compared with S(+)-ketamine was seen (Geisslinger et al. 1993). By hepatic biotransformation cytochrome P450 (CYP) 3A4 is the primary enzyme responsible for *N*-demethylation (metabolite I) of ketamine to norketamine, with minor contributions from CYP2B6 and CYP2C9 isoforms. The unconjugated *N*-demethylated metabolite was found to be less than one-sixth as potent as ketamine. Potential inhibitors of these isoenzymes could decrease the rate of ketamine elimination if administered concurrently; in contrast, potential inducers could increase the rate of elimination.

Additional breakdown via hydroxylation of the cyclohexanone ring results in hydroxyl-ketamine with a 0.1% anaesthetic potency. Ketamine and its metabolites undergo hydroxylation and conjugation with the water-soluble conjugates which are excreted in the urine. Metabolism half-life is 2.5–3 h. The plasma clearance is 15–20 ml/kg per minute in adults and higher for S(+)-ketamine than for the enantiomer (Geisslinger et al. 1993). There are no other significant differences between the pharmacokinetic properties of the S-(+) and R-(−)-isomers. Even repeated doses of ketamine administered to animals did not produce any detectable increase in microsomal enzyme activity.

The urinary excretion of unmetabolized drug is approx. 4%. In forensic medicine, ketamine use can be detected in the urine for about 3 days. Concentration ranges for ketamine in urine have been reported as low as 10 ng/ml and up to 25 μg/ml.

2.2 *Dosage*

The therapeutic range of ketamine or S(+)-ketamine makes them one of the safest sedative agents for most emergency clinical and preclinical situations. Distinct and useful effects are obtained when the drugs are administered at different doses. Low-dose ketamine infusion provides potent analgesia, which is useful in conjunction with sedation or as a narcotic in areas with scarce resources.

2.2.1 Racemic Ketamine

Intravenously administered, the induction dose for general anaesthesia is 1–2 mg/kg; after induction, a continuous dose of 1–6 mg/kg per hour is necessary. In lower concentrations of 0.25–0.5 mg/kg an adequate analgesia can be seen. The same concentration is necessary for sedation, whereby a permanent dose of 0.4–1 mg/kg per hour is required for continuous sedation. To get the same effects by intramuscular injections 2–4 times higher doses have to be injected. Higher doses are also necessary for rectal (8–10 mg/kg) and nasal admission (5 mg/kg).

2.2.2 S(+)-Ketamine

The purely optical S(+)-isomer of ketamine is characterized by a higher affinity or potency to specific receptors, so that lower doses are required. For general anaesthesia 0.5–1 mg/kg followed by a continuous infusion of 0.5–3 mg/kg are necessary. For analgesia, doses of 0.125–0.25 mg/kg are helpful, whereby using these doses an additional sedation can be observed. In parallel to racemic mixtures for rectal as well as nasal administered, a dose reduction of 50% is recommended. These results are in a wide spread of plasma concentrations and absorption times. Rapid and high-level drug absorption after nasal drug administration is possible.

2.3 *Ketamine Binding Sites*

2.3.1 Glutamate Receptors

The major excitatory synaptic transmission in the mammalian CNS is mainly mediated by L-glutamate. This amino acid acts via ligand-gated ion channels: ionotropic glutamate receptors (iGluRs) and G protein-coupled (metabotropic) receptors (Hirota and Lambert 1996b). The iGluRs are ubiquitously expressed in the brain and spinal cord. Mammalian iGluRs are encoded by 18 genes which constitute three families of ionotropic glutamate receptors: *N*-Methyl-d-aspartate (NMDA), α-amino-3-hydroxy-5-methyl-4-isoxazole propionic acid (AMPA) and kainate.

Seven genes encode for the NMDA receptors (*NR1, NR2A–D, NR3A–NR3B*), four genes encode for the AMPA receptor (*GluR 1–4*) and five for the kainate (*GluR 5–7, KA1* and *KA2*) receptor. They can either exist as homomeric or heteromeric assemblies. Co-assembly of iGluRs within but not between families generates a large number of receptor subtypes. KA subunits are capable of forming channels when co-assembled with members of the GluR5–7 family (McBain and Mayer 1994; Mori and Mishina 1995; Mayer and Armstrong 2004).

iGluRs consist of multimeric assemblies of four or five subunits. Each subunit consists of three membrane-spanning segments with a pore loop forming the ion channel, a cytoplasm domain of variable length, the binding core, which consists of two domains, and the amino-terminal domain located on the cell surface. There is a great variety among the glutamate receptors. Multiple receptor isoforms with distinct brain distributions and functional properties emerge by selective RNA splicing of the NR1 transcripts and differential expression of the NR2 subunits.

2.3.2 NMDA Receptor

The NMDA receptor (Fig. 3) consists of a heterodimer formation between NR1 and one form of NR2 (NR2A-D). The glutamate-binding domain is located at the junction of the NR1 and NR2 subunits. The receptor contains binding places for glutamate, NMDA and, in the spinal cord and the lower brain regions, glycine. They allosterically influence the activity of the receptor. The NMDA receptor is a trans-membrane protein and forms an ion channel for Na^+, K^+ and Ca^{2+}. Thereby it spans the electric field generated by the membrane potential. Depending on agonist binding, the channel has different conducting states. The magnesium blockade of the open NMDA receptor channel is voltage-dependent. The magnesium binding site within the receptor is physically located within this electric field. The magnesium ion carries a double positive charge. When the cell is hyperpolarized, magnesium is stabilized inside the negative charged channels. At resting membrane potentials the NMDA receptor is inactive because of a voltage-dependent block of the channel pore by magnesium ions. As the cell is depolarized, the negative field effect weakens and the magnesium ions are released out of the channel and are rapidly substituted by another magnesium ion during repolarization. During the

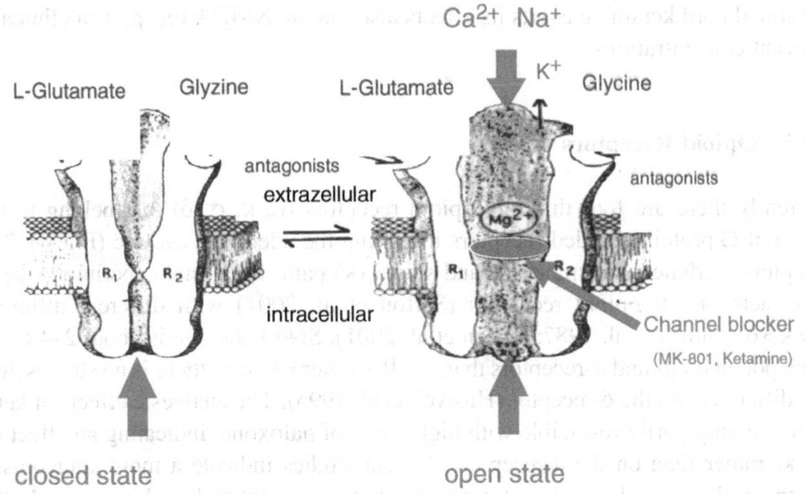

Fig. 3 *N*-Methyl-d-aspartate receptor

brief phase in which magnesium is absent from the open channel, Ca^{2+}-, Na^{+}- and K^{+}-ions flow through the channel. The Ca^{2+} influx is crucial for the induction of the NMDA receptor-dependent long-term potentiation (LTP), which is thought to underlie neuronal plasticity, learning and memory. NMDA receptors are included in the wind-up phenomenon, which is the result of central sensitization causing hyperalgesia and hyperexcitability and seems to be responsible for the development of chronic pain syndromes.

The activation of the NMDA receptor leads to a Ca^{2+}/calmodulin-mediated activation of NO synthetase, which plays a crucial role in nociception and neurotoxicity. NMDA receptors are involved in global and focal ischaemia and in various neurological diseases such as schizophrenia (Lindsley et al. 2006). While the NMDAR channel itself displays no voltage-dependency, the magnesium block confers voltage dependency to the channel. Effectively, the NMDA receptor is both a ligand-gated and voltage-gated ion channel.

Ketamine acts as an antagonist on the glutamate receptors (Irifune et al. 1992). Primarily like PCP, ketamine blocks the NMDA receptor non-competitively resulting in a use-dependent block. The binding site is located within the receptor at the PCP binding site. The PCP binding site is localized within the receptor and partially overlaps with the Mg^{2+} binding site. Ketamine blocks the open channel and reduces channel mean open time. Ketamine also decreases the frequency of channel opening by allosteric mechanisms. Both ketamine stereoisomers act via the same binding sites but with different affinities and potencies. The S(+)-isomer has a 3–4 times higher affinity than the R-enantiomer (Zeilhofer et al. 1992). As the NMDA receptor consists of various subunits, ketamine isomers possess different affinities to the various subunit compositions, resulting in different clinical effects. In addition, in the spinal cord ketamine exerts its effects also via the NMDA receptor in clinically relevant concentrations.

2.3.3 Opioid Receptors

Currently there are four different opioid receptors (μ, κ, σ, δ) that belong to the group of G protein-coupled receptors inhibiting the adenylate cyclase (Fig. 4). The receptors mediate supraspinal (μ) and spinal (κ) pain. In animal experiments ketamine acts on all opioid receptors (Sarton et al. 2001) with different affinities (μ>κ>δ) (Smith et al. 1987; Sarton et al. 2001). S(+)-ketamine is about 2–4 times more potent on μ- and κ-receptors than the R-isomer whereas there is no stereoselective difference on the δ-receptor (Hustveit et al. 1995). The analgesic effects of ketamine are only partly reversible with high doses of naloxone, indicating an effect on the κ- rather than on the μ-receptors. Recent studies indicate a more antagonistic action on the μ- and an agonistic action on the κ-receptor. In a human study the analgesic and the sedative effects of ketamine could not be reversed by naloxone (Mikkelsen et al. 1999). κ-Agonists are known to induce psycho-mimetic reactions, which resemble the phenomenon observed during ketamine anaesthesia.

The role of the σ-opioid receptor is not yet clear. There are two types of σ-binding places: the naloxone-sensible σ1 binding place and the non-naloxone-sensible σ2 binding place. The R(–)-enantiomer has a higher affinity for both receptors than the S(+)-ketamine. Both isomers seem to induce negative inotropic (σ-1) and excitatory (σ-2) effects via σ-receptors.

In conclusion, ketamine has an analgesic effect on the spinal cord level but this probably does not involve opioid receptors (Hao et al. 1998) since the effects of

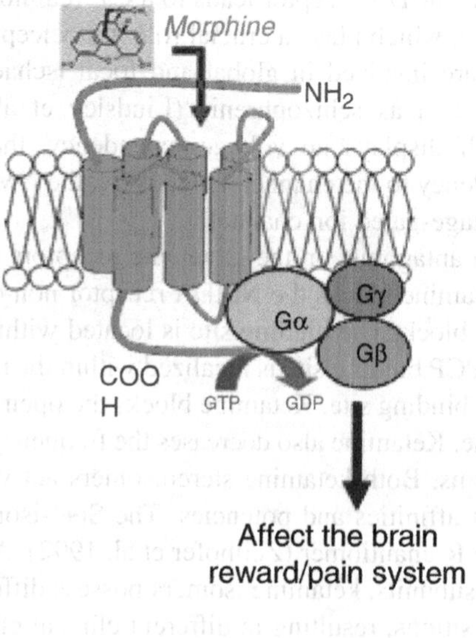

Fig. 4 Opioid receptor

ketamine on spinal or supraspinal opioid receptors play only a minor role in analgesia.

2.3.4 Nicotinic Acetylcholine Receptors

Human nicotinic acetylcholine receptors (nAch) consist of different α- and β-subunits of various compositions. Ketamine antagonizes nAch receptors non-competitively; receptors with mainly β-subunits are especially sensitive vs α-subunits (Yamakura et al. 2000). Ketamine lacks a stereoisomeric effect on the nicotinergic acetylcholine receptors at concentrations necessary for anaesthesia (Sasaki 2000) but interacts stereo-specifically with nAch receptors in human sympathetic ganglion cells (Friederich et al. 2000). This effect is antagonized by the central activating enhancement of the sympathetic nervous system.

2.3.5 Muscarinic Acetylcholine Receptors

Ketamine profoundly inhibits muscarinic signalling via m1 muscarinic receptors . This effect might explain some of the anti-cholinergic clinical effects of ketamine, both central (effects on memory and consciousness) as well as peripheral (prominent sympathetic tone, bronchodilation, mydriasis) (Durieux 1995; Fisher and Durieux 1996). Ketamine also affects m2 and m3 muscarinic receptors. This might contribute to amnesia and mydriasis bronchodilatation, and at least partly explains the increase of bronchial and mucus secretion.

2.3.6 $GABA_A$ Receptors

γ-Aminobutyric acid (GABA) is the major inhibitory transmitter system in the mammalian brain. The $GABA_A$ receptor (Fig. 5) is a pentameric structure consisting of five subunits which incorporates a Cl^- channel. The activation results in hyperpolarization of the neuronal membrane. Ketamine has only a very weak affinity to the $GABA_A$ receptor, leading to an increase in Cl^--permeability. In addition, GABA reuptake is attenuated by ketamine. In conclusion, the effects of ketamine on $GABA_A$ receptor do not significantly contribute to its clinical effect.

2.3.7 Local Anaesthetic Effects/Sodium Channels

Ketamine, similar to local anaesthetics, reduces sodium permeability in isolated neurons in clinically relevant concentrations (Dowdy et al. 1973; Arhem and Rydqvist 1986). After spinal or epidural application in rats, ketamine induces a decrease in blood pressure and an increase in heart rate comparable to the sympathicolysis and limb weakness that results from increasing the dosages of classical

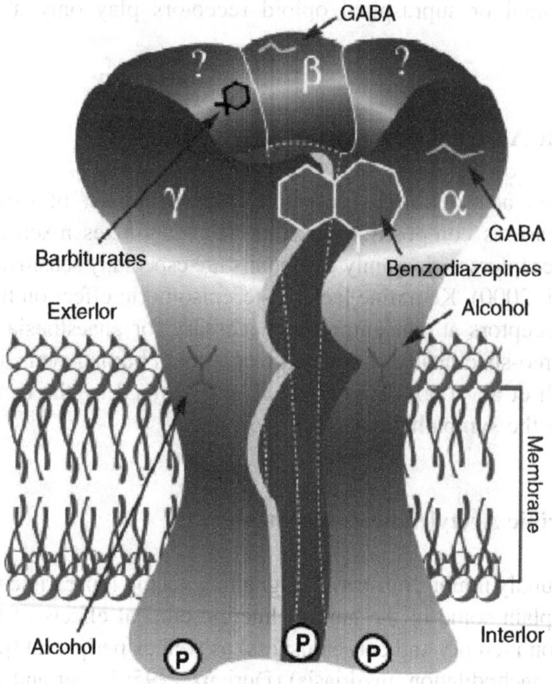

Fig. 5 Model of the γ-aminobutyric acid $(GABA)_A$ receptor

sodium channel blockers. Moreover, Durrani and colleagues reported that ketamine (>0.3%) produced adequate i.v. regional anaesthesia with complete sympathetic, sensory and motor block (Durrani et al. 1989). So far, systematic effects have not been observed.

2.3.8 Calcium Channels

In neurons, L-type Ca^{2+} channels are mainly involved in neurotransmitter release. Pharmacologically the L-type Ca^{2+} channel can be blocked by dihydropyridine or verapamil at different binding sites. Neither binding site is a target for ketamine as both binding sites could only be blocked in concentrations exceeding those required to produce general anaesthesia (Hirota and Lambert 1996a, b). The anaesthetic effects of ketamine are not supposed to be mediated via Ca^{2+} channels. In large concentrations ketamine blocks T-type Ca^{2+} channels in rat sensory neurons (Todorovic and Lingle 1998). In muscles and in the myocardium, ketamine affects the Ca^{2+} influx by blocking the L-type Ca^{2+} channels. This explains the vasodilatation, bronchodilatation and negative inotropic effects of ketamine (Baum and Tecson 1991; Yamakage et al. 1996).

3 Clinical Effects

3.1 Intracranial Pressure and Cerebral Blood Flow

Ketamine can be used safely in neurologically impaired patients under conditions of controlled ventilation, co-administration of a $GABA_A$ receptor agonist (such as benzodiazepines) and avoidance of nitrous oxide. Ketamine increases cerebral blood flow (CBF) and metabolism in spontaneously breathing patients. Under controlled ventilation, however, ketamine does not increase intracranial pressure (ICP) (Himmelseher and Durieux 2005). In combination with isoflurane/nitrous oxide, ketamine reduces ICP and middle cerebral artery blood flow but has no impact on mean arterial blood pressure (Mayberg et al. 1995). By maintaining a greater cerebral perfusion pressure, the application of ketamine is associated with a reduction in catecholamine treatment.

3.2 Neuroprotection

Numerous in vitro studies have reported neuroprotective effects of ketamine when applied prior, during or after the induction of neuronal damage. This might be related to a reduction in glutamate-induced neurotoxicity which results from the blockade of the NMDA receptor (Himmelseher et al. 1996). There is evidence that neuronal damage leads to an increase in NMDA receptor density resulting in an increased neuronal glutamate input. This input activates the up-regulation of further NMDA receptors and finally induces cell death. Ketamine seems to reduce the effects of this vicious cycle (Himmelseher and Durieux 2005). Additionally, a decrease in DNA fragmentation and apoptotic protein activation might be responsible (Chang et al. 2002; Engelhard et al. 2003).

Although a great variety of animal studies reveal neuroprotective effects of ketamine, the animal data cannot be extrapolated to human brains. Future clinical studies will have to show short- and long-term benefits from ketamine treatment associated with neuronal damage.

3.3 Neurotoxicity

The neurodegenerative properties of ketamine were first noted in adult rats 2 h after exposure to ketamine (Olney 1989). Extending these observations on the developing brain, a series of repeated ketamine injections resulted in extensive neuronal apoptosis (Ikonomidou et al. 1999). These observations are also detectable in mammals. After exposing pregnant or newborn rhesus monkeys to ketamine for 24 h, extensive neuronal cell death could be detected, depending on the development stage

(Slikker et al. 2007). In addition to its apoptotic effects, ketamine also affects dendritic arbour development (Vutskits et al. 2006). And in addition to the effects on the developing brain, in the ageing brain experimental data reveal ketamine-induced apoptosis (Jevtovic-Todorovic et al. 2003; Jevtovic-Todorovic and Carter 2005). There are also clinical and experimental data concerning the neurotoxicity of ketamine on the spinal cord (Vranken et al 2005). Single doses applied intrathecally were without neurotoxic properties. In contrast, the repeated application of ketamine in adult rabbits resulted in extensive neuronal necrosis. In a patient with chronic cancer pain the continuous application of ketamine in combination with bupivacaine, morphine, and clonidine revealed severe histological abnormalities (Vranken et al. 2006). It is not clear, however, whether the results from the animal experiments can be directly transferred to humans. Further research is therefore absolutely necessary.

3.4 Cardiovascular Effects

On the isolated heart, ketamine and both ketamine stereoisomers possess negative inotrope, chronotrope and dromotrope effects. These effects are highly stereoselective because the R(−)-isomer is significantly more cardio-depressive and shows negative chronotropy vs the S(+)-isomer, which in low concentrations even possesses positive inotrope qualities. These effects are diminished after complete depletion of the catecholamine storage, which leads to the conclusion that the stereoselective effects are dependent on the presence of catecholamines (Graf et al. 1995). Neuronal catecholamine reuptake is inhibited by both ketamine isomers, with S(+) being more potent than R(−)-ketamine. The S(+)-isomer also inhibits the extra neuronal uptake whereas R(−)-ketamine is without any effect (Lundy et al. 1986). Consistent with the results from mechanical experiments, electrophysiological experiments using whole cell voltage clamp techniques revealed that both isomers suppressed identically the trans-sarcolemmal Ca^{2+} current (ICa^{2+}), which plays a role in the generation of the force of contraction and the spontaneous firing of sinoatrial node cells (Sekino et al. 1996). In the isolated heart, ketamine increases coronary perfusion and coronary oxygen supply. Although the increase in heart rate and contractility increases oxygen demand, the coronary reserve is not restricted (Graf et al. 1995).

Racemic ketamine has been reported to block ischaemic preconditioning, and this effect was attributed more to the R(−)- than the S(−)-isomer (Molojavyi et al. 2001). However, in vitro experiments have demonstrated preconditioning properties for racemic and S(+)-ketamine (Hanouz et al. 2005). The activation of adenosine triphosphate-sensitive potassium channels and stimulation of α- and β-adrenergic receptors seem to be at least in part involved.

Ketamine also possesses significant and stereoselective vasodilator activity in the pulmonary vascular bed (Kaye et al. 2000). The vasodilator responses are mediated via the L-type calcium channel (Kaye et al. 1998). The effect of S(+)-ketamine is significantly weaker compared with that of the racemate and R(−)-ketamine. This stereoselective difference is not due to nitric oxide release, activation of adenosine triphosphate-sensitive potassium channels, or differential inhibition of L-type calcium channels in rat isolated aortic rings (Kanellopoulos et al. 1998).

3.5 Bronchopulmonary Effects

Racemic ketamine relaxes tracheal smooth muscle. This effect, mediated probably via the L-type Ca^{2+} channel, is not stereoselective. In contrast, the Ach-induced bronchodilatation is more enhanced by the R(−)-isomer than the S(+)-isomer (Pabelick et al. 1997). In bronchial epithelium of asthmatic patients, endothelin 1 is detectable in the serum during severe asthmatic attacks. Ketamine attenuates the endothelin 1-induced bronchial smooth muscle constriction (Sato et al. 1997). Histamine-induced bronchoconstriction is not attenuated stereo-specifically, but the potentiation of the adrenalin-induced dilatation is, however, more enhanced by the S(+)-isomer (Graf et al. 1995). Clinically, ketamine reduces bronchoconstriction via antagonistic effects on the vagal nerve and attenuates opioid-induced hypoventilation (Brown and Wagner 1999). Limited evidence is available in the literature to support administration of ketamine in severely exacerbated asthma.

4 Clinical Application

4.1 Analgosedation

Ketamine and S(+)-ketamine are suitable drugs for analgosedation for diagnostic and surgical procedures due to its acceptable analgesic quality and mild deactivation of the consciousness. Both drugs preserve respiratory activity, in contrast to other anaesthetics, and increase blood pressure and heart rate by sympathetic activation. The dissociative properties of ketamine disallow its application as a sole analgosedative drug. Psychotomimetic reactions can be blunted by co-application of sedatives or hypnotics as benzodiazepines or propofol in subclinical concentrations (Adams et al. 2001).

The sympathomimetic effects on the cardiovascular and respiratory system characterize the position as an adjunctive in analgosedation of cardiovascular- or pulmonary-compromised adults and paediatric patients in intensive care and emergency medicine. By stimulating the sympathetic nervous system, ketamine reduces the exogenous catecholamine demand. In contrast to opioids, ketamine has no negative impact on gut motility. This is independent of the combination with either propofol or midazolam. During continuous haemodiafiltration only 0.5% of the administrated ketamine and a minimal fraction of norketamine is eliminated. Ketamine has been shown to reduce the need for inotropic support in septic patients, an effect that may be related to inhibition of catecholamine uptake. In addition, infusion of ketamine resulted in better sedation, increased arterial pressure and diminution of bronchospasm in a patient with acute lymphatic leukaemia who developed bilateral fulminating pneumonia with marked agitation, hypotension and bronchospasm (Park et al. 1987; Yli-Hankala et al. 1992).

In long-term exposure, high tolerance, drug craving and flashbacks have been described. There is, however, little evidence of a physiological withdrawal syndrome, except with abrupt discontinuation in chronic users.

4.2 Anaesthesia

Because of the favourable cardiovascular profile related to central sympathetic stimulation and inhibition of neuronal catecholamine uptake, ketamine is preferred in haemodynamically unstable patients. The sympathetic activation counteracts its direct negative inotropic effect. In patients with a failing myocardium, however, the negative inotropic effects may be unmasked, resulting in deterioration in cardiac performance and cardiovascular instability (Bovill 2006). The bronchodilatory properties of ketamine make it a possible drug for the induction and maintenance of anaesthesia in patience with asthma and life-threatening acute bronchial exacerbation. Although a few cases suggest possible benefits from ketamine, controlled clinical trials to demonstrate that such benefits outweigh the risks are missing (Brown and Wagner 1999).

Ketamine also belongs to the small group of drugs approved for the induction of caesarean section. In concentrations exceeding 2 mg/kg or 1 mg/kg S(+)-ketamine, respiratory depression of the newborn must be anticipated.

4.2.1 Neuromonitoring

Ketamine/S(+)-ketamine produces high-amplitude θ-activity in the EEG, with an accompanying increase in β-activity that appears to represent activation of thalamic and limbic structures. It has been reported to provoke seizure activity in persons with epilepsy but not in normal subjects. Ketamine in doses of 0.25–0.5 mg/kg sufficient to produce anaesthesia has no impact on Bispectral Index value (BIS) (Aspect Medical Systems, Norwood, MA) monitoring. In combination with propofol, BIS changes are attributed to propofol (Sakai et al. 1999). Like etomidate, ketamine increases cortical somatosensory evoked potentials (SSEP) amplitude, with the maximum effect occurring within 2–10 min of bolus administration (Schubert et al. 1990; Stone et al. 1992). No effect on cortical latency or subcortical waveforms is evident so far. However, the addition of nitrous oxide or 1.0 MAC (minimal alveolar concentration) enflurane to a ketamine background anaesthetic depressed SSEP amplitude by approximately 50%. An increase in amplitude of muscle and spinal recorded responses after spinal stimulation was also observed (Kano and Shimoji 1974). Similarly, ketamine does not suppress the mid-latency auditory evoked potential (Schwender et al. 1993).

4.3 *Pain Therapy*

The analgesic effects of ketamine are mediated primarily via NMDA receptors and the opioid receptors.

4.3.1 Acute Pain

To treat acute post-operative pain, opioids are traditionally an integral part of therapy. Unfortunately, opioids produce hyperalgesia, resulting in increased analgesic requirements. The neurophysiological mechanisms are alterations in inhibitory and excitatory pathways mediated by wind-up phenomena, neurokinins and the NMDA receptor (Ali 1986; De Conno et al. 1991; Mao et al. 1995). Blockade of these mechanisms by subanaesthetic and repeated doses of ketamine has been shown to prevent the development of increased pain sensitivity and opioid tolerance (Laulin et al. 2002). For post-operative pain, subanaesthetic doses of ketamine are effective at reducing morphine requirements in the first 24 h after surgery and reducing post-operative nausea and vomiting. To date, the optimal route of administration and dosing regimen is unclear.

4.3.2 Chronic Pain

Ketamine can be a suitable option for pain therapy in patients with chronic pain where standard analgesics such as opioids, anti-depressants and anti-convulsants are insufficient. This includes the reduction of allodynia and hyperpathia in cancer pain, fibromyalgia, ischaemic, phantom or orofacial pain and in complex regional pain syndromes (Hocking and Cousins 2003).

The possible route of application can be i.v., subcutaneous (0.125–0.3 mg/kg per hour), epidural (20–30 mg per day), oral (30 mg-1 g per day, mean 200 mg), or i.m. The rate of non-responders is variable and can be as high as 70%. Psychomotor side-effects result in a reduced acceptance of ketamine as an analgesic. The incidence can be influenced by co-application of midazolam, increasing of the dose slowly, creating a quiet and relaxed atmosphere or application at night rather than during the day.

Currently the most widely accepted indication for ketamine is the acute aggravation of chronic neuropathic pain. These patients are often afflicted by hyperalgesia resulting from large opioid dosages for pain control (Mao et al. 1995). Ketamine is supposed to reduce the hyperalgesia by blocking the NMDA receptor, which seems to be partly involved in the development of opioid tolerance (Hocking and Cousins 2003).

4.4 *Neuroanaesthesia*

Ketamine racemate can increase ICP especially when the ICP is already increased and when the dose exceeds 1 mg/kg i.v. Two reasons seem to be responsible:

increased cerebral perfusion as a result of accelerated arterial pressure and increased $PaCO_2$ due to hypoventilation and concomitantly increased cerebral volume. Independent of pre-existing ICP, ketamine does not increase ICP when normocapnia is maintained by controlled ventilation (Bourgoin et al. 2003). A mild increase in ICP during controlled ventilation can be attenuated by hyperventilation or the co-administration of benzodiazepines or propofol (Albanese et al. 1997).

Ketamine increases CBF when administered in combination with nitrous oxide or in cases of pre-existing increased cerebral vascular resistance (Takeshita et al. 1972). Mechanisms involved seem to be hypercapnia, regional metabolic demand and L-Type Ca^{2+} channel-mediated vasodilatation. In summary, cerebral autoregulation is not affected by S(+)-ketamine (Engelhard et al. 2001).

5 Side-Effects of Ketamine/S(+)-Ketamine

Ketamine has a wide therapeutic range, making overdose difficult or even impossible. Patients have recovered uneventfully after receiving 10 times the normal dose. The median lethal dose (LD_{50}) observed in animals is approximately 100 times the average human intravenous dose and 20 times the average human intramuscular dose.

Other potential adverse effects of ketamine administration include hypersalivation, hyperreflexia, muscle hypertonicity, transient clonus, increased intraocular pressure, emesis, transient rash and agitation. Hypertension, tachycardia, increase pulmonary pressures and even pulmonary oedema can also be seen as an effect of sympathomimetic stimulation by ketamine. In combination with halothane, catecholamine or thyroid hormones, hypertension and arrhythmias can be aggravated.

Although continuous of spontaneous breathing is a positive effect of ketamine, in higher concentrations respiratory depression is seen and artificial ventilation is necessary. Laryngospasm is frequently cited as an adverse effect of ketamine, but it is rarely observed. Especially in children (who are more susceptible), it is usually caused by stimulation of the vocal cords by instrumentation or secretions. Based on pooled data, the previous literature shows the risk of laryngospasm that required intubation during ketamine anaesthesia at 1 per 5,000 individuals (0.02%), which is nearly 100 times lower compared to other anaesthetic agents (Green and Krauss 2004).

Psychotomimetic reactions include anxiety, chest pain, palpitations, agitation, rhabdomyolysis, flashbacks, delirium, dystonia, psychosis, schizophrenic-like symptoms, dizziness, seizures, and paranoia.

6 Contraindications

Ketamine/S(+)-ketamine is appropriate for painful procedures; however, there are a few contraindications which should be considered using ketamine:

- Severe cardiovascular disease, such as angina, heart failure, or malignant hypertension (because of cardio stimulant effects of ketamine; however, this is controversial, particularly in combination with other anaesthetic agents) or during preclampsia
- CSF obstructive states (e.g. severe head injury, central congenital, or mass lesions; however, this is also controversial particularly in combination with artificial ventilation)
- Intraocular pressure pathology (e.g. glaucoma or acute globe injury; however, so far only seen in animal studies)
- Previous psychotic illness (because of potential activation of psychoses)
- Hyperthyroidism or thyroid medication use (because of potential for severe tachycardia or hypertension)
- Porphyries (because of possibility of triggering a porphyric reaction)
- First trimester, since ketamine is ranked category B for pregnancy. Animal reproduction studies have not demonstrated a risk to the foetus and there are no adequate and well-controlled studies in pregnant women or animal studies which have shown an adverse effect. Adequate and well-controlled studies in pregnant women have failed to demonstrate a risk to the foetus in any trimester.

7 Abuse

Ketamine psychedelic side-effects prompted its first recreational abuse in 1965; today ketamine is used as a party drug with the following synonyms:
- K, Ket, Special K, Lady K, Jet, Super Acid, Bump, Special LA Coke, KitKat, Cat Valium, Vitamin K, Keller, Barry Keddle, HOSS, The Hoos, Hossalar, kurdamin and tranq
- Users have likened the physical effects of ketamine to those of PCP, and the visual effects to LSD.

Decreased awareness of the general environment, sedation, a dream-like state, vivid dreams, feelings of invulnerability, increased distractibility, and disorientation are common, and subjects are generally uncommunicative. Intense hallucinations, impaired thought processes, out-of-body experiences, and changes in perception about body, surroundings, time and sounds have been reported. Similarly, delirium and hallucinations can be experienced after awakening from anaesthesia.

References

Adams HA, Brausch M, Schmitz CS, Meyer MC, Hecker H (2001) Analgosedation with (S)-ketamine/propofol vs. (S)-ketamine/midazolam: control and quality of sedation, stress response and haemodynamic reactions [in German]. Anasthesiol Intensivmed Notfallmed Schmerzther 36:417–424

Albanèse J, Arnaud S, Rey M, Thomachot L, Alliez B, Martin C (1997) Ketamine decreases intracranial pressure and electroencephalographic activity in traumatic brain injury patients during propofol sedation. Anesthesiology 87:1328–1334

Ali N (1986) Hyperalgesic response in a patient receiving high concentrations of spinal morphine. Anesthesiology 65:449

Arhem P, Rydqvist B (1986) The mechanism of action of ketamine on the myelinated nerve membrane. Eur J Pharmacol 126:245–251

Baum V, Tecson M (1991) Ketamine inhibits transsarcolemmal calcium entry in guinea pig myocardium: direct evidence by single cell voltage clamp. Anesth Analg 73:804–807

Bourgoin A, Albanèse J, Wereszczynski N, Charbit M, Vialet R, Martin C (2003) Safety of sedation with ketamine in severe head injury patients: comparison with sufentanil. Crit Care Med 31:711–717

Bovill J (2006) Intravenous anaesthesia for the patient with left ventricular dysfunction. Semin Cardiothorac Vasc Anesth 10:43–48

Brown R, Wagner E (1999) Mechanisms of bronchoprotection by anaesthetic induction agents: propofol versus ketamine. Anesthesiology 90:822–828

Chang ML, Yang J, Kem S, Klaidman L, Sugawara T, Chan PH, Adams JD (2002) Nicotinamide and ketamine reduce infarct volume and DNA fragmentation in rats after brain ischemia and reperfusion. Neurosci Lett 322:137–140

De Conno F, Caraceni A, Martini C, Spoldi E, Salvetti M, Ventafridda V (1991) Hyperalgesia and myoclonus with intrathecal infusion of high-dose morphine. Pain 47:337–339

Domino E, Chodoff P, Corssen G (1965) Pharmacologic effects of CI-581, a new dissociative anaesthetic in human. Clin Pharmacol Ther 6:279–291

Dowdy EG, Kaya K, Gocho Y (1973) Some pharmacologic similarities of ketamine, lidocaine, and procaine. Anesth Analg 52:839–842

Durieux M (1995) Inhibition by ketamine of muscarinic acetylcholine receptor function. Anesth Analg 81:57–62

Durrani Z, Winnie AP, Zsigmond EK, Burnett ML (1989) Ketamine for intravenous regional anaesthesia. Anesth Analg 68:328–332

Engelhard K, Werner C, Möllenberg O, Kochs E (2001) S(+)-Ketamine/propofol maintain dynamic cerebrovascular autoregulation in humans. Can J Anaesth 48:1034–1039

Engelhard K, Werner C, Eberspächer E, Bachl M, Blobner M, Hildt E, Hutzler P, Kochs E (2003) The effect of the α2-agonist dexmedetomidine and the NMDA antagonist S(+)ketamine on the expression of apoptosis-regulating proteins after incomplete cerebral ischemia and reperfusion in rats. Anesth Analg 96:524–531

Fisher D, Durieux ME (1996) Muscarinic signaling in the central nervous system: recent developments and anaesthetic implications. Anesthesiology 84:173–189

Friederich P, Dybek A, Urban BW (2000) Stereospecific Interaction of ketamine with nicotinic acetylcholine receptors in human sympathetic ganglion-like SH-SY5Y cells. Anesthesiology 93:818–824

Geisslinger G, Hering W, Thomann P, Knoll R, Kamp HD, Brune K (1993) Pharmacokinetics and pharmacodynamics of ketamine enantiomers in surgical patients using a stereoselective analytical method. Br J Anaesth 70:666–671

Graf BM, Vicenzi MN, Martin E, Bosnjak ZJ, Stowe DF (1995) Ketamine has stereospecific effects in the isolated perfused guinea pig heart. Anesthesiology 82:1426–1437

Green S, Krauss B (2004) Ketamine is a safe, effective, and appropriate technique for emergency department paediatric procedural sedation. Emerg Med J 21:271–272

Hanouz JL, Zhu L, Persehaye E, Massetti M, Babatasi G, Khayat A, Ducouret P, Plaud B, Gérard JL (2005) Ketamine preconditions isolated human right atrial myocardium: roles of adenosine triphosphate-sensitive potassium channels and adrenoceptors. Anesthesiology 102:1190–1196

Hao JX, Sjölund BH, Wiesenfeld-Hallin Z (1998) Electrophysiological evidence for an antinociceptive effect of ketamine in the rat spinal cord. Acta Anaesthesiol Scand 42:435–441

Himmelseher S, Durieux M (2005) Revising a dogma: ketamine for patients with neurological injury? Anesth Analg 101:524–534

Himmelseher S, Pfenninger E, Georgieff M (1996) The effects of ketamine-isomers on neuronal injury and regeneration in rat hippocampal neurons. Anesth Analg 83:505–512

Hirota K, Lambert DG (1996a) I. v anaesthetic agents do not interact with the verapamil binding site on L-type voltage-sensitive Ca^{2+} channels. Br J Anaesth 77:385–386

Hirota K, Lambert DG (1996b) Ketamine: its mechanism(s) of action and unusual clinical uses. Br J Anaesth 77:441–444

Hocking G, Cousins M (2003) Ketamine in chronic pain management: an evidence-based review. Anesth Analg 97:1730–1739

Hustveit O, Maurset A, Oye I (1995) Interaction of the chiral forms of ketamine with opioid, phencyclidine, and muscarinic receptors. Pharmacol Toxicol 77:355–359

Ikonomidou C, Bosch F, Miksa M, Bittigau P, Vöckler J, Dikranian K, Tenkova TI, Stefovska V, Turski L, Olney JW (1999) Blockade of the NMDA receptors and apoptotic neurodegeneration in the developing brain. Science 283:70–74

Irifune M, Shimizu T, Nomoto M, Fukuda T (1992) Ketamine-induced anaesthesia involves the N-methyl-D-aspartate receptor-channel complex in mice. Brain Res 596:1–9

Jevtovic-Todorovic V, Carter L (2005) The anaesthetic nitrous oxide and ketamine are more neurotoxic to old than to young rat brain. Neurobiol Aging 26:947–956

Jevtovic-Todorovic V, Hartman RE, Izumi Y, Benshoff ND, Dikranian K, Zorumski CF, Olney JW, Wozniak DF (2003) Early exposure to common anaesthetics agents causes widespread neurodegeneration in the developing rat brain and persistent learning deficits. J Neurosci 23:876–882

Johnson M (1959) Sernyl (CI-395) in clinical anaesthesia. Br J Anaesth 31:433–439

Kanellopoulos A, Lenz G, Mühlbauer B (1998) Stereoselective differences in the vasorelaxing effects of S(+) and R(−) ketamine on rat isolated aorta. Anesthesiology 88:718–724

Kano T, Shimoji K (1974) The effects of ketamine and neuroleptanalgesia on the evoked electrospinogram and electromyogram in man. Anesthesiology 40:241–246

Kaye AD, Banister RE, Anwar M, Feng CJ, Kadowitz PJ, Nossaman BD (1998) Pulmonary vasodilation by ketamine is mediated in part by L-type calcium channels. Anesth Analg 87:956–962

Kaye AD, Banister RE, Fox CJ, Ibrahim IN, Nossaman BD (2000) Analysis of ketamine responses in the pulmonary vascular bed of the cat. Crit Care Med 28:1077–1082

Larenza MP, Landoni MF, Levionnois OL, Knobloch M, Kronen PW, Theurillat R, Schatzmann U, Thormann W (2007) Stereoselective pharmacokinetics of ketamine and norketamine after racemic ketamine or S-ketamine administration during isoflurane anaesthesia in Shetland ponies. Br J Anaesth 98:204–212

Laulin JP, Maurette P, Corcuff JB, Rivat C, Chauvin M, Simonnet G (2002) The role of ketamine in preventing fentanyl-induced hyperalgesia and subsequent acute morphine tolerance. Anesth Analg 94:1263–1269

Lindsley CW, Shipe WD, Wolkenberg SE, Theberge CR, Williams DL, Sur C, Kinney GG (2006) Progress towards validating the NMDA receptor hypofunction hypothesis of schizophrenia. Curr Top Med Chem 6:771–785

Lundy PM, Lockwood PA, Thompson G, Frew R (1986) Differential effects of ketamine isomers on neuronal and extraneuronal catecholamine uptake mechanisms. Anesthesiology 64:359–363

Mao J, Price DD, Mayer DJ (1995) Mechanisms of hyperalgesia and morphine tolerance: a current view of their possible interactions. Pain 62:259–274

Mayberg TS, Lam AM, Matta BF, Domino KB, Winn HR (1995) Ketamine does not increase blood flow velocity or intracranial pressure during isoflurane/nitrous oxide anaesthesia in patients undergoing craniotomy. Anesth Analg 81:84 –9

Mayer M, Armstrong N (2004) Structure and function of glutamate receptor ion channels. Annu Rev Physiol 66:161–181

McBain C, Mayer M (1994) N-methyl-D-aspartic acid receptor structure and function. Physiol Rev 74:723–760

Mikkelsen S, Ilkjaer S, Brennum J, Borgbjerg FM, Dahl JB (1999) The effect of naloxone on ketamine-induced effects on hyperalgesia and ketamine-induced side effects in humans. Anesthesiology 90:1539–1545

Molojavyi A, Preckel B, Comfère T, Müllenheim J, Thämer V, Schlack W (2001) Effects of ketamine and its isomers on ischemic preconditioning in the isolated rat heart. Anesthesiology 94:623–629

Mori H, Mishina M (1995) Neurotransmitter receptors VIII. Structure and function of the NMDA receptor channel. Neuropharmacology 34:219–237

Olney JW, Labruyere J, Price MT (1989) Pathological changes induced in cerebrocortical neurons by phencyclidine and related drugs. Science 244:1360–1362

Pabelick CM, Jones KA, Street K, Lorenz RR, Warner DO (1997) Calcium concentration-dependent mechanisms through which ketamine relaxes canine airway smooth muscle. Anesthesiology 86:1104–1111

Park GR, Manara AR, Mendel L, Bateman PE (1987) Ketamine infusion. Its use as a sedative, inotrope and bronchodilator in a critically ill patient. Anaesthesia 42:980–983

Sakai T, Singh H, Mi WD, Kudo T, Matsuki A (1999) The effect of ketamine on clinical endpoint of hypnosis and EEC variables during propofol infusion. Acta Anaesthesiol Scand 43:212–216

Sarton E, Teppema LJ, Olievier C, Nieuwenhuijs D, Matthes HW, Kieffer BL, Dahan A (2001) The involvement of the μ-opioid receptor in ketamine-induced respiratory depression and antinociception. Anesth Analg 93:1495–1500

Sasaki T, Andoh T, Watanabe I, Kamiya Y, Itoh H, Higashi T, Matsuura T (2000) Nonstereoselective inhibition of neuronal nicotinic acetylcholine receptors by ketamine isomers. Anesth Analg 91:741–748

Sato T, Hirota K, Matsuki A, Zsigmond EK, Rabito SF (1997) The relaxant effect of ketamine on guinea pig airway smooth muscle is epithelium-independent. Anesth Analg 84:641–647

Schubert A, Licina MG, Lineberry PJ (1990) The effect of ketamine on human somatosensory evoked potentials and its modification by nitrous oxide. Anesthesiology 72:33–90

Schwender D, Klasing S, Madler C, Poppel E, Peter K (1993) Mid-latency auditory evoked potentials during ketamine anaesthesia in humans. Br J Anaesth 71:629–632

Sekino N, Endou M, Hajiri E, Okumura F (1996) Nonstereospecific actions of ketamine isomers on the force of contraction, spontaneous beating rate, and Ca^{2+} current in the guinea pig heart. Anesth Analg 83:75–80

Slikker W, Zou X, Hotchkiss CE, Divine RL, Sadovova N, Twaddle NC, Doerge DR, Scallet AC, Patterson TA, Hanig JP, Paule MG, Wang C (2007) Ketamine-induced neuronal cell death in the perinatal rhesus monkey. Toxicol Sci 98:145–158

Smith DJ, Bouchal RL, deSanctis CA, Monroe PJ, Amedro JB, Perrotti JM, Crisp T (1987) Properties of the interaction between ketamine and opiate binding sites in vivo and in vitro. Neuropharmacology 26:1253–1260

Stone JL, Ghaly RF, Levy WJ, Kartha R, Krinsky L, Roccaforte P (1992) A comparative analysis of enflurane anaesthesia on primate motor and somatosensory evoked potentials. Electroencephalogr Clin Neurophysiol 84:180–187

Takeshita H, Okuda Y, Sari A (1972) The effects of ketamine on cerebral circulation and metabolism in man. Anesthesiology 36:69 –75

Todorovic S, Lingle C (1998) Pharmacological properties of T-type Ca^{2+} current in adult rate sensory neurons: effects of anticonvulsant and anaesthetic agents. J Neurophysiol 79:240–252

Vranken JH, Troost D, Wegener JT, Kruis MR, van der Vegt MH (2005) Neuropathological findings after continuous intrathecal administration of S(+)-ketamine for the management of neuropathic cancer pain. Pain 117:231–235

Vranken JH, Troost D, de Haan P, Pennings FA, van der Vegt MH, Dijkgraaf mg, Hollmann MW (2006) Severe toxic damage to the rabbit spinal cord after intrathecal administration of preservative-free S(+)-ketamine. Anesthesiology 105:813–818

White P, Ham J, Way WL, et al (1980) Pharmacology of ketamine isomers in surgical patients. Anesthesiology 52:231–239

Yamakage M, Hirshman CA, Croxton TL (1996) Inhibitory effects of thiopental, ketamine, and propofol on voltage-dependent Ca^{2+} channels in porcine tracheal smooth muscle cells. Anesthesiology 83:1274–1282

Yamakura T, Chavez-Noriega LE, Harris RA (2000) Subunit-dependent inhibition of human neuronal nicotinic acetylcholine receptors and other ligand-gated ion channels by dissociative anaesthetics ketamine and dizocilpine. Anesthesiology 92:1144–1153

Yli-Hankala A, Kirvel M, Randell T, Lindgren L (1992) Ketamine anaesthesia in a patient with septic shock. Acta Anaesthesiol Scand 36:483–485

Zeilhofer HU, Swandulla D, Geisslinger G, Brune K (1992) Differential effects of ketamine enantiomers on NMDA receptor currents in cultured neurons. Eur J Pharmacol 213:155–158

Midazolam and Other Benzodiazepines

K.T. Olkkola(✉) and J. Ahonen

Abstract The actions of benzodiazepines are due to the potentiation of the neural inhibition that is mediated by gamma-aminobutyric acid (GABA). Practically all effects of the benzodiazepines result from their actions on the ionotropic $GABA_A$ receptors in the central nervous system. Benzodiazepines do not activate $GABA_A$ receptors directly but they require GABA. The main effects of benzodiazepines are sedation, hypnosis, decreased anxiety, anterograde amnesia, centrally mediated

K.T. Olkkola
Department of Anaesthesiology, Intensive Care, Emergency Care and Pain Medicine, Turku University Hospital, PO Box 52 (kiinamyllynkatu 4–8), FI-20521 Turku, Finland
klaus.olkkola@utu.fi

J. Schüttler and H. Schwilden (eds.) *Modern Anesthetics.*
Handbook of Experimental Pharmacology 182.

muscle relaxation and anti-convulsant activity. In addition to their action on the central nervous system, benzodiazepines have a dose-dependent ventilatory depressant effect and they also cause a modest reduction in arterial blood pressure and an increase in heart rate as a result of a decrease of systemic vascular resistance. The four benzodiazepines, widely used in clinical anaesthesia, are the agonists midazolam, diazepam and lorazepam and the antagonist flumazenil. Midazolam, diazepam and flumazenil are metabolized by cytochrome P450 (CYP) enzymes and by glucuronide conjugation whereas lorazepam directly undergoes glucuronide conjugation. CYP3A4 is important in the biotransformation of both midazolam and diazepam. CYP2C19 is important in the biotransformation of diazepam. Liver and renal dysfunction have only a minor effect on the pharmacokinetics of lorazepam but they slow down the elimination of the other benzodiazepines used in clinical anaesthesia. The duration of action of all benzodiazepines is strongly dependent on the duration of their administration. Based on clinical studies and computer simulations, midazolam has the shortest recovery profile followed by lorazepam and diazepam. Being metabolized by CYP enzymes, midazolam and diazepam have many clinically significant interactions with inhibitors and inducers of CYP3A4 and 2C19. In addition to pharmacokinetic interactions, benzodiazepines have synergistic interactions with other hypnotics and opioids. Midazolam, diazepam and lorazepam are widely used for sedation and to some extent also for induction and maintenance of anaesthesia. Flumazenil is very useful in reversing benzodiazepine-induced sedation as well as to diagnose or treat benzodiazepine overdose.

1 Introduction

The first benzodiazepines were synthesized already in the 1950s (Greenblatt and Shader 1974) but the intravenous use of benzodiazepines did not begin until 1960s when intravenous diazepam was used for induction of anaesthesia (Stovner and Endresen 1965). To date, thousands of different benzodiazepines have been synthesized and about 30 are in clinical use in various parts of the world. However, only four benzodiazepines, the agonists midazolam, diazepam and lorazepam and the antagonist flumazenil are widely used in clinical anaesthesia. This chapter will focus on the basic and clinical pharmacology of these four benzodiazepines. In addition, the chapter will review the pharmacology of the new benzodiazepine agonist Ro 48-6791 which was developed for anaesthesia but which so far has not been registered for clinical use (Dingemanse et al. 1997a, b).

2 Chemical Structure and Physicochemical Characteristics

The four benzodiazepines commonly used in clinical anaesthesia are rather small molecules with molecular weights ranging from 284.7 to 325.8 daltons. Their structures and the structure of Ro 48-6791 are shown in Fig. 1.

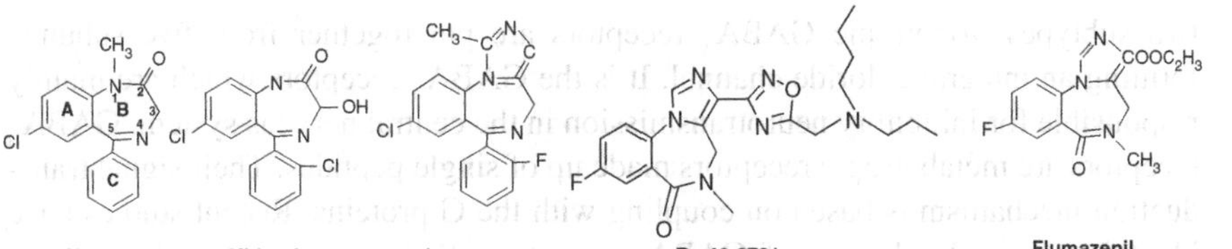

Fig. 1 The structure of Ro 48-6791 and the four benzodiazepines used in clinical anaesthesia. They are all composed of a benzene ring (*A*) fused to a seven-membered 1,4-diazepine ring (*B*). Anaesthesiologically relevant benzodiazepine agonists also contain a 5-aryl substituent (ring *C*), which enhances the pharmacological potency. However, the benzodiazepine antagonist flumazenil has two important structural differences as compared to the above agonists. Flumazenil has a keto function at position *5* instead of ring *C* and a methyl substituent at position *4*

Table 1 Physicochemical characteristics of four benzodiazepines used in clinical anaesthesia

	Molecular weight (daltons)	pK_a	Water solubility	Lipid solubility
Midazolam	325.8 (hydrochloride 392.3)	6.2	Good at pH<4	Good at pH>4
Diazepam	284.7	3.2	Poor	Good
Lorazepam	321.2	1.3, 11.5	Poor	Moderate
Flumazenil	303.3	1.7	Moderate	Poor

Data from Dollery (1991)

The physicochemical characteristics of midazolam, diazepam, lorazepam and flumazenil are summarized in Table 1. Unlike the other benzodiazepines, midazolam is used clinically as a hydrochloride salt which is essential for the physicochemical characteristics desirable in clinical anaesthesia. Interestingly, midazolam hydrochloride displays pH-dependent solubility. The pH of the commercial midazolam hydrochloride preparation is adjusted to 3 with hydrochloride acid and sodium hydroxide. As midazolam is injected into patients, pH is increased and the seven-membered 1,4-diazepine ring is closed thus increasing the lipid solubility (Gerecke 1983).

3 Pharmacology

3.1 Pharmacological Action at Receptor Level

Practically all effects of the benzodiazepines result from their actions on the central nervous system. Compared to other intravenous anaesthetics, the mechanism of action of benzodiazepines is rather well understood (Möhler et al. 2002). The main effects of benzodiazepines are sedation, hypnosis, decreased anxiety, anterograde amnesia, centrally mediated muscle relaxation and anti-convulsant activity. The current view is that the actions of benzodiazepines are due to the potentiation of the neural inhibition that is mediated by gamma-aminobutyric acid (GABA). GABA receptors are membrane-bound proteins which can be divided into two subtypes. Ionotropic $GABA_A$ receptors are put together from five subunits forming an integral chloride channel. It is the $GABA_A$ receptors which are mainly responsible for inhibitory neurotransmission in the central nervous system. $GABA_B$ receptors are metabotropic receptors made up of single peptides. Their signal transduction mechanism is based on coupling with the G proteins. Recent studies have identified several subtypes of $GABA_A$ receptors. Sedation, anterograde amnesia and anti-convulsant activity are mediated through α_1 receptors whereas anxiolysis and muscle relaxation seem to be mediated by the α_2 $GABA_A$ receptor (Möhler et al. 2002).

Benzodiazepines exert their action by binding to a specific site that is distinct from that of GABA binding on the $GABA_A$ receptors. Benzodiazepines do not act at $GABA_B$ receptors. The chemical structure of the each benzodiazepine is closely linked to its receptor binding properties and also pharmacokinetics. The order of receptor affinity of the three agonists is lorazepam > midazolam > diazepam. Thus, midazolam is more potent than diazepam and lorazepam is more potent than midazolam (Mould et al. 1995). Benzodiazepines do not activate $GABA_A$ receptors directly but they require GABA. The ligands binding to the benzodiazepine-receptor have different effects depending on the ligand in question. They can act as agonists, antagonists or inverse agonists. Agonists increase the $GABA_A$-produced chloride current at the benzodiazepine receptor while the antagonists have an opposite effect. Thus, benzodiazepine agonists shift the GABA concentration-response curve to the left. Inverse agonists shift the curve to the right. The actions of both agonists and inverse agonists can be inhibited by benzodiazepine antagonists which themselves do not affect the function of $GABA_A$ receptors.

3.2 *Central Nervous System*

Compared to barbiturates, propofol and inhalational anaesthetics, the benzodiazepines are not able to produce the same degree of neuronal depression. At low doses the benzodiazepines have anxiolytic and anti-convulsive effects. As the dose increases, the benzodiazepines produce sedation, amnesia and finally sleep. The effect of the benzodiazepines is clearly dose-related but there seems to be a ceiling effect where increasing the dose does not increase the effect (Hall et al. 1988). Benzodiazepines reduce cerebral metabolism ($CMRO_2$) and cerebral blood flow (CBF) without disturbing the normal CBF/$CMRO_2$ ratio (Forster et al. 1982). Although the benzodiazepines may be used as hypnotics during the intravenous induction of anaesthesia, they are not optimally suited for this purpose. Induction of sleep requires relatively high doses, meaning that recovery from all the effects of benzodiazepines takes a long time because, for instance, amnesia and sedation are produced at much lower concentrations than the hypnotic effects. If benzodiazepines are used also for the maintenance of anaesthesia, the recovery is even slower because during and after long-lasting infusions, it is the elimination of the drug from the body which is of vital importance for the recovery. Following bolus injection of benzodiazepines, recovery from anaesthesia is enhanced by the redistribution of the drug within the body from the receptors to non-specific sites of action. Thus, it is understandable that the postoperative period of sedation can be rather long (Fig. 2).

The development of tolerance to benzodiazepines seems to be a controversial issue. While some authors have observed tolerance to benzodiazepines, others have been unable to confirm these findings (Coldwell et al. 1998; Fiset et al. 1995; Greenblatt and Shader 1978; Ihmsen et al. 2004; Shafer 1998; Shelly et al. 1991; Somma et al. 1998). Additionally, different mechanisms for tolerance have been suggested. A popular explanation for tolerance is the downregulation of the benzodiazepine-$GABA_A$ receptor complex (Miller 1991). However, Tietz et al. (1989) suggested that the prolonged exposure to benzodiazepines results in an altered effect of the benzodiazepine agonists on the GABA concentration-response relationship.

There is some evidence in experimental animals that benzodiazepines would have a neuroprotective effect in brain (de Jong and Bonin 1981; Ito et al. 1999). Furthermore, midazolam, diazepam and lorazepam also decrease the local anaesthetic-induced mortality in mice (de Jong and Bonin 1981). Unfortunately, studies in other animals have not been able to confirm the usefulness of benzodiazepines in neuroprotection (Hall et al. 1998). There is no evidence that benzodiazepines would have neuroprotective effects in man.

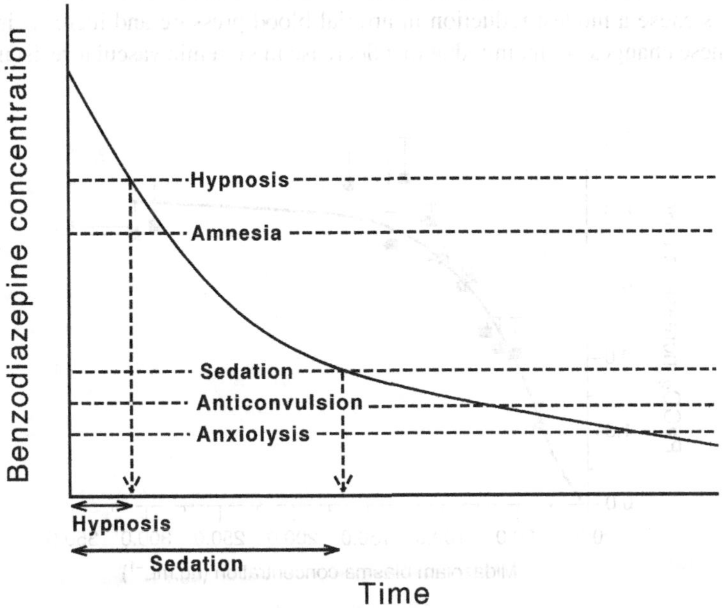

Fig. 2 Schematic presentation on the relationship between benzodiazepine concentration and clinical effect

3.3 Respiration

Normal oral hypnotic doses of benzodiazepines have essentially no effect on respiration in normal subjects. At higher doses, the benzodiazepines do influence respiration. The benzodiazepines affect respiration in two different ways. First, they have an effect on the muscular tone leading to an increased risk of upper airway obstruction (Norton et al. 2006). Thus, benzodiazepines are not recommended and are considered even contraindicated in patients suffering from obstructive sleep apnoea. Second, they also affect the ventilatory response curve to carbon dioxide by flattening the response (Fig. 3). However, unlike opioids, benzodiazepines do not shift the curve to the right (Sunzel et al. 1988). A typical reaction to benzodiazepines is a decrease in tidal volume. If the patient is given benzodiazepine together with an opioid, the risk of clinically significant ventilatory depression is increased markedly (Tverskoy et al. 1989). An important factor contributing to the ventilatory depressant effect of benzodiazepines is their ability to depress the reaction to hypoxia under hypercapnic conditions (Alexander and Gross 1988). Especially patients suffering from chronic obstructive pulmonary disease should be closely monitored.

3.4 Cardiovascular System

The intravenous administration of sedative or anaesthetic doses of the benzodiazepines cause a modest reduction in arterial blood pressure and increase in heart rate. These changes are mainly due to a decrease in systemic vascular resistance. In

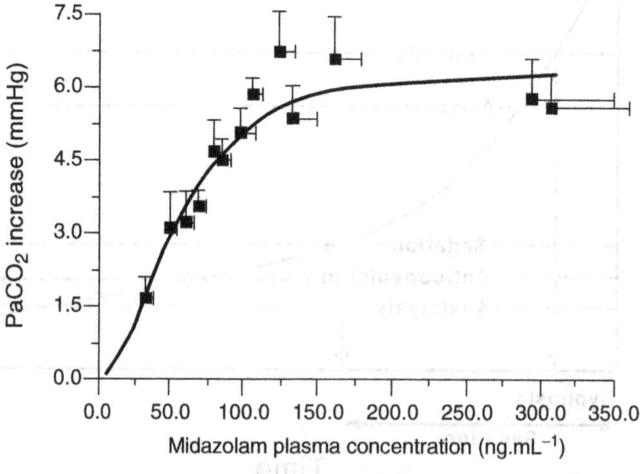

Fig. 3 Increase in $PaCO_2$ from baseline versus the midazolam plasma concentration after three intravenous bolus doses of midazolam (0.05 mg/kg) given at 20-min intervals. Mean values ± standard error of mean (SEM) are given. (Modified with permission from Sunzel et al. 1988)

addition, they induce a minor reduction of cardiac output (Samuelson et al. 1981; Ruff and Reves 1990). Midazolam and diazepam have also been shown to depress the baroreflex. This occurrence means that both midazolam and diazepam induce a limited ability to compensate for haemodynamic alterations related to hypovolemia (Marty et al. 1986).

4 Pharmacokinetics and Biotransformation

The pharmacokinetic variables of intravenous benzodiazepines are summarized in Table 2. The two principal pathways of the benzodiazepine biotransformation involve hepatic microsomal oxidation (*N*-dealkylation or aliphatic hydroxylation) and glucuronide conjugation (Fig. 4). Microsomal oxidation reactions are catalysed by cytochrome P450 (CYP) isoenzymes 3A4/3A5 and 2C19. Unlike glucuronide conjugation, oxidation may be affected, e.g. by age, disease states and concurrent

Table 2 Pharmacokinetic variables of midazolam, diazepam, lorazepam, Ro 48–6971, and flumazenil

	Elimination half-life (h)	Clearance (ml/kg/min)	V_{ss} (l/kg)	Plasma protein binding (%)	Reference(s)
Midazolam	1.7–2.6	5.8–9.0	1.1–1.7	96	Dundee et al. 1984a
Diazepam	20–50	0.2–0.5	0.7–1.7	98	Greenblatt et al. 1980
Lorazepam	11–22	0.8–1.8	0.8–1.3	90	Greenblatt et al. 1979
Ro 48–6791	3.8	18–44	1.5–3.4		Dingemanse et al. 1997a, b
Flumazenil	0.7–1.3	13–17	0.9–1.1	40	Klotz and Kanto 1988; Breimer et al. 1991

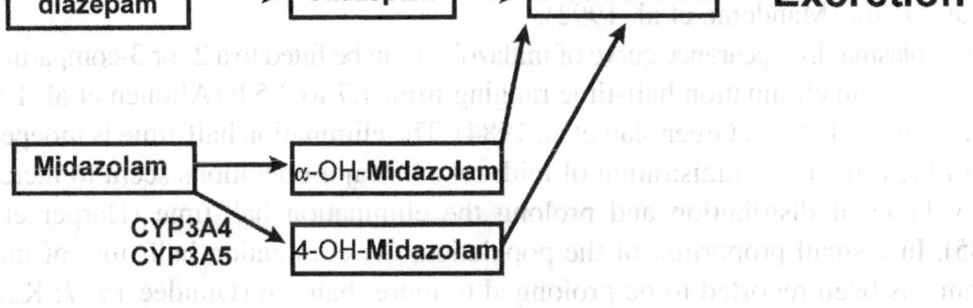

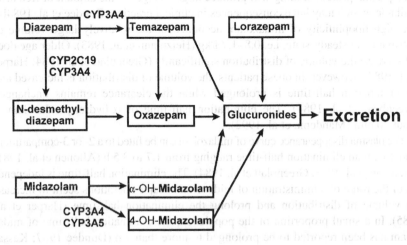

Fig. 4 Metabolic pathways of midazolam, diazepam and lorazepam

intake of other drugs (Elliott 1976; Klotz and Reimann 1980; Heizmann et al. 1983; Inaba et al. 1988; Park et al. 1989; Wandel et al. 1994).

4.1 Midazolam

The first step in the metabolism of midazolam is hydroxylation by CYP3A4 and CYP3A5 (Wandel et al. 1994). The two metabolites formed are α-hydroxymidazolam and 4-hydroxymidazolam, which both are pharmacologically active (Heizmann et al. 1983; Ziegler et al. 1983). The α-hydroxymidazolam is as potent as the parent compound and may contribute significantly to the effects of the parent drug when present in sufficiently high concentrations. 4-Hydroxymidazolam is quantitatively unimportant (Mandema et al. 1992). Both metabolites are rapidly conjugated by glucuronic acid to form products which have been considered to be pharmacologically inactive (Heizmann et al. 1983).

Following intravenous administration, midazolam is rapidly distributed and the distribution half-time is 6–15 min (Allonen et al. 1981). The fused imidazole ring of midazolam is oxidized much more rapidly than the methylene group of the diazepine ring of other benzodiazepines, which accounts for the greater plasma clearance of midazolam ranging from 5.8 to 9.0 ml/kg per minute as compared with diazepam, 0.2–0.5 ml/kg per minute and lorazepam, 0.8–1.8 ml/kg per minute (Greenblatt et al. 1979, 1980; Dundee et al. 1984a; Bailey et al. 1994). In elderly men, the clearance of midazolam is reduced and the elimination half-time is prolonged as compared to young males. Between elderly and young women, however, no significant differences were detected in the clearance or the elimination half-time of midazolam (Greenblatt et al. 1984).

Midazolam is extensively bound to plasma proteins (94%–98%). Small changes in its plasma protein binding will produce large changes in the amount of free drug available, which may have consequences in clinical practice (Dundee et al. 1984b). The high lipophilicity of midazolam accounts for the relatively large volume of distribution at steady-state, i.e. 0.8–1.7 l/kg (Heizmann et al. 1983). Older age does not increase the volume of distribution significantly (Greenblatt et al. 1984; Harper et al. 1985). However, in obese patients, the volume of distribution is increased and the elimination half-time is prolonged while the clearance remains unchanged (Greenblatt et al. 1984). The elimination half-time of α-hydroxymidazolam is about 70 min (Mandema et al. 1992).

The plasma disappearance curve of midazolam can be fitted to a 2- or 3-compartment model with an elimination half-time ranging from 1.7 to 3.5 h (Allonen et al. 1981; Heizmann et al. 1983; Greenblatt et al. 1984). The elimination half-time is independent of the route of administration of midazolam. Major operations seem to increase the volume of distribution and prolong the elimination half-time (Harper et al. 1985). In a small proportion of the population, the elimination half-time of midazolam has been reported to be prolonged to more than 7 h (Dundee 1987; Kassai et al. 1988). In five out of 90 subjects (46 healthy volunteers, 17 surgical patients, and

12 patients with stabilized cirrhosis), the volume of distribution was clearly increased without a change in clearance. Thus, the prolonged elimination half-time was secondary to an increase in the volume of distribution (Wills et al. 1990).

In addition to the liver, midazolam is also metabolized at extrahepatic sites. This has been demonstrated by the discovery of metabolites following intravenous injection of midazolam during the anhepatic period of liver transplantation (Park et al. 1989). In patients with advanced cirrhosis of the liver, the plasma clearance is reduced and the elimination half-time is prolonged as compared to healthy volunteers, while the volume of distribution remains unchanged (Pentikäinen et al. 1989).

Glucuronidated α-hydroxymidazolam, the main metabolite of midazolam, has a substantial pharmacological effect and can penetrate the intact blood–brain barrier. It can accumulate in patients with renal failure (Fig. 5). Furthermore, in vitro binding studies show that the affinity of glucuronidated α-hydroxymidazolam to the cerebral benzodiazepine receptor is only about ten times weaker than that of midazolam or unconjugated α-hydroxymidazolam (Bauer et al. 1995).

4.2 *Diazepam*

Diazepam is metabolized in the liver with only traces of the unchanged drug being excreted in urine. The two major pathways of diazepam metabolism, the formation of *N*-desmethyldiazepam and temazepam, are catalysed by different CYP isoforms (Inaba et al. 1988). The third potential metabolite, 4-hydroxydiazepam,

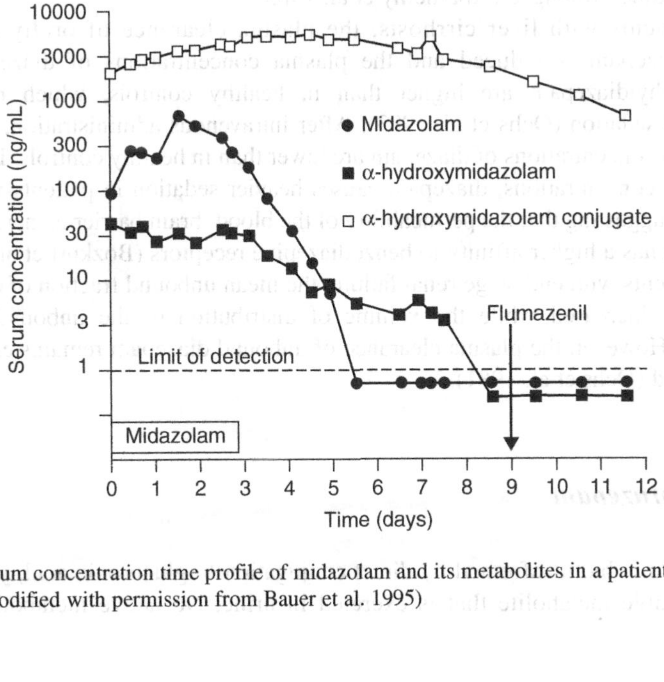

Fig. 5 Serum concentration time profile of midazolam and its metabolites in a patient with renal failure. (Modified with permission from Bauer et al. 1995)

seems to be less important. Studies with a series of CYP isoform-selective inhibitors and an inhibitory anti-CYP2C antibody indicate that temazepam formation is carried out mainly by CYP3A isoforms, whereas the formation of *N*-desmethyldiazepam is mediated by both CYP3A isoenzymes and *S*-mephenytoin hydroxylase, CYP2C19 (Andersson et al. 1994; Kato and Yamazoe 1994). *N*-Desmethyldiazepam has a similar pharmacodynamic profile to diazepam but its elimination half-time is longer. *N*-Desmethyldiazepam is hydroxylated to oxazepam, which is also active. Oxazepam has a shorter elimination half-time and it is conjugated with glucuronic acid (Greenblatt 1981). Temazepam and oxazepam do not appear to contribute much to the effects of diazepam since they have shorter half-times than the parent drug.

Due to the redistribution of diazepam, the concentrations considerably decrease during the first 2–3 h after administration. Thereafter the rate of disappearance from plasma slows down (Greenblatt et al. 1989). The distribution half-time of diazepam, 30–66 min (Mandelli et al. 1978; Greenblatt et al. 1980), is significantly longer than that of midazolam or lorazepam. In healthy volunteers, the clearance of diazepam ranges from 0.2 to 0.5 ml/kg per minute (Greenblatt et al. 1979) but older age tends to reduce the clearance (MacLeod et al. 1979). The formation of *N*-desmethyldiazepam accounts for 50%–60% of total diazepam clearance. The mean elimination half-time of diazepam is 30 h with a range of 20–100 h while that of *N*-desmethyldiazepam is even longer with a range of 30–200 h (Mandelli et al. 1978). During the elimination phase following single or multiple doses, the plasma concentration of *N*-desmethyldiazepam can be higher than that of diazepam. Plasma protein binding of diazepam averages 98% and the volume of distribution is 0.7–1.7 l/kg (Dasberg 1975; Jack and Colburn 1983; Greenblatt et al. 1988). In obese patients, the volume of distribution of diazepam is increased and the elimination half-time prolonged (Abernethy et al. 1983).

In patients with liver cirrhosis, the plasma clearance of orally administered diazepam is reduced and the plasma concentrations of diazepam and *N*-desmethyldiazepam are higher than in healthy controls, which results in increased sedation (Ochs et al. 1983). After intravenous administration, however, the serum concentrations of diazepam are lower than in healthy controls. In spite of the lower concentrations, diazepam causes heavier sedation in patients with liver disease, suggesting that the permeability of the blood–brain barrier is increased and diazepam has a higher affinity to benzodiazepine receptors (Bozkurt et al. 1996).

In patients with end-stage renal failure, the mean unbound fraction of diazepam is greatly increased while the volume of distribution of the unbound drug is reduced. However, the plasma clearance of unbound diazepam remains essentially unchanged (Ochs et al. 1981).

4.3 *Lorazepam*

Lorazepam is biotransformed by direct conjugation to glucuronic acid, yielding a water-soluble metabolite that is excreted in urine. No active metabolites have been identified. The mean elimination half-time is 15 h with a range of 8–25 h (Greenblatt et al. 1979). The plasma protein binding of lorazepam is about 90%. The clearance varies from 0.8 to 1.8 ml/kg per minute and the volume of distribution from 0.8 to 1.3 l/kg (Greenblatt 1981).

The elimination half-time of lorazepam is increased in patients with alcoholic cirrhosis as compared to healthy controls but the systemic plasma clearance remains unchanged. Acute viral hepatitis has no effect on the disposition kinetics of lorazepam with the exception of a modest decrease in plasma protein binding (Kraus et al. 1978). In renal impairment, the elimination half-time and the volume of distribution of lorazepam are increased but the clearance does not differ significantly from that in healthy controls (Morrison et al. 1984).

4.4 *Ro 48-6791*

Ro 48-6791 was developed in the search for a benzodiazepine with a faster recovery profile than that of midazolam, while retaining the favourable physicochemical and pharmacodynamic properties of the latter (Dingemanse et al. 1997a, b). Ro 48-6791, 3-(5-dipropylaminomethyl-1, 2,4-oxadiazol-3-yl)-8-fluoro-5-methyl-5, 6-dihydro-4H-imidazo [1, 5-a] [1,4] benzodiazepin-6-one, is a water-soluble full agonist at the benzodiazepine receptor. In two studies with healthy volunteers, the pharmacokinetics of Ro 48-6791 was described with a 2- or 3-compartment model (Dingemanse et al. 1997a, b). The volume of distribution at steady-state and plasma clearance were four- to fivefold higher for Ro 48-6791 than for midazolam. The distribution and the elimination half-times of Ro 48-6791 and midazolam were similar, because both the volume of distribution and the clearance changed in the same direction (Dingemanse et al. 1997a).

Following intravenous administration to man, Ro 48-6791 undergoes rapid biotransformation to form the monopropyl derivate Ro 48-6792. In animals, Ro 48-6792 is at least tenfold less potent a sedative than the parent compound, and the maximum plasma concentration of Ro 48-6792 attained in the study by Dingemanse et al. (1997a) was unlikely to have contributed significantly to the effects of Ro 48-6791. However, the plasma concentrations indicated that the elimination half-time of Ro 48-6792 was markedly longer than that of the parent compound, suggesting that the metabolite could accumulate during prolonged sedation with Ro 48-6791.

4.5 *Flumazenil*

The plasma protein binding of flumazenil is about 40%, and the elimination half-time is reported to be about 40–80 min. The steady-state volume of distribution is 0.9–1.1 l/kg, and the plasma clearance ranges 13–17 ml/kg per minute. After intravenous administration, flumazenil is extensively metabolized in the liver to the inactive carboxylic acid form, which is excreted predominantly in the urine (Klotz and Kanto 1988; Breimer et al. 1991).

Licensed drug information states that in patients with hepatic failure, the elimination half-time of flumazenil is prolonged and the systemic clearance is reduced compared with healthy subjects. However, the pharmacokinetics of flumazenil is not significantly affected by renal disease or haemodialysis.

5 Pharmacokinetic-Dynamic Relationship

In a multicompartment pharmacokinetic model, the distribution of the drug between the central and peripheral compartments is a significant contributor to drug disposition in the central compartment. The traditional elimination half-time is inadequate to describe the various drug concentration decrements observed after different dosing schemes (Shafer and Varvel 1991). Computer simulations based on pharmacokinetic models can be used to describe the decay of plasma drug concentrations after discontinuation of drug administration. Specifically, it has been suggested that context-sensitive half-times (Hughes et al. 1992) or other decrement times (Bailey 1995) can be used to describe the decay of drug concentration after discontinuation of drug administration and thus better describe the cessation of drug effect. The context-sensitive half-time (50% decrement time) is the time required for blood or plasma concentrations of a drug to decrease by 50% after stopping the drug administration. Correspondingly, 80% decrement time is the time required for drug concentrations to decrease by 80%. In many cases it is the 50% decrement of the drug concentration that is useful for the prediction of the duration of drug action. However, the duration of drug effect is a function of both pharmacokinetic and pharmacodynamic properties. Other variables include an inconsistent relationship between concentration and response, variable response characteristics for different patients, and the variable effect of concomitantly administered drugs (Keifer and Glass 1999). Figure 6 shows the context-sensitive half-times for commonly used intravenous anaesthetics.

Midazolam has been used as a continuous intravenous infusion with a supplemental volatile agent (Ahonen et al. 1996a) or as the sole hypnotic agent (Theil et al. 1993) in cardiac surgery. More often, continuous infusions of midazolam and lorazepam are administered to intensive care patients for sedation during mechanical ventilation. A recent study shows that midazolam and lorazepam have substantial pharmacokinetic and pharmacodynamic differences when given during intensive care. Barr et al. (2001) have observed that the pharmacodynamic model can predict the depth of sedation for both midazolam and lorazepam with 76% accuracy. The estimated sedative potency of lorazepam is twice that of midazolam and the relative amnestic potency of lorazepam fourfold that of midazolam. The predicted emergence times from sedation after a 72-h benzodiazepine infusion for light and deep sedation in a typical patient are 3.6 and 14.9 h for midazolam infusions and 11.9 and 31.1 h for lorazepam infusions, respectively (Fig. 7). Since both formal modelling

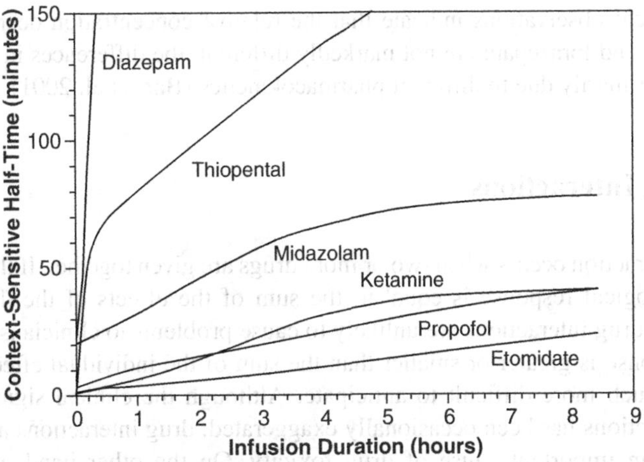

Fig. 6 The context-sensitive half-times for commonly used intravenous anaesthetic drugs. (Modified with permission from Reves et al. 1994)

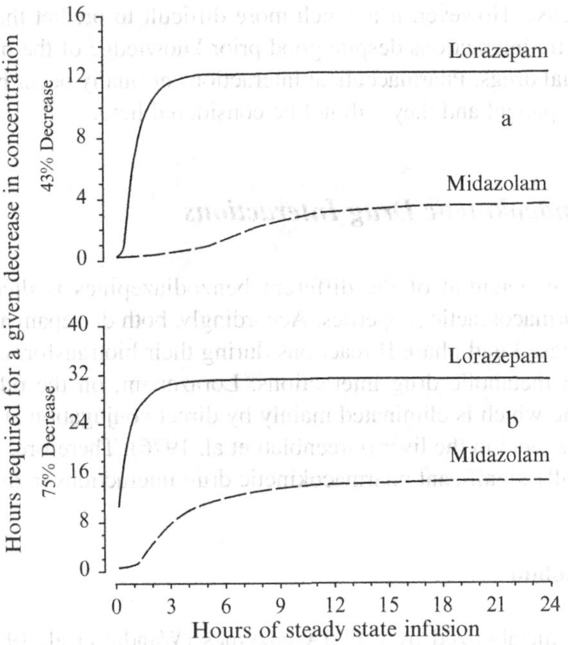

Fig. 7 Predicted time required for (*a*) a 43% decrease and (*b*) a 75% decrease in plasma benzodiazepine concentration as a function of the duration of the benzodiazepine infusion corresponding to the benzodiazepine concentration change required to emerge from light and deep sedation, respectively. (Modified with permission from Barr et al. 2001)

and empirical observations indicate that the relative concentration decrements for midazolam and lorazepam are not markedly different, the differences in emergence times are primarily due to different pharmacokinetics (Barr et al. 2001).

6 Drug Interactions

A drug interaction occurs when two or more drugs are given together. If the resulting pharmacological response is equal to the sum of the effects of the drugs given separately, drug interactions are unlikely to cause problems to clinicians. However, if the response is greater or smaller than the sum of the individual effects, the net result is much more difficult to anticipate. Although the clinical significance of drug interactions has been occasionally exaggerated, drug interactions are in some instances an important cause of drug toxicity. On the other hand, many drug interactions are beneficial and modern anaesthetic techniques depend on the utilization of such drug interactions. A sound combination of drugs helps clinicians to increase the efficacy and safety of drug treatment.

Drugs may interact on a pharmaceutical, pharmacokinetic or pharmacodynamic basis. A number of drugs may also interact simultaneously at several different sites. Many pharmacodynamic interactions are predictable and can be avoided by the use of common sense. However, it is much more difficult to predict the likelihood of pharmacokinetic interactions despite good prior knowledge of the pharmacokinetics of individual drugs. Pharmaceutical interactions normally occur before the drug is given to the patient and they will not be considered here.

6.1 Pharmacokinetic Drug Interactions

The interaction potential of the different benzodiazepines is dictated by their individual pharmacokinetic properties. Accordingly, both diazepam and midazolam undergoing phase I and phase II reactions during their biotransformation are more likely to have metabolic drug interactions. Lorazepam, on the other hand, is a benzodiazepine which is eliminated mainly by direct conjugation at the 3 position with glucuronic acid in the liver (Greenblatt et al. 1976). Therefore, it is less likely to have clinically significant pharmacokinetic drug interactions in man.

6.1.1 Midazolam

Midazolam is metabolized by CYP3A enzymes (Wandel et al. 1994) and it has been shown to have numerous clinically significant interactions with inhibitors and inducers of CYP3A4. It has a rather low oral bioavailability and therefore it is the oral route which is especially susceptible to metabolic drug interactions. However, inhibitors and inducers of CYP3A4 affect also intravenous midazolam. Erythromycin, fluconazole, itraconazole, saquinavir and voriconazole have been shown to reduce the clearance of intravenous midazolam in healthy volunteers by 50%–70% (Fig. 8). Accordingly, during continuous infusion, the concentrations of midazolam are expected to increase two- to threefold by strong inhibitors of CYP3A4 (Olkkola et al. 1993, 1996; Palkama et al. 1999; Saari et al. 2006). Long-term infusions of midazolam to patients receiving these inhibitors, e.g. during intensive care treatment, may result in undesirably long-lasting hypnotic effects if the dose is not titrated according to the effect. Propofol, an intravenous hypnotic used for the induction and maintenance of anaesthesia, also reduces the clearance of intravenous midazolam by 37% by inhibition of hepatic CYP3A4 (Hamaoka et al. 1999). Correspondingly, fentanyl decreases midazolam clearance by 30% (Hase et al. 1997). These interactions appear to be of minor clinical significance.

The data obtained from healthy volunteers is supported also by data in patients undergoing coronary artery bypass grafting and patients in intensive care (Ahonen et al. 1996a, 1999). Thirty patients undergoing coronary artery bypass grafting were randomly assigned to receive either diltiazem (60 mg orally and an infusion of 0.1 mg/kg per hour for 23 h) or placebo in a double-blind manner. Anaesthesia was induced with midazolam 0.1 mg/kg, alfentanil 50 μg/kg and propofol 20–80 mg and maintained with infusions of 1.0 μg/kg per minute of both midazolam and alfentanil supplemented with isoflurane until skin closure. Diltiazem increased the area under the midazolam concentration-time curve by 25% and that of alfentanil by 40%. Delayed elimination of midazolam and alfentanil was reflected also in pharmacodynamic variables because patients receiving diltiazem were extubated on the average 2.5 h later than those receiving placebo (Fig. 9).

Since the inhibitors change the pharmacokinetics of oral midazolam both by reducing the first-pass metabolism and by reducing elimination, they affect the pharmacokinetics of oral midazolam more than that of intravenous midazolam. Previous studies have shown that the above-mentioned inhibitors may cause up to a tenfold increase in the area under the midazolam concentration-time curve (Olkkola et al.

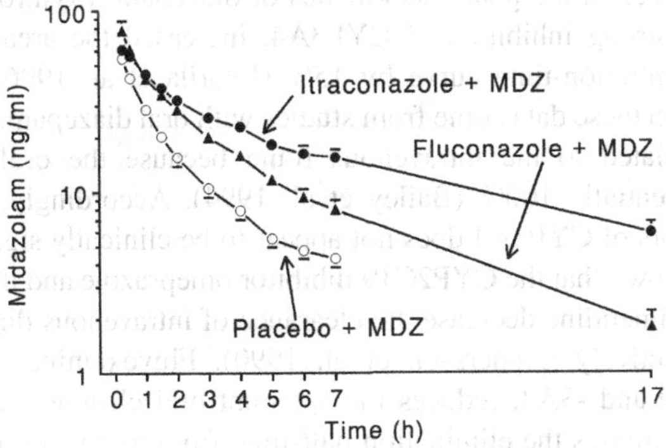

Fig. 8 Concentrations (mean±SEM) of midazolam (*MDZ*) in plasma after an intravenous dose of 0.05 mg/kg after pretreatment with itraconazole (200 mg), fluconazole (400 mg on the first day and then 200 mg), or placebo for 6 days to 12 healthy volunteers. The intravenous dose of midazolam was given on the fourth day of pretreatment. (Modified with permission from Olkkola et al. 1996)

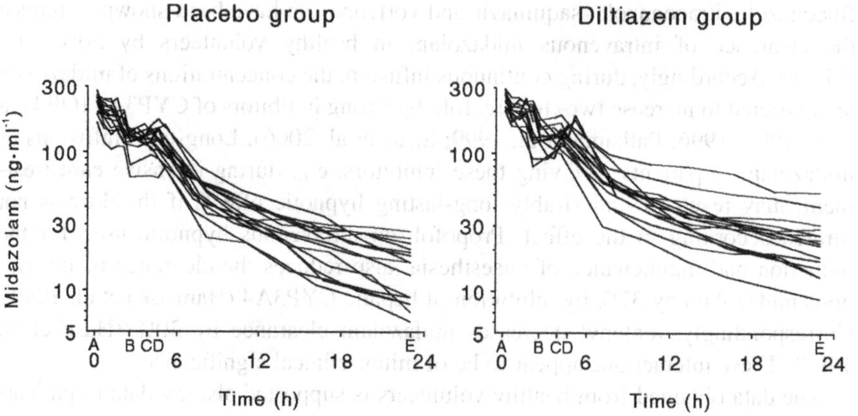

Fig. 9 Midazolam and alfentanil plasma concentrations during and after anaesthesia in 15 coronary artery bypass grafting (CPB) patients receiving diltiazem and in 15 patients receiving placebo. *A*, induction of anaesthesia; *B*, initiation of CPB (average); *C*, end of CPB (average); *D*, end of anaesthesia (average); and *E*, end of diltiazem or placebo infusion. (Modified with permission from Ahonen et al. 1996a)

1993, 1996; Palkama et al. 1999; Saari et al. 2006). The inducers of CYP3A4 cause a profound increase in the elimination midazolam (Backman et al. 1996, 1998). Midazolam is also susceptible to interact with other drugs affecting CYP3A4.

6.1.2 Diazepam

Diazepam is metabolized primarily by CYP2C19 and -3A4 isoenzymes (Bertz and Granneman 1997) and on theoretical basis it is likely to interact with drugs affecting the activity of these isoenzymes. Even strong inhibitors of CYP3A4 appear to have only a minor effect on the pharmacokinetics of diazepam. Erythromycin and itraconazole, both strong inhibitors of CYP3A4, increased the area under the oral diazepam concentration-time curve by 15% (Luurila et al. 1996; Ahonen et al. 1996b). Although these data come from studies with oral diazepam, the results may also be extrapolated to the intravenous route because the oral bioavailability diazepam is essentially 100% (Bailey et al. 1994). Accordingly, the interaction between inhibitors of CYP3A4 does not appear to be clinically significant.

It has been shown that the CYP2C19 inhibitor omeprazole and the CYP1A2 and -3A4 inhibitor cimetidine decrease the clearance of intravenous diazepam by 27% and 38%, respectively (Andersson et al. 1990). Fluvoxamine, an inhibitor of CYP1A2, -2C19 and -3A4, reduces the apparent oral clearance of diazepam by 65% and also increases the elimination half-time from 51 to 118 h (Perucca et al. 1994). Thus, the interactions of the strong inhibitors of CYP2C19 and diazepam seem to be clinically significant when diazepam is administered for a longer period. When single bolus doses of intravenous diazepam are used, these interactions are unlikely to be clinically significant.

Interestingly, ciprofloxacin, an inhibitor of CYP1A2, also delays the elimination of intravenous diazepam. Seven-day treatment with ciprofloxacin reduced diazepam clearance by 37% and prolonged the elimination half-time from 37 to 71 h (Kamali et al. 1993). No changes in drug effect were observed. In contrast, rifampicin, an inducer of many cytochromal enzymes increased diazepam clearance by 200%. Thus, the diazepam dose must be increased in patients on rifampicin (Ohnhaus et al. 1987).

6.1.3 Lorazepam

Unlike the other two benzodiazepine agonists, lorazepam is mainly eliminated by direct conjugation with glucuronic acid. It is therefore plausible that it has few pharmacokinetic interactions with other drugs. Probenecid decreases lorazepam clearance by 50% by decreasing the formation clearance of lorazepam-glucuronide (Abernethy et al. 1985). Valproic acid seems to affect the pharmacokinetics of lorazepam with the same mechanism (Samara et al. 1997).

6.1.4 Flumazenil

So far no pharmacokinetic interactions have been reported with flumazenil.

6.2 Pharmacodynamic Drug Interactions

Although pharmacokinetic drug interactions are of academic interest and are also in some cases clinically significant, pharmacodynamic interactions are far more common and have greater significance in anaesthetic practice. Many pharmacodynamic interactions are predictable and can be avoided by the use of common sense and good knowledge of pharmacology. However, in most cases pharmacodynamic drug interactions can be regarded as desirable because a sound combination of drugs having synergistic effects may facilitate the use of smaller and less toxic doses of the individual drugs.

All benzodiazepines act on the central nervous system and they interact with other drugs acting on the central nervous system too. When the interaction between morphine and midazolam is quantified by their sedative effect, the effects of these two drugs are additive (Tverskoy et al. 1989). However, the interactions between the benzodiazepines and opioids are usually considered synergistic. Vinik et al. (1994) studied the hypnotic effects of propofol, midazolam, alfentanil and their binary and triple combinations. The ratios of a single-drug fractional dose (ED_{50}=1.0) to a combined fractional dose (in fractions of single-drug ED_{50} values). thus indicating the degree of supra-additivity (synergism), were: 1.4 for propofol–alfentanil, 1.8 for midazolam–propofol, 2.8 for midazolam–alfentanil, and 2.6 for propofol–midazolam–alfentanil (Fig. 10). Accordingly, the propofol–midazolam–alfentanil

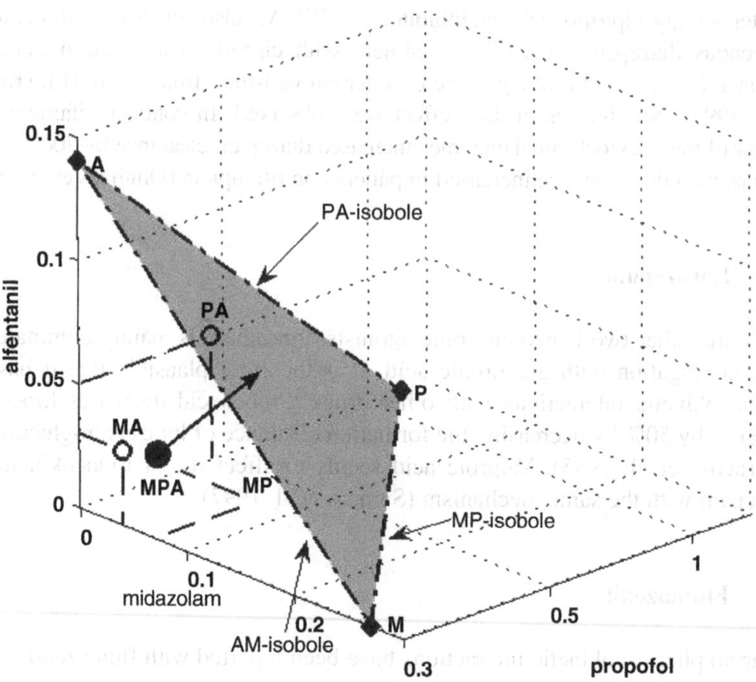

Fig. 10 Binary versus triple synergism: ED_{50} isobolograms for the hypnotic interactions among midazolam (M), alfentanil and propofol (P). The shaded area shows the additive plane passing through three single drug ED_{50} (solid diamonds A,M,P). The boundaries of the plane are binary additive isoboles. The open circles are measured ED_{50} points for the binary combinations (MA, MP, PA) and the solid circle is the measured ED_{50} point for the triple combination (MPA). The ratio (*R*) of the single-drug dose (ED_{50}=1) to combined fractional dose (in fractions of single-drug ED_{50} values), reflects the degree of synergism. All measured interaction values are significantly different from the additive effect. (Data from Vinik HR, Bradley EL Jr, Kissin I (1994) Triple anesthetic combination: propofolmidazolam-alfentanil. Anesth Analg 78:354-358).

interaction produced a profound hypnotic synergism which is not significantly different from that of the binary midazolam–alfentanil combination.

The interaction between midazolam and ketamine is additive (Hong et al. 1993). The lack of synergism has been regarded as most likely due to the different mechanisms of action of ketamine and midazolam. Ketamine inhibits excitatory transmission by decreasing the depolarization through the blockade of *N*-methyl-d-aspartate (NMDA) receptors. Thiopental, propofol and midazolam exert their general effects by the allosteric modulation of the $GABA_A$ receptors. Thus, the interactions between the hypnotic effects of midazolam and thiopental (Short et al. 1991) and propofol and midazolam are synergistic (McClune et al. 1992).

Xanthines are mainly used for asthma and chronic obstructive pulmonary disease. Besides bronchodilating effects, they also stimulate the central nervous system. Intravenous aminophylline is able to reverse at least partially the sedation from intravenous diazepam (Arvidsson et al. 1982). This interaction appears to be due to the blockade of adenosine receptors by aminophylline (Niemand et al. 1984).

7 Clinical Use

7.1 Midazolam

Midazolam is mainly used for sedation in minor investigative or surgical procedures, premedication, induction of general anaesthesia, and sedation in intensive care unit (ICU) patients. Anxiolysis, amnesia, sedation and hypnosis are desirable benzodiazepine properties (de Jong and Bonin 1981; Reves et al. 1985). The ability of midazolam to reduce anxiety and to provide amnesia has been demonstrated reliably over a range of doses administered by various routes (Reinhart et al. 1985; Barker et al. 1986; Forrest et al. 1987). The effects of midazolam and other benzodiazepines on memory are anterograde; the retrograde memory is not affected. It is desirable that the duration of amnesia is not much longer than the duration of the procedure and the period of sedation or anaesthesia. The intensity and duration of amnesia following intravenous administration of midazolam appears to be dose-dependent. After an anaesthetic induction dose the amnestic period is 1–2 h (Langlois et al. 1987; Miller et al. 1989). Typical of benzodiazepines, during sedation the volunteers or the patients seem conscious and coherent, yet they are amnestic for events and procedures (George and Dundee 1977). Compared with intravenously administered midazolam, at identical plasma concentrations of the drug, an oral dose produces more marked effects due to the higher plasma concentrations of the active metabolite alpha-hydroxymidazolam (Crevoisier et al. 1983; Mandema et al. 1992).

A usual total dose for sedation in minor surgical and other procedures in adults varies between 2.5 and 7.5 mg intravenously. An initial dose of 2 mg over 30 s has been suggested supplemented with incremental doses of 0.5–1 mg at intervals of about 2 min if required. The usual dose for induction of anaesthesia is between 0.1 and 0.2 mg/kg in pre-medicated patients and 0.3 mg/kg in patients with no premedication. After intravenous administration, the onset of action of midazolam occurs usually within 30–60 s. The half-time of equilibration between the plasma concentration and the EEG effects is approximately 2–3 min (Breimer et al. 1990). In well pre-medicated patients, an induction dose of 0.2 mg/kg of midazolam given in 5–15 s induced anaesthesia in 28 s, whereas when diazepam at 0.5 mg/kg was also given in 5–15 s induction occurred in 39 s (Samuelson et al. 1981). Due to a synergistic interaction, concurrent administration of other intravenous anaesthetics reduces the induction dose of midazolam and vice versa; even sub-hypnotic doses of midazolam reduce the induction dose of thiopental, for example, by more than 50%. Synergism is strongest in patients who are relatively insensitive to thiopental (Vinik and Kissin 1990; Vinik 1995). Administration of midazolam for premedication and induction of anaesthesia should be undertaken cautiously in the elderly, who are more sensitive to the sedative effects than younger individuals (Gamble et al. 1981; Jacobs et al. 1995).

Emergence from anaesthesia depends on the dose of midazolam and on the administration of adjuvant anaesthetics (Reves et al. 1985). The emergence from a midazolam dose of 0.32 mg/kg supplemented with fentanyl is about 10 min longer than from a thiopental dose of 4.75 mg/kg supplemented with fentanyl (Reves et al. 1979). Maintenance infusions of midazolam have been used for anaesthesia or sedation (Theil et al. 1993; Barvais et al. 1994; Barr et al. 2001). The termination of action of the benzodiazepines is primarily a result of their redistribution from the central nervous system to other tissues (Greenblatt et al. 1983). After a continuous infusion, however, blood levels of midazolam will decrease more rapidly than those of the other benzodiazepines due to the greater clearance of midazolam. As stated above, the context-sensitive decrement times rather than the elimination half-time can be used to assess the emergence from an infusion anaesthetic (Hughes et al. 1992; Bailey 1995; Keifer and Glass 1999).

7.2 *Diazepam*

Diazepam is very effective in relieving anxiety before surgery. Diazepam has amnestic properties but it is less effective in this regard than midazolam (Pandit et al. 1971). However, amnesia is more profound when diazepam is combined with other drugs, e.g. with opioids (Dundee and Pandit 1972).

For sedation in minor investigative or surgical procedures, an intravenous dose of 0.1–0.2 mg/kg of diazepam is recommended. At equal plasma levels of diazepam, elderly patients are more sensitive to the depressant effects of diazepam than younger individuals (Reidenberg et al. 1978). The effects of various doses of intravenous diazepam and midazolam on clinical sedation and psychomotor performance have been studied in healthy volunteers. The maximal effects seen after 0.3 mg/kg of diazepam do not reach those of 0.1 mg/kg of midazolam. The effects of midazolam, however, disappear sooner than those of diazepam (Nuotto et al. 1992). After intravenous administration of 0.15 mg/kg of diazepam in healthy volunteers, the duration of diazepam effect, based on a statistically significant difference over the predrug baseline EEG values, is 5–6 h compared with 2.5 h after administration of 0.1 mg/kg of midazolam. When the effect of benzodiazepines is quantified by EEG, diazepam has an EC_{50} value of 269 ng/ml and midazolam 35 ng/ml, respectively (Greenblatt et al. 1989). This difference indicates a greater potency of midazolam compared with diazepam, which is in good agreement with the results of different pharmacodynamic tests (Nuotto et al. 1992). Due to the extremely long context-sensitive half-time of diazepam, it is not suitable to be administered by continuous infusion for the maintenance of anaesthesia or sedation (Reves et al. 1994).

7.3 *Lorazepam*

Lorazepam has been shown to be an effective anxiolytic and amnestic agent (Fragen and Caldwell 1976). A dose of 2–3 mg may be useful for anxious patients given the night before the operation followed by a smaller dose before the procedure.

Alternatively, 2–4 mg may be given about 2 h before surgery. A dose of 0.05 mg/kg may be administered 30–45 min before the operation if given intravenously. With doses of 4 mg, amnesia persists for 4 h (Pandit et al. 1976). Due to the long-lasting amnestic effect of lorazepam, it is widely used for oral premedication and as an intravenous anaesthetic adjuvant in coronary artery bypass graft surgery. In intensive care, continuous infusions of lorazepam are used for sedation during mechanical ventilation (Barr et al. 2001). Using a target-controlled infusion pump, the initial target plasma concentration of 50 ng/ml has been used. Subsequently, the infusion is titrated according to the level of sedation sought (Barr et al. 2001).

7.4 Flumazenil

A slow intravenous injection of flumazenil can be used to reverse the benzodiazepine-induced sedation as well as to diagnose or treat benzodiazepine overdose. The initial dose for the reversal of benzodiazepine-induced sedation is 0.2 mg, followed by further doses of 0.1–0.2 mg at intervals of 60 s if needed. The total dose should be not more than 1 mg or occasionally 2 mg. If drowsiness recurs, an intravenous infusion of 0.1–0.4 mg per hour may be used (Brogden and Goa 1991).

References

Abernethy DR, Greenblatt DJ, Divoll M, Shader RI (1983) Prolonged accumulation of diazepam in obesity. J Clin Pharmacol 23:369–376

Abernethy DR, Greenblatt DJ, Ameer B, Shader RI (1985) Probenecid impairment of acetaminophen and lorazepam clearance: direct inhibition of ether glucuronide formation. J Pharmacol Exp Ther 234:345–349

Ahonen J, Olkkola KT, Hynynen M, Salmenperä M, Neuvonen PJ (1996a) Effect of diltiazem on midazolam and alfentanil disposition in patients undergoing coronary artery bypass grafting. Anesthesiology 85:1246–1252

Ahonen J, Olkkola KT, Neuvonen PJ (1996b) The effect of the anti-mycotic itraconazole on the pharmacokinetics and pharmacodynamics of diazepam. Fundam Clin Pharmacol 10:314–318

Ahonen J, Olkkola KT, Takala A, Neuvonen PJ (1999) Interaction between fluconazole and midazolam in intensive care patients. Acta Anaesthesiol Scand 43:509–514

Alexander CM, Gross JB (1988) Sedative doses of midazolam depress hypoxic ventilatory responses in humans. Anesth Analg 67:377–382

Allonen H, Ziegler G, Klotz U (1981) Midazolam kinetics. Clin Pharmacol Ther 30:653–661

Andersson T, Andren K, Cederberg C, Edvardsson G, Heggelund A, Lundborg P (1990) Effect of omeprazole and cimetidine on plasma diazepam levels. Eur J Clin Pharmacol 39:51–54

Andersson T, Miners JO, Veronese ME, Birkett DJ (1994) Diazepam metabolism by human liver microsomes is mediated both by S-mephenytoin hydroxylase and CYP3A isoforms. Br J Clin Pharmacol 38:131–137

Arvidsson SB, Ekstrom-Jodal B, Martinell SA, Niemand D (1982) Aminophylline antagonises diazepam sedation. Lancet 2:1467

Backman JT, Olkkola KT, Ojala M, Laaksovirta H, Neuvonen PJ (1996) Concentrations and effects of oral midazolam are greatly reduced in patients treated with carbamazepine or phenytoin. Epilepsia 37:253–257

Backman JT, Kivistö KT, Olkkola KT, Neuvonen PJ (1998) The area under the plasma concentration-time curve for oral midazolam is 400-fold larger during treatment with itraconazole than with rifampicin. Eur J Clin Pharmacol 54:53–58

Bailey JM (1995) Technique for quantifying the duration of intravenous anesthetic effect. Anesthesiology 83:1095–1103

Bailey L, Ward M, Musa MN (1994) Clinical pharmacokinetics of benzodiazepines. J Clin Pharmacol 34:804–811

Barker I, Butchart DGM, Gibson J, Lawson JIM, Mackenzie N (1986) IV sedation for conservative dentistry. A comparison of midazolam and diazepam. Br J Anaesth 58:371–377

Barr J, Zomorodi K, Bertaccini EJ, Shafer SL (2001) A double-blind, randomized comparison of IV lorazepam versus midazolam for sedation of ICU patients via a pharmacologic model. Anesthesiology 95:286–298

Barvais L, D'Hollander AA, Cantraine F, Coussaert E, Diamon G (1994) Predictive accuracy of midazolam in adult patients scheduled for coronary surgery. J Clin Anesth 6:297–302

Bauer TM, Haberthür C, Ha HR, Hunkeler W, Sleight AJ, Scollo-Lavizarri G, Haefeli WE (1995) Prolonged sedation due to accumulation of conjugated metabolites of midazolam. Lancet 346:145–147

Bertz RJ, Granneman GR (1997) Use of in vitro and in vivo data to estimate the likelihood of metabolic pharmacokinetic interactions. Clin Pharmacokinet 32:210–258

Bozkurt P, Kaya G, Suzer O, Senturk H (1996) Diazepam serum concentration-sedative effect relationship in patients with liver disease. Middle East J Anesthesiol 13:405–413

Breimer LTM, Hennis PJ, Burm AGL, Danhof M, Bovill JG, Spierdijk J, Vletter AA (1990) Quantification of the EEG effects of midazolam by a periodic analysis in volunteers. Pharmacokinetic/pharmacodynamic modelling. Clin Pharmacokinet 18:245–253

Breimer LTM, Hennis PJ, Burm AGL, Danhof M, Bovill JG, Spierdijk J, Vletter AA (1991) Pharmacokinetics and EEG effects of flumazenil in volunteers. Clin Pharmacokinet 20:491–496

Brogden RN, Goa KL (1991) Flumazenil: a reappraisal of its pharmacological properties and therapeutic efficacy as a benzodiazepine antagonist. Drugs 42:1061–1089

Coldwell SE, Kaufman E, Milgrom P, Kharasch ED, Chen P, Mautz D, Ramsay DS (1998) Acute tolerance and reversal of the motor control effects of midazolam. Pharmacol Biochem Behav 59:537–545

Crevoisier CH, Ziegler WH, Eckert M, Heizmann P (1983) Relationship between plasma concentration and effect of midazolam after oral and intravenous administration. Br J Clin Pharmacol 16:S51–S61

Dasberg HM (1975) Effects and plasma concentrations of desmethyldiazepam after oral administration in normal volunteers. Psychopharmacologia 43:191–198

de Jong RH, Bonin JD (1981) Benzodiazepines protect mice from local anaesthetic convulsions and deaths. Anesth Analg 60:385–389

Dingemanse J, van Gerven JMA, Schoemaker RC, Roncari G, Oberyé JJL, van Oostenbruggen MF, Massarella J, Segala P, Zell M, Cohen AF (1997a) Integrated pharmacokinetics and pharmacodynamics of Ro 48-6791, a new benzodiazepine, in comparison with midazolam during first administration to healthy male subjects. Br J Clin Pharmacol 44:477–486

Dingemanse J, Häussler J, Hering W, Ihmsen H, Albrecht S, Zell M, Schwilden H, Schüttler J (1997b) Pharmacokinetic-pharmacodynamic modelling of the EEG effects of Ro 48-6791, a new short-acting benzodiazepine, in young and elderly subjects. Br J Anaesth 79:567–574

Dollery C (1991) Therapeutic drugs. Churchill Livingstone, London

Dundee JW (1987) Pharmacokinetics of midazolam. Br J Clin Pharmacol 23:591–592

Dundee JW, Pandit SK (1972) Anterograde amnesic effects of pethidine, hyoscine and diazepam in adults. Br J Pharmacol 44:140–144

Dundee JW, Halliday NJ, Harper KW, Brogden RN (1984a) Midazolam. A review of its pharmacological properties and therapeutic use. Drugs 28:519–554

Dundee JW, Halliday NJ, Loughran PG (1984b) Variance in response to midazolam. Br J Clin Pharmacol 17:645–646

Elliott HW (1976) Metabolism of lorazepam. Br J Anaesth 48:1017–1023
Fiset P, Lemmens HL, Egan TE, Shafer SL, Stanski DR (1995) Pharmacodynamic modeling of the electroencephalographic effects of flumazenil in healthy volunteers sedated with midazolam. Clin Pharmacol Ther 58:567–582
Forrest P, Galletly DC, Yee P (1987) Placebo controlled comparison of midazolam, triazolam, and diazepam as oral premedicants for outpatient anesthesia. Anaesth Intensive Care 15:296–304
Forster A, Juge O, Morel D (1982) Effects of midazolam on cerebral blood flow in human volunteers. Anesthesiology 56:453–455
Fragen RJ, Caldwell N (1976) Lorazepam premedication: lack of recall and relief of anxiety. Anesth Analg 55:792–796
Gamble JAS, Kawar P, Dundee JW, Moore J, Briggs LP (1981) Evaluation of midazolam as an intravenous induction agent. Anesthesiology 36:868–873
George KA, Dundee JW (1977) Relative amnestic actions of diazepam, flunitrazepam, and lorazepam in man. Br J Clin Pharmacol 4:45–50
Gerecke M (1983) Chemical structure and properties of midazolam compared with other benzodiazepines. Br J Clin Pharmacol 16:11S–16S
Greenblatt D, Shader R (1974) Benzodiazepines in clinical practice. Raven Press, New York
Greenblatt DJ (1981) Clinical pharmacokinetics of oxazepam and lorazepam. Clin Pharmacokinet 6:89–105
Greenblatt DJ, Shader RI (1978) Dependence, tolerance, and addiction to benzodiazepines: clinical and pharmacokinetic considerations. Drug Metab Rev 8:13–28
Greenblatt DJ, Schillings RT, Kyriakopoulos AA, Shader RI, Sisenwine SF, Knowles JA, Ruelius HW (1976) Clinical pharmacokinetics of lorazepam. I. Absorption and disposition of oral 14C-lorazepam. Clin Pharmacol Ther 20:329–341
Greenblatt DJ, Shader RI, Franke K (1979) Pharmacokinetics and bioavailability of intravenous, intramuscular, and oral lorazepam in humans. J Pharm Sci 68:57–63
Greenblatt DJ, Allen MD, Harmatz JS, Shader RI (1980) Diazepam disposition determinants. Clin Pharmacol Ther 27:301–312
Greenblatt DJ, Shader RI, Abernethy DR (1983) Drug therapy. Current status of benzodiazepines. N Engl J Med 309:410–416
Greenblatt DJ, Abernethy DR, Locniskar A, Harmatz JS, Limjuco RA, Shader RI (1984) Effect of age, gender, and obesity in midazolam kinetics. Anesthesiology 61:27–35
Greenblatt DJ, Divoll MK, Soong MH, Boxenbaum HG, Harmatz JS, Shader RI (1988) Desmethyldiazepam pharmacokinetics: studies following intravenous and oral desmethyldiazepam and clorazepate, and intravenous diazepam. J Clin Pharmacol 28:853–859
Greenblatt DJ, Ehrenberg BL, Gunderman J, Locniskar A, Scavone JM, Harmatz JS, Shader RI (1989) Pharmacokinetic and electroencephalographic study of intravenous diazepam, midazolam, and placebo. Clin Pharmacol Ther 45:356–365
Hall ED, Fleck TJ, Oostveen JA (1998) Comparative neuroprotective properties of the benzodiazepine receptor full agonist diazepam and the partial agonist PNU-101017 in the gerbil forebrain ischemia model. Brain Res 798:325–329
Hall RI, Schwieger IM, Hug CC (1988) The anesthetic efficacy of midazolam in enflurane-anesthetized dog. Anesthesiology 68:862–866
Hamaoka N, Oda Y, Hase I, Mizutani K, Nakamoto T, Ishizaki T, Asada A (1999) Propofol decreases the clearance of midazolam by inhibiting CYP3A4: an in vivo and in vitro study. Clin Pharmacol Ther 66:110–117
Harper KW, Collier PS, Dundee JW, Elliott P, Halliday NJ, Lowry KG (1985) Age and nature of operation influence the pharmacokinetics of midazolam. Br J Anaesth 57:866–871
Hase I, Oda Y, Tanaka K, Mizutani K, Nakamoto T, Asada A (1997) I.v. fentanyl decreases the clearance of midazolam. Br J Anaesth 79:740–743
Heizmann P, Eckert M, Ziegler WH (1983) Pharmacokinetics and bioavailability of midazolam in man. Br J Clin Pharmacol 16:S43–S49
Hong W, Short TG, Hui TW (1993) Hypnotic and anesthetic interactions between ketamine and midazolam in female patients. Anesthesiology 79:1227–1232

Hughes MA, Glass PSA, Jacobs JR (1992) Context-sensitive half-time in multicompartment pharmacokinetic model for intravenous anesthetic drugs. Anesthesiology 76:334–341

Ihmsen H, Albrecht S, Hering W, Schuttler J, Schwilden H (2004) Modelling acute tolerance to the EEG effect of two benzodiazepines. Br J Clin Pharmacol 57:153–161

Inaba T, Tait A, Nakano M, Mahon WA, Kalow W (1988) Metabolism of diazepam in vitro by human liver: independent variability of N-demethylation and C3-hydroxylation. Drug Metab Dispos 16:605–608

Ito H, Watanabe Y, Isshiki A, Uchino H (1999) Neuroprotective properties of propofol and midazolam, but not pentobarbital, on neuronal damage induced by forebrain ischemia, based on the $GABA_A$ receptors. Acta Anaesthesiol Scand 43:153–162

Jack ML, Colburn WA (1983) Pharmacokinetic model for diazepam and its major metabolite desmethyldiazepam following diazepam administration. J Pharm Sci 73:1318–1323

Jacobs JR, Reves JG, Marty J, White WD, Bai SA, Smith LR (1995) Aging increases pharmacodynamic sensitivity to the hypnotic effects of midazolam. Anesth Analg 80:143–148

Kamali F, Thomas SH, Edwards C (1993) The influence of steady-state ciprofloxacin on the pharmacokinetics and pharmacodynamics of a single dose of diazepam in healthy volunteers. Eur J Clin Pharmacol 44:365–367

Kassai A, Toth G, Eichelbaum M, Klotz U (1988) No evidence of a genetic polymorphism in the oxidative metabolism of midazolam. Clin Pharmacokinet 15:319–325

Kato R, Yamazoe Y (1994) The importance of substrate concentration in determining cytochromes P450 therapeutically relevant in vivo. Pharmacogenetics 4:359–362

Keifer J, Glass PSA (1999) Context-sensitive half-time and anesthesia: how does theory match reality? Curr Opin Anaesthesiol 12:443–448

Klotz U, Kanto J (1988) Pharmacokinetics and clinical use of flumazenil (Ro 15–1788). Clin Pharmacokinet 14:1–12

Klotz U, Reimann I (1980) Delayed clearance of diazepam due to cimetidine. N Engl J Med 302:1012–1014

Kraus JW, Desmond PV, Marshall JP, Johnson RF, Schenker S, Wilkinson GR (1978) Effects of aging and liver disease on disposition of lorazepam. Clin Pharmacol Ther 24:411–419

Luurila H, Olkkola KT, Neuvonen PJ (1996) An interaction between erythromycin and the benzodiazepines diazepam and flunitrazepam. Pharmacol Toxicol 78:117–122

MacLeod SM, Giles HG, Bengert B (1979) Age- and gender-related differences in diazepam pharmacokinetics. J Clin Pharmacol 19:15–19

Mandelli M, Tognoni G, Garattini S (1978) Clinical pharmacokinetics of diazepam. Clin Pharmacokinet 3:72–91

Mandema JW, Tuk B, van Stevenick AL, Breimer DD, Cohen AF, Danhof M (1992) Pharmacokinetic-pharmacodynamic modelling of the central nervous system effects of midazolam and its main metabolite α-hydroxymidazolam in healthy volunteers. Clin Pharmacol Ther 51:715–728

Marty J, Gauzit R, Lefevre P, Couderc E, Farinotti R, Henzel C, Desmonts JM (1986) Effects of diazepam and midazolam on baroreflex control of heart rate and on sympathetic activity in humans. Anesth Analg 65:113–119

McClune S, McKay AC, Wright PM, Patterson CC, Clarke RS (1992) Synergistic interaction between midazolam and propofol. Br J Anaesth 69:240–245

Miller LG (1991) Chronic benzodiazepine administration: from the patient to the gene. J Clin Pharmacol 31:492–495

Miller RI, Bullard DE, Patrissi GA (1989) Duration of amnesia associated with midazolam/fentanyl intravenous sedation. J Oral Maxillofac Surg 47:155–158

Möhler H, Fritschy JM, Rudolp U (2002) A new benzodiazepine pharmacology. J Pharmacol Exp Ther 300:2–8

Morrison G, Chiang ST, Koepke HH, Walker BR (1984) Effect of renal impairment and hemodialysis on lorazepam kinetics. Clin Pharmacol Ther 35:646–652

Mould DR, DeFeo TM, Reele S, Milla G, Limjuco R, Crews T, Choma N, Patel IH (1995) Simultaneous modeling of the pharmacokinetics and pharmacodynamics of midazolam and diazepam. Clin Pharmacol Ther 58:35–43

Niemand D, Martinell S, Arvidsson S, Svedmyr N, Ekstrom-Jodal B (1984) Aminophylline inhibition of diazepam sedation: is adenosine blockade of GABA-receptors the mechanism? Lancet 1:463–464

Norton JR, Ward DS, Karan S, Voter WA, Palmer L, Varlese A, Rackovsky O, Bailey P (2006) Differences between midazolam and propofol sedation on upper airway collapsibility using dynamic negative airway pressure. Anesthesiology 104:1155–1164

Nuotto EJ, Korttila KT, Lichtor JL, Östman PL, Rupani G (1992) Sedation and recovery of psychomotor function after intravenous administration of various doses of midazolam and diazepam. Anesth Analg 74:265–271

Ochs HR, Greenblatt DJ, Kaschell HJ, Klehr U, Divoll M, Abernethy DR (1981) Diazepam kinetics in patients with renal insufficiency or hyperthyroidism. Br J Clin Pharmacol 12:829–832

Ochs HR, Greenblatt DJ, Eckardt B, Harmatz JS, Shader RI (1983) Repeated diazepam dosing in cirrhotic patients: cumulation and sedation. Clin Pharmacol Ther 33:471–476

Ohnhaus EE, Brockmeyer N, Dylewicz P, Habicht H (1987) The effect of antipyrine and rifampin on the metabolism of diazepam. Clin Pharmacol Ther 42:148–156

Olkkola KT, Aranko K, Luurila H, Hiller A, Saarnivaara L, Himberg JJ, Neuvonen PJ (1993) A potentially hazardous interaction between erythromycin and midazolam. Clin Pharmacol Ther 53:298–305

Olkkola KT, Ahonen J, Neuvonen PJ (1996) The effect of the systemic antimycotics, itraconazole and fluconazole, on the pharmacokinetics and pharmacodynamics of intravenous and oral midazolam. Anesth Analg 82:511–516

Palkama V, Neuvonen PJ, Olkkola KT (1999) Effect of saquinavir on the pharmacokinetics and -dynamics of oral and intravenous midazolam. Clin Pharmacol Ther 66:33–39

Pandit GR, Heisterkamp DV, Cohen PJ (1976) Further studies on the antirecall effect of lorazepam: a dose dose-time-effect relationship. Anesthesiology 45:495–500

Pandit SK, Dundee JW, Keilly SR (1971) Amnesia studies with intravenous premedication. Anaesthesia 26:421–428

Park GR, Manara AR, Dawling S (1989) Extra-hepatic metabolism of midazolam. Br J Clin Pharmacol 27:634–637

Pentikäinen PJ, Välisalmi L, Himberg JJ, Crevoicier C (1989) Pharmacokinetics of midazolam following intravenous and oral administration in patients with chronic liver disease and in healthy subjects. J Clin Pharmacol 29:272–277

Perucca E, Gatti G, Cipolla G, Spina E, Barel S, Soback S, Gips M, Bialer M (1994) Inhibition of diazepam metabolism by fluvoxamine: a pharmacokinetic study in normal volunteers. Clin Pharmacol Ther 56:471–476

Reidenberg MM, Levy M, Warner H, Coutinho CP, Schwartz MA, Yu G, Cheripko J (1978) Relationship between diazepam dose, plasma level, age, and central nervous system depression. Clin Pharmacol Ther 23:371–374

Reinhart K, Dallinger-Stiller G, Dennhardt R, Heinemeyer G, Eyrich K (1985) Comparison of midazolam, diazepam and placebo IM as premedication for regional anaesthesia: a randomized double-blind study. Br J Anaesth 57:294–299

Reves JG, Vinik R, Hirschfield AM, Holcomb C, Strong S (1979) Midazolam compared with thiopentone as a hypnotic component in balanced anesthesia: a randomized, double-blind study. Can Anaesth Soc J 26:42–49

Reves JG, Fragen RJ, Vinik HR, Greenblatt DJ (1985) Midazolam: pharmacology and uses. Anesthesiology 62:310–324

Reves JG, Glass PSA, Lubarsky DA (1994) Nonbarbiturate intravenous anesthetics. In: Miller RD (ed) Anesthesia. Churchill Livingstone, New York, p 250

Ruff R, Reves JG (1990) Hemodynamic effects of lorazepam-fentanyl anesthetic induction for coronary artery bypass surgery. J Cardiothorac Anesth 4:314–317

Saari TI, Laine K, Leino K, Valtonen M, Neuvonen PJ, Olkkola KT (2006) Effect of voriconazole on the pharmacokinetics of oral and intravenous midazolam. Clin Pharmacol Ther 794:362–370

Samara EE, Granneman RG, Witt GF, Cavanaugh JH (1997) Effect of valproate on the pharmacokinetics and pharmacodynamics of lorazepam. J Clin Pharmacol 37:442–450

Samuelson PN, Reves JG, Kouchoukos NT, Smith LR, Dole KM (1981) Hemodynamic responses to anesthetic induction with midazolam or diazepam in patients with ischemic heart disease. Anesth Analg 60:802–809
Shafer A (1998) Complications of sedation with midazolam in the intensive care unit and a comparison with other sedative regimens. Crit Care Med 26:947–956
Shafer SL, Varvel JR (1991) Pharmacokinetics, pharmacodynamics, and rational opioid selection. Anesthesiology 74:53–63
Shelly MP, Sultan MA, Bodenham A, Park GR (1991) Midazolam infusions in critically ill patients. Eur J Anaesthesiol 8:21–27
Short TG, Galletly DC, Plummer JL (1991) Hypnotic and anaesthetic action of thiopentone and midazolam alone and in combination. Br J Anaesth 66:13–19
Somma J, Donner A, Zomorodi K, Sladen R, Ramsay J, Geller E, Shafer SL (1998) Population pharmacodynamics of midazolam administered by target controlled infusion in SICU patients after CABG surgery. Anesthesiology 89:1430–1443
Stovner J, Endresen R (1965) Diazepam in intravenous anaesthesia. Lancet 2:1298–1299
Sunzel M, Paalzow L, Berggren L, Eriksson I (1988) Respiratory and cardiovascular effects in relation to plasma levels of midazolam and diazepam. Br J Clin Pharmacol 25:561–569
Theil DR, Stanley TE, White WD, Goodman DK, Glass PS, Bai SA, Jacobs JR, Reves JG (1993) Midazolam and fentanyl continuous infusion anesthesia for cardiac surgery: a comparison of computer-assisted versus manual infusion systems. J Cardiothorac Vasc Anesth 7:300–306
Tietz EI, Chiu TH, Rosenberg HC (1989) Regional GABA/benzodiazepine receptor/chloride channel coupling after acute and chronic benzodiazepine treatment. Eur J Pharmacol 167:57–65
Tverskoy M, Fleyshman G, Ezry J, Bradley EL Jr, Kissin I (1989) Midazolam-morphine sedative interaction in patients. Anesth Analg 68:282–285
Vinik HR (1995) Intravenous anesthetic drug interactions: practical applications. Eur J Anaesthesiol 12:S13–S19
Vinik HR, Kissin I (1990) Midazolam for coinduction of thiopental anesthesia. Anesthesiology 73:A1216
Vinik HR, Bradley EL Jr, Kissin I (1994) Triple anesthetic combination: propofol-midazolam-alfentanil. Anesth Analg 78:354–358
Wandel C, Böcker R, Böhrer H, Browne A, Rügheimer E, Martin E (1994) Midazolam is metabolized by at least three different cytochrome P450 enzymes. Br J Anaesth 73:658–661
Wills RJ, Khoo KC, Soni PP, Patel IH (1990) Increased volume of distribution prolongs midazolam half-life. Br J Clin Pharmacol 29:269–272
Ziegler WH, Schalch E, Leishman B, Eckert M (1983) Comparison of the effects of intravenously administered midazolam, triazolam and their hydroxyl metabolites. Br J Clin Pharmacol 16:S63–S69

Part IV
Pharmacokinetics-Pharmacodynamics Based Administration of Anesthetics

Section Editor: D.R. Stanski

The Effect of Altered Physiological States on Intravenous Anesthetics

T.K. Henthorn

Abstract This chapter begins with the rationale for the intense interest in how altered physiologic states change the effect seen following administration of similar doses of intravenous anesthetic drugs. It then traces the development of two types of pharmacokinetic models that have been used to understand the relationship between pharmacokinetics and cardiovascular physiology. Physiologic pharmacokinetic models are constructed from detailed knowledge of tissue blood flow, tissue weight, and blood:tissue partitioning characteristics. The invasive methods involved are often destructive of the subjects being studied. Rodent models are developed and scaled to simulate human subjects under a variety of physiologic conditions. Traditional pharmacokinetic models, based on drug concentration versus time data from easily obtained blood samples, can also be plumbed for physiologic information. Whereas the physiologic estimates obtained are less detailed than those from physiologic models, they do represent the actual pharmacokinetics for the subjects studied and give sufficient physiological detail to delineate the basis for the changed pharmacokinetics of intravenous pharmacokinetics.

1 Introduction

The effect of altered physiologic states on intravenous anesthetics has been a subject of interest since the observation in the 1940s of fatalities resulting from the use of standard doses of thiopental to otherwise healthy young patients suffering from

T.K. Henthorn
Department of Anesthesiology, University of Colorado Health Sciences Center,
4200 E. 9th Avenue, Denver, CO 80262, USA
thomas.henthorn@uchsc.edu

J. Schüttler and H. Schwilden (eds.) *Modern Anesthetics*.
Handbook of Experimental Pharmacology 182.

trauma and blood loss (Halford 1943). These catastrophic results with the first widely used intravenous anesthetic represented a significant departure from the expected dose–response relationship, triggering some of the earliest pharmacokinetic studies of interindividual dose–response variation. Assuming that vital organs did not suddenly become more sensitive to the effects of thiopental, investigators examined the concentration–response relationship, hypothesizing that hypovolemia and low cardiac output resulted in higher than normal plasma thiopental concentrations.

The pharmacokinetic (or disposition) processes of drug distribution to body tissues and drug metabolism or elimination determine the time course of plasma drug concentrations following intravenous administration. If distribution and elimination are reduced, plasma drug concentrations will be elevated longer, thus exposing effector organs to more drug. Conversely, if distribution and elimination are both increased, the end organs see less drug. Whether increases or decreases in end organ drug exposure are sufficient to affect the pharmacologic effect seen depends on the nature of the concentration–response relationship or pharmacodynamics.

The degree to which drugs are distributed to both pharmacologically active and inert tissues is related to tissue perfusion and the affinity or binding of the drug to various tissues. A drug with high affinity for a pharmacologically inert tissue such as muscle will exhibit lower plasma concentrations during distribution than a drug with a low affinity for this tissue. Drug elimination is related to the efficiency of metabolism and/or excretion carried out by the organs of drug elimination (e.g., liver, kidney, lungs), as well as the blood flow to these organs.

Much of the research aimed at understanding interindividual differences in the dose–response relationship for intravenous anesthetics has been to connect changes in pharmacokinetics to specific physiologic alterations by devising mathematical models. Other research, aimed at understanding pharmacodynamic changes, is the subject the chapter by P. Bischoff et al. in this volume. Pharmacokinetic models can be constructed with physiologic factors such as cardiac output, regional blood flow and drug-eliminating organ function as variables in order to predict the time course of plasma drug concentrations under various physiologic conditions. The two basic approaches for analyzing the effects of physiology on pharmacokinetics are the so-called forward and inverse models.

2 Physiologic Pharmacokinetic Models

With the forward model or problem, investigators estimate or measure the blood flow to each of the major organs (e.g., lungs, heart, brain, kidneys, liver, intestines) and tissue types (e.g., muscle, fat, skin) as well as the organ and tissue affinities of the drug relative to blood (i.e., tissue:blood partition coefficients) (Bischoff and Dedrick 1968). With these physiologic parameters tissue blood flow roughly represents transfer clearances between the central circulation and the tissue. The product of the tissue:blood partition coefficient and tissue masses roughly equals the volume of distribution of the drug for that tissue. Once the physiologic pharmacokinetic model is constructed it is possible to simulate the effect of changes in tissue blood flow or cardiac output on the time course of plasma drug concentrations. Thus, physiologic models allow extrapolation outside the range of data and the existing physiologic conditions as well as interspecies scaling if the mechanisms of transport are understood and valid (Dedrick 1973).

In the 1950s and 1960s while organ mass, blood flow, and drug affinity could be measured, methods for precise measurement of drug concentrations were not widely available. Physiologic models were the only modeling techniques available to study the effects of altered blood volume and regional blood flow on the pharmacokinetics of intravenous anesthetics. Price was the first to describe thiopental plasma concentrations using such a physiologic-based pharmacokinetic model (Price 1960); the rate of fall of plasma as well as brain thiopental concentrations following intravenous administration was shown to be the result of ongoing distribution of drug to pharmacologically inert tissues, initially to the vessel-rich splanchnic tissues and later to the vessel-poor but much larger skeletal muscles. Later Price et al. (1960) determined that a reduction in cardiac output would result in elevated plasma thiopental concentrations in the few minutes following its intravenous injection as well as a slower rate of decline. This provided the scientific basis for utilizing smaller doses of thiopental in reduced cardiac output states. Conversely, their results indicated that larger doses would be necessary when the cardiac output was increased from normal.

Although the work by Price's group explained why altered physiologic conditions could produce large differences in drug effect from identical doses in the same individual under different circumstances, they were unable to correlate results derived from physiologic pharmacokinetic model simulations with actual thiopental concentration measurements in patients with varying cardiac outputs. Sensitive thiopental drug assays were not available when Price was doing his work, and even if such assays were available, it is not practical to obtain timed tissue samples from multiple organs and tissues in human patients or to obtain precise estimates of regional blood flow.

Small animal studies can be performed in which tissue and body fluid samples can be assayed for drug content. In 1968 Bischoff and Dedrick reported a physiologic pharmacokinetic model of thiopental in rats based on blood:tissue drug partitioning, tissue and organ weights, and blood flow estimates (Bischoff and Dedrick 1968). Their results were quite predictive of blood thiopental concentrations. These investigators expanded their work to a variety of other drugs and developed the principles for interspecies scaling (Dedrick 1973). They cited the well-documented similarities in the anatomy and physiology of mammalian species and tendency of the equilibrium distribution of foreign chemicals in the body to follow basic principles of thermodynamic partitioning across species. In vitro systems can also provide information on metabolic pathways and their kinetic characteristics. These investigators showed how these data can then be used to develop physiologic pharmacokinetic models that incorporate existing knowledge about other species in a variety of physiologic conditions to predict pharmacokinetics in intact animals including man.

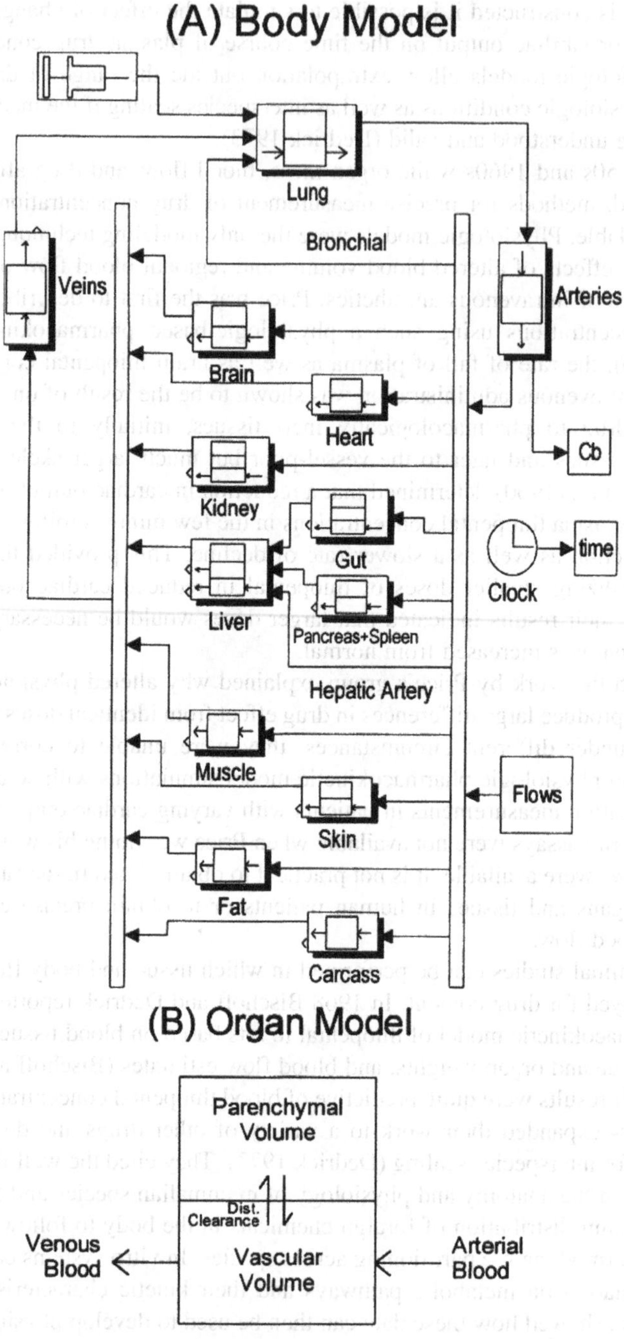

Fig. 1 **A** The total body pharmacokinetic model describing thiopental disposition in humans. The model consists of multiple tissues and blood pools connected via the vasculature, and assumes venous injection and arterial blood sampling. The "clock" generates simulation times corresponding

In the 1990s the group led by Stanski and Ebling advanced the Bischoff and Dedrick approach by developing a modeling approach in rats in which each organ or tissue had its own disposition function, determined by a numerical deconvolution technique from the arterial and tissue drug concentration data, in addition to organ weights, drug partitioning, blood flows, and vascular volumes (see Fig. 1; Ebling et al. 1994). Their approach of deriving detailed tissue disposition functions gave increased fidelity to the pharmacokinetic events during the critical first few minutes after intravenous administration, when anesthetic drugs such as thiopental have their peak effect. Through the principles of interspecies scaling (Dedrick 1973), this investigative team was able to create detailed human pharmacokinetic models which examined the effects of increased and decreased cardiac output, age, and body weight as well as gender on predicted arterial blood thiopental concentrations during the first 5 min after a 1-min intravenous infusion of a standard dose (Wada et al. 1997). They showed that changing cardiac output had the largest effect on thiopental kinetics, producing a twofold difference in peak plasma thiopental concentration between the low and the high cardiac output conditions, even more of an effect than produced by extremes of body weight (see Fig. 2). Thus a patient with a 50% decrement from a normal cardiac output will require 35% less drug, while the same individual with a 50% increase in cardiac output would require 30% more drug than normal.

Regarding body weight, a twofold increase in body weight only required a 46% increase in thiopental dose. This suggests that dose adjustments for increased weight should probably be based on a percentage of the weight above the predicted ideal body weight rather than on a more conventional milligram-per-kilogram basis.

Similar scaling of rat pharmacokinetic models were performed for fentanyl and alfentanil to humans, again with varying cardiac output and ages (Björkman et al. 1990, 1998). The physiologic pharmacokinetic models were able to predict plasma concentrations of fentanyl and alfentanil in surgical patients. As opposed to thiopental, the kinetics of the opioids appeared to be only modestly influenced by changes in physiologic state; compensatory dose adjustments would not seem to be necessary when administering these drugs over the short term. Since opioids, unlike thiopental, are often given continuously over hours or even days, cardiac output-induced changes in clearance, volume of distribution, and terminal half-life could warrant dose adjustments under these circumstances.

Upton, Runciman, and Mather developed a chronically instrumented sheep model to determine the effects of physiologic changes on the systemic and regional pharmacokinetics of intravenous anesthetic drugs (Runciman et al. 1984a, b). The

Fig. 1 (continued) to the simulated blood concentrations. Regional blood flows are generated in the *box* in the *lower right corner*, and sum to cardiac output. **B** A typical pharmacokinetic model for an organ. Organs such as the brain or heart consist of two compartments representing vasculature and parenchyma. The rate of mass transfer between compartments is proportional to the concentration gradient; this proportionality constant is the distribution clearance. (Wada et al. 1997)

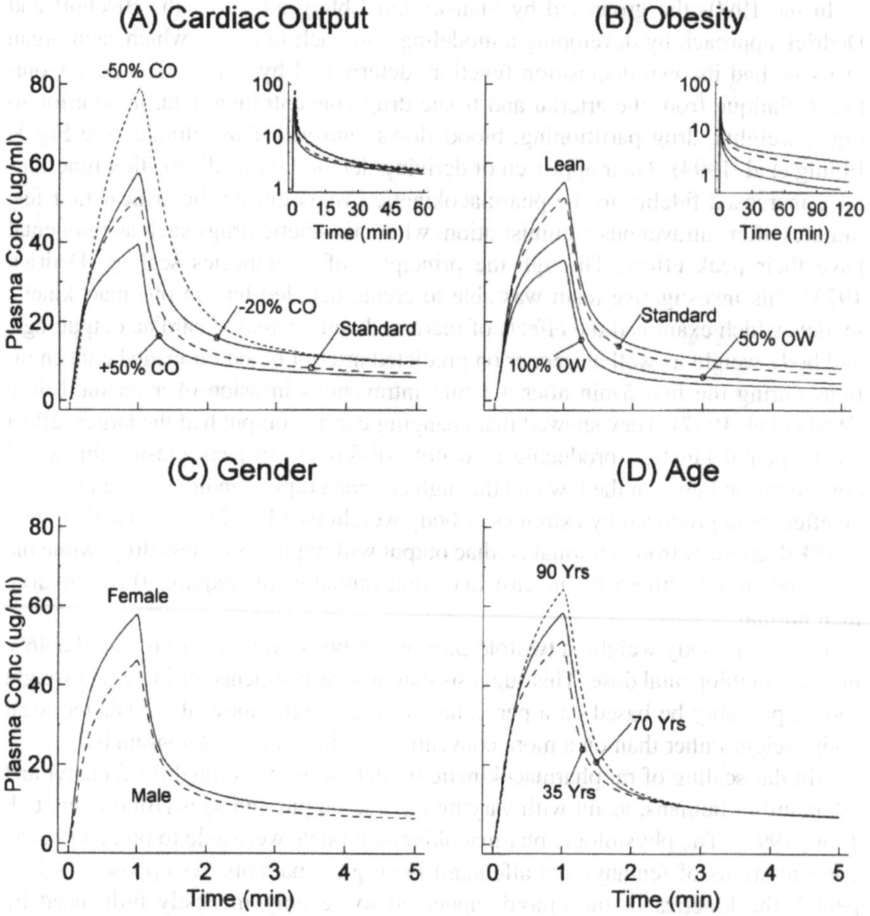

Fig. 2 Model predictions of arterial plasma concentrations after a 1-min intravenous thiopental infusion (250 mg). **A** Cardiac output (*CO*). Blood flows are increased or decreased 50% relative to the standard human, or altered as thiopental is administered to produce a 20% thiopental-induced decrease in cardiac output. The inset displays the predictions over 60 min. **B** Obesity. Organ masses are increased or decreased relative to the standard human. The inset displays the predictions over 120 min. **C** Gender. Blood flows and body compositions are changed for females or males. **D** Age. Blood flows and body compositions are changed for subjects of age 35, 70, and 90 years. (From Wada et al. 1997)

investigators conducted high-resolution blood sampling on both arterial and venous sides of several organs and tissues while also measuring cardiac output and regional blood flow, giving unique insights into the effects of physiologic changes on pharmacokinetics. In one study, they demonstrated a doubling of arterial blood meperidine concentrations during a continuous infusion when propofol or thiopental

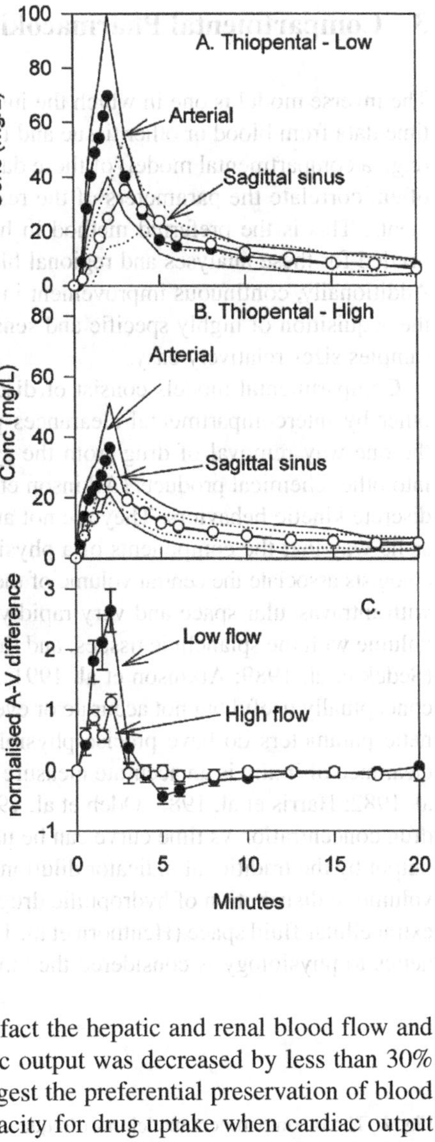

Fig. 3 The arterial and sagittal sinus concentrations (mean and 95% confidence limits) observed for the low cerebral blood flow (**A**) and high cerebral blood flow (**B**) states (produced by hyper- and hypoventilation, respectively) for thiopental. The time course of the normalized arteriovenous difference for each state is shown for comparison on the same graph (**C**); data are shown as the mean and SEM for clarity. (Upton et al. 2000)

anesthesia was induced, this despite the fact the hepatic and renal blood flow and clearance were little changed and cardiac output was decreased by less than 30% (Mather et al. 1990). These findings suggest the preferential preservation of blood flow to tissues and organs with little capacity for drug uptake when cardiac output is decreased by propofol or thiopental.

This experimental model can also be used to examine other physiologic effects on drug disposition. For instance, cerebral uptake of thiopental and propofol following a 10-s injection was studied as a function of variable cerebral blood flow (Ludbrook and Upton 1997; Upton et al. 2000). Their data showed both a delayed peak and decreased cerebral uptake of anesthetic drug when cerebral blood flow, but not cardiac output, is reduced by hyperventilation (Fig. 3). Thus the speed of the onset of anesthetic effect and its intensity can be affected by subtle physiologic effects.

3 Compartmental Pharmacokinetics

The inverse model is one in which the investigator uses only drug concentration vs time data from blood or other tissue and fluids to create a mathematical description (e.g., a compartmental model) of these data and then seeks to either derive or, more often, correlate the parameters of the resulting model with physiologic measurements. This is the preferred method in humans, as only timed blood samples are needed for these analyses and regional blood flow measurements are not required. Additionally, continuous improvement in drug measurement technology has made the acquisition of highly specific and sensitive drug concentration data from small samples sizes relatively easy.

Compartmental models consist of discrete distribution volumes linked to each other by intercompartmental clearances plus an elimination clearance describing the one-way removal of drug from the system by its excretion or its metabolism into other chemical products (Atkinson et al. 1991). The volumes have statistically discrete kinetic behaviors. They are not anatomically discrete or identifiable in the same way that the components of a physiologic model are. Nevertheless, pharmacologists associate the central volume of the typical three-compartment model (Fig. 4) with intravascular space and very rapidly equilibrating tissues, the fast peripheral volume with the splanchnic tissues, and the slow compartment with skeletal muscle (Sedek et al. 1989; Atkinson et al. 1991). These are very rough estimates that are conceptually useful but not accurate or even rigorously testable. Some pharmacokinetic parameters do have precise physiologic meaning. For instance, elimination clearance of inulin is an accurate measure of glomerular filtration rate (Henthorn et al. 1982; Harris et al. 1988; Odeh et al. 1993). The area under the first pass arterial drug concentration vs time curve can be used in many instances to estimate cardiac output by the traditional indicator dilution technique (Meier and Zierler 1954). The volume of distribution of hydrophilic drugs or indicators (e.g., inulin) estimates the extracellular fluid space (Henthorn et al. 1982). This progression from pharmacokinetics to physiology is considered the "inverse" of the "forward" model of taking

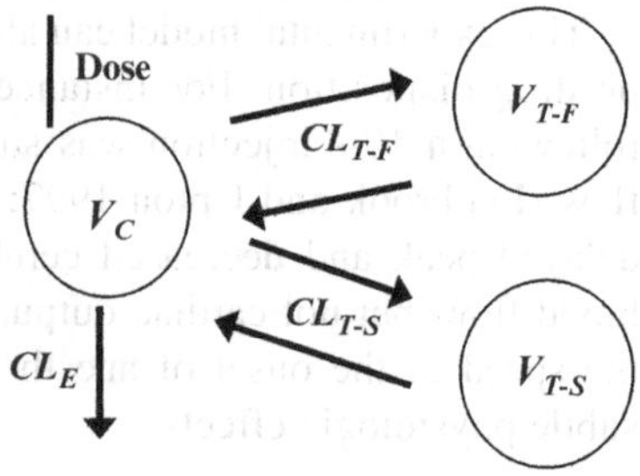

Fig. 4 Three-compartment model most frequently used to characterize the pharmacokinetics of intravenous anesthetic drugs. V_C is the central compartment distribution volume which includes the intravascular volume into which the drug is administered and which is assumed to mix instantaneously. From this central volume drug is cleared from the body by the elimination clearance (CL_E) or exchanges bidirectionally with fast and slow equilibrating peripheral tissue distribution volumes ($V_{T\text{-}F}$ and $V_{T\text{-}S}$, respectively) via distribution clearances ($CL_{T\text{-}F}$ and $V_{T\text{-}S}$)

physiologic principles and estimates to derive pharmacokinetics. Whichever way you look at it, pharmacokinetics and physiology are intertwined.

One of the earliest demonstrations of the relationship between anesthetic drug pharmacokinetics and physiologic changes came with the observation that intercompartmental clearance of thiopental to the rapidly equilibrating peripheral compartment was decreased in elderly patients, possibly explaining their increased sensitivity to the drug (Avram et al. 1990; Stanski and Maitre 1990). While it was tempting to attribute this change in clearance to a reduction in cardiac output with age, cardiac output was not measured in these studies. Subsequent studies were able to make this connection. The intercompartmental clearance of alfentanil was subsequently demonstrated to be closely correlated with cardiac output in healthy human subjects (Henthorn et al. 1992b). Later, porcine hemorrhagic shock models directly linked decreases in intercompartmental clearances of etomidate, propofol, fentanyl, and remifentanil to decreased cardiac output and elevated blood drug concentrations (Egan et al. 1999; Johnson et al. 2001, 2003a, b).

The development of recirculatory pharmacokinetic models has more directly linked blood flow to intercompartmental clearances (Krejcie et al. 1994, 1996, 1997). With frequent arterial sampling following rapid intravenous drug or physiologic marker injection these models permit estimation of cardiac output and its distribution. Consider the pharmacokinetics of an intravascular marker such as indocyanine green (ICG) (Henthorn et al. 1992a). The arterial ICG concentration history following a nearly instantaneous central venous bolus is shown in Fig. 5 in

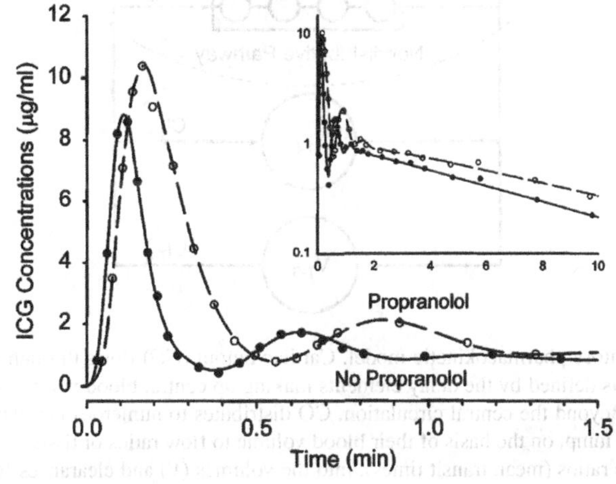

Fig. 5 Arterial blood indocyanine green concentration histories for the first 1.5 min (illustrating the first- and second-pass peaks of the intravascular mixing phase) and for 10 min (*inset* illustrating the elimination phase) after rapid intravenous injection in one of the four subjects without propranolol (*solid line* and *solid symbols*) and during the propranolol infusion (*broken line* and *open symbols*). The *symbols* represent indocyanine green concentrations, whereas the *lines* represent concentrations predicted by the models. (Niemann et al. 2000)

the same subject under control conditions and during a propranolol infusion to reduce cardiac output (Niemann et al. 2000). The first seven arterial ICG concentrations in the control condition and nine when propranolol was being administered represent the so-called first-pass. The Stewart–Hamilton indicator-dilution cardiac output principle can thus be employed by simply dividing the ICG dose by the first-pass AUC to derive the cardiac output (Meier and Zierler 1954). The anatomical volumes involved in the first-pass portion would encompass the central venous injection site, the heart-lung segment, and the arterial tree extending to points temporally equivalent to the arterial sampling site. The first recirculatory (secondary) peak is caused by the initial recirculation of only a minority of the total blood flow returning from the periphery; if it were all of the blood a much larger second peak would be seen. Thus, the circulation needs to be viewed in terms of two peripheral blood circuits, one with a short time constant (low blood volume relative to blood flow) and one with a long time constant (large blood volume relative to its blood flow) in order to characterize the complete arterial blood ICG concentration history.

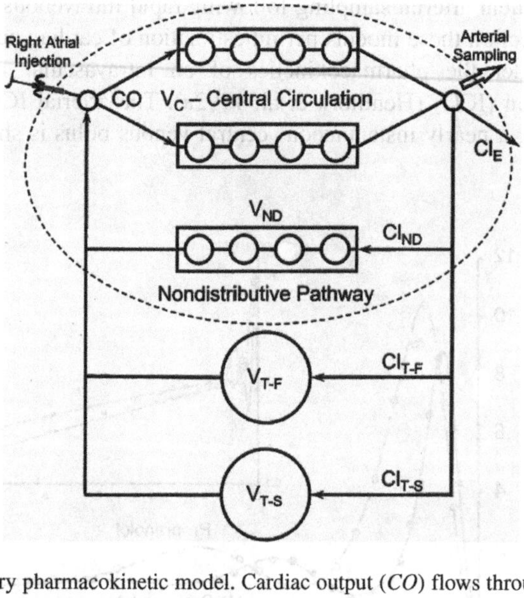

Fig. 6 Recirculatory pharmacokinetic model. Cardiac output (*CO*) flows through the central circulation, which is defined by the delay elements making up central blood volume and pulmonary tissue volume. Beyond the central circulation, CO distributes to numerous circulatory and tissue pathways which lump, on the basis of their blood volume to flow ratios or tissue volume to distribution clearance ratios (mean transit times), into the volumes (*V*) and clearances (*Cl*) of the nondistributive peripheral pathway (V_{ND}, Cl_{ND}) and the fast ($V_{T\text{-}F}$, $Cl_{T\text{-}F}$) and slow ($V_{T\text{-}S}$, $Cl_{T\text{-}S}$) tissue volume groups. The parallel rapidly and slowly equilibrating tissues are no more than the fast and slow compartments, respectively, of traditional three-compartment pharmacokinetic models, whereas the central circulation and nondistributive peripheral pathway(s) are detailed representations of the ideal instantaneously mixing central volume (V_C) of the traditional multicompartment mammillary model (Fig. 3). The *dotted ellipse* surrounds the components of the ideal central volume of a three-compartment model. (From Avram and Krejcie 2003)

This pharmacokinetic model is consistent with physiologic models of the circulation in which the slow peripheral circuit is thought to represent mainly splanchnic circulation and the fast circuit most of the remaining circulation (Caldini et al. 1974).

Moving beyond a purely intravascular marker such as ICG to a drug, the recirculatory model must expand to include additional compartments that characterize drug distribution to tissues. These additions are actually nothing more than the peripheral compartments of traditional pharmacokinetic models. The main difference is that the tissue compartments are connected as parallel circuits in the recirculatory model (Fig. 6), more closely resembling the structure of a physiologic model (Fig. 1). In addition, the intercompartmental clearances become components of the overall cardiac output. Preservation of the cardiac output in a recirculatory model is vital to our ability to examine how physiologic covariates affect pharmacokinetics.

To summarize, a recirculatory model uses only measured arterial drug concentration vs time data. Thus, it is a pharmacokinetic, as opposed to a physiologic, model. However, a recirculatory model has elements of a physiologic model in that (1) cardiac output is retained, (2) tissue distribution is modeled by compartments in parallel circuits, and (3) the model delineates the disproportionate distribution of cardiac output to various statistically grouped tissues.

The recirculatory model is essentially a three-compartment pharmacokinetic model with a central compartment that includes both the first pass through the heart-lung segment and the quick recirculation through a peripheral circuit in which there is little or no exchange of drug with tissue (Krejcie and Avram 1999). This rapid recirculation of drug has variously been called a pharmacokinetic shunt or nondistributive blood flow (Krejcie et al. 1994; Henthorn et al. 1999). It may represent flow to tissues with little distributive capacity relative to blood flow such as kidney, skin, and brain, or it may be the manifestation of distribution that is not flow-limited, i.e., where distribution is diffusion-limited. The latter is certainly the case for the hydrophilic muscle relaxants (Kuipers et al. 2001). In either case, physiologic change in the proportion of cardiac output that makes up this quick nondistributive circuit directly affects the early blood drug concentrations and thus the exposure of the effect site to drug.

To further demonstrate the dependence of intercompartmental clearance on cardiac output, Kuipers et al. showed a significant correlation between tissue distribution clearance of alfentanil and cardiac output in a recirculatory model (Kuipers et al. 1999), corroborating the earlier findings using less detailed pharmacokinetic analyses (Henthorn et al. 1992b).

Lipid-soluble drug markers have been used as surrogates to study the effects of covariates of drug distribution so that anesthetic drugs such as thiopental and propofol, with known physiologic effects, can be studied without affecting the physiologic state of the test subject (Avram et al. 2002; Weiss et al. 2007a, b). Antipyrine is a lipid-soluble drug that distributes to tissue in a flow-limited fashion with no discernable effects on physiology or consciousness. Avram et al. recently demonstrated that the pharmacokinetics of antipyrine closely resemble those of thiopental (Avram et al. 2002). In a study of the recirculatory kinetics of antipyrine performed in conscious dogs treated with vasoactive drugs, Krejcie et al. found

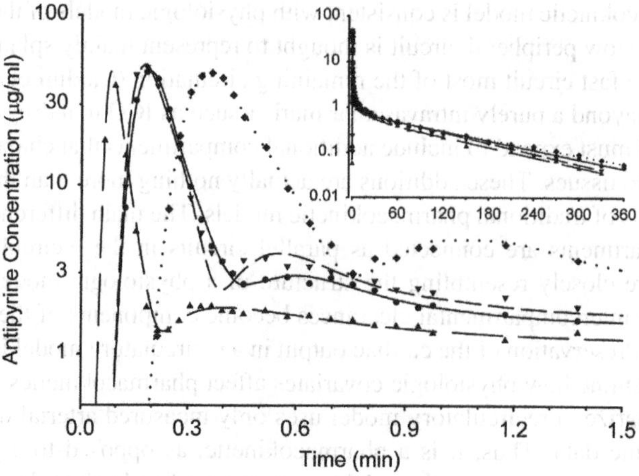

Fig. 7 Arterial blood antipyrine concentration histories for the first 1.5 min (illustrating the first- and second-pass peaks) and for 360 min (*inset*), following right atrial injection in one dog under four conditions: (1) when it received no vasoactive drug (control, *closed circles, solid line*), (2) during an isoproterenol infusion (*upright triangles, long dashed line*), (3) during a nitroprusside infusion (*inverted triangles, short dashed line*), and (4) during a phenylephrine infusion (*diamonds, dotted line*). The *symbols* represent drug concentrations; the *lines* represent concentrations predicted by the recirculatory models. (Krejcie et al. 2001)

that phenylephrine approximately doubled the antipyrine area under the arterial drug concentration-time curve (AUC) from 0–3 min (Fig. 7), while isoproterenol halved it over control (Krejcie et al. 2001). The increase in AUC with phenylephrine was a direct result of an increased fraction of the cardiac output going to the nondistributive circuit. In contrast, the lower AUC for isoproterenol was a result of a much larger fraction of cardiac output going to tissues that rapidly equilibrated antipyrine with blood. That phenylephrine caused a disproportionate preservation of nondistributive blood flow nicely points out that changes in tissue blood flow are not simply proportional to cardiac output as others have assumed. A similar effect on AUC from 0 to 3 min following treatment with isoflurane was also caused by the combined effects of a decreased cardiac output and preservation of the nondistributive blood flow (Avram et al. 2000). Presumably, had a drug with rapid action on the central nervous system been administered instead of antipyrine, a much greater peak effect would have been seen in the phenylephrine and isoflurane-treated subjects vs control and a lesser one in the those treated with isoproterenol.

Doses of intravenous anesthetic drugs are administered rapidly in order to deliver sufficient drug concentrations to the brain to produce loss of consciousness and/or analgesia, but in doses not so large or by infusions not so rapid as to result in arterial drug concentrations that might produce toxicity such as cardiovascular collapse.

Interindividual differences in the pharmacokinetics of intravenous anesthetic drugs, over the first several minutes after their rapid administration, are mostly due to alterations in the cardiovascular physiologic state in existence prior to anesthetic drug administration. These physiologic changes to cardiac output and the circulation have many causes (e.g., hemorrhagic shock, disease, concomitantly administered drugs), but a more thorough understanding of how these physiologic changes affect early anesthetic drug pharmacokinetics should lead to the selection of safer and more effective drug doses and administration rates.

References

Atkinson AJ Jr, Ruo TI, Frederiksen MC (1991) Physiological basis of multicompartmental models of drug distribution. Trends Pharmacol Sci 12:96–101

Avram MJ, Krejcie TC (2003) Using front-end kinetics to optimize target-controlled drug infusions. Anesthesiology 99:1078–1086

Avram MJ, Krejcie TC, Henthorn TK (1990) The relationship of age to the pharmacokinetics of early drug distribution: the concurrent disposition of thiopental and indocyanine green. Anesthesiology 72:403–411

Avram MJ, Krejcie TC, Niemann CU, Enders-Klein C, Shanks CA, Henthorn TK (2000) Isoflurane alters the recirculatory pharmacokinetics of physiologic markers. Anesthesiology 92:1757–1768

Avram MJ, Krejcie TC, Henthorn TK (2002) The concordance of early antipyrine and thiopental distribution kinetics. J Pharmacol Exp Ther 302:594–600

Bischoff KB, Dedrick RL (1968) Thiopental pharmacokinetics. J Pharm Sci 57:1346–1351

Björkman S, Stanski DR, Verotta D, Harashima H (1990) Comparative tissue concentration profiles of fentanyl and alfentanil in humans predicted from tissue/blood partition data obtained in rats. Anesthesiology 72:865–873

Björkman S, Wada DR, Stanski DR (1998) Application of physiologic models to predict the influence of changes in body composition and blood flows on the pharmacokinetics of fentanyl and alfentanil in patients. Anesthesiology 88:657–667

Caldini P, Permutt S, Waddell JA, Riley RL (1974) Effect of epinephrine on pressure, flow, and volume relationships in the systemic circulation of dogs. Circ Res 34:606–623

Dedrick RL (1973) Animal scale-up. J Pharmacokinet Biopharm 1:435–461

Ebling WF, Wada DR, Stanski DR (1994) From piecewise to full physiologic pharmacokinetic modeling: applied to thiopental disposition in the rat. J Pharmacokinet Biopharm 22:259–292

Egan TD, Kuramkote S, Gong G, Zhang J, McJames SW, Bailey PL (1999) Fentanyl pharmacokinetics in hemorrhagic shock: a porcine model. Anesthesiology 91:156–166

Halford FJ (1943) A critique of intravenous anesthesia in war surgery. Anesthesiology 4:67–69

Harris DC, Chan L, Schrier RW (1988) Remnant kidney hypermetabolism and progression of chronic renal failure. Am J Physiol 254:F267–F276

Henthorn TK, Avram MJ, Frederiksen MC, Atkinson AJ Jr (1982) Heterogeneity of interstitial fluid space demonstrated by simultaneous kinetic analysis of the distribution and elimination of inulin and gallamine. J Pharmacol Exp Ther 222:389–394

Henthorn TK, Avram MJ, Krejcie TC, Shanks CA, Asada A, Kaczynski DA (1992a) Minimal compartmental model of circulatory mixing of indocyanine green. Am J Physiol 262: H903–H910

Henthorn TK, Krejcie TC, Avram MJ (1992b) The relationship between alfentanil distribution kinetics and cardiac output. Clin Pharmacol Ther 52:190–196

Henthorn TK, Krejcie TC, Niemann CU, Enders-Klein C, Shanks CA, Avram MJ (1999) Ketamine distribution described by a recirculatory pharmacokinetic model is not stereoselective. Anesthesiology 91:1733–1743

Johnson KB, Kern SE, Hamber EA, McJames SW, Kohnstamm KM, Egan TD (2001) Influence of hemorrhagic shock on remifentanil: a pharmacokinetic and pharmacodynamic analysis. Anesthesiology 94:322–332

Johnson KB, Egan TD, Kern SE, White JL, McJames SW, Syroid N, Whiddon D, Church T (2003a) The influence of hemorrhagic shock on propofol: a pharmacokinetic and pharmacodynamic analysis. Anesthesiology 99:409–420

Johnson KB, Egan TD, Layman J, Kern SE, White JL, McJames SW (2003b) The influence of hemorrhagic shock on etomidate: a pharmacokinetic and pharmacodynamic analysis. Anesth Analg 96:1360–1368

Krejcie TC, Avram MJ (1999) What determines anesthetic induction dose? It's the front-end kinetics, doctor! Anesth Analg 89:541–544

Krejcie TC, Henthorn TK, Shanks CA, Avram MJ (1994) A recirculatory pharmacokinetic model describing the circulatory mixing, tissue distribution and elimination of antipyrine in dogs. J Pharmacol Exp Ther 269:609–616

Krejcie TC, Henthorn TK, Niemann CU, Klein C, Gupta DK, Gentry WB, Shanks CA, Avram MJ (1996) Recirculatory pharmacokinetic models of markers of blood, extracellular fluid and total body water administered concomitantly. J Pharmacol Exp Ther 278:1050–1057

Krejcie TC, Avram MJ, Gentry WB, Niemann CU, Janowski MP, Henthorn TK (1997) A recirculatory model of the pulmonary uptake and pharmacokinetics of lidocaine based on analysis of arterial and mixed venous data from dogs. J Pharmacokinet Biopharm 25:169–190

Krejcie TC, Wang Z, Avram MJ (2001) Drug-induced hemodynamic perturbations alter the disposition of markers of blood volume, extracellular fluid, and total body water. J Pharmacol Exp Ther 296:922–930

Kuipers JA, Boer F, Olofsen E, Olieman W, Vletter AA, Burm AG, Bovill JG (1999) Recirculatory and compartmental pharmacokinetic modeling of alfentanil in pigs: the influence of cardiac output. Anesthesiology 90:1146–1157

Kuipers JA, Boer F, Olofsen E, Bovill JG, Burm AG (2001) Recirculatory pharmacokinetics and pharmacodynamics of rocuronium in patients: the influence of cardiac output. Anesthesiology 94:47–55

Ludbrook GL, Upton RN (1997) A physiological model of induction of anaesthesia with propofol in sheep. 2. Model analysis and implications for dose requirements. Br J Anaesth 79:505–513

Mather LE, Selby DG, Runciman WB (1990) Effects of propofol and of thiopentone anaesthesia on the regional kinetics of pethidine in the sheep. Br J Anaesth 65:365–372

Meier P, Zierler KL (1954) On the theory of the indicator-dilution method for measurement of blood flow and volume. J Appl Physiol 6:731–744

Niemann CU, Henthorn TK, Krejcie TC, Shanks CA, Enders-Klein C, Avram MJ (2000) Indocyanine green kinetics characterize blood volume and flow distribution and their alteration by propranolol. Clin Pharmacol Ther 67:342–350

Odeh YK, Wang Z, Ruo TI, Wang T, Frederiksen MC, Pospisil PA, Atkinson AJ Jr (1993) Simultaneous analysis of inulin and 15N2-urea kinetics in humans. Clin Pharmacol Ther 53:419–425

Price HL (1960) A dynamic concept of the distribution of thiopental in the human body. Anesthesiology 21:40–45

Price HL, Kovnat PJ, Safer JN, Conner EH, Price ML (1960) The uptake of thiopental by body tissues and its relation to the duration of narcosis. Clin Pharmacol Ther 1:16–22

Runciman WB, Ilsley AH, Mather LE, Carapetis R, Rao MM (1984a) A sheep preparation for studying interactions between blood flow and drug disposition. I. Physiological profile. Br J Anaesth 56:1015–1028

Runciman WB, Mather LE, Ilsley AH, Carapetis RJ, Upton RN (1984b) A sheep preparation for studying interactions between blood flow and drug disposition. III. Effects of general and spinal anaesthesia on regional blood flow and oxygen tensions. Br J Anaesth 56:1247–1258

Sedek GS, Ruo TI, Frederiksen MC, Frederiksen JW, Shih SR, Atkinson AJ Jr (1989) Splanchnic tissues are a major part of the rapid distribution spaces of inulin, urea and theophylline. J Pharmacol Exp Ther 251:1026–1031

Stanski DR, Maitre PO (1990) Population pharmacokinetics and pharmacodynamics of thiopental: the effect of age revisited. Anesthesiology 72:412–422

Upton RN, Ludbrook GL, Grant C, Doolette DJ (2000) The effect of altered cerebral blood flow on the cerebral kinetics of thiopental and propofol in sheep. Anesthesiology 93:1085–1094

Wada DR, Björkman S, Ebling WF, Harashima H, Harapat SR, Stanski DR (1997) Computer simulation of the effects of alterations in blood flows and body composition on thiopental pharmacokinetics in humans. Anesthesiology 87:884–899

Weiss M, Krejcie TC, Avram MJ (2007a) Circulatory transport and capillary-tissue exchange as determinants of the distribution kinetics of inulin and antipyrine in dog. J Pharm Sci 96:913–926

Weiss M, Krejcie TC, Avram MJ (2007b) A minimal physiological model of thiopental distribution kinetics based on a multiple indicator approach. Drug Metab Dispos 35:1525–1532

Anesthetics Drug Pharmacodynamics

P. Bischoff, G. Schneider, and E. Kochs(✉)

Abstract Anesthesia cannot be defined in an unambiguous manner. The essential components of general anesthesia are absence of consciousness and pain. This translates into two particular qualities: (1) sedation and hypnosis, i.e., mental blockade and (2) analgesia/antinociception, i.e., sensory blockade. Anesthetic actions on these two subcomponents are difficult to separate. On the one hand, very few anesthetics act exclusively on one of these components. On the other hand, these components are closely related to each other. Unconsciousness prevents (conscious) perception of pain, and nociception may serve as an arousal stimulus and change the level of sedation and hypnosis. The art of anesthesia lies in adequate dosing of drugs to reach both mental and sensory blockade. Drug administration can be based on pharmacokinetic considerations. Pharmacokinetic models allow an estimation of what happens to the administered drug in the body. Models with an effect site compartment may facilitate a tailored administration of anesthetic drugs. Finally, the quantification of pharmacodynamic effects allows a precise titration of drugs. Clinical assessment

E. Kochs
Klinik für Anästhesiologie, Klinikum rechts der isar, Technische Universität München Ismaningerstr. 22, D-81675 München, Germany
E.F.Kochs@lrz.tu-muenchen.de

J. Schüttler and H. Schwilden (eds.) *Modern Anesthetics.*
Handbook of Experimental Pharmacology 182.

of mental blockade is often dichotomous, and therefore not very helpful to guide drug administration. Several scoring systems exist, but once consciousness is lost they become less reliable, in particular because reaction to stimuli is assessed, which mixes assessment of mental blockade with assessment of sensory blockade. Clinical assessment of analgesia requires a conscious patient, so antinociception is difficult to measure. Several methods of objective quantification on the basis of electrical brain activity are discussed including EEG and evoked potentials. Despite numerous indexes of the hypnotic component of anesthesia, there is no parameter that unambiguously quantifies the level of mental or sensory blockade.

1 Introduction

General anesthesia cannot be defined in an unambiguous manner. Anesthetic actions at subcellular and cellular levels, and in neuronal networks within the brain and the spinal cord contribute to a clinical state of unresponsiveness and unconsciousness that clinically presents as anesthesia. It is composed of numerous components of which sedation/hypnosis, antinociception, and altered autonomous reactivity are some of the most prominent features. From the patient's point of view, the crucial main effects of general anesthesia are absence of consciousness and pain. This translates into two particular qualities of both general anesthesia and anesthetics:

1. Sedation and reduction of voluntary responsiveness (hypnosis)—mental blockade
2. Analgesia/antinociception—sensory blockade

These components are closely related to each other, and it may not always be possible to separate these components from each other by objective measurements. Consequently, the influence of drugs on these components may not easily be separated. This can be illustrated with the clinical effects of opioids. Considered to be potent analgesic drugs, in higher doses they also induce sedation. On the other hand, experimental results suggest that propofol, a sedative, also has analgesic properties. This may be explained in part by the fact that both main pharmacodynamic effects lead to a decrease of pain perception and pain sensation, but due to different mechanisms. Sedation is defined as a (possibly unspecific) suppression of the central nervous system and cortical function, whereas analgesia is mediated by a more specific modulation of nociceptive pathways. Still, both lead to analgesia, as analgesia refers to perception of pain, which implies consciousness. In contrast to analgesic effects, antinociceptive mechanisms refer to a pathway-specific reduction of stimulus responses, i.e., not only conscious perception of painful stimuli but modulation of afferent noxious stimulation. Unfortunately, in the clinical setting antinociceptive effects are even harder to quantify than analgesia.

During the awake state, the level of sedation and analgesia can be assessed by clinical evaluation. During general anesthesia, with loss of response to stimuli, no parameter reliably indicates "deepening" or "lightening" of hypnosis or analgesia.

Only unspecific "surrogate" parameters such as heart rate, blood pressure, sweating, tearing, etc., may indirectly indicate changes of the anesthetic level.

In daily clinical practice of general anesthesia, the goal is an individually tailored dosing of drugs, resulting in the "optimal" anesthetic level that is neither too light nor too deep. On the one side of the spectrum, excessively high drug doses (and inadequately "deep" levels of anesthesia) should be avoided to reach short recovery times and prevent excessive depression of the cardiovascular system. On the other side of the spectrum, inadequately low doses of anesthetics (and inadequately "light" levels of anesthesia) must be avoided to guarantee unconsciousness and prevent memory formation for intraoperative traumatic procedures (awareness). Underdosage of anesthetics leads to conscious perception or even awareness (conscious perception with explicit memory) during anesthesia. As large multicenter studies in Scandinavia and the United States have shown, the incidence of this event is between 0.1% and 0.2% in an average patient population (Sandin et al. 2000; Sebel et al. 2004). This implies the risk of clinical consequences, e.g., pain flashbacks (Salomons et al. 2004), or—in the worst case—post-traumatic stress disorder (PTSD) (Schneider 2003). It is important to know that by the time of discharge from the hospital, patients may report that they are not suffering from any consequences of the awareness and yet experience consequences after a symptom-free interval. This latency is rather characteristic for PTSD and has also been reported on patients of the Scandinavian multicenter study (Lennmarken et al. 2002).

Besides efforts to optimize anesthesia to shield the patient from the stress and consequences of surgery, cost saving and issues of economy may be an issue for dosing strategies (Song et al. 1998; White et al. 2004). Management of anesthesia aimed at early recovery of the patient has been addressed as so-called "fast track anesthesia," which nevertheless comprises much more than optimized dosing of anesthetic drugs. In this context, one challenge for the anesthesiologist is to avoid both over- and underdosage. Therefore, knowledge of pharmacokinetic and pharmacodynamic properties of anesthetic drugs is imperative.

For perioperative management of general anesthesia techniques, the following main drug classes are widely used in clinical practice and of particular interest: These are hypnotic (propofol, etomidate, barbiturates, ketamine, and inhaled anesthetic agents), analgesic, and narcotic drugs (morphine, opioids), sometimes supplemented by benzodiazepines and α_2 agonists.

2 Pharmacokinetics

2.1 Pharmacokinetic Principles

Pharmacokinetics describe the relationship between drug dose and drug concentration in plasma or the effect site. This relationship is described by processes of absorption, distribution, and clearance. For intravenous drugs, absorption is irrelevant, so pharmacokinetic properties are described by distribution and clearance alone.

2.1.1 Volume of Distribution

The distribution of a drug in the plasma can be seen as a process of dilution. The dilution results from the injection of a drug into a larger volume. The change of the known concentration in the syringe to the measured concentration in the larger volume allows a calculation of this volume. The volume of distribution depends on the specific drug and on the individual.

Central Volume of Distribution

For calculation of the central volume of distribution, a drug is injected into an arm vein, and the concentration is measured in an artery. The central volume of distribution includes the volume in the heart, great vessels, upper arm, and the drug uptake by the lungs. The central volume of distribution also reflects any metabolism that occurs between injection and arterial sampling. The concept of the central volume of distribution has its limitations. It is based on the erroneous assumption that the drug is instantaneously mixed in the volume. In practice, the peak concentration is seen within 30–40 s. The mathematics of the corresponding time course are of particular interest during induction of anesthesia and have been examined in detail, including recirculatory concentration peaks. For anesthetic drugs, the analysis of the central volume of distribution remains difficult and is highly influenced by the study design (moment of blood sampling).

Peripheral Volumes of Distribution

Anesthetic drugs do not remain in the central compartment but are widely distributed into peripheral tissues. Pharmacologically, these tissues are additional volumes of distribution (peripheral compartments). Blood flow connects peripheral compartments with the central compartment. The size of the peripheral volumes of distribution reflects the solubility of the drug in the specific compartment (tissue). The better a drug is soluble in peripheral tissues, the higher is the volume of peripheral tissues. Usually the exact solubility of a drug in peripheral tissues is unknown. For calculation of a drug dose, a small mass with high solubility cannot be differentiated from a large mass with low solubility. By convention in pharmacokinetics, solubility of drugs in peripheral tissues is the same as in plasma. This assumption allows a characterization of drug distribution into tissues, but leads to very large volumes of distribution for drugs with high solubility (up to several thousands of liters).

The volume of distribution at steady state relates the plasma drug concentration at steady state (e.g., a long lasting intravenous infusion) to the total amount of drug in the body. It is composed from central volume plus peripheral volumes.

2.1.2 Clearance

Hepatic, Renal, Tissue Clearance

Clearance refers to the process of elimination of a substance from a volume. It is defined as the volume that is completely cleared of drug per unit of time.

The main organs of clearance are the liver, kidneys, and, in some particular cases, the lungs. Some substances are cleared in the plasma and tissue. Clearance involves biotransformation and filtration/elimination of drugs. Hepatic clearance is mainly based on enzymatic processes, which produce (with a few exceptions) less active or inactive metabolites. The clearance rate depends on the blood flow to the liver. Clearance of drugs that are completely extracted by the organ are "flow limited." Not every drug is 100% extracted from the volume, i.e., some residual drug is still in the plasma after circulation through the clearing organ. The extraction ratio depends on the capacity of the liver to take up and metabolize the drug. Such drugs are "capacity limited." Renal clearance is characterized by filtration (glomerulus) and transport (tubulus). Renal clearance decreases with age, and the dose of (mainly) renally cleared drugs should be reduced in the elderly. Tissue clearance plays an important role for a small subset of anesthetics. Tissues include blood, muscle, and lungs. An example is remifentanil, which is cleared by nonspecific esterases in muscle, intestines, and, to a minor degree, lungs, liver, muscles, and blood.

Distribution Clearance

Distribution clearance describes the transfer of the drug between blood or plasma and the peripheral tissues. Unlike metabolic clearance, in distribution clearance the drug is not removed from the body. It is influenced by cardiac output, tissue and organ blood flow, and the capillary permeability of the drug.

2.2 *Pharmacokinetic Models*

2.2.1 Physiologic Pharmacokinetic Models

In animal studies it is possible to analyze volumes and clearances for all organs in the body and to construct physiologically and anatomically correct models of pharmacokinetics. Several studies have demonstrated that tissue volumes and clearances can be scaled up and applied to humans. The resulting models are typically complex. As an example, an animal model for propofol induction has already been constructed from six compartments (Upton and Ludbrook 1997). The physiologic description of longer lasting infusions will require even more compartments. Interestingly, these complex models do not allow a more precise description of pharmacokinetics than simplified compartmental models.

2.2.2 Compartmental Pharmacokinetic Models

Compartmental models are grossly simplified models of volumes and clearances in the body. The simplest model is a one-compartment model. It contains a single volume and a single clearance (Fig. 1a–c), as if the human body were a pot. For anesthetic drugs, compartmental models are built from several pots (compartments), which are connected by tubes to a central pot (central compartment) allowing flow from and to the peripheral pots (peripheral compartments). The volume of the central compartment and the sum of the volumes of the peripheral compartments are the volume of distribution at steady state. The clearing that leaves the central volume to the outside is the central (metabolic) clearance; the clearance between the central compartment and the peripheral compartments are intercompartmental clearances.

For many drugs, three distinct phases of drug distribution can be distinguished. The rapid distribution phase begins immediately after bolus injection and describes drug distribution to rapidly equilibrating tissues, followed by the slow distribution phase, which describes flow from plasma to slowly equilibrating tissues (usually with low blood flow) and redistribution from rapidly equilibrating tissues. The terminal phase (elimination phase) is characterized by a constant relative proportion of drug in plasma and peripheral volumes with a (slow) removal of drug from the body. A three-compartment model best describes this characteristic behavior after bolus injection.

2.2.3 Plasma Concentration: Effect Site Concentration

The plasma is not the site where anesthetic drugs unfold their clinical effect. As mentioned above, the main effect of anesthetics can objectively be assessed by EEG or evoked potentials. By doing so, it becomes obvious that the main effect at the brain (effect site) is delayed when compared to the plasma peak concentration. There is a time delay between drug concentration in the plasma and drug concentration at the effect site. For the purpose of pharmacokinetic modeling, an effect site compartment can be added (Fig. 2). The effect site compartment is connected to the central compartment by a first order process. The constant K_{eo} is the rate constant for elimination of drug from the effect site. It has a large influence on the rate of rise and offset of drug effect, and the dose required to produce a certain drug effect.

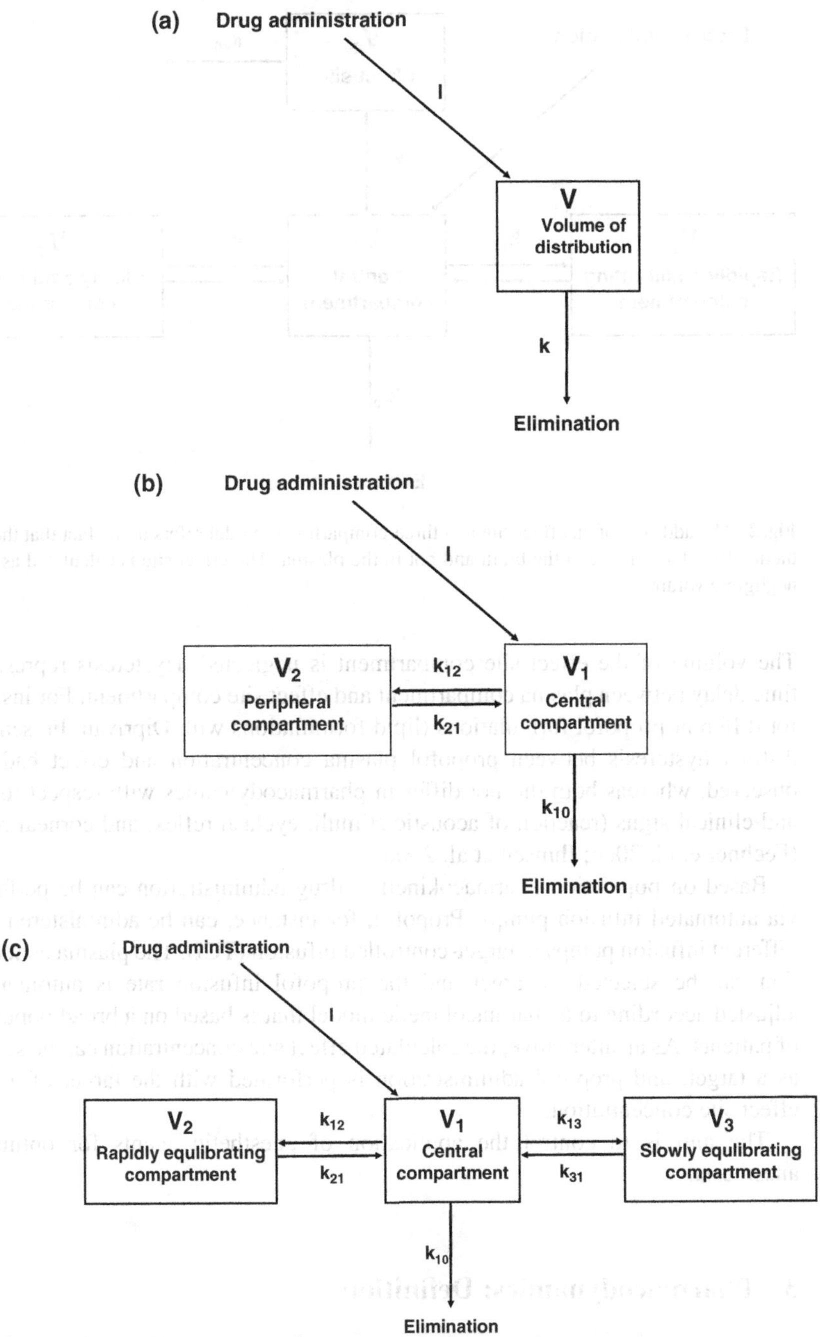

Fig. 1 Pharmacokinetic models. **a** A pharmacokinetic model with a single compartment. **b** One peripheral compartment is added to the central compartment. **c** A three-compartment model with one rapidly and one slowly equilibrating compartment is shown

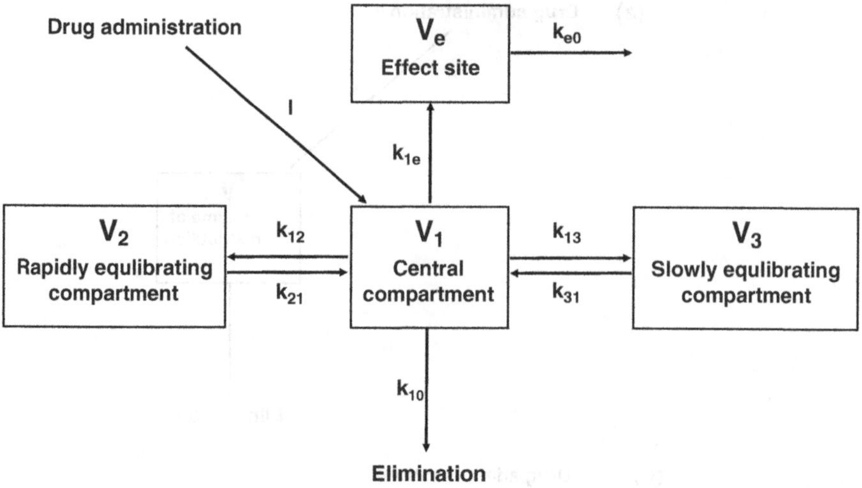

Fig. 2 The addition of an effect site to a three-compartment model refers to the fact that the anesthetic effect takes place in the brain and not in the plasma. The effect site is calculated as with a negligible volume

The volume of the effect site compartment is neglected. Hysteresis represents a time delay between plasma compartment and effect site compartment. For instance, for different propofol formulations (lipid formulations with Diprivan, Fresenius) a distinct hysteresis between propofol plasma concentration and effect had been observed, whereas both did not differ in pharmacodynamics with respect to EEG and clinical signs (reaction of acoustic stimuli, eyelash reflex, and corneal reflex) (Fechner et al. 2004; Ihmsen et al. 2006).

Based on population pharmacokinetics, drug administration can be performed via automated infusion pumps. Propofol, for instance, can be administered using different infusion pumps in target-controlled infusion (TCI). The plasma concentration can be selected as target and the propofol infusion rate is automatically adjusted according to a pharmacokinetic model that is based on a broad population of patients. As an alternative, the calculated effect site concentration can be selected as a target, and propofol administration is performed with the target of a given effect site concentration.

The aim is to control the application of anesthetic agents for optimizing anesthesia.

3 Pharmacodynamics: Definition

In contrast to the definition of pharmacokinetics (i.e., description of "What does the organism do with the drug?"), pharmacodynamics refers to the (physiologic) response of the organism to the drug (i.e., description of "What does the drug do to the organism?"). In a simplified way, pharmacodynamics may be seen as drug-mediated effects represented by biologic signal transmission. Many general anesthetic agents produce anesthesia by interaction with receptors, e.g., by increasing the activity of inhibitory receptors or systems and/or decreasing the activity of disinhibitory functions. In an experimental setup, this can be revealed by the observation of reactions to agonists, partial antagonist, and antagonists.

Furthermore, another focus for the study of anesthetic drug action is on molecular mechanisms in structures and "second messenger" processes. Yet, when drug-associated receptor stimulation results in physiologic responses, the evaluation of the most important pharmacodynamic effect (anesthesia, sedation, hypnosis, analgesia) is primarily based on clinical responses. This can be achieved by clinical assessment, e.g., application of sedation scores, grading of voluntarily movement on command, etc., and within some limits also with the EEG. The main target organ of anesthetics is the brain, thus change in brain electrical activity can be visualized and quantified by the EEG or derived parameters (indexes, evoked potentials).

The classical tool to assess effects of anesthetic agents with respect to their clinical effect is the establishment of a dose–effect relationship. For this purpose, the drug concentration or dose is plotted versus an absolute or relative effect on the target parameter. The statistical connection of both is usually a sigmoid curve. This procedure allows qualitative and quantitative comparison of different drugs or drug effects. Many studies have shown a close dose–response relationship between effect site concentration of hypnotics and derived EEG parameters.

4 Pharmacodynamic Components of Anesthesia

General anesthesia, which has not yet been defined precisely, is composed of different subcomponents. The respective grading and interaction of these components to guarantee optimal conditions is, to a certain degree, unknown.

Optimized general anesthesia is represented by four components:

1. Mental blockade: providing unconsciousness during anesthesia
2. Sensory blockade: avoiding perception of (painful) stimuli and reactions of the nociceptive system during anesthesia
3. Motoric blockade: avoiding movement to provide optimal surgical conditions, mostly by muscle relaxants (neuromuscular monitoring)
4. Autonomic blockade and stress shielding by blocking neurovegetative and cardio circulatory responses (cardio circulatory monitoring)

Unfortunately, the effect of anesthetic drugs on these components is not easy to quantify. To begin with, there is no 100% reliable parameter for each of the subcomponents. Furthermore, there are very few drugs that act exclusively on only one subcomponent. Monitoring of components 3 and 4, motoric and autonomic blockade, by neuromuscular and hemodynamic monitoring is common in clinical practice. The sensitivity and specificity of standard hemodynamic parameters (blood pressure, heart rate) that have no good correlation to anesthetic depth can be increased by additional (calculated) parameters, e.g., pulse transit time or heart rate variability. However, the main components (1 and 2), namely mental and sensory blockade, are hard to separate and to quantify.

This difficulty can be illustrated by the following clinical example. After induction of anesthesia, in the relatively stimulus-free interval of waiting for skin incision, anesthesia may seem excessively "deep." With the stimulus of skin incision, the level of anesthesia may change, because skin incision may be seen as an arousal stimulus by induction of increased afferent nociceptive signal transmission. Subsequently, anesthesia becomes "too light." This change of the anesthetic level is due to insufficient blockade of the sensory pathway (component 2). This may also induce changes in components 1 (mental blockade) and 4 (autonomic blockade).

This overlap of the effects of different components of anesthesia may in part be the reason that no satisfactory monitoring for components 1 and 2 has been defined so far (see the chapter by T.K. Henthorn, this volume). Finally, the components are not independent from each other and are hard to separate. Several attempts to quantify specific requirements in analgesia or hypnosis failed because there is no valid parameter available.

In daily clinical practice, the administration of anesthetic agents is mainly based on pharmacodynamic side effects. Decreases in hemodynamic parameters with hypotension and bradycardia are common side effects of excessively high doses of anesthetics (both mainly hypnotic and mainly analgesic agents). On the other end of the spectrum, increases in hemodynamic parameters with hypertension and tachycardia (directly) reflect insufficient sensory blockade, but this may be caused by insufficient mental blockade (leading to stress reaction to unintended consciousness) or insufficient sensory blockade (leading to stress reaction to pain).

4.1 Mental Blockade

The term mental blockade refers to the goal of unconsciousness during general anesthesia. If defined as not being a dichotomous parameter, it implies a gradation. The corresponding anesthetic effect is referred to as the sedative and hypnotic component.

In particular if "lighter levels" of mental blockade are considered, an additional component of mental block must be kept in mind, namely the amnesic component. By definition, (complete) unconsciousness prevents memory formation because lack of consciousness prevents perception of events. If events are unperceived they cannot be remembered. With levels of anesthesia insufficient to produce complete unconsciousness, memory formation becomes possible. Again, it may be extremely difficult to detect and quantify these memories, because they may be implicit ("unconscious memory") and not voluntarily accessible. Still, traces of collected material have been stored and may subsequently influence a person or his/her behavior (see below, clinical evaluation). Generally, hypnotic and amnesic components are phenomena that are independent from each other (Veselis et al. 2001). By and large, explicit recall is already prevented by subanesthetic (sedative) concentrations of anesthetics, but the required level of consciousness for implicit memory formation is unclear. Recent data suggest that perceptual priming may occur in deeper levels of sedation and hypnosis than conceptual priming. A higher probability of memory formation is expected for events and contents that refer to the particular situation of a patient (when compared to unrelated or non-sense information). In addition, it is assumed that catecholamine promotes learning and memory during anesthesia.

Given the described phenomena of consciousness and amnesia, it may not be sufficient to aim for prevention of awareness (consciousness with subsequent explicit recall), but to prevent consciousness itself during anesthesia.

4.2 Sensory Blockade

The International Association for Study of Pain defines pain as "an unpleasant sensory and emotional experience associated with actual or potential tissue damage, or described in terms of such damage". Pain involves conscious perception of a noxious stimulus; it is a combination of sensory (discriminative) and affective (emotional) components. The sensory component of pain is defined as nociception. The term analgesia refers to absence of pain. As the definition of pain refers to both the state of consciousness (component 1, mental blockade) and reaction to a noxious stimulus, it must be avoided if a separation between component 1 (mental blockade) and component 2 (sensory blockade) is the goal.

While analgesia refers to (conscious) perception of pain (and can thus be reached by blockade of pain pathways and consciousness), antinociception is specifically mediated by drug modulation of signal transmission within the nociceptive system. Therefore, antinociception does not only prevent conscious (or unconscious) perception, but will also prevent neuronal or spinal effects related to nociceptive input (e.g., changes in protein or gene expression), which have been shown to induce long-term effects of insufficient analgesia (and insufficient antinociception).

5 Quantification of Anesthetic Drug Pharmacodynamics

In general, responses to anesthetics are associated with depression of the cardio-circulatory system, resulting in hypotension or bradycardia. In daily clinical practice, these parameters are predominantly used to assess the level of general anesthesia. As mentioned before, such a strategy uses side effects of anesthetics rather than specific main effects to assess their effect. Quantification of drug effects on the basis of hemodynamic reactions uses only indirect and nonspecific parameters—so-called surrogate parameters, which are not only affected by the drug that is to be quantified, but are influenced by several unspecific effects (e.g., antihypertensive medication, lack of nociceptive stimulation, individual variability).

It is very unlikely that the concentration–effect relationship between main effect and surrogate parameters is constant for all anesthetics. Therefore, parameters that reflect directly and specifically anesthetic main effects are required to assess pharmacodynamic responses to these drugs. Several parameters and clinical methods are available to assess the level of sedation/hypnosis and analgesia/antinociception. Most of these methods are to some degree helpful in daily clinical practice, but each of the methods has its limitations.

Clinical assessment of the specific drug effect can only be performed during the awake state (see Sect. 4.1). During deeper levels of sedation and during general anesthesia itself, (specific) patient reactions have ceased and monitoring methods can be based on changes of (electrical) brain activity using EEG, EP, or calculated anesthesia indexes (see Sect. 4.2).

5.1 Clinical Assessment of Mental and Sensory Blockade

5.1.1 Clinical Assessment of Mental Blockade: OAA/S, MOAA/S, Scoring Systems of Sedation

Limitations of surrogate parameters to assess the anesthetic pharmacodynamics of mental blockade have been demonstrated. In a closed claims analysis for awareness during anesthesia, awareness was not conclusively indicated by respective surrogate parameters: increases in blood pressure (only 10% of all cases), tachycardia (only 7% of all cases), or movement (only 2% of all cases) (Domino et al. 1999). There have been other attempts to assess the mental blockade more specifically. Different approaches to the clinical assessment of mental blockade reflect the differences in the underlying definition of mental blockade. First, mental blockade can be seen as a dichotomous "all or none" phenomenon, i.e., the patient is conscious or unconscious. The assessment accordingly is usually performed during induction of and emergence from anesthesia. The assessment refers to patient responsiveness, i.e., the patient is asked to follow a command, e.g., to open his/her eyes or squeeze the assessor's hand (Brice et al. 1970). This approach refers to a very distinctive clinical feature but does not allow investigators to differentiate anesthetic effects beyond the loss of consciousness or at "lighter levels," i.e., before loss of consciousness. In other clinical settings, absence/presence of awareness, i.e., consciousness with explicit memory, serves as a dichotomous clinical measure (Myles et al. 2004). Unfortunately, in contrast to consciousness, awareness cannot be detected while it occurs. As it involves storage (and explicit recall) of events, it can only be detected after the cessation of anesthesia, i.e., too late. Further dichotomous measures include eyelash reflex, corneal reflex, or other reflexes. Unfortunately, these are only surrogate parameters of the level of consciousness, and are not necessarily directly related to the level of sedation and hypnosis. As dichotomous measures only separate into two different stages, they are not very helpful with respect to a graduation of anesthetic effects. For this purpose, a more detailed assessment is required. As with any subjective assessment, the quantification of pharmacodynamic drug effects on vigilance bears the risk of subjectivity and bias. In 1990, Chernik et al. introduced a standardized questionnaire with a scale to assess the effects of midazolam on vigilance, the so-called OAA/S (observers assessment of alertness/sedation scale) (Chernik et al. 1990). The OAA/S is based on a combination of observations of the resting patient (expression, eyes) and patient responses (responsiveness, speech) to verbal commands with increasing intensity. In the original work, it was developed and validated to assess the sedative effect of midazolam.

The OAA/S scale has never been validated for drugs other than midazolam; nevertheless it has been treated as a pseudo gold standard, and several studies used the OAA/S to quantify pharmacodynamic effects of drug-induced sedation (Table 1).

Several characteristics of the OAA/S assessment require particular attention. First, it quantifies reactions of a patient to commands. By definition, this requires

Table 1 OAA/S score. The subcomponent with the lowest numerical score equals the OAA/S composite score

Clinical assessment				Composite score level
Responsiveness[1]	Speech[2]	Facial expression[3]	Eyes[4]	
Responds readily to name spoken in normal tone	Normal	Normal	Clear, no ptosis	5
Lethargic response to name spoken in normal tone	Mild slowing or thickening	Mild relaxation	Glazed or mild ptosis (less than half the eye)	4
Responds only after name is called loudly and/or repeatedly	Slurring or prominent slowing	Marked relaxation (slack jaw)	Glazed and marked ptosis (half the eye or more)	3
Responds only after mild prodding or shaking	Few recognizable words	–	–	2
Does not respond to mild prodding or shaking	–	–	–	1

[1]Responsiveness is assessed by calling the subject's name once or twice in normal tone

[2]Speech is assessed by asking the subject to repeat the sentence "The quick brown fox jumps over the lazy dog"

[3]Facial expression

[4]The subject's ability to focus and ptosis are assessed

a patient who remains, to some degree, responsive, i.e., OAA/S can only be used to quantify sedation, i.e., subanesthetic effects, because anesthetic effects render a patient unconscious and unresponsive. Second, the assessment itself changes the level of sedation because arousal stimuli are used to quantify pharmacodynamic effects. In an attempt to extend the assessment to "deeper" levels of anesthesia, a modification of the OAA/S score (MOAAS) has been developed. The MOAAS is an extension of the OAA/S with assessment of reaction to painful stimuli. As reactions to painful stimuli are still possible at anesthetic levels that block reactions to verbal command, prodding, or shaking, the MOAAS can be used to assess "deeper" levels of anesthesia. The tradeoff of this advantage is a mixed assessment of a combination of mental and sensory blockade.

Analgesia and sedation are essential elements of intensive care treatment and relevant for patient outcome. There is a need to monitor and define the level of sedation and pain to provide patients with adequate analgesia and sedation. The development of several scoring systems has provided tools to evaluate a patient's state and to assess respective pharmacodynamic effects of concepts for sedation, analgesia, and anxiolysis. For the assessment of the level of sedation in intensive care patients, clinical assessment of sedation is most often performed by the Ramsay scale, the sedation agitation scale, or the Richmond agitation sedation scale (Table 2).

Information about pharmacodynamic effects from clinical evaluation during very deep sedation resulting in Ramsay sedation scale 5 and 6 and/or neuromuscular blockade is far from sufficient. Again, clinical evaluation using scoring systems is restricted to the awake state. In the unconscious or unresponsive patient, monitoring of brain electrical activity (and neuromonitoring) may provide more information about increasing pharmacodynamic effects, i.e., mental blockade and sensory blockade. Thus, anesthetic drug pharmacodynamics has been evaluated for years by different monitoring systems that derived their information from EEG or the evoked potentials (Fig. 3).

5.1.2 Clinical Assessment of Sensory Blockade: Visual Analog Scale

Standard clinical assessment in awake subjects refers to analgesia, i.e., subjective pain perception. The visual or numerical analog scale allows an estimation of pain intensity by asking the patient to rate his current pain level. The method can be used to assess pain and the effects of analgesia, i.e., conscious perception of a noxious stimulus. Both pain and the visual analog scale (VAS) require responsiveness and consciousness of the patient and are therefore not useful constructs during anesthesia. At the latest stage, after loss of consciousness, a measure of nociception is required. United States guidelines for the application of analgesic and sedative drugs in critically ill patients call for constant and systematic assessment and documentation of pain symptoms. The most valid and reliable criterion for pain rating is the self-assessment of the patient via numerical or VAS. Assessment of pain and analgesia/antinociception in patients with limited communication or unconsciousness require

Table 2 Overview: scores for the assessment of sedation/agitation of ICU patients

Ramsay sedation score		Sedation agitation scale (SAS)		Motor activity assessment scale		Vancouver interaction and calmness scale		Richmond agitation sedation scale	
Score	Awake levels	Score	Degree of sedation	Score	Degree of sedation	Score		Score	Degree of sedation
1	Patient anxious and agitated or restless, or both	7	Dangerous agitation	0	Unresponsive	Interaction score/30	+4	Combative	
2	Patient cooperative, oriented and tranquil	6	Very agitated	1	Responsive only to noxious stimuli	1–6	Patient interacts	+3	Very agitated
3	Patient responds to command only	5	Agitated	2	Responsive to touch or name	1–6	Patient communicates	+2	Agitated
4	Brisk response	4	Calm and Cooperative	3	Calm and coo perative	1–6	Information communicated by patient is reliable	+1	Restless
5	Sluggish response	3	Sedated	4	Restless and cooperative	1–6	Patient cooperates	0	Alert and calm
6	No response	2	Very sedated	5	Agitated	6–1	Patient needs encouragement to respond to questions	−1	Drowsy
		1	Unarousable	6	Dangerously agitated, uncooperative	Calmness score/30		−2	Light sedation
						1–6	Patient appears calm	−3	Moderate sedation

(continued)

Table 2 (continued)

Ramsay sedation score		Sedation agitation scale (SAS)		Motor activity assessment scale		Vancouver interaction and calmness scale		Richmond agitation sedation scale	
Score	Awake levels	Score	Degree of sedation	Score	Degree of sedation	Score		Score	Degree of sedation
						6–1	Patient appears restless	–4	Deep sedation
						6–1	Patient appears distressed	–5	Unarousable
						6–1	Patient is moving uneasily around in bed		
						6–1	Patient is pulling at lines/tubes		
Most widely used		Validity/reliability tested in ICU patients		Adapted from SAS			Reliable and valid score for quality of sedation in adult ICU patients		Reliable and valid assessment of sedation and changes over time
Never tested for validity or reliability		Detailed assessment of agitation		Validated/reliable assessment of ventilated patients Better assessment of analgesia than VAS			Correlation with analgesic and sedative drugs		

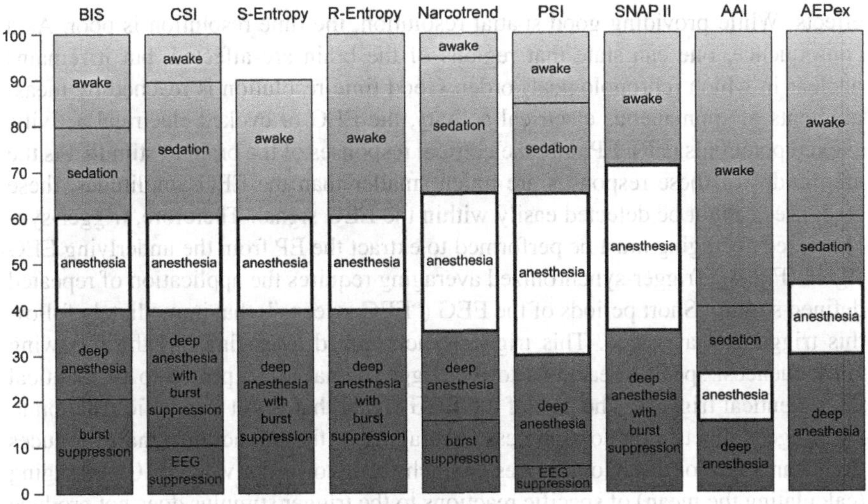

Fig. 3 Indexes of the hypnotic component of anesthesia. The figure shows currently available monitors of the hypnotic component of anesthesia and manufacturers' recommendations for index ranges. The fact that different indexes use different scaling may make direct comparisons difficult

the use of subjective parameters such as movement, facial expression, and physiologic parameters such as heart rate, respiratory rate, and blood pressure and requires gauging their change after analgesic therapy (Jacobi et al. 2002).

Adequacy of analgesia and antinociception during anesthesia and surgery is complex. With insufficient analgesia/antinociception, noxious stimuli are perceived and lead to a (subcortical) stress response. With adequate analgesia/antinociception, the perception of a noxious stimulus and the subcortical stress response are blocked. With increasing stimulus intensity, a higher dose of analgesic drugs is required to reach adequate analgesia/antinociception. With a lower level of noxious stimuli, less analgesic drugs are required to reach adequate analgesia and antinociception. It remains uncertain if, in the absence of stimuli, adequate analgesia and antinociception may be reached even without analgesic drugs. After all, adequacy of analgesia and antinociception is dependent on stimulus intensity, the level of analgesic drugs, and the individual drug response. In addition, the level of analgesia is dependent on the degree of mental blockade (the hypnotic component of anesthesia).

5.2 *Objective Assessment of Mental and Sensory Blockade*

Because the main target organ of anesthetic procedures is the brain, the pharmacodynamics of anesthetics may be assessed by parameters that reflect brain activity. For experimental purposes, this can be reached with positron emission tomography (PET) or functional MRI (fMRI). Both methods allow localization of drug main effects. While providing good spatial resolution, the time resolution is poor. As a consequence, one can state that regions of the brain are affected, but it remains unclear in which (chronological) order. Good time resolution is reached by measurements of spontaneous electrical activity, the EEG or evoked electrical activity, evoked potentials (EP). EP reflect electrical responses of the brain to stimuli. As the amplitudes of these responses are much smaller than the EEG amplitudes, these responses cannot be detected easily within the EEG signal. Therefore, trigger-synchronized averaging must be performed to extract the EP from the underlying EEG signal (Fig. 4). Trigger-synchronized averaging requires the application of repeated defined stimuli. Short periods of the EEG ("EEG sweeps") that immediately follow this trigger are averaged. This trigger-synchronized averaging has the following consequences: specific reactions to the trigger signal are expected to be identical after identical triggers. The part of the EEG signal that is not a specific reaction to the trigger reflects a random process. Averaging of these random signals produces the mean value of a random process, which tends toward a value of 0. Averaging (calculating the mean) of specific reactions to the trigger stimulus does not produce a value of 0, but the specific amplitude value of the reaction to this stimulus. As such, the trigger-related (specific) characteristic evoked potential curve develops while the trigger-unrelated (unspecific) background EEG disappears. Different stimuli can be used to produce EP. For the assessment of mental block, auditory stimuli have been suggested. The resulting signals are auditory evoked potentials (AEP). For the assessment of sensory blockade, different stimuli have been suggested, e.g., electrical stimuli (somatosensory EP, SSEP), painful stimuli [electrical stimulation to pain fibers (pain EP), painful laser stimuli (laser pain EP), or painful heat stimuli (contact heat-evoked potential stimuli, CHEPS)].

5.2.1 Monitoring of Mental Blockade: Spontaneous and Auditory Evoked Brain Activity—EEG and AEP

Anesthetics mediate inhibition of cerebral neuronal activity. The EEG is a noninvasive method to assess electrical activity of the (cortical) brain. Scalp electrodes capture cortical electrical activity, especially when clinical neurologic evaluation during anesthesia is impossible. During anesthesia, the EEG shows characteristic drug-induced changes. These changes are drug-specific, complex, and hard to quantify for the nonexpert. Classically, the EEG signal is analyzed with respect to localization (spatial distribution of the signal on the cortical surface). Several analytical approaches have been described that are based on different characteristics of the EEG signal.

Analysis of the EEG Frequency Spectrum

The EEG can be described with respect to frequency and amplitude. If Fourier transformation is used the EEG is seen as a periodic function that is reasonably

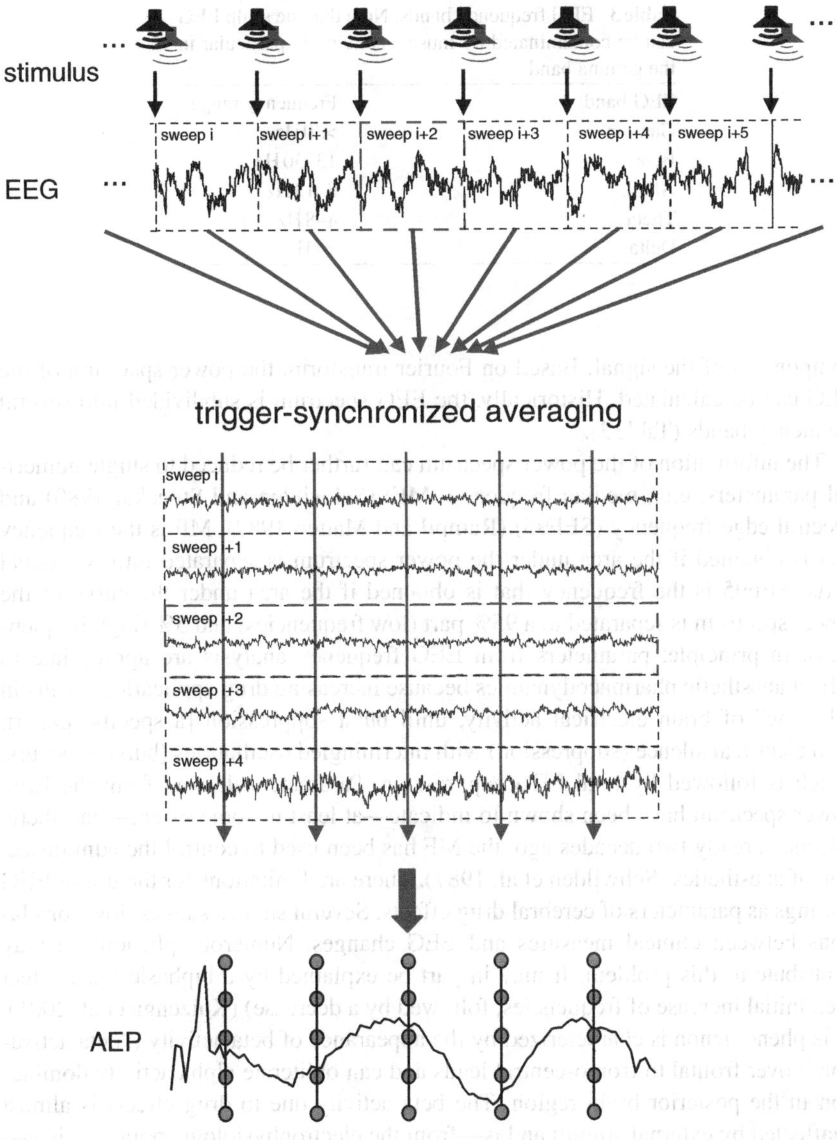

Fig. 4 Generation of an auditory evoked potential (*AEP*). Repeated auditory stimuli (*trigger*) are given (*above*) and the EEG is recorded together with the trigger stimulation (*second line*). Trigger-synchronized averaging (*middle*) reduces nontrigger-related EEG components as background noise, and leads to the averaged AEP (*below*). (Modified from Kochs et al. 2004)

continuous, and can therefore be expressed as the sum of a series of sine and cosine terms, each of which is defined by frequency, amplitude, and phase characteristics. The decomposition of a signal by Fourier transform leads to coefficients quantifying the fractional amount of each test function that describes specific frequency

Table 3 EEG frequency bands. Note that the scalp EEG can be contaminated by muscle activity, in particular in the gamma band

EEG band	Frequency range
Gamma	>30 Hz
Beta	13–30 Hz
Alpha	8–13 Hz
Theta	4–8 Hz
Delta	<4 Hz

components of the signal. Based on Fourier transform, the power spectrum of the EEG can be calculated. Historically, the EEG spectrum is subdivided into several frequency bands (Table 3).

The information of the power spectrum can further be reduced to single numerical parameters, e.g., median frequency (MF) (Schwilden and Stoeckel 1980) and spectral edge frequency (SEF95) (Rampil and Matteo 1987). MF is the frequency that is obtained if the area under the power spectrum is separated into two equal parts. SEF95 is the frequency that is obtained if the area under the curve of the power spectrum is separated to a 95% part (low frequencies) and 5% (high frequencies). In principle, parameters from EEG frequency analysis are appropriate to reflect anesthetic pharmacodynamics because increasing drug application results in "slowing" of brain electrical activity, until burst suppression [a specific pattern with electrical silence (suppression) with intermingled oscillations (bursts)] occurs, which is followed by total EEG suppression. Parameters derived from the EEG power spectrum have been shown to indicate—at least to some extent—anesthetic effects. Already two decades ago, the MF has been used to control the administration of anesthetics (Schwilden et al. 1987). There are limitations for the use of EEG findings as parameters of cerebral drug effects. Several studies suggest low correlations between clinical measures and EEG changes. Numerous phenomena may contribute to this problem. It may in part be explained by a biphasic EEG effect (i.e., initial increase of frequencies, followed by a decrease) (Kuizenga et al. 2001). This phenomenon is characterized by the appearance of beta activity ("beta activation") over frontal to fronto-central leads and can obliterate alpha activity domination in the posterior brain region. The beta activity due to drug effects is almost unaffected by external stimuli and is—from the electrophysiologic point of view—in contrast to the clinical picture, which reflects the onset of tiredness/sleepiness.

In addition, potential sources of error include inappropriate parameters calculated from the EEG, high intra- or interindividual variability, age-related alterations of the EEG, or insufficient artifact detection. Drug-specific effects can further impede the clinical applicability of the EEG (disinhibition, excitation of cerebral neuronal activity following ketamine or etomidate).

MF and SEF reflect frequency and power (=amplitude^2) of the EEG spectrum, but phase information (which describes the time relation between single frequencies) is lost. Phase information of the EEG is described by the bispectrum or the bicoherence. An excellent description of principles of frequency-based EEG analysis has been published by Rampil (1998). Parameters of the bispectrum have been shown to detect inadequate anesthesia (Abke et al. 1996). However, their contribution to the EEG in the anesthetized state has been challenged recently by the finding that during propofol/alfentanil anesthesia the bicoherence is zero or a constant (Jeleazcov et al. 2005). It was concluded that in this case the EEG can be considered as a linear random process, suggesting that during anesthesia the spectral information in the frequency domain is mostly contained in the power spectrum. Nevertheless, EEG measures for quantification of nonlinear characteristics of the signal have been developed recently.

Analysis of the EEG Order/Disorder

EEG parameters that quantify the order or disorder of the EEG have been suggested as measures of anesthetic effects, such as approximate entropy (ApEn) (Pincus et al. 1991), spectral entropy (SpEn) (Zhang et al. 2001), and Lempel-Ziv complexity (LZC) (Zhang et al. 2001). These nonlinear measures may quantify characteristics of the EEG signal that are not assessed by (linear) spectral analysis, which considers the EEG signal as a sum of harmonic oscillations. Permutation entropy (PeEn) is an alternative measure of complexity. In contrast to ApEn, PeEn is not limited to the prerequisite of low dimensionality. Because the order of EEG signals may be of higher dimensions and superposed with noise, PeEn can provide better results than other complexity parameters (Jordan et al. 2006).

ApEn considers the EEG signal generated by a low-dimensional dynamic system, which should reflect complementary properties of EEG signals. Basically, it describes the regularity of signals but is not an estimation of the entropy, since the EEG is assumed to be high dimensional (Thakor and Tong 2004). ApEn seems to be an appropriate measure indicating depth of anesthesia, because the EEG signal shows more "order" and less "random" with increasing depth of anesthesia, and the values of ApEn correlates with the anesthetic concentration (Bruhn et al. 2000). SpEn is based on the spectrum of the EEG and computes the Shannon entropy of the frequency distribution of the EEG. EEG containing more frequency components leads to a higher entropy than signals with focused frequency content.

The LZC is based on a coarse graining of the EEG data, where the signal is first transformed into a binary sequence. The parameter gives a measure that counts the number of distinct subsequences in the analyzed sequence. It belongs to the class of nonlinear parameters and may reflect properties of the EEG signal similar to the properties represented by ApEn.

The PeEn analyzes consecutive subvectors of constant length n in the EEG signal interval. The order of samples in every subvector according to their amplitudes is computed and defines a permutation group of order n. The parameter value is given by the entropy of the distribution of the obtained permutations and quantifies the monotonic behavior of adjacent signal amplitudes.

While the parameters ApEn, LZC, and PeEn are rather independent of absolute amplitudes of the EEG and quantify the structure of the signal, SpEn is based on analysis of amplitudes.

Visual Analysis of AEP

For visual analysis of the AEP, characteristic peaks and troughs of the signal must be identified. Once identified, these peaks and troughs are analyzed with respect to amplitude (height of peak/trough) and latency (time from stimulus to peak/trough). The early components of the AEP (BAEP) reflect the response of the brainstem to auditory stimuli and are relatively unaffected by general anesthesia. Long latency components (LLAEP) reflect conscious processing and associations of the auditory signal. These components are unstable and tend to vanish during sedation and anesthesia. Assessment of the mental blockade may be reached by analysis of the mid-latency component of the AEP (MLAEP), which has by numerous research groups been suggested to reflect amnesia and unresponsiveness. In general, increasing anesthetic administration decreases amplitudes and increases latencies. A review about the application of evoked potentials in anesthesia has been published by Thornton and Sharpe (1998). Unfortunately, numerous artifact sources are present during surgical anesthesia and it is difficult to identify AEP signal components (Schneider et al. 2004). As there is no gold standard for artifact rejection and signal smoothing, and visual analysis is not only time-consuming but may also be subjective and biased, several methods for automated analysis have been suggested.

Frequency-Based Analysis of AEP: Fourier Transform

In principle, peaks and troughs of the AEP may also be seen as waves. As described in the EEG section, waves can be analyzed by Fourier transform, which—in the case of AEP analysis—may detect longer latencies and lower amplitudes as "slower" waves, i.e., decrease of frequencies. Nevertheless, the application of Fourier transform to AEP analysis has several limitations. In principle, Fourier transform can be applied to a continuous periodic function, but may not be applied to transient signals (e.g., the AEP, a limited sequence of waves). Still, Fourier transform detects a change of the waveforms in general. Unfortunately, Fourier transform may loose information on the specific frequency contents of each component, i.e., the exact localization of this change within the AEP cannot be detected. Thus, it remains unclear whether the changes occur in the MLAEP (indicating mental blockade) or other components. The Fourier transform uses sinusoids of infinite length to evaluate the spectrum of a signal. With the simple spectrum, the information about the time is lost. Several techniques can be applied to compensate this disadvantage of Fourier transform. With the short-term Fourier transform the signal is broken into small pieces, the windowed Fourier transform uses a windowing function (e.g., a Hanning window) to limit the length of the sinusoidal wave.

With these modifications of Fourier analysis, time frequency resolution is possible to a certain degree, but restricted to the frequency of the sinusoidal wave compared to the length of the analysis window. The use of Fourier transform may limit the detection capability to a periodic component of the AEP signal.

Time–Frequency-Based Analysis of AEP: Wavelet Transform

Wavelet transform allows a time–frequency transformation of the AEP signal. Fourier transform decomposes a waveform into a sine wave and a family of harmonics. Wavelet transform is analogous to Fourier transform, but the fundamental unit of decomposition is not a sine waves of infinite duration, but a transient signal from a set of functions called "mother-wavelets." A wavelet is a finite function, is locally defined, and has an integral of 0. For wavelet analysis of the AEP, a specific mother-wavelet with the best approximation of the signal characteristics (i.e., peaks and troughs, frequencies) must be selected. For analysis of different frequencies of the signal, the wavelet is modified for each analysis step. These modifications include dilation of the mother-wavelet (broadening or narrowing of the wavelet along the time axis) to extract the information about the underlying frequencies. Wavelets are shifted along the x-axis to extract information about time with respect to the different peaks and troughs of each AEP component. Wavelet analysis of the AEP can been used to separate consciousness from unconsciousness during general anesthesia—either alone (Kochs et al. 2001; Scheller et al. 2005) or in combination with EEG parameters (Schneider et al. 2005).

EEG-/AEP-Based Indexes of the Hypnotic Component of Anesthesia

In the last decade, several indexes of the hypnotic component of anesthesia have been developed. These indexes combine parameters from EEG (and in part AEP) analysis. In contrast to conventional parameters of EEG signal analysis, these indexes are designed by statistical or mathematical methods and nonphysiologic parameters.

Often, these indexes do not only analyze the "classical" EEG range (up to 30 Hz), but also high-frequency components. High-frequency components of the signal may not only reflect neuronal activity, but also muscle signal (electromyogram, EMG). Muscle activity is in the high-frequency range and overlaps with or obscures the EEG signal. This is in particular the case if signals are derived from the forehead, because the frontal muscle is a very prominent source of signal activity. Table 4 gives an overview of currently available indexes and their subcomponents.

Usually they are expressed as dimensionless numbers in the range of 0–100 and are designed to correlate inversely with the level of sedation and hypnosis during anesthesia. For each commercial index monitor, target ranges for sedation, general anesthesia, "deep" hypnosis, "near" suppression, and increasing burst suppression are recommended (Fig. 3).

Table 4 Indexes of the hypnotic level of anesthesia and their subcomponents. These indexes are mostly taken from several subcomponents. The table shows subcomponents that are currently on the market and contains information that has been published. As the algorithms are mostly proprietary, the information may be incomplete

Index	Subcomponents			
BIS	Spectral component: relative beta ratio= $\log \frac{P_{30\text{-}47Hz}}{P_{11-20Hz}}$	Bispectral component: SynchFastSlow= $\log \frac{B_{0.5-47Hz}}{B_{40-47Hz}}$	QUAZI suppression	Burst suppression ratio
CSI	Beta ratio = $S_N[f_1, f_2] = \sum_{f_i=f_1}^{f_2} P_n(f_i) \log\left(\frac{1}{P_n(f_i)}\right)$	Alpha ratio = $\log \frac{E_{30-42.5Hz}}{E_{11-21Hz}}$	(Beta-alpha) ratio = $\log \frac{E_{6-12Hz}}{E_{11-21Hz}}$	Burst suppression ratio
S-Entropy	Shannon entropy of the power spectrum 0.8–32 Hz:			
R-Entropy	Shannon entropy of the power spectrum 0.8–47 Hz:			
Narcotrend	Spectral parameters	Amplitude measures	Parameters of autoregressive modeling	
PSI	Absolute power gradient fronto polar—vertex regions (gamma band, up to 50 Hz)	Absolute power changes midline frontal—central regions (beta band)	Absolute delta power (vertex)	Mean frequency (midline frontal region)
	Total spectral power (frontopolar)	Absolute power changes midline frontal—parietal regions (alpha band)	Relative power slow delta (posterior)	Others (?)
SNAP II	High-frequency signal analysis (80–420 Hz)	Low frequency EEG analysis (0.1–18 Hz)		
AAI	"AEP" (via autoregressive modeling)	EEG analysis: $\log \frac{E_{30-47Hz}}{E_{10-20Hz}}$	Functions of the signal-noise-ratio	Burst suppression
AEPex	Morphology: $\text{Morph} = \sum_{t=0}^{N-2} \sqrt{\lvert s(t+1) - s(t) \rvert}$			

P, sum of spectral power; B, sum of bispectrum activity; E, sum of spectral energy

This correlation and the simple numerical structure would make these indexes an ideal measure of the pharmacodynamic effects of general anesthesia. In numerous studies, it has been suggested that these indexes are suitable for this purpose. Unfortunately, there are still some limitations. As already mentioned, these indexes are not physiologic measures, but statistical constructs. They are generally developed from databases of patients under general anesthesia. As the dataset is critical during the design of such an index, errors in this early stage may have fatal consequences, e.g., inadequate classification of the mental blockade by such an index. Unfortunately, the databases for the development of different indexes are proprietary and not freely accessible to the user. In addition, the algorithms of these indexes are mainly proprietary. Even when detailed algorithms of subcomponents have been described, the exact mode of combination of these subcomponents is still proprietary and inaccessible to the public. In addition, the calculation of these indexes requires some time. EEG has to be measured, analyzed, combined, and an index must be calculated. The resulting time delay before the actual index number is presented to the user is unknown. A recent study showed that this delay is not only different for different indexes, but varies even within a single index. Depending on both the direction and level of anesthetic change, the interval is widely variable and may last more than 2 min (Pilge et al. 2006). All these factors make it difficult to identify the reasons underlying results that seem unreasonable or hard to explain, even more so when different indexes lead to different assumptions of pharmacodynamic properties of drugs.

Indexes might be better suited to grading sedative or hypnotic effects than classical EEG parameters such as median or spectral edge frequency, but they are less than ideal for assessment of anesthetic depth. Nevertheless, monitors for depth of anesthesia provide additional information about anesthetic effects on the brain (and possibly frontal muscle). Due to the problems of contamination with muscle activity and unknown algorithms, the various monitors on the basis of processed EEG or AEP parameters should be treated as surrogate measures of mental blockade.

5.2.2 Monitoring of Sensory Blockade: Current Approaches and Potential Candidates

Monitoring of sensory blockade is even more complex than monitoring of mental blockade. One of the main problems is the relative lack of reliable clinical assessment. A good measure of sensory blockade should detect nociception and assess the level of antinociception. Assessment of adequacy of antinociception is characteristically a stimulus–response type of measurement. The according clinical questions are:

- Will the patient *respond* to a given noxious *stimulus*? (prediction)
- Did the patient *respond* (nociception) to a noxious *stimulus*? (detection)

Analysis of Evoked Potentials

SSEP may reflect the analgesic component. Several findings and theoretical aspects suggest that changes in pain perception or the modulation of nociceptive transmission in response to drug application can be assessed by cortical SSEP components. In particular, the pontine thalamic components of the SSEP can measure the analgesic component of balanced anesthesia (Thornton et al. 1998). Unfortunately, SSEP are not only influenced by antinociception, but also by sedation and hypnotic drugs. There are two main problems to assess qualitative SSEP signal changes:

1. Electrical surface stimulation does not specifically stimulate the nociceptive system, i.e., Aδ- and C-fibers, but generally (and mainly) sensory pathways. There may be more information from findings with an intradermal electrical stimulation technique, which specifically stimulates nociceptive pathways. Obviously, such an approach, which requires invasive preparation of the skin, must remain experimental. A further limitation is habituation, i.e., decrease of nociceptive responses after repeated stimuli. An alternative approach is the application of laser-evoked heat stimuli. Selection of the appropriate wavelength allows for stimulation under the surface of the skin, with an optimum depth in the region of nociceptors (Arendt-Nielsen 1994; Bromm and Treede 1991). Due to its noninvasive character, the laser stimulus can be moved over the surface and habituation is avoided. Unfortunately, even laser-evoked potentials—which use a specific stimulus for the nociceptive pathway—decrease to both analgesic and hypnotic/sedative drugs. As the stimulus specificity does not allow a reliable differentiation between mental blockade and sensory blockade, the assessment of laser-induced evoked potentials has not become the standard assessment of the sensory blockade of anesthesia. Lately, a nonspecific approach has been studied, the application of fast heating surface electrodes to apply CHEPS. The first observations seem promising, but a separation between mental and sensory blockade may also not be reached (unpublished data from the first observations in a volunteer study performed by P. Bischoff, G. Schneider, E. Kochs).
2. Differentiation of SSEP signal changes (components) induced by antinociceptive drug effects cannot currently be separated from signal changes induced by sedative/hypnotic drug effects.

Decreases of brain electrical activity until loss of consciousness also suppresses evoked potentials. This may be due to either a direct depressant effect or an indirect general effect on the central nervous system. As the application of specific stimuli may not allow a separation between mental and sensory blockade, it has been suggested that specific parts of the changes of the EP may indicate mental, other parts sensory, blockade. It seems a reasonable assumption that specific signal components may be separated by signal analysis methods. The main problem in this context is the lack of a specific clinical measure of antinociception. Without this clinical assessment, it may be hard to identify such a component in the mixed reaction of the EP.

Several studies suggest that evoked potential responses to anesthetics are complex and not uniform. The literature indicates a high variability in responses to anesthetics. Findings range from decrease to increase, some drugs do not seem to affect signal generation, and therefore SSEP changes may not indicate a simple suppression of neural activity. In general, EP parameters cannot be easily correlated with the functional state of the brain.

The Combined Index Approach to the Quantification of Sensory Blockade

Similar to the development of a combined EEG (AEP) index, an index composed from different parameters may indicate the level of antinociception. During the development of such an index, one must control the input (noxious stimulus) and the level of antinociception (level of analgesic drug) in individuals and measure the response to this stimulus. Unfortunately, the assessment of the response remains difficult for this approach also. In addition, as daily clinical practice shows, there is a wide interindividual variability in the requirements of analgesic drugs. One of the potential parameters is blood pressure, in particular the arterial pressure curve, because it reflects not only the pressure reaction of stimulation, but also details of vasomotor responses. Unfortunately, continuous blood pressure is seldom available. In addition, there are many confounding factors. It has been suggested that changes of the heart rate reflects reactions to noxious stimuli. Sudden acceleration indicates sympathetic activation, which is potentially caused by nociception. Again, this parameter is sensitive to various confounding factors and difficult to interpret individually. In addition, heart rate variability and respiratory sinus arrhythmia have been suggested as more robust measures, but they may rather reflect the level of activation of the autonomic nervous system. Various influences on sympathetic and parasympathetic factors indicate sensitivity to confounding factors. In addition, a very large inter- and intraindividual variability has been observed, which makes results difficult to interpret on an individual basis. Skin vasomotor response (SVmR) may also be a promising parameter. It is based on vasoconstriction due to sympathetic activation. This sympathetic activation may be caused by nociception and can be measured on the skin surface by laser Doppler. Unfortunately, all the parameters mentioned are not specific for sensory blockade, but rather reflect autonomic blockade. They may be altered as a consequence of insufficient sensory blockade, but again, they are only surrogate parameters of sensory blockade.

In principle, the search for a quantification of sensory blockade must be performed on the basis of clearly defined prerequisites.

The response approach may allow a sensitive and to some degree specific detection of nociception (stress reaction due to noxious stimulus). In immobilized patients with adequate levels of hypnosis, this may serve as a detection or warning of insufficient antinociception.

The state approach may allow an assessment of the effect of analgesic drugs on an ongoing stimulus and bears the potential of prediction.

Unfortunately, both approaches currently seem to be based on autonomic blockade as a surrogate target for sensory blockade. Therefore, the basic requirement is the development of a reliable clinical reference score that remains valid once consciousness is lost.

5.3 Closing Remarks About the Assessment of Mental and Sensory Blockade

So far, our knowledge about multimodal complex mechanisms in the brain is unsatisfactory. Findings from several studies are controversial, and findings from animals are not necessarily transferable to humans. Even if numerous approaches tend to develop specific measures of the defined subcomponents (mental, sensory, motor, and autonomic blockade), no specific parameter has been found. In addition, while the separation into these four subcomponents may be a helpful construct, the general mechanisms are more complex and it may be impossible to clearly separate the subcomponents. As of today, there is no parameter available reliably reflecting the qualitative or quantitative pharmacodynamics of anesthetic drugs.

References

Abke J, Nahm W, Stockmanns G, Kalkman C, Kochs E (1996) Detection of inadequate anesthesia by EEG power and bispectral analysis. Anesthesiology 85:A477

Arendt-Nielsen L (1994) Characteristics, detection, and modulation of laser-evoked vertex potentials. Acta Anaesthesiol Scand 101:7–44

Brice DD, Hetherington RR, Utting JE (1970) A simple study of awareness and dreaming during anaesthesia. Br J Anaesth 42:535–542

Bromm B, Treede RD (1991) Laser-evoked cerebral potentials in the assessment of cutaneous pain sensitivity in normal subjects and patients. Rev Neurol (Paris) 147:625–643

Bruhn J, Röpcke H, Hoeft A (2000) Approximate entropy as an electroencephalographic measure of anesthetic drug effect during desflurane anesthesia. Anesthesiology 92:715–726

Chernik DA, Gillings D, Laine H, Hendler J, Silver JM, Davidson AB, Schwam EM, Siegel JL (1990) Validity and reliability of the Observer's Assessment of Alertness/Sedation Scale: study with intravenous midazolam. J Clin Psychopharmacol 10:244–251

Domino KB, Posner KL, Caplan RA, Cheney FW (1999) Awareness during anesthesia: a closed claims analysis. Anesthesiology 90:1053–1061

Fechner J, Ihmsen H, Hatterscheid D, Jeleazcov C, Schiessl C, Vornov JJ, Schwilden H, Schüttler J (2004) Comparative pharmacokinetics and pharmacodynamics of the new propofol prodrug GPI 15715 and propofol emulsion. Anesthesiology 101:626–639

Ihmsen H, Jeleazcov C, Schüttler J, Schwilden H, Bremer F (2006) Pharmacodynamics of two different propofol formulations. Anaesthesist 55:635–642

Jacobi J, Fraser GL, Coursin DB, Riker RR, Fontaine D, Wittbrodt ET, Chalfin DB, Masica MF, Bjerke HS, Coplin WM, Crippen DW, Fuchs BD, Kelleher RM, Marik PE, Nasraway SA Jr, Murray MJ, Peruzzi WT, Lumb PD (2002) Clinical practice guidelines for the sustained use of sedatives and analgesics in the critically ill adult. Crit Care Med 30:119–141

Jeleazcov C, Fechner J, Schwilden H (2005) Electroencephalogram monitoring during anesthesia with propofol and alfentanil: the impact of second order spectral analysis. Anesth Analg 102:1365–1369

Jordan D, Schneider G, Kochs EF (2006) EEG Permutation entropy separates consciousness from unconsciousness during anesthesia. ASA abstracts A-1551

Kochs E, Stockmanns G, Thornton C, Nahm W, Kalkman CJ (2001) Wavelet analysis of middle latency auditory evoked responses: calculation of an index for detection of awareness during propofol administration. Anesthesiology 95:1141–1150

Kochs HD, Stockmanns G, Lücke D, Kochs E, Schneider G, Jordan D (2004) Tiefschlaf garantiert. Neue Technick für mehr Sicherheit bei Narkosen. Forum Forschung. http://www.forum-forschung.de/2004/pdf/fofo2004_13_kochs.pdf. Cited 5 Sep 2007

Kuizenga K, Wierda JM, Kalkman CJ (2001) Biphasic EEG changes in relation to loss of consciousness during induction with thiopental, propofol, etomidate, midazolam or sevoflurane. Br J Anaesth 86:354–360

Lennmarken C, Bildfors K, Enlund G, Samuelsson P, Sandin R (2002) Victims of awareness. Acta Anaesthesiol Scand 46:229–231

Myles PS, Leslie K, McNeil J, Forbes A, Chan MT (2004) Bispectral Index monitoring to prevent awareness during anaesthesia: the B-Aware randomised controlled trial. Lancet 363:1757–1763

Pilge S, Zanner R, Schneider G, Blum J, Kreuzer M, Kochs EF (2006) Time delay of index calculation: analysis of cerebral state, bispectral, and narcotrend indices. Anesthesiology 104:488–494

Pincus SM, Gladstone IM, Ehrenkranz RA (1991) A regularity statistic for medical data analysis. J Clin Monit 7:335–345

Rampil IJ (1998) A primer for EEG signal processing in anesthesia. Anesthesiology 89:980–1002

Rampil IJ, Matteo RS (1987) Changes in EEG spectral edge frequency correlate with the hemodynamic response to laryngoscopy and intubation. Anesthesiology 67:139–142

Salomons TV, Osterman JE, Gagliese L, Katz J (2004) Pain flashbacks in posttraumatic stress disorder. Clin J Pain 20:83–87

Sandin RH, Enlund G, Samuelsson P, Lennmarken C (2000) Awareness during anaesthesia: a prospective case study. Lancet 355:707–711

Scheller B, Schneider G, Daunderer M, Kochs EF, Zwissler B (2005) High-frequency components of auditory evoked potentials are detected in responsive but not in unconscious patients. Anesthesiology 103:944–950

Schneider G (2003) Intraoperative Wachheit. Anesthesiol Intensivmed Notfallmed Schmerzther 38:75–84

Schneider G, Kochs EF, Arenbeck H, Gallinat M, Stockmanns G (2004) Signal verification of middle latency auditory evoked potentials by automated detection of the brainstem response. Anesthesiology 101:321–326

Schneider G, Hollweck R, Ningler M, Stockmanns G, Kochs EF (2005) Detection of consciousness by electroencephalogram and auditory evoked potentials. Anesthesiology 103:934–943

Schwilden H, Stoeckel H (1980) Investigations on several EEG-parameters as indicators of the state of anaesthesia the median—a quantitative measure of the depth of anaesthesiol. Anesthesiol Intensivther Notfallmed 15:279–286

Schwilden H, Schüttler J, Stoeckel H (1987) Closed-loop feedback control of methohexital anesthesia by quantitative EEG analysis in humans. Anesthesiology 67:341–347

Sebel PS, Bowdle TA, Ghoneim MM, Rampil IJ, Padilla RE, Gan TJ, Domino KB (2004) The incidence of awareness during anesthesia: a multicenter United States study. Anesth Analg 99:833–839

Song D, van Vlymen J, White PF (1998) Is the Bispectral Index useful in predicting fast-track eligibility after ambulatory anesthesia with propofol and desflurane? Anesth Analg 87:1245–1248

Thakor NV, Tong S (2004) Advances in quantitative electroencephalogram analysis methods. Annu Rev Biomed Eng 6:453–495

Thornton C, Sharpe RM (1998) Evoked responses in anaesthesia. Br J Anaesth 81:771–781

Upton RN, Ludbrook GL (1997) A physiological model of induction of anaesthesia with propofol in sheep. 1. Structure and estimation of variables. Br J Anaesth 79:497–504

Veselis RA, Reinsel RA, Feshchenko VA (2001) Drug-induced amnesia is a separate phenomenon from sedation: electrophysiologic evidence. Anesthesiology 95:896–907
White PF, Ma H, Tang J, Wender RH, Sloninsky A, Kariger R (2004) Does the use of electroencephalographic Bispectral Index or auditory evoked potential index monitoring facilitate recovery after desflurane anesthesia in the ambulatory setting? Anesthesiology 100:811–817
Zhang XS, Roy RJ, Jensen EW (2001) EEG complexity as a measure of depth of anesthesia for patients. IEEE Trans Biomed Eng 48:1424–1433

Defining Depth of Anesthesia

S.L. Shafer and D.R. Stanski(✉)

Abstract In this chapter, drawn largely from the synthesis of material that we first presented in the sixth edition of *Miller's Anesthesia*, Chap 31 (Stanski and Shafer 2005; used by permission of the publisher), we have defined anesthetic depth as the probability of non-response to stimulation, calibrated against the strength of the stimulus, the difficulty of suppressing the response, and the drug-induced probability of non-responsiveness at defined effect site concentrations. This definition requires measurement of multiple different stimuli and responses at well-defined drug concentrations. There is no one stimulus and response measurement that will capture depth of anesthesia in a clinically or scientifically meaningful manner. The "clinical art" of anesthesia requires calibration of these observations of stimuli and responses (verbal responses, movement, tachycardia) against the dose and concentration of anesthetic drugs used to reduce the probability of response, constantly adjusting the administered dose to achieve the desired anesthetic depth. In our definition of "depth of anesthesia" we define the need for two components to create the anesthetic state: hypnosis created with drugs such as propofol or the inhalational anesthetics and analgesia created with the opioids or nitrous oxide. We demonstrate the scientific evidence that profound degrees of hypnosis in the absence of analgesia will not prevent the hemodynamic responses to profoundly noxious stimuli. Also, profound degrees of analgesia do not guarantee unconsciousness. However, the combination of hypnosis and analgesia suppresses hemodynamic response to noxious stimuli and guarantees unconsciousness.

D.R. Stanski
3903 Albemarle St. NW, Washington, DC 20016, USA
drstanski@prodigy.net

J. Schüttler and H. Schwilden (eds.) *Modern Anesthetics*.
Handbook of Experimental Pharmacology 182.

1 Introduction

Anesthesiologists have offered multiple, and sometimes inconsistent, views on quantitative measures of the anesthetic state. Fortunately, an integrated, quantitative concept of the anesthetic state can now be built on the incremental knowledge developed since the introduction of anesthesia over a century ago. The history of attempts to define "depth of anesthesia" make one realize that our knowledge of the specific attributes of the drugs used in clinical practice has to be incorporated into our understanding of anesthetic depth. In this chapter we draw largely from the synthesis of material that we first presented in the sixth edition of *Miller's Anesthesia*, Chap. 31 (Stanski and Shafer 2005).

Depth of anesthesia is the interaction of two drug effects fundamental to clinical anesthesia. One drug effect involves the hypnotic component that creates unconsciousness. The second effect involves the analgesic component that decreases the body's reflex response to noxious stimuli. Finally, the judicious titration of these two components by the anesthesiologist produces clinical anesthesia in a safe and effective manner over a broad range of clinical situations.

2 What Is Anesthesia? A Modern Definition

The *sine qua non* of the anesthetized state is unconsciousness, the lack of conscious processing of thoughts. The crux of the difficulty in defining "anesthetic depth" is that unconsciousness cannot be measured directly. What can be measured is response to stimulation. Does the patient move when his name is called? Does the response to incision suggest conscious perception? Does the heart rate or blood pressure go up in response to surgical manipulation? Does the patient remember events, conversations, or pain? As observed by Prys-Roberts, anesthesia is non-responsiveness, broadly defined (Prys-Roberts 1987). The "depth" of anesthesia is determined by the applied stimulus, the observed response, and the drug concentration at the site of action that blunts responsiveness.

The state of consciousness can also be inferred, although not directly measured, by analysis of electroencephalographic information. This can be done using either spectral-based techniques, such as the "Bispectral Index" (BIS) (Aspect Medical Systems, Norwood, MA, USA) or using evoked potentials, such as auditory evoked potentials. These indices do not directly measure unconsciousness or unresponsiveness. However, through extensive clinical validation it is clear that these measures are predictive of the likelihood of response, provided that the anesthetic state has been induced with the drugs used to calibrate the electrophysiological measure.

Non-responsiveness can be introduced by deep natural sleep or 2% isoflurane. What distinguishes the non-reponsiveness of the anesthetic state from the non-responsiveness of normal sleep is the differential in stimulus that can penetrate the state of non-responsiveness and rouse the brain to conscious perception. The hypnotic drugs used in anesthesia (propofol, thiopental, inhaled anesthetics, ketamine) are each capable of producing such profound CNS depression that even the most painful surgical stimulus cannot rouse patients from a state of near total non-responsiveness. However, if the surgical stimulus can be attenuated before reaching the cortical level, then lower concentrations of drug are required to maintain the state of non-responsiveness.

Attenuation of surgical stimulation is the function of analgesic drugs (e.g., opioids) and local anesthetics. The interaction between analgesics and hypnotics is thus fundamental to understanding and defining anesthetic depth. Table 1 indicates the components of defining depth of anesthesia in the remainder of this chapter.

Extending ideas proposed by Glass (1998), consciousness is the balance within the cortex between depression and excitation (Fig. 1, upper right). The cortex is primarily

Table 1 Components needed to define depth of anesthesia

1. Afferent stimulus
2. Efferent response
3. Equilibrated concentrations of analgesic components
4. Equilibrated concentrations of hypnotic components
5. Equilibrated concentrations of other relevant drugs (e.g., beta blockers, muscle relaxants, local anesthetics)
6. Interaction surface relating the drug concentrations to the probability of the given response to the given stimulus

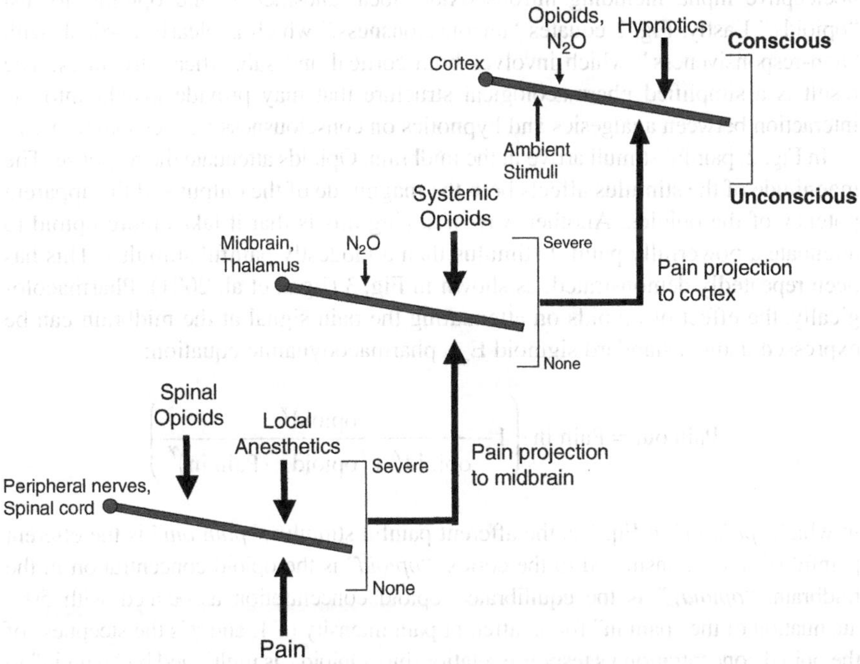

Fig. 1 Stylized view of the interaction between hypnotics, which depress consciousness, and analgesics, which suppress noxious stimuli

depressed by hypnotics, although opioids and nitrous oxide also have sedating properties. Cortical depression promotes unconsciousness. These effects are opposed by both ambient stimulation (e.g., music, a hard cold mattress) and the excitatory effects of pain projected from the thalamus and midbrain upon the cortex.

Figure 1 also shows the influence of opioids, nitrous oxide, and local anesthetics at preventing noxious stimulation from reaching the cortex. Opioids act primarily on the midbrain thalamus (Bencherif et al. 2002) and spinal cord. Local anesthetics act either at the spinal cord (for neuraxial blocks) or on peripheral nerves (e.g., nerve blocks and local infiltration). Nitrous oxide exerts some of its analgesic effects through spinal mechanisms (Fukuhara et al. 1998; Quock et al. 1990) as well as midbrain, (Fang et al. 1997), but for simplicity we will lump it together with opioids at the midbrain. The net effect of analgesics and local anesthetics is to attenuate the transmission of painful sensation to the cortex, reducing the amount of hypnotic required to obtain a state of non-responsiveness.

3 The Pharmacological View of the Anesthetic State

Figure 2 reduces the model in Fig. 1 to a highly simplified pharmacological view. The subcortical actions in Fig. 1 have been compressed to a single site of action, the midbrain. Similarly, Fig. 2 compresses all drugs that attenuate transmission of nociceptive input, including nitrous oxide, local anesthetics, and opioids, to just "opioids." Lastly, Fig. 2 equates "unconsciousness," which is clearly cortical, with "non-responsiveness," which involves both cortical and subcortical structures. The result is a simplified pharmacological structure that may provide insight into the interaction between analgesics and hypnotics on consciousness and responsiveness.

In Fig. 2, painful stimuli arrive in the midbrain. Opioids attenuate the response. The magnitude of the stimulus affects both the magnitude of the output and the apparent potency of the opioids. Another way of saying this is that it takes more opioid to attenuate a powerfully painful stimulus than a modestly painful stimulus. This has been repeatedly demonstrated, as shown in Fig. 3 (Egan et al. 2001). Pharmacologically, the effect of opioids on attenuating the pain signal at the midbrain can be expressed using a standard sigmoid E_{max} pharmacodynamic equation:

$$\text{Pain out} = \text{Pain in} \cdot \left(1 - \frac{\text{opioid}^{\gamma}}{\text{opioid}^{\gamma} + (\text{opioid}_{50} \cdot \text{Pain in})^{\gamma}}\right)$$

in which "*pain in*" in Eq. 1 is the afferent painful stimulus, "*pain out*" is the efferent painful stimulus transmitted to the cortex, "*opioid*" is the opioid concentration in the midbrain, "$opioid_{50}$" is the equilibrated opioid concentration associated with 50% attenuation of the "pain in" for an afferent pain intensity of 1, and γ is the steepness of the opioid concentration vs response relationship. Opioid_{50} is multiplied by "pain in" to reflect the decreased potency of opioids in attenuating severe pain, as shown in Fig. 3.

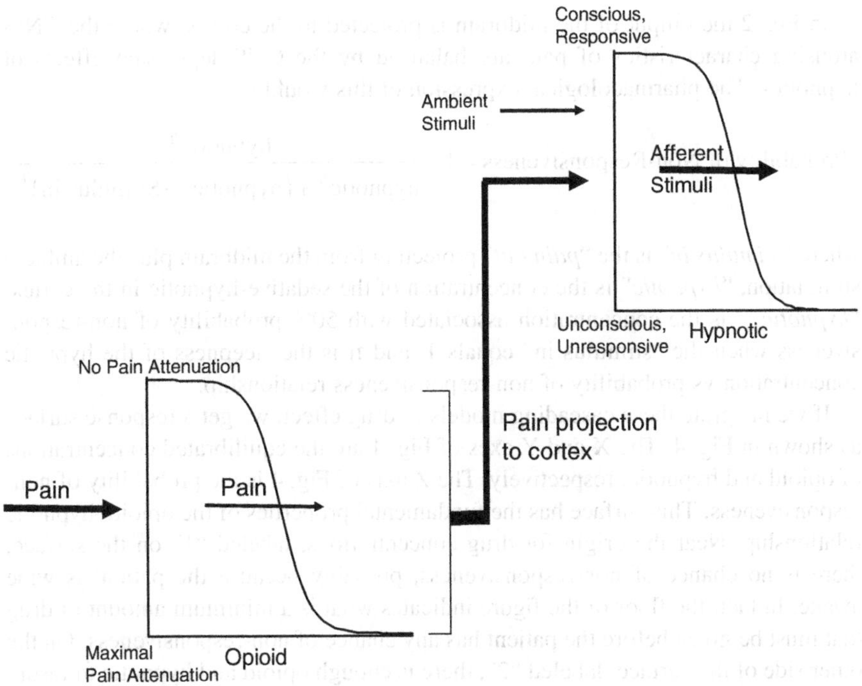

Fig. 2 Pharmacological interpretation of the interaction between hypnotics and analgesics

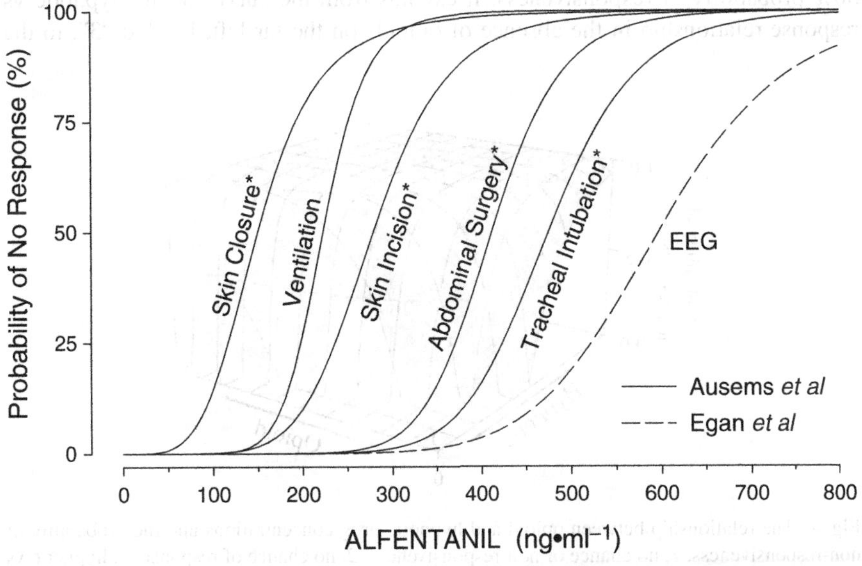

Fig. 3 The effect of increasingly painful stimulation on the opioid concentration vs response relationship (Egan et al. 2001). As the pain intensity increases, the apparent potency of the opioids decreases

In Fig. 2 the output of the midbrain is projected to the cortex, where the CNS-arousing characteristics of pain are balanced by the CNS-depressant effects of hypnotics. The pharmacological expression of this would be:

$$\text{Probability of Non-Responsiveness} = 1 - \frac{\text{hypnotic}^{\eta}}{\text{hypnotic}^{\eta} + \left(\text{hypnotic}_{50} \cdot \text{Stimulus in}\right)^{\eta}}$$

where "*stimulus in*" is the "*pain out*" projecting from the midbrain plus the ambient stimulation, "*hypnotic*" is the concentration of the sedative-hypnotic in the cortex, "$hypnotic_{50}$" is the concentration associated with 50% probability of non-responsiveness when the "stimulus in" equals 1, and η is the steepness of the hypnotic concentration vs probability of non-responsiveness relationship.

If we integrate these cascading models of drug effect, we get a response surface as shown in Fig. 4. The X and Y axes of Fig. 4 are the equilibrated concentrations of opioid and hypnotic, respectively, The Z axis of Fig. 4 is the probability of non-responsiveness. This surface has the fundamental properties of the opioid–hypnotic relationship. Near the origin for drug concentrations, labeled "1" on the surface, there is no chance of non-responsiveness, probably because the patient is wide awake. In fact, the floor of the figure indicates what is a minimum amount of drug that must be given before the patient has any chance of non-responsiveness. On the other side of the surface, labeled "2", there is enough opioid and hypnotic to insure virtually no chance of response. The gray line in the middle of the surface is the 50% isobole. This line shows the opioid and hypnotic concentrations associated with 50% probability of responsiveness. It extends from the curve for the hypnotic vs response relationship in the absence of opioids on the far left, labeled "3", to the

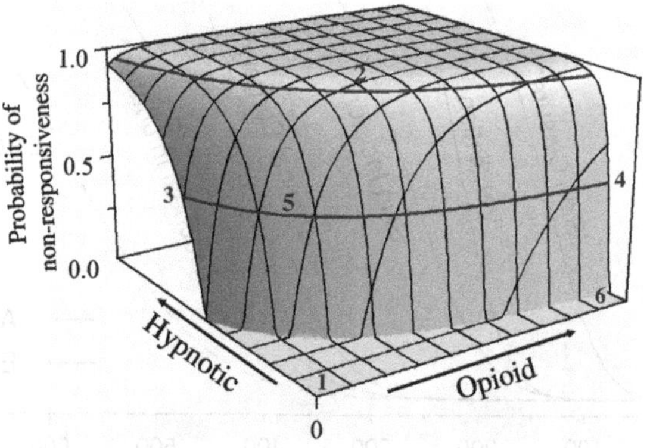

Fig. 4 The relationship between opioid and hypnotic drug concentrations and the probability of non-responsiveness. *1*, no chance of non-responsiveness; *2*, no chance of response; *3*, hypnotic vs response relationship in the absence of opioids; *4*, hypnotic vs response relationship in the presence of large doses of opioids; *5*, area of maximum synergy between opioids and hypnotics; *6*, in the absence of opioids even profound levels of opioids cannot suppress response; *gray line in the middle of the surface*, the 50% isobole; *gray curve at the top of the surface*, 95% isobole

hypnotic vs response relationship in the presence of large quantities of opioids on the right, labeled "4". The relationship between hypnotics and opioids is highly synergistic, in that when the drugs are used in combination (for example, at the point labeled "5"), it takes far less of either drug than would be the case were the opioids or hypnotics used alone. Notice how some hypnotic is required to achieve the anesthetized state. In the absence of a hypnotic, even profound levels of opioids are unable to produce a state of non-responsiveness, as can be seen at point "6" on the surface (Wynands et al. 1984; Sebel et al. 1992; McEwan et al. 1993; Vuyk et al. 1995). However, a modest amount of opioid profoundly reduces the concentration of hypnotic necessary for non-responsiveness, as seen at point "5". Beyond this, additional opioid has only modest effect at further reducing the hypnotic dose required for drug effect. The corollary is that large doses of hypnotic are required in the absence of an opioid (Smith et al. 1994; Kazama et al. 1997, 1998a). The gray curve at the top of the surface is the 95% isobole. This curve defines the opioid and hypnotic combinations associated with 95% probability of non-responsiveness. Because the surface is very steep, once there is a modest probability of non-responsiveness, a modest increase in drug concentration is all that is required to move from a 50% chance of non-responsiveness to 95% chance of non-responsiveness.

Figure 4 is intentionally left unit-less to illustrate that a very simple model of the anesthetic state, as shown in Fig. 2, generates a pharmacological response surface that is very much like those seen in virtually all drug interaction trials (Minto et al. 2000).

The ability of inhaled anesthetics to induce immobility in response to noxious stimulation is mediated by the spinal cord, not the cortex (Rampil et al. 1993; Rampil 1994; Antognini and Schwartz 1993). We also know that intravenous opioids primarily work at the level of the spinal cord and midbrain. Experimentally, the interaction between inhaled anesthetics and opioids in preventing movement response to noxious stimulation looks very close to Fig. 4. Thus, it seems logical that downward projections from the midbrain to the spinal cord (Fields and Anderson 1978) are responsible for the minimum alveolar concentration (MAC)-sparing properties of opioids. As such, a pharmacological model of the effect of opioids on MAC would resemble Fig. 1, with a few changes to reflect opioids attenuating the signal at the dorsal horn, and the response endpoint (movement) mediated by the spinal cord rather than the cortex.

4 Experimental Characterization of the Anesthetic State

To quantify anesthetic depth, we must be rigorous about the definition of the Z axis of Fig. 4, non-responsiveness. We consider a complex matrix of stimuli and responses, as shown in Fig. 5. Stimuli can be roughly divided into benign and noxious. Benign stimuli are not physically painful. Thus, responses to benign stimuli are readily suppressed by hypnotics alone, with minimal need for analgesic drugs. Noxious stimuli are physically painful, and thus responses to noxious stimuli are more readily suppressed in the presence of analgesics. Among the noxious stimuli,

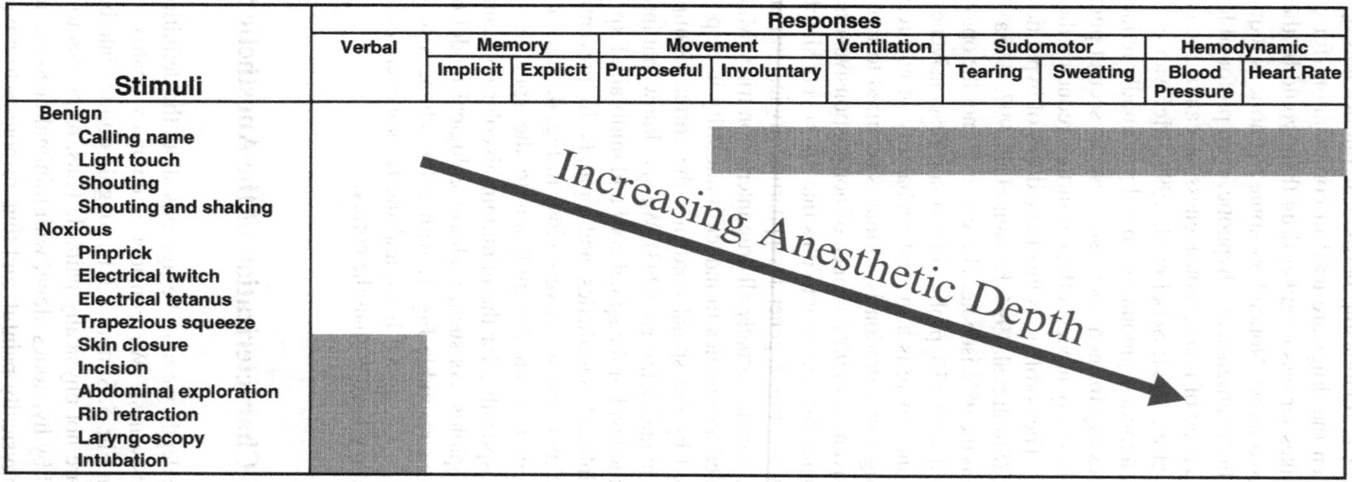

Fig. 5 Matrix of relevant stimuli and responses. Stimuli are in approximately increasing order of noxiousness. Responses are in approximately increasing order of difficulty of suppression. As the cells progress from *left to right*, and from *top to bottom*, increasingly larger doses of anesthetic drug are required to suppress the given response to the given stimulus

skin incision appears somewhat in the middle, being more stimulating than electrical pain, but much less stimulating than laryngoscopy and intubation. Figure 5 represents the noxious stimuli in approximately increasing order.

Responses can be categorized as verbal, purposeful movement, involuntary movement, ventilation, hemodynamic response, sudomotor response, formation of implicit and explicit memories, and electroencephalographic responses, as shown in Fig. 5. The responses follow a rank order, in that loss of verbal response precedes loss of purposeful movement, which proceeds loss of involuntary movement. Opioids tend to ablate hemodynamic response before movement, while hypnotics tend to ablate movement response before hemodynamic response (Kazama et al. 1998b). Given this, we would anticipate that the interaction surfaces between opioids and hypnotics for hemodynamic response and movement response would have several intersections. Frequently the responses are grouped. For example, the responses that suggest conscious perception: verbal, voluntary movement, and memory might be grouped together. Responses that are autonomic in nature, such as hemodynamic and sudomotor responses, are logically grouped together.

For simplicity we will consider complete non-responsiveness to be a lack of any of these responses. If we were only interested in consciousness, then we might not include involuntary movement, ventilation response, hemodynamic response, or sudomotor response in our list of important responses, since these can still occur in the absence of any conscious perception.

Figure 5 shows a matrix of stimuli and responses with 140 cells. Not all of the cells are clinically relevant. For example, people rarely have involuntary movements, hyperventilate, or show autonomic responses to hearing their name. On the converse side, anesthesia should never be so inadequate that patients scream on incision. Thus, some cells in Fig. 5 have been removed as being clinically uninteresting, leaving 122 cells to define anesthetic depth. If we wanted to fully characterize the ability of isoflurane and fentanyl to create a state of non-responsiveness for each the listed responses to any of the listed stimuli, we would need to characterize the response surface (Fig. 4) for each clinically relevant cell. With so many choices of stimuli and interactions, it is not surprising that anesthesiologists cannot agree on a simple definition of anesthetic depth. Fortunately, it is not really necessary to characterize the response to every stimulus. If we characterize the response to a benign stimulus, such as shaking and shouting, and several noxious stimuli, such as electrical tetanus, incision, laryngoscopy, and intubation, then we will have captured the clinically relevant range of benign and noxious stimulation.

To this we must add the matrix of hypnotics vs opioids. The commonly used hypnotics include the anesthetic gases halothane, isoflurane, sevoflurane, and desflurane, and the intravenous hypnotics propofol, thiopental, etomidate, and midazolam. The commonly used opioids include fentanyl, alfentanil, sufentanil, remifentanil, morphine, meperidine, hydromorphone, methadone, and (in Europe) tramadol and piritramide. With 8 hypnotics and 10 opioids, there are 80 combinations. Eighty combinations times 122 interactions yields 9,760 combinations of opioids, hypnotics, stimuli, and responses. To this we must then add the influence of age, disease, genetics, etc. Clearly, it is impractical to create response surfaces to characterize how opioids and hypnotics produce a state of non-responsiveness for all possible combinations of drugs, patients, stimuli, and responses.

Fortunately, there are powerful generalizations that provide both clinical insight and tractable experimental design. The most important is that for any stimulus–response pair, depth of anesthesia is the probability of non-response. More generally, *depth of anesthesia is the probability of non-response to stimulation, calibrated against the strength of the stimulus, the difficulty of suppressing the response, and the drug-induced probability of non-responsiveness.* Anesthetic depth ranges from 100% probability of an easily suppressed response (verbal answer) to a mild stimulus (e.g., calling name) and readily suppressed responses (e.g., verbal answer), to 100% probability of non-response to profoundly noxious stimuli (e.g., intubation) and responses that are difficult to suppress (e.g., tachycardia). Table 1 lists the components needed to define anesthetic depth.

Figure 6 integrates the role of anesthetic drugs into the stimulus–response relationship. It shows three stimuli of increasing intensity: calling name, incision, and intubation. It also shows three responses of increasing difficulty to suppress: verbal, movement, and hemodynamic response. Within three of the cells are representative opioid-hypnotic interactions. As seen in the cells, verbal response to name calling is readily suppressed by hypnotics, with only modest effect from opioids. Movement to incision requires more hypnotic and opioid to suppress. Additionally, the "Z" probability axis has been stretched vertically to indicate that 100% chance of

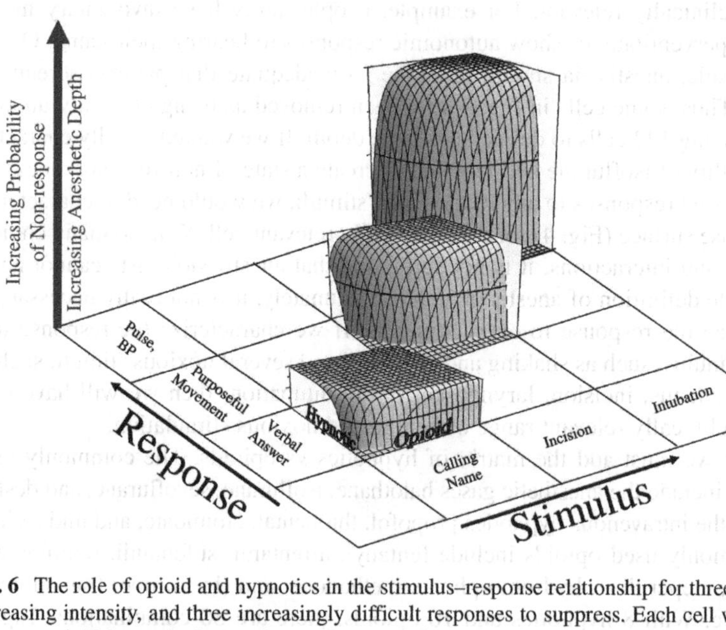

Fig. 6 The role of opioid and hypnotics in the stimulus–response relationship for three stimuli of increasing intensity, and three increasingly difficult responses to suppress. Each cell would have its own opioid–hypnotic interaction surface, and three are displayed. The *vertical axis* is the probability of non-response. Verbal non-responsiveness to name calling is readily suppressed, even at light levels of anesthesia. In contrast, profound levels of anesthesia are required to suppress homodynamic response to intubation

non-response to incision is a more profound level of drug effect than 100% chance of non-response to name calling. Suppressing the most difficult response, hypertension and tachycardia, to the most profound stimulus, intubation, requires even more opioid and hypnotic. Additionally, the probability axis is further elongated vertically, indicating that suppression of hemodynamic response to intubation requires a more profound drug effect than suppressing movement to incision. The distant response surface in Fig. 6 demonstrates a profound anesthetic depth, based on the stimulus, the response, and the drug-induced probability of non-response. As demonstrated by Fig. 5, anesthetic depth ranges from 100% chance of a verbal response to a verbal command (wide awake, no drug) to enough opioid and hypnotic to provide 100% chance of no hemodynamic response to intubation.

For the inhaled anesthetics, MAC creates a unifying principle. Although each inhaled anesthetic has some pharmacological peculiarities, in general they have parallel dose–response curves across drugs (e.g., isoflurane vs sevoflurane vs desflurane) and across stimuli–response pairs [MAC_{awake}, MAC, MAC_{bar} (Stoelting et al. 1970; Eger 2001; Roizen et al. 1981; Daniel et al. 1998)]. Thus, by knowing the relative values of MAC, one can infer the relative values of the other stimulus–response relationships. There is less similarity among the intravenous hypnotics. Fortunately, only propofol and midazolam are commonly used to induce and maintain the anesthetic state, which limits the number of clinically interesting intravenous anesthetic combinations.

Although there are conflicting reports of pharmacological idiosyncrasies with each member of the fentanyl series, fentanyl, alfentanil, sufentanil, and remifentanil appear to mainly differ in potency, with otherwise parallel concentration vs response relationships. Morphine, meperidine, hydromorphone, and methadone appear to differ both in potency and intrinsic efficacy, having slightly reduced maximum analgesic effect than the fentanyl series of opioids. These latter four also have their own pharmacological quirks, particularly meperidine.

Nitrous oxide is not only the oldest of the anesthetic drugs still in common use, but remains one of the least well understood. It has properties of both hypnotics, with an identifiable MAC slightly greater than 1 atmosphere (Hornbein et al. 1982), and analgesic (of which it is potent as well). Although the interaction of nitrous oxide with opioids (Ausems et al. 1986), inhaled anesthetics (Ghouri and White 1991; Rampil et al. 1991), and propofol (Stuart et al. 2000; Ichinohe et al. 2000) have been characterized, no studies have gathered enough data to generate the response surfaces needed to fully understand the interactions of this nearly ubiquitous anesthetic drug.

5 Fundamental Relationships That Characterize the Anesthetic State

Based on the simplifying assumptions, we need to understand a limited number of prototypical drug combinations: isoflurane–fentanyl, isoflurane–nitrous oxide, nitrous oxide–fentanyl, propofol–fentanyl, propofol–nitrous oxide, midazolam–nitrous oxide, and midazolam–fentanyl. For each of these, characterization of the response surface for a handful of stimuli and responses would allow understanding of current clinical practice, and provide for definition of the full range of anesthetic depth:

1. Loss of response to shouting and shaking
   a. Any response is considered (i.e., "MAC_{awake}")
2. Loss of response to electrical tetanus
   a. Verbal response or purposeful movement
   b. Any autonomic (hemodynamic or sudomotor) response
   c. Any memory response
3. Loss of response to an intermediate stimulus (incision, trapezius muscle squeeze)
   a. Purposeful movement (i.e., "MAC")
   b. Any autonomic (hemodynamic or sudomotor) response, (i.e., "MAC_{bar}")
   c. Any memory response
4. Loss of response to laryngoscopy/intubation
   a. Purposeful movement
   b. Any autonomic (hemodynamic or sudomotor) response
   c. Any memory response
5. The unstimulated concentration vs EEG response relationship

We now have a matrix of just 11 stimulus-vs-response relationships. Multiplied by our 7 prototypical drug combinations yields 77 response surfaces, from which we can infer the rest of the surfaces through scaling based on MAC for inhaled drugs and C_{50} for intravenous drugs, and the relative rankings of stimuli and responses. Moreover, the combinations range from light anesthesia, with modest stimulation and easily attenuated responses found in the upper right corner of Fig. 5, to deep anesthesia, with profound stimuli and very difficult to ablate responses found in the lower right corner of Fig. 5.

Figure 7 shows examples of response surfaces for a modest stimulus on the left (withdrawal to electrical tetanus), and a profound stimulus on the right (movement response to intubation). These interaction surfaces are based on the same model as the interaction surface shown in Fig. 2, differing only in the intensity of the afferent painful signal. We find the same pattern when we examine real data. The left image in Fig. 8 shows the response surface for MAC reduction of isoflurane by fentanyl (McEwan et al. 1993). The right image of Fig. 8 shows the interaction of propofol with alfentanil on blunting all responses to intubation (Vuyk et al. 1995). The shapes of these curves are not exactly like the shapes derived from our hypnotic–opioid interaction model because (1) the investigators were only interested in characterizing the interaction at the level of 50% response and thus did not gather enough data to characterize the upper and lower edges of either curve, and (2) the mathematical function used was multiple logistic regression, which has several shortcomings as a

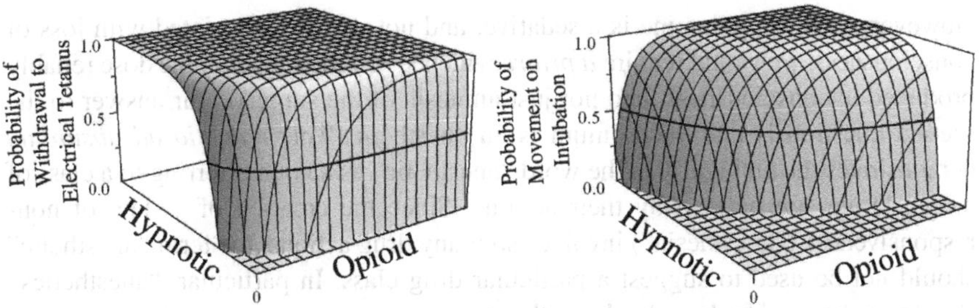

Fig. 7 Examples of response surfaces for a modest stimulus on the *left* (withdrawal to electrical tetanus), and a profound stimulus on the *right* (movement response to intubation), based on model shown in Fig. 5 with differing intensity of the afferent painful signal. The figure on the *left* shows a relatively mild stimulus–response combination, while the figure on the *right* shows a profoundly noxious stimulus–response combination

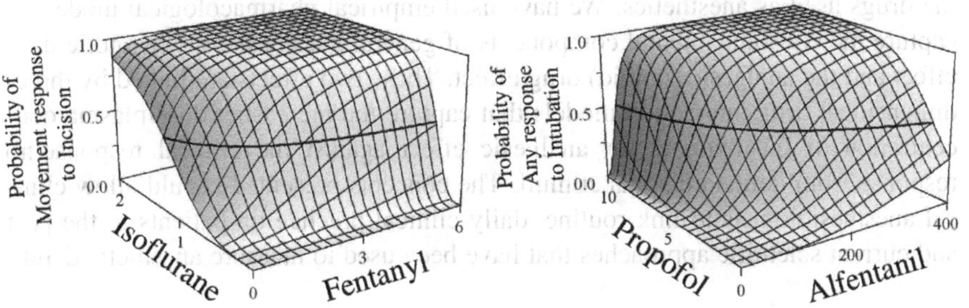

Fig. 8 The *left image* shows the response surface for MAC reduction of isoflurane by fentanyl (McEwan et al. 1993). The *right image* shows the interaction of propofol with alfentanil on blunting all responses to intubation (Vuyk et al. 1995). Both figures demonstrate the intrinsic synergy between opioids and hypnotics in producing unresponsiveness

model of drug interaction. Nevertheless, the figures demonstrate the intrinsic synergy between opioids and hypnotics in producing unresponsiveness, as well as the tendency for more profoundly noxious stimulation (e.g., intubation) to generate more synergy between the analgesic and hypnotic components of anesthesia.

Given our broad definition of anesthetic depth as providing non-responsiveness to a wide range of stimuli and response pairs (Fig. 5), one might wonder what drugs constitute anesthetics. For example, one can envision an anesthetic consisting of beta-blockers to blunt hemodynamic response, trimethaphan to prevent tearing, a ventilator to control respiration, vecuronium to prevent movement, and scopolamine to prevent memory. There is no chance of any response to any stimulation, so: (1) is the patient deeply anesthetized, and (2) are beta-blockers, trimethaphan, ventilators, muscle relaxants, scopolamine, and vecuronium anesthetics?

The answer to both questions is "yes." For the first question, if the proposed technique could truly provide for 100% chance of non-response (and we haven't tried this personally) then it would be clinically indistinguishable from a conventional hypnotic–opioid technique that produced a similar state of non-responsiveness.

However, since scopolamine is a sedative, and not usually associated with loss of consciousness, we would require *a priori* evidence that the scopolamine dose reliably produced unconsciousness, and not just amnesia of the surgery. Our answer to the second question is that vecuronium is an anesthetic. This *reductio ad absurdum* demonstrates the ambiguity in the word "anesthetic" as a noun referring to a class of drugs. Drugs are defined by their actions. Since the creation of a state of non-responsiveness ("anesthesia") involves so many drug actions, the term "anesthetic" should not be used to suggest a particular drug class. In particular, "anesthetics" should not be used to describe drugs that suppress consciousness, as these are more accurately termed "hypnotics."

In summary, this chapter has presented a current/modern approach to conceptualizing depth of anesthesia. We have not treated anesthetic depth as a single pharmacological process, rather we have approached the concept as a pragmatic, empirical approach that links both the basic and clinical sciences associated with the drugs used as anesthetics. We have used empirical pharmacological models to capture the two fundamental components of general anesthesia, the hypnotic drug effect and the analgesic (opioid) drug effect. These two effects are linked by three-dimensional drug interaction models that capture the increasing dose/plasma concentration of the hypnotic or analgesic effect against the clinical response/no response from defined clinical stimuli. The concepts presented should allow clinical anesthesiologists to link routine, daily clinical practice on patients to the past and current scientific approaches that have been used to measure anesthetic depth.

References

Antognini JF, Schwartz K (1993) Exaggerated anesthetic requirements in the preferentially anesthetized brain. Anesthesiology 79:1244–1249

Ausems ME, Hug CC Jr, Stanski DR, Burm AGL (1986) Plasma concentrations of alfentanil required to supplement nitrous oxide anesthesia for general surgery. Anesthesiology 65:362–373

Bencherif B, Fuchs PN, Sheth R, Dannals RF, Campbell JN, Frost JJ (2002) Pain activation of human supraspinal opioid pathways as demonstrated by [11C]-carfentanil and positron emission tomography (PET). Pain 99:589–598

Daniel M, Weiskopf RB, Noorani M, Eger EI (1998) Fentanyl augments the blockade of the sympathetic response to incision (MAC-BAR) produced by desflurane and isoflurane: desflurane and isoflurane MAC-BAR without and with fentanyl. Anesthesiology 88:43–49

Egan TD, Muir KT, Hermann DJ, Stanski DR, Shafer S (2001) The electroencephalogram (EEG) and clinical measure of opioid potency: defining the EEG-clinical potency relationship ("fingerprint") with application to remifentanil. Int J Pharm Med 15:1–9

Eger EI (2001) Age, minimum alveolar anesthetic concentration, and minimum alveolar anesthetic concentration-awake. Anesth Analg 93:947–953

Fang F, Guo TZ, Davies MF, Maze M (1997) Opiate receptors in the periaqueductal gray mediate analgesic effect of nitrous oxide in rats. Eur J Pharmacol 336:137–141

Fields HL, Anderson SD (1978) Evidence that raphe-spinal neurons mediate opiate and midbrain stimulation-produced analgesia. Pain 5:333–349

Fukuhara N, Ishikawa T, Kinoshita H, Xiong L, Nakanishi O (1998) Central noradrenergic mediation of nitrous oxide-induced analgesia in rats. Can J Anaesth 45:1123–1129

Ghouri AF, White PF (1991) Effect of fentanyl and nitrous oxide on the desflurane anesthetic requirement. Anesth Analg 72:377–381
Glass PS (1998) Anesthetic drug interactions: an insight into general anesthesia—its mechanism and dosing strategies. Anesthesiology 88:5–6
Hornbein TF, Eger EI, Winter PM, Smith G, Wetstone D, Smith KH (1982) The minimum alveolar concentration of nitrous oxide in man. Anesth Analg 61:553–556
Ichinohe T, Aida H, Kaneko Y (2000) Interaction of nitrous oxide and propofol to reduce hypertensive response to stimulation. Can J Anaesth 47:699–704
Kazama T, Ikeda K, Morita K (1997) Reduction by fentanyl of the Cp50 values of propofol and hemodynamic responses to various noxious stimuli. Anesthesiology 87:213–227
Kazama T, Ikeda K, Morita K (1998a) The pharmacodynamic interaction between propofol and fentanyl with respect to the suppression of somatic or hemodynamic responses to skin incision, peritoneum incision, and abdominal wall retraction. Anesthesiology 89:894–906
Kazama T, Ikeda K, Morita K, Katoh T, Kikura M (1998b) Propofol concentration required for endotracheal intubation with a laryngoscope or fiberscope and its interaction with fentanyl. Anesth Analg 86:872–879
McEwan AI, Smith C, Dyar O, Smith LR, Goodman D, Glass P (1993) Isoflurane minimum alveolar concentration reduction by fentanyl. Anesthesiology 78:864–869
Minto CF, Schnider TW, Short TG, Gregg KM, Gentilini A, Shafer SL (2000) Response surface model for anesthetic drug interactions. Anesthesiology 92:1603–1816
Prys-Roberts C (1987) Anaesthesia: a practical or impossible construct? Br J Anaesth 59:1341–1345
Quock RM, Best JA, Chen DC, Vaughn LK, Portoghese PS, Takemori AE (1990) Mediation of nitrous oxide analgesia in mice by spinal and supraspinal kappa-opioid receptors. Eur J Pharmacol 175:97–100
Rampil IJ (1994) Anesthetic potency is not altered after hypothermic spinal cord transactions in rats. Anesthesiology 80:606–610
Rampil IJ, Lockhart SH, Zwass MS, Peterson N, Yasuda N, Eger EI, Weiskopf RB, Damask MC (1991) Clinical characteristics of desflurane in surgical patients: minimum alveolar concentration. Anesthesiology 74:429–433
Rampil IJ, Mason P, Singh H (1993) Anesthetic potency (MAC) is independent of forebrain structures in the rat. Anesthesiology 78:707–712
Roizen MF, Horrigan RW, Frazer BM (1981) Anesthetic doses blocking adrenergic (stress) and cardiovascular responses to incision—MAC BAR. Anesthesiology 54:390–398
Sebel PS, Glass PS, Fletcher JE, Murphy MR, Gallagher C, Quill T (1992) Reduction of the MAC of desflurane with fentanyl. Anesthesiology 76:52–59
Smith C, McEwan AI, Jhaveri R, Wilkinson M, Goodman D, Smith LR, Canada AT, Glass PS (1994) The interaction of fentanyl on the Cp50 of propofol for loss of consciousness and skin incision. Anesthesiology 81:820–828
Stanski DR, Shafer SL (2005) Measuring depth of anesthesia. In: Miller RD (ed) Miller's anesthesia, 6th edn. Elsevier Churchill Livingston, Philadelphia, pp 1227–1264
Stoelting RK, Longnecker DE, Eger EI (1970) Minimum alveolar concentrations in man on awakening from methoxyflurane, halothane, ether and fluroxene anesthesia: MAC awake. Anesthesiology 33:5–9
Stuart PC, Stott SM, Millar A, Kenny GN, Russell D (2000) CP50 of propofol with and without nitrous oxide 67%. Br J Anaesth 84:638–649
Vuyk J, Lim T, Engbers FH, Burm AG, Vletter AA, Bovill JJ (1995) The pharmacodynamic interaction of propofol and alfentanil during lower abdominal surgery in women. Anesthesiology 83:8–22
Wynands JE, Wong P, Townsend GE, Sprigge JS, Whalley DG (1984) Narcotic requirements for intravenous anesthesia. Anesth Analg 63:101–105

Target Controlled Anaesthetic Drug Dosing

H. Schwilden(✉) and J. Schüttler

Abstract It belongs to the particularities of anaesthesia that the conscious response of the patient to drug therapy is not available for the adjustment of drug therapy and that the side-effects of anaesthetic drug therapy would be in general lethal if no special measures were taken such as artificial ventilation. Both conditions do not allow for a slow, time-consuming titration of drug effect towards the therapeutically effective window, but measures have to be taken to reach a therapeutic target fast (within seconds to a few minutes), reliably, and with precision. Integrated pharmacokinetic–pharmacodynamic models have proved to be a useful mathematical framework to institute such drug delivery to patients. The theory of model-based interactive drug dosing on the basis of common pharmacokinetic–pharmacodynamic (pk–pd) models is outlined and the target-controlled infusion system (TCI) is presented as a new anaesthetic dosing technique that has developed during the last decade. Whereas TCI presents an open-loop dosing strategy (the past output does not influence the future input), current research deals with the model-based adaptive closed-loop administration of anaesthetics. In these systems the past output is used to adapt and individualize the initial pk–pd model to the patients and thus has an influence on future drug dosing which is based on the adapted model.

H. Schwilden
Klinik für Anästhesiologie, Universität Erlangen-Nürnberg, Krankenhausstr.12, 91054 Erlangen, Germany
Schwilden@kfa.imed.uni-erlangen.de

J. Schüttler and H. Schwilden (eds.) *Modern Anesthetics.*
Handbook of Experimental Pharmacology 182.

1 Particularities of Anaesthetic Drug Dosing

Anaesthesia regarded from the aspect of drug therapy has a number of particularities as compared to other medical specialties, to these belong:

- Duration of therapy is confined from a few minutes to a couple of hours and the onset of therapeutic effects such as loss of consciousness or neuromuscular blockade should occur within seconds to very few minutes.
- The effects and side-effects of the drugs used are lethal if special measures, e.g. artificial ventilation, are not taken.
- The conscious response of the patient to drug delivery is not available and cannot be used to guide drug therapy.

As a consequence of these particularities it appears natural that a dosing strategy which requires a time-consuming careful titration of drug dose to drug effect is obsolete; instead, short-acting drugs with a quick onset of action and a high degree of 'predictability' (Stanski and Hug 1982) are required. Predictability in this context means that the laws governing the time course of drug action after the delivery of drug into the central circulation of the human body are reliable and have a reasonably limited interindividual variability. Given the knowledge of such laws they may be used to construct drug delivery schemes which aim at the appropriate targets. As has become clear, however, from the previous chapters, there seems to be no unique target for anaesthesia (Kissin and Gelman 1988; Kissin 1993), nor can a target be identified, such as a cancer cell, as an anatomical or physical entity, as is the case in other specialties, nor does one actually know what the necessary conditions are to establish the state of surgical anaesthesia in patients. The only things which seem to be apparent from clinical practice and research are some sufficient conditions for the establishment of anaesthesia. It is for those reasons that the formulation of targets for surgical anaesthesia is based on surrogate parameters. A long-standing tradition in identifying targets for anaesthetic drug dosing has been the exhaled concentration or vapour pressure of inhalational anaesthetics (Eger et al. 1965) which in turn might, under suitable conditions, serve as an estimation of the vapour pressure or concentration of the anaesthetic at the brain.

In the past three decades blood concentrations of intravenous anaesthetics served as targets which give rise to so-called target-controlled infusion (TCI) (Glass et al. 1997) systems for the delivery of intravenous anaesthetics. As for many anaesthetic drugs including muscle relaxants, there is a hysteresis between drug effect and blood concentration. Hull developed the notion of the biophase (Hull et al. 1978), also known as effect compartment (Sheiner et al. 1979), as a virtual site of drug action which shows up no hysteresis to effect. More recent TCI systems use the biophase concentration as the target. In most cases neither blood concentration nor biophase concentration can be actually measured in real time. It is understandable therefore that measurable drug effects such as alterations of the EEG (Schwilden et al. 1985; Kochs et al. 1994; Katoh et al. 1998; Bruhn et al. 2003) or the spontaneous contractility of the lower oesophagus (Ghouri et al. 1993) have been used as targets. Again, these targets have to be considered as surrogates (Schuttler and Schwilden 1999) with respect to the final goal of anaesthetic effectiveness. Only in the field of muscle relaxants is the measurable effect close to the therapeutic effectiveness.

2 Model-Based Open Loop Drug Dosing

2.1 Pharmacokinetics–Pharmacodynamics

Figure 1 depicts today's conceptual understanding of the relationship between drug dosing and ultimate clinical effect (Camu et al. 1998) and the possible targets which are currently used in the clinical practice of anaesthesia. It is common sense to subdivide this pathway into 'pharmacokinetics' and 'pharmacodynamics'. These terms are often explained by the aphorism that pharmacodynamics is what the drug does to the body, and pharmacokinetics is what the body does to the drug.

If one considers the patient as a black box system (Fig. 2) into which an anaesthetic drug (input) is administered, and some output is determined as a therapeutic surrogate end-point, one may distinguish between the following four modes of drug dosing:

- Input is independent of all previous outputs and all previous inputs: naïve dosing
- Input is independent of all outputs, but may depend on previous inputs: TCI
- Input is independent of all previous inputs but may depend on previous outputs: naïve feedback (e.g. proportional–integral–differential, or PID, control)
- Input depends on previous inputs and previous outputs: e.g. model-based closed loop

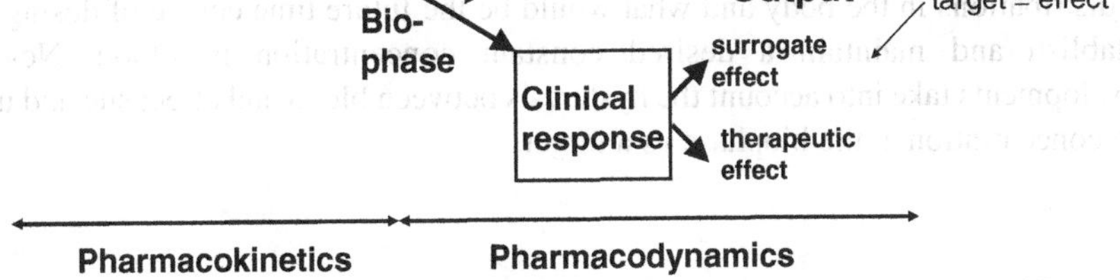

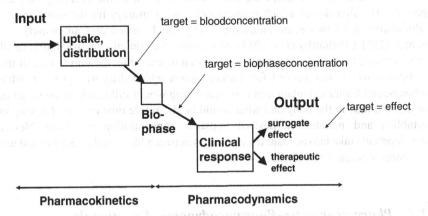

Fig. 1 Conceptual pathway from anaesthetic drug dosing to ultimate clinical effect of anaesthesia as estimated by surrogate effects (e.g. slowing of EEG frequency) or direct measurable therapeutic effects (e.g. neuromuscular blockade). Model-based anaesthetic drug dosing has at present three different targets: (1) the drug concentration in the central circulation, (2) the drug concentration at some virtual site of drug action called the biophase or (3) a measurable parameter which can be a surrogate for a direct measurable therapeutic effect or (in rare cases) the effect itself

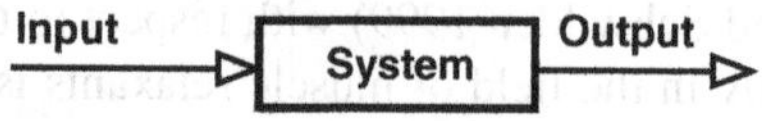

Fig. 2 From a systemic theoretical point of view, the mapping of the drug input function on the ultimate therapeutic effect as the output is, in the first instance, a black box. Pharmacokinetic and pharmacodynamic models give the black box some structure

The traditional form of target-controlled dosing is by target-controlled *infusion* (TCI) (Glen 1998) which was developed in the context of the development of the induction and maintenance of general anaesthesia by administration of i.v. agents only, without the use of volatile or gaseous anaesthetics, so-called total intravenous anaesthesia (TIVA) (Hengstmann et al. 1980; Schuttler et al. 1988; Visser et al. 2001). From the above scheme it becomes evident that target-controlled dosing was the first formalized step that went beyond naïve dosing and incorporated the dosing history into the actual dosing scheme. Thereby pharmacokinetic–pharmacodynamic models were used to estimate the present impact of doses given even far in the past on the present state of the system.

TCI aims at the control of the time course of the anaesthetic drug concentration in blood, especially in plasma. As the varying surgical phases require different drug concentrations to appropriately suppress adverse responses to the varying painful stimuli, programmed (as of the early 1970s; Salamonsen 1978; Mapleson 1979) or pre-programmed dosing techniques (Crankshaw et al. 1993; Blake et al. 1998) were inadequate at handling this dosing problem. TCI was developed on the grounds of the pharmacokinetic models (Schwilden 1981; Schuttler et al. 1983; Schwilden et al. 1983; Alvis et al. 1985; Ausems et al. 1985; Kenny and White 1990) of the drugs in order to interactively adapt the blood concentration to the changing surgical periods. The first device which realized this dosing strategy for the simultaneous administration of two intravenous drugs (e.g. an hypnotic and an opioid) was named CATIA (Schuttler et al. 1983), an acronym for computer-assisted titration of intravenous anaesthesia. The name was chosen to underline the importance of the computer, which was needed for tracking when which drug was given in what amount, and for the calculation of how much drug would still reside in the volumes of distributions in the body and what would be the future time course of dosing to establish and maintain a desired constant concentration in blood. Newer developments take into account the hysteresis between blood and effect site and use the concentration at the biophase as a target.

2.2 *Pharmacokinetic–Pharmacodynamic Functionals*

This chapter outlines some aspects of the theory of model-based dosing of anaesthetics, which is not actually confined to anaesthetics but may be also applied to other drugs and specialties.

Pharmacokinetics relates the time course of drug dosing to the time course of drug concentration in some tissues. Most often the chosen tissue is blood. In mathematical terms this relation may be considered as a functional *K* which maps the time course of drug dosing onto the time course of drug concentration. Let *I(t)* denote the function of time of drug dosing, which is the amount of drug delivered per unit time at the specified moment in time *t*, in the same way let *c(t)* denote the drug concentration in the selected tissue at time *t*; then one may write

$$c(t) = K(I(\ ), t, pk)$$

which specifies the concentration value at time *t* as a functional of the entire function *I()* (not only the function value at a specific time *t'*, but at all times), the time *t* itself and a set of model specifying parameters *pk*.

In a similar manner pharmacodynamics may be considered as a function D which maps the time course of drug concentration onto the time course of drug effect. Let *E(t)* denote the numeric value of the measured effect at time *t*; then one may write

$$E(t) = D(c(\ ), t, pd)$$

whereby again *c()* denotes the entire function *c(t)* for all *t*, and *pd* denotes a set of model specifying parameters.

2.2.1 Linear, Time-Invariant Pharmacokinetics

It has been shown in numerous investigations that for many drugs the functional *K* is linear with respect to drug dosing (Gepts et al. 1995), when the concentration is within the therapeutic window. There are only very few examples of anaesthetics which may show deviations from linear and time-invariant pharmacokinetics (Stoeckel et al. 1979; Cordato et al. 1999). This means especially that multiplying the drug dosing function *I()* by number λ will multiply the concentration (doubling the dose doubles the concentration) in formula $K(\lambda I(), t, pd) = \lambda c(t)$. This finding reduces the possible space of functionals dramatically, namely to linear functionals. The most general ansatz for a general linear functional is

$$c(t) = K(I(\ ), t, pd) = \int_{-\infty}^{+\infty} H(t, t'; pk) I(t') dt'$$

where by *H(t,t';pk)* is a suitable function of the arguments *t* and *t'* and of the set of parameters *pk*. In this formula the time *t'* is the moment in time when the amount *I(t')dt'* is given and *t* denotes the time at which the concentration is determined. Causality requires that some dose in the future may not affect the concentrations in the past, one has therefore to require

$$H(t,t';pk)=0, for; t<t'(causality); hence$$

$$c(t)=\int_{-\infty}^{t} H(t,t';pk)I(t')dt'$$

The next assumption which is commonly made for the last equation to be useful is the assumption that the pharmacokinetic mechanisms do not vary with time. This is probably a very simplistic assumption; it rules out, for instance, circadian and other rhythms, but this assumption keeps the equation as a rather useful one for studying pharmacokinetic properties. In mathematical terms this assumption says that *H(t,t';pk)* does not depend on *t* and *t'* separately but only on their difference *t−t'*. Let us denote the resulting function as *G(t−t',pk)*, assuming further that drug administration starts at *t*=0, then the pharmacokinetic equation results in

$$c(t)=\int_{0}^{t} G(t-t',pk)I(t')dt' \tag{1}$$

The meaning of the function *G* becomes immediately clear if one administers a bolus of unit dose (I(t)=δ(t) whereby *δ(t)* denotes Dirac's δ-function). Inserting this function into the last equation yields

$$c(t)=\int_{0}^{t} G(t-t',pk)\delta(t')dt'=G(t;pk)$$

That is to say *G(t;pk)* is just the concentration course after a bolus of unit dose.

Equation 1 is a relation between the three functions *I(t)*=drug delivery, *c(t)*=drug concentration and *G(t,pk)*=the drug-specific disposition function. Given two of these functions, the third may be determined by using the equation. Given *G* and *I* one may determine the resulting concentration, this is a straightforward task and widely used in pharmacokinetic simulation computer programmes. Given discrete measured concentrations and the drug administration scheme *I(t)*, one may determine the disposition function *G(t,pk)*. There are two big approaches for the determination of *G(t,pk)*; one is by non-linear least-square curve fitting (Sheiner and Steimer 2000). This approach requires an idea about the type of the function—very often a polyexponential function is used—and fits only the limited number of parameters *pk*. An entirely different approach is the model-independent determination of the function itself (Schwilden et al. 1993), not in terms of an analytical expression but as the set of all function values *(t,G(t))* for arbitrary *t*. As this problem is largely underdetermined, regularization methods have been developed since the 1970s to attack such problems (Groetsch 1984).

2.2.2 From Disposition Function to Dosing Function

Finally, if the disposition is known and the time course of drug concentration *c(t)* is given as 'target', one may determine the drug dosing scheme *I(t)* which approximates the time course *c(t)* best. The approach originally used in pharmacokinetic model-based dosing systems such as CATIA was to determine some kind of inverse function $G^{-1}(t;pk)$ (Schwilden 1981) such that

$$\int_{-\infty}^{+\infty} dt' G^{-1}(t-t';pk)\,G(t'-t'';pk) = \delta(t-t'')$$

If such function can be determined then the dosing function *I(t)* is immediately given by

$$I(t) = \int_0^t dt' G^{-1}(t-t';pk)\,c(t') \qquad (2)$$

For many drugs one finds that the function *G(t;pk)* can be approximated by a sum of exponential functions

$$G(t;pk) = Ae^{-\alpha t} + Be^{-\beta t} + Ce^{-\gamma t} + \ldots$$

whereby the parameter set $pk=\{A, \alpha, B, \beta, C, \gamma, \ldots\}$.

In the following we will no longer specify the parameter set *pk* in the function *G* but only write *G(t)*. The number of exponentials *n* is commonly confined for most intravenous anaesthetics to 3. For the purpose of simplicity we will stick for further theoretical investigations to $n=2$, which exhibits all the principal features which are also valid for $n>2$. Given the two-exponential disposition function $G(t)=Ae^{-\alpha t}+Be^{-\beta t}$ it can be shown that its inverse $G^{-1}(t)$ is given be the following formula

$$G^{-1}(t) = \frac{1}{A+B}\left(\delta'(t) + (\alpha+\beta-p_2)\delta(t) - p_1 p_2 e^{-p_2 t}\Theta(t)\right)$$

whereby $\delta(t)$ denotes Dirac's δ-function, which may be interpreted as bolus injection; $\Theta(t)$ is the Heaviside function being zero for negative *t* and 1 for positive *t* and p_1, p_2 are abbreviations for the following expressions

$$p_2 = \frac{A\beta + B\alpha}{A+B};\ p_1 = \alpha + \beta - p_2 - \alpha\beta / p_2$$

If one inserts the expression for $G^{-1}(t)$ into Eq. 2 one ends up with

$$\begin{aligned} I(t) &= \int_0^t dt' G^{-1}(t-t')c(t') \\ &= \frac{1}{A+B}\left(c'(t) + (\alpha+\beta-p_2)c(t) - p_1 p_2 \int_0^t dt' e^{-p_2(t-t')}c(t')\right) \end{aligned}$$

One realizes immediately that the dosing function *I(t)* consists of three parts: a term proportional to the derivative of the concentration *c(t)*, a term proportional to *c(t)* and a term proportional to the weighted integral over *c(t)*. It should be emphasized that this result is achieved without any reference to differential equations or compartment models; it is solely based on the principles of linearity and time-invariance and the analytical expression for the bolus disposition function.

A rather simple application would be the establishment of a constant concentration c_0 of an anaesthetic drug from time t=0 onwards, i.e. $c(t)=c_0\Theta(t)$. Inserting this expression in the formula above yields

$$I(t)=\frac{c_0}{A+B}\left(\delta(t)+\left(\alpha+\beta-p_2-p_1\right)+p_1e^{-p_2t}\right) \tag{3}$$

The dosing scheme consists of three parts: an initial bolus at time t=0, a constant rate infusion and an infusion rate which declines exponentially towards 0. Though this result has been entirely generated without any reference to differential equations and compartment models the interpretation of these dosing formulae becomes very vivid if one interprets it in the framework of classical compartment models. Figure 3 shows a two-compartment model and the set of differential equations associated with it

$$\frac{dm_1}{dt}=-\left(k_{10}+k_{12}\right)m_1+k_{21}m_2+I(t)$$
$$\frac{dm_2}{dt}=k_{12}m_1-k_{21}m_2$$

whereby $m_1(t)$ and $m_2(t)$ denote the amount of drug (as mass) in the compartment '1' or '2' at time t which is sought to be a volume with instantaneous homogeneous distribution. One assumes that compartment '1', the volume of distribution of which is denoted by V_1, includes the blood. Given this assumption the concentration formed by the expression $m_1(t)/V_1$ has to be equated with the concentration term *c(t)* in the previous formulae. Thus maintaining a constant concentration c_0

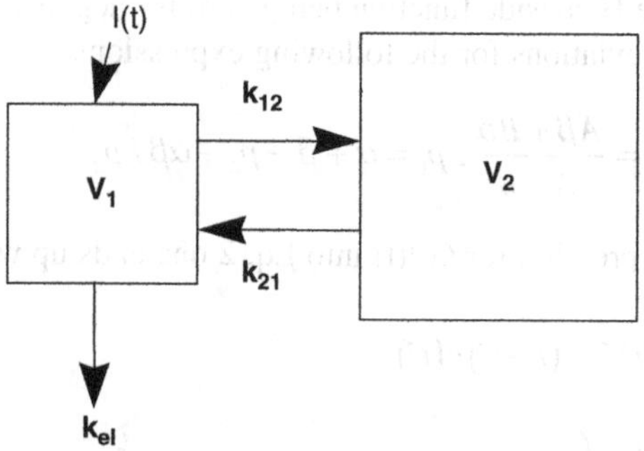

Fig. 3 Multicompartment models are popular tools to visualize the distribution processes of anaesthetics within the body. As shown above, however, they are absolutely unnecessary for the determination of appropriate dosing strategies to achieve a desired concentration, because only the drug disposition function has to be known and not its interpretation in terms of idealized diagrams

beginning at time t=0 is thus equivalent to have constant mass in volume V_1 $m_1(t)=c_0V_1\Theta(t)$. Inserting this expression into the first differential equation and solving for $I(t)$ yields

$$I(t)=c_0V_1\delta(t)+(k_{10}+k_{12})c_0V_1-k_{21}m_2$$

From the second differential equation one concludes

$$m_2(t)=k_{12}\int_0^t dt\, e^{-k_{21}(t-t')}m_1(t)=\frac{k_{12}}{k_{21}}c_0V_1\left(1-e^{-k_{21}t}\right)$$

leading after insertion in the above formula to

$$I(t)=c_0V_1\left(\delta(t)+k_{10}+k_{12}e^{-k_{21}t}\right) \tag{5}$$

This formula has become familiar as the "BET" (bolus, elimination, transfer) infusion scheme, because it is easily interpreted in terms of the two-compartment model. Namely, to establish initially the amount c_0V_1 in compartment '1' one has to administer a bolus of this into the volume of distribution, subsequently one has to substitute those amounts of drug which are removed from the volume V_1, this is elimination of the constant amount of $k_{10}c_0V_1$ per unit time and the net transfer of drug from volume V_1 to volume V_2. Most of today's TCI systems used in clinical practice are based on these or similar formulae. Figure 4 depicts the theoretical dosing scheme to establish a constant concentration for the opioid alfentanil. After

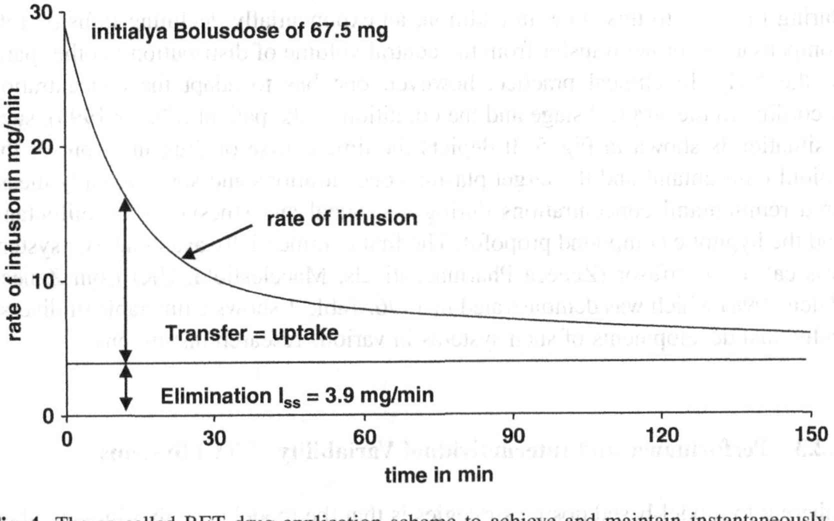

Fig. 4 The so-called BET drug application scheme to achieve and maintain instantaneously a constant drug concentration in blood. An initial bolus to reach the initial concentration is followed by a constant rate infusion substituting the constant amount of drug per unit time which is eliminated from the body, if the concentration is kept constant. The transfer of drug by the distribution to other tissues in the body than blood is a process which eventually declines to zero

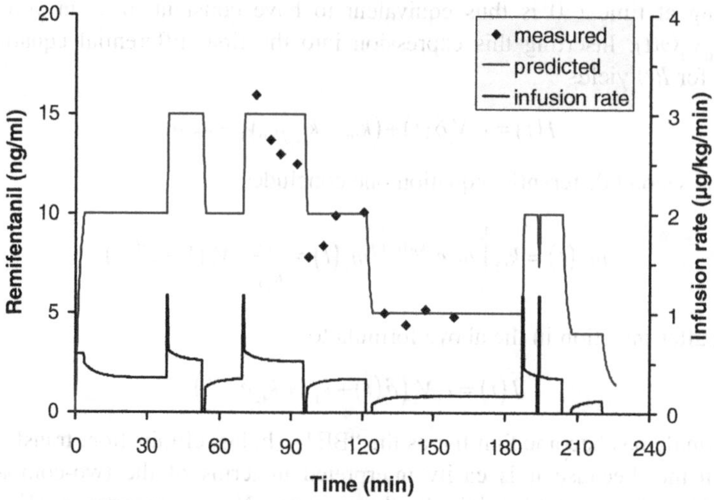

Fig. 5 TCI dosing systems for anaesthesia must allow them to be operated interactively in order to adapt dosing to the individual patient and to the varying conditions the surgical procedure imposes on the patient. The figure depicts the actual rate of infusion of the opioid remifentanil during a surgical anaesthesia and the anticipated remifentanil concentration based on an assumed pharmacokinetic model. The *dots* mark actually measured plasma concentrations of remifentanil

the initial bolus the rate of infusion is composed of two parts: the constant rate infusion to maintain the concentration after steady-state has been achieved, and during the time to this state, in addition, an exponentially declining infusion rate compensating for net transfer from the central volume of distribution to other parts of the body. In clinical practice, however, one has to adapt the concentration according to the surgical stage and the condition of the patient (Shafer 1993), such a situation is shown in Fig. 5. It depicts the time course of drug infusion for the opioid remifentanil and the target plasma concentrations and some actually measured remifentanil concentrations during a surgical anaesthesia with remifentanil and the hypnotic compound propofol. The first commercially available TCI system was called Diprifusor (Zeneca Pharmaceuticals, Macclesfield, UK) from Zeneca (Glen 1998) which was demonstrated in 1996. Table 1 shows a timetable of diverse individual developments of such systems in various research institutions.

2.2.3 Performance and Interindividual Variability of TCI Systems

Inherent to model-based dosing strategies is that the model describes in general an average or 'typical' patient. As the individual patient actually treated on the basis of this model will deviate from the average, this will translate into prediction errors with respect to the target concentrations. One approach to reduce systematic individual deviations is to take into account the dependence of the pharmacokinetic

Table 1 Forerunners of today's target-controlled infusion systems

CATIA: computer-assisted titration of intravenous anaesthesia
Schüttler J., Schwilden H., Stoeckel, Bonn University, Bonn, Germany, 1981–1983
CACI: computer-assisted continuous infusion
Alvis J.M., Reves J.G., Govier A.V., Duke University, North Carolina, USA, 1985
TIAC: titration of intravenous agents by computer
Ausems J.M., Stanski D.R., Hug C.C., Stanford University, California, USA, 1985
Diprifusor: a portable target-controlled propofol infusion system
Kenny G.N.C., White M., University of Glasgow, Scotland, 1992
Commercial Diprifusor
By Zeneca, Sydney, 1996

parameters on anthropometric data such as sex, age, weight, etc. by population pharmacokinetics (e.g. Schuttler and Ihmsen 2000), and to consider special pathophysiological conditions of the patient or the specific anaesthetic procedure and its co-medication (Servin et al. 2003; Billard et al. 2004). To characterize the performance of TCI systems one measures blood concentrations and compares them with the corresponding predictions (Varvel et al. 1992; Mertens et al. 2003; Li et al. 2005). In technical terms one determines as prediction error *PE* the relative deviation from the target:

$$PE_{ij} = \frac{C_{ij} - C_{Target}}{C_{Target}}$$

where C_{ij} is the jth measured concentration in the ith patient. Figure 6 depicts for 12 individual patients undergoing intravenous anaesthesia with propofol and an opioid (fentanyl or alfentanil) the box whisker diagrams of PE for each patient and for the total of n=114 measured blood concentrations of propofol (Fechner et al. 1998).

As a quantitative measure of bias in each patient the median prediction error

$$MDPE_i = \text{median}\left\{ PE_{ij}, j = 1, \ldots N_i \right\}$$

is determined, and as a quantitative measure of inaccuracy the median absolute prediction error

$$MDAPE_i = \text{median}\left\{ \left| PE_{ij} \right|, j = 1, \ldots N_i \right\},$$

where N_i is the number of measurements in the ith patient. Furthermore, linear regression of

$$\left| PE_{ij} \right|$$

versus time yields the divergence D_i as the slope of the regression line which is a measure for a time-related trend of the prediction error.

$$W_i = \text{median}\left\{ \left| PE_{ij} - MDPE_i \right|, j = 1, \ldots N_i \right\}$$

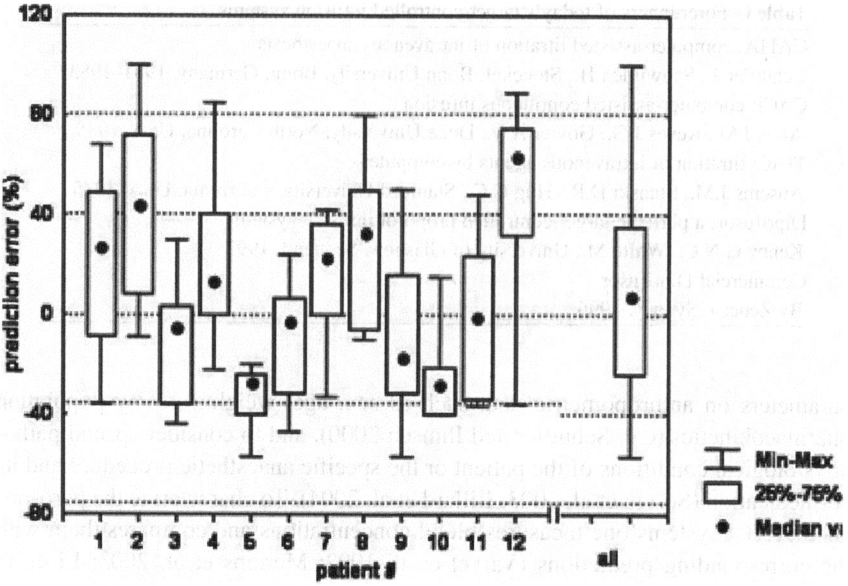

Fig. 6 The pharmacokinetic models used for the target-controlled delivery of anaesthetic drugs are models for an "average" patient. It is therefore that this model will not describe exactly the individual patient treated. This will lead to deviations of measured blood concentrations from the target concentrations aimed at. The quantitation of this deviation is generally done by comprising measured concentrations with model predictions. The figure depicts whisker-box plots of the ration of measured/predicted concentrations in 12 patients treated with a TCI system for propofol

is defined as a measure for the intraindividual variability of the prediction error. Table 2 compares these measures as given for TCI dosing systems in the literature (Glass et al. 1989; Coetzee et al. 1995; Vuyk et al. 1995; Fechner et al. 1998) and also for manual dosing (Fechner et al. 1998).

2.2.4 Target-Controlled Dosing for the Effect Site

In many cases the relation between drug concentration and induced drug effect is given by monotonic relationship between a baseline value E_0 and a maximum effect value $E_{max}>E_0$. Given this fact, the concentration–effect relationship *E(c)* can be modelled by

$$E(c) = E_0 + (E_{max} - E_0)R(c) \tag{6}$$

whereby *R(c)* is a continuous, monotonic increasing function defined for *c*>=0 with minimum value 0 and maximum value 1. That is to say *R(c)* has all properties of a distribution in the statistical sense over the range [0, ∞]. It is therefore natural to write Eq. 6 as

Table 2 Typical bias and precision values of target-controlled drug delivery from various research centres

Authors	Bias (mdpe)	Precision (mdape)
Coetzee et al.	-17.9%	27.7%
Glass et al.	-26.0%	41.0%
Vuyk et al.	26.0%	28.0%
Fechner et al.	6.7%	27.5%
Manual control	44.2%	50.0%

$$E(c) = E_0 + (E_{\max} - E_0)\int_0^c dc'\rho(c')$$

whereby the function $\rho(c)$ is any distribution density such as the Gaussian distribution or any other one. A particularly suited distribution which has been proved to be reasonably valid in many investigations is the density h with the distribution H (the so-called Hill function)

$$h(c) = \frac{\gamma}{c}\frac{(c/c_0)^\gamma}{\left(1+(c/c_0)^\gamma\right)^2},\ H(c) = \frac{(c/c_0)^\gamma}{1+(c/c_0)^\gamma} \qquad (7)$$

The practical aspect of this ansatz from a computational point of view is that unlike other distributions (e.g. Gaussian distribution) this one can be easily given in an explicit form without integral expression.

It appears, however, that the concentration which has to be inserted into Eq. 7 is in general not identical to the concentration in blood or plasma but that there is some hysteresis between the effect and the plasma concentration (Hull et al. 1978; Sheiner et al. 1979) which appears as if the blood concentrations are smeared out and damped. Heuristically this may be interpreted as a distribution to a fictitious site of action. This picture of the biophase summarizes, however, a multitude of physiological processes including distribution processes to receptive structures but also relaxation times of receptors, further signalling pathways, gene and proteome expression. Choosing the normalization that at steady-state all concentrations (or all partial pressures) at each tissue in the body are identical, one might determine the biophase concentration c_B to be inserted into the concentration–response relationship by

$$c_B(t) = \int_{-\infty}^{t} dt'\rho_B(t-t')c(t')$$

whereby $\rho_B(t)$ is a suitable distribution density. An often chosen function for ρ_B is given by the exponential distribution which has the advantage of being interpretable in the simplistic terms of diffusion

$$\rho_B(t) = \kappa e^{-\kappa t}\Theta(t),\ hence\ \frac{dc_B(t)}{dt} = \kappa(c - c_B)$$

There are data which suggest that even on the macroscopic level of clinical effects this choice of ρ_B might be too simplistic (Mandema et al. 1991).

Hysteresis between drug effect and drug concentration in blood implies that one cannot achieve a desired effect immediately but one has to wait until maximum effect is achieved. One can shorten the time needed to achieve a therapeutic effect level within a shorter time but only by giving higher initial doses which will, however, lead to overshooting (Mortier and Struys 2003; Van Poucke et al. 2004) concentrations at the biophase and even higher overshooting in the initial volume of distribution. That is to say, such systems need to balance between time to onset and degree of overshoot with concomitant adverse side-effects.

2.4 TCI Devices

At present (2007) three TCI systems are approved in Germany. Disoprifusor is approved for the infusion of the special propofol formulation 'Disoprivan' (AstraZeneca, Wedel, Germany). This device uses plasma concentrations as the target and is based on the pharmacokinetic model of Marsh et al. (1991) for propofol. Another system is Fresenius Base Primea (Fresenius Kabi, Bad Homburg, Germany), one of the first TCI systems which is neither confined to a special propofol formulation nor to propofol at all. This device also allows effect site concentrations as the target; for propofol the models of Marsh et al. and Schnider et al. are offered. The Braun Controller fm (B. Braun, Melsungen, Germany) uses so-called optimized TCI (OTCI) which maintains as target the current predicted effect site concentration in plasma. Beside its use in clinical practice, pharmacokinetic model-based drug infusion has been primarily used in drug research and drug development, especially to combine phase I/II (Dingemanse et al. 1997; Fechner et al. 2004, 2005) studies as well as phase II/III (Hering et al. 1996; Ihmsen et al. 2001) studies.

Actually, target-controlled dosing using biophase concentrations is a somewhat virtual target, and one may consider controlling drug administration by measuring the drug effect directly instead of using a biophase concentration as a surrogate variable constructed out of the time course of drug effect. If one measures, however, the drug effect, it is natural to consider the direct feedback of the measured drug effect onto the drug delivery algorithm. This leads to the concept of feedback-controlled anaesthetic drug delivery, which is in the field of anaesthesia not yet ready for routine clinical application but has been shown to be an excellent research tool for experimental and clinical studies.

3 Feedback Controlled Drug Dosing

Although closed-loop systems have a long tradition in engineering, their continued use for patients care is limited to the last 20 years, with the exception of Bickford's and others pioneering work in the 1950s (Bickford 1950; Mayo et al. 1950; Bickford

1951; Belleville and Attura 1957; Belleville et al. 1960). It has been shown that automated closed-loop systems for drug delivery can provide unique study designs for clinical research (Schüttler and Schwilden 1997; Albrecht et al. 1999) allowing experimental set-ups not realizable by traditional means. It is, however, evident that a lot of research and development has to be done on therapeutic closed-loop systems to solve the many questions related to reliability and safety that the use of therapeutic closed systems in the routine clinical setting imposes on an automatic system.

3.1 Introduction

The human body provides a rich plethora of feedback controlled systems to maintain its homeostasis under changing environmental conditions. Well known, for instance, are the diverse servo-loops for adjusting blood pressure or body temperature. Simple mechanical artificial feedback systems have been used for thousands of years. Artificial feedback control methods in anaesthesiology and intensive care medicine have been investigated and applied for nearly 50 years. It is likely that the publication of Bickford's paper, 'Automatic electroencephalographic control of general anaesthesia', in 1950 marks the beginning of research on and application of feedback systems in anaesthesia. Bickford's work dealt with the control of the delivery of ether and thiopentone. Besides the automatic control of drug delivery to maintain anaesthesia, neuromuscular blockade (Asbury et al. 1980; Linkens et al. 1981; Webster and Cohen 1987; O'Hara et al. 1991; Schwilden and Olkkola 1991; Kansanaho and Olkkola 1996a), blood pressure (Sheppard and Kouchoukos 1977; Cosgrove et al. 1989; Ruiz et al. 1993; Kwok et al. 1995; Hoeksel et al. 1996; Meijers et al. 1997; Gentilini et al. 2002) or blood glucose (Pfeiffer et al. 1974; Jaremko and Rorstad 1998; Chee et al. 2002; Chee et al. 2003; Schiel 2003; Hanaire 2006), there have been investigations on non-drug delivery systems such as feedback control of artificial ventilation (Bates et al. 2001; Brunner 2001; Dojat and Brochard 2001; Anderson and East 2002; Branson et al. 2002; Tehrani et al. 2004). This review will deal primarily with the feedback control of drug delivery.

3.2 Concept of Closed-Loop Control

Control theory distinguishes between open-loop control and closed-loop control (Vozeh and Steimer 1985). In open-loop control the input to the system (e.g. drug dosage) is independent of the output (e.g. depth of anaesthesia), whereby in closed-loop control systems the input at a given moment in time is a function of the previous output. Both control systems require a controller to determine the optimum dosage strategy. This might be the anaesthesiologist and/or a model of the process to be controlled (e.g. the anaesthetic depth of the patient). When the input to the system is controlled by a model, this is commonly referred to as model-based control. Model-based closed-loop control systems may use the measured output of the system not only to determine the next input but to update the model describing the relationship between input and output. This method is called model-based and adaptive. Among the models used, one can distinguish between heuristic and deterministic models. PID is a frequently used heuristic model for feedback control (Hayes et al. 1984; Westenskow 1997). In this case it is assumed that the input to the system needed to correct for a difference between measured output and set-point is related to the output itself, the integral of the output as well as its derivative. Pharmacokinetic/-dynamic models are an example for deterministic models when controlling drug dosage. In more recent years other knowledge-based or rule-based approaches to automatic control have been used especially in conjunction with fuzzy logic, so called fuzzy control (Westenskow 1997; Bates et al. 2001; Dojat and Brochard 2001).

3.3 *Model-Based Adaptive Closed-Loop Control*

The control system consists of five parts (Fig. 7) the patient, as the system to be controlled; the response, which is considered as a measurable representation of the process to be controlled; a model of the input–output relationship; an adapter; and a controller. The model is some formalized representation of the input–output relationship; most often this is a mathematical model. The model will in general depend on certain parameters, for example, body weight of the patient, clearance of the drug administered, etc. The adaptor is a tool to adapt the initial estimates of the parameters, whereby the controller transforms the error signal into commands for dosing. The core of the feedback system is a model of the patient with respect to the relationship between drug dosing and drug effect. Such models can be used in two directions. Using the forward direction it can give a prediction of the measured

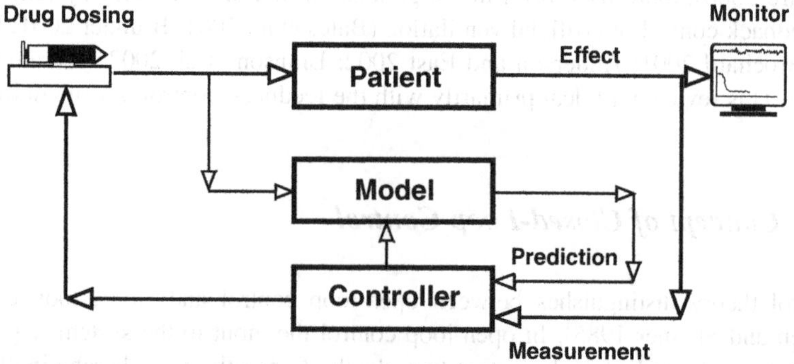

Fig. 7 Block diagram of a model-based adaptive closed-loop system for automatic drug delivery. The closed-loop system consists of five parts: the patient, as the system to be controlled; the response that is considered as a measurable representation of the process to be controlled; a model of the input–output relationship, for instance a mathematical formula; an adapter, which provides an updating of the initial estimates of the values of the parameters of the model; and a controller, which transforms the error signal and the set-point to a drug delivery scheme

output. In the backwards direction is can be used to determine the necessary input to achieve and maintain a certain level of the output. Given such a model, the system incorporates three values for the effect. Let E_m denote the effect that is actually measured, E_p the effect that is predicted by the model and E_s the chosen set-point. Ideally, all three values coincide:

$$E_m = E_p = E_s$$

De facto, these three values will differ from each other, allowing us to construct two differences, for instance $E_m - E_p$ and $E_m - E_s$. A non-zero difference, $E_m - E_p$, states that the measured effect is different from the predicted effect, thus stating that the model does not precisely describe the actual patient (Fig. 7).

The difference $E_m - E_s$ states that the measured effect is not at the set-point. These two differences can be used in the following way: the difference between E_m and E_p is used to adapt the model to the patient. That is to say, the parameter values are modified such that the model prediction will coincide with the measured value. On the basis of the updated model a new dosing scheme is calculated that should bring the measured output to the set-point and maintain it.

For the development of an EEG-based feedback controlled administration of intravenous anaesthetics one can combine the pharmacokinetic-based TCI approach with a target selection as determined from the pharmacodynamics. The relationship between the concentration *c(t)* and the measured EEG, effect *E*, can be modelled according to a Hill function (see Eq. 7)

$$E = E_0 - E_{\max} \frac{c^\gamma}{c_0^\gamma + c^\gamma}$$

The first paper on pharmacokinetic–pharmacodynamic model-based anaesthetics closed-loop control by the EEG used as effect *E* the median EEG frequency of the EEG power spectrum (Schwilden et al. 1987). Hereby E_0 denotes the baseline median EEG frequency, a typical value of which is 9 Hz, E_{max} denotes the maximum dynamic range of the signal, a typical value of which is 8 Hz. c_0 denotes the concentration at which the signal is at the half of the maximum dynamic range and γ is an index of the steepness of the concentration–response curve. In the past few years model-based feedback systems using the Bispectral Index (Aspect Medical Systems, Norwood, MA) as the EEG parameter have been investigated in more detail with respect to performance and in comparison to 'standard clinical practice' (Mortier et al. 1998; Struys et al. 2001; Struys et al. 2004).

3.4 Closed-Loop Systems as Research Tools

A common study design of pharmacological studies is to give a dose of a drug and to follow the time course of drug effects. Thus, in typical studies such as dose finding studies or the determination of ED_{50}, minimum alveolar concentration or the characterization of drug–drug interactions will inevitably require or produce conditions during which the patients or volunteers are over- or underdosed with respect to the therapeutic window. This is because for any pre-specified dose there is always some likelihood that this dose will over- or undershoot the therapeutic window, especially if the common bracketing techniques in case of quantal responses are used (Quasha et al. 1980). Given feedback systems these problems can be resolved. Closed-loop systems allow users to invert the classic handling of the dose–effect relationship (Schüttler and Schwilden 1997); instead of giving a dose and observing the resultant effect, feedback systems allow the specification of an effect and observation of the dose necessary to achieve and maintain that effect.

3.4.1 Effective Therapeutic Infusions

Figure 8(upper panel) depicts a typical cumulative curve of drug needed to maintain median EEG frequency at a preset value. The figure refers to a closed-loop feedback control of alfentanil during surgical anaesthesia (Schwilden and Stoeckel 1993).

Given the theoretical framework as described above, one has to assume that at a fixed pharmacodynamic effect the concentration is maintained constant. Given the time course of the concentration one may use Eq. 5 to determine $I(t)$.

Obviously the integral

$$D(t)=\int_0^t dt'I(t') \tag{8}$$

is nothing else but the cumulative dose. Inserting Eq. 5 into Eq. 8 and assuming that the time course $c(t)$ is constant, that is $c(t)=c$, one obtains

$$D(t)=\frac{c}{A+B}\left(1+k_{el}t+\frac{k_{12}}{k_{21}}\left(1-e^{-k_{21}t}\right)\right) \tag{9}$$

which is the theoretical time course of cumulative drug requirement during feedback-controlled drug delivery.

The general form of Eq. 9 looks like

$$D(t)=M_1+M_2\left(1-e^{-kt}\right)+I_{as}t$$

as depicted in Fig. 8 (lower panel).

Besides the cumulative curve, the figure represents also the asymptote to this curve. The asymptote is given by the formula $D_{as}(t)=M_1+M_2+I_{as}t$. The asymptote is uniquely defined by its value at $t=0$ and the slope. $D_{as}(0)=M_1+M_2$ and is nothing but the amount of drug in the body at steady-state, which is the so-called body load. The slope has the dimension of amount per unit time, and it represents an infusion

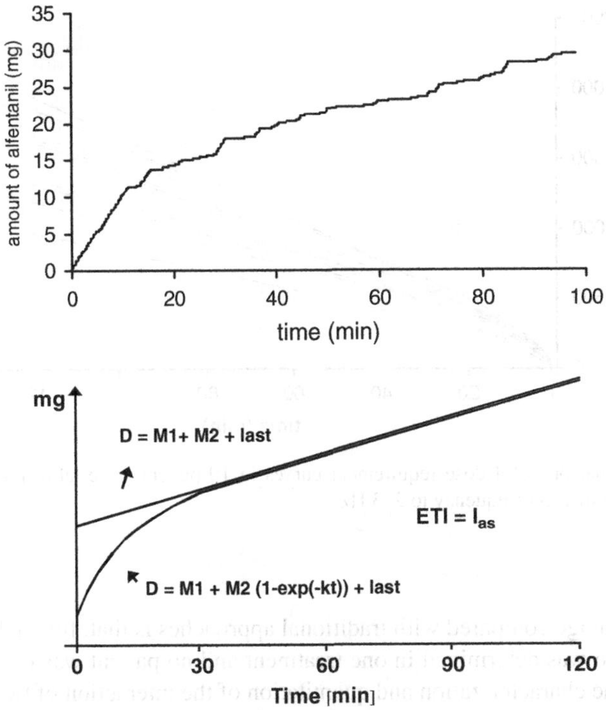

Fig. 8 Automatic feedback dosing systems generate cumulative drug requirement curves, which represent the minimum amount of drug to maintain the desired therapeutic state as measured by the corresponding target of drug effect as a surrogate parameter. From the cumulative curve one can derive the effective therapeutic infusion needed to maintain the effect as the slope of the asymptotic straight line. Feedback systems thus offer the chance to study interindividual variability of drug requirement without forcing patients to be underdosed or overdosed, as is commonly the case in the bracketing techniques of dose finding

rate. Obviously this rate of infusion is effective in maintaining the preset effect; we therefore call it effective infusion rate. Moreover, if one chooses the effect to be therapeutically adequate it is an effective therapeutic infusion (ETI). Thus, the slope of the asymptote of the cumulative drug requirement curve represents an effective therapeutic infusion. Given an experimental cumulative curve one may apply non-linear least-square fitting to obtain the coefficients M_1, M_2 and I_{as}. Especially in clinical research, feedback systems can provide rather practical and convenient conditions; for example, the study of interindividual variability in maintenance dose requirements for a given therapeutic effect. Instead of treating numerous patients with several doses, one might use a feedback system, which obtains for each patient during one treatment the exact dose requirement for this patient. Given these effective doses in a group of patients one can now study the variability. Figure 9 shows individual fitted cumulative dose requirement curves in a group of 10 volunteers together with their mean.

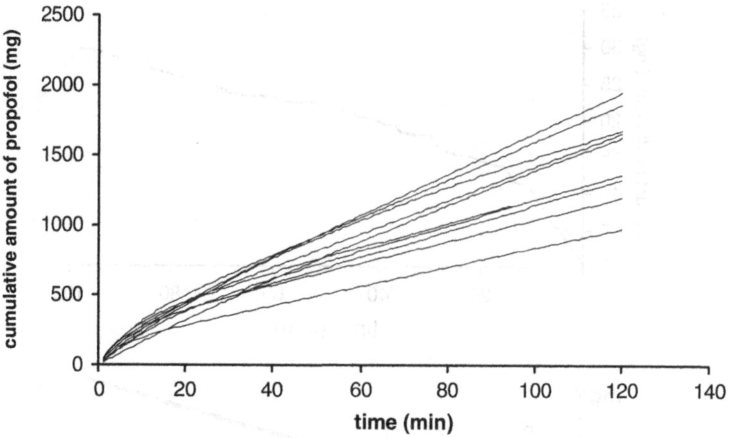

Fig. 9 Individual propofol dose requirement curves in 10 patients to establish and maintain a typical slowing of EEG frequency to 2–3 Hz

The advantage compared with traditional approaches is that, for each patient, an effective dose was determined in one treatment and no patient was over- or underdosed. For the characterization and quantitation of the interaction of two drugs, one can show that the use of the closed-loop approach can reduce the number of required investigations from n^2 to n. That is, feedback systems have the potential to be more practical, more effective, more economical and more patient-friendly than traditional approaches in clinical research. Olkkola and his group have extensively used these advantages of feedback control to quantitate the interaction of various muscle relaxants with other muscle relaxants and volatile and intravenous anaesthetics (Olkkola and Tammisto 1994a, b, c; Kansanaho and Olkkola 1995, 1996b; Olkkola and Kansanaho 1995).

It is interesting to note that there are essentially two different approaches to closed-loop drug administrations that differ in their control algorithms, namely model-based and knowledge-based feedback systems. Obviously model-based systems require some explicit understanding of the input–output relationship in terms of some mathematical formula. PID controllers are such a type. However, no general method exists to select the relative weights of the three terms (proportional, integral, differential) when the physiological response is unknown. Because physiological systems are often poorly characterized and may change with time, it is desirable to use controllers that automatically adapt their operation to changes in the system characteristics (model-based adaptive controllers). Knowledge-based systems, such as fuzzy control, have the ability to control a process without the determination of an explicit mathematical model of the input–output relationship. It is therefore a suitable system when little is known about the patient. The two presented closed-loop systems for the control of neuromuscular blockade and arterial blood pressure follow this reasoning. Neuromuscular blockade is induced by substances that are generally 'not known' to the body (xenobiotics). It is therefore likely that there are only few or no internal mechanisms that may interfere with the action of the xenobiotic. Thus, the input–output relationship between the xenobiotic and the neuromuscular blockade can be modelled easily by some mathematical formulae. This is in contrast to the case of the control of blood pressure. Numerous internal feedback systems are known that participate in the control of blood pressure. It is therefore virtually impossible to establish a valid model between one drug and the blood pressure without incorporating the action of the diverse internal feedback loops. In such case a knowledge-based control algorithm might be obviously more successful.

If closed-loop systems are superior to manual control, one should expect a widespread use of such devices, which is obviously not the case. The reason is that this technology is not fully developed (Jastremski et al. 1995). So far, all applications in clinical anaesthesia have been used in a research environment, and it has been shown that feedback systems can he very powerful research tools. But the development of systems which work under daily routine conditions is several orders magnitude more difficult than developing a research tool.

It remains to be shown that closed-loop systems will safely operate under common daily clinical conditions and provide a better control of drug administration. To this end, additional research and development is needed, especially in two areas: sensor technology and artefact detection and elimination. Both areas constitute the weak links in most closed-loop systems. The use of monitors in anaesthesia seems to indicate that redundancy could be a successful approach to tackle this problem. Redundancy brings the focus to the other major area of research and development in closed-loop system in clinical anaesthesia, namely multiple input–multiple output control. All feedback systems discussed used a specific drug as one input and one specific signal as output. This approach, however, represents an oversimplification of anaesthetic management. In the general clinical setting, several drugs are given and several physiological variables are measured and monitored. To mimic this situation by an automated closed-loop system one needs to control several drug inputs on the basis of several measured effects. For closed-loop systems, which are based on model-based control algorithms, this indicates that some future research has to be done in the field of quantitating drug–drug interactions in anaesthesiology. For knowledge-based fuzzy control systems, one might consider the integration of artificial neural net technology.

3.5 Conclusion

The use of automated closed-loop systems in clinical anaesthesia is currently restricted to research projects in clinical anaesthesia. For the expansion of such automated closed-loop systems, the ongoing research projects will have to demonstrate real-world efficacy.

References

Albrecht S, Frenkel C, Ihmsen H, Schuttler J (1999) A rational approach to the control of sedation in intensive care unit patients based on closed-loop control. Eur J Anaesthesiol 16:678–687

Alvis JM, Reves JG, Spain JA, Sheppard LC (1985) Computer-assisted continuous infusion of the intravenous analgesic fentanyl during general anesthesia—an interactive system. IEEE Trans Biomed Eng 32:323–329

Anderson JR, East TD (2002) A closed-loop controller for mechanical ventilation of patients with ARDS. Biomed Sci Instrum 38:289–294

Asbury AJ, Brown BH, Linkens DA (1980) Control of neuromuscular blockade by external feedback mechanisms. Br J Anaesth 52:633P

Ausems ME, Stanski DR, Hug CC (1985) An evaluation of the accuracy of pharmacokinetic data for the computer assisted infusion of alfentanil. Br J Anaesth 57:1217–1225

Bates JH, Hatzakis GE, Olivenstein R (2001) Fuzzy logic and mechanical ventilation. Respir Care Clin N Am 7:363–377, vii

Belleville JW, Attura GM (1957) Servo control of general anesthesia. Science 126:827–830

Belleville JW, Fennel PJ, Murphy T, Howland WS (1960) The relative potencies of methohexital and thiopental. J Pharmacol Exp Ther 129:108–114

Bickford RG (1950) Automatic electroencephalographic control of general anesthesia. Electroencephalogr Clin Neurophysiol 2:93–96

Bickford RG (1951) Use of frequency discrimination in the automatic electroencephalographic control of anesthesia (servo-anesthesia). Electroencephalogr Clin Neurophysiol 3:83–86

Billard V, Servin F, Guignard B, Junke E, Bouverne MN, Hedouin M, Chauvin M (2004) Desflurane-remifentanil-nitrous oxide anaesthesia for abdominal surgery: optimal concentrations and recovery features. Acta Anaesthesiol Scand 48:355–364

Blake DW, Hogg MN, Hackman CH, Pang J, Bjorksten AR (1998) Induction of anaesthesia with sevoflurane, preprogrammed propofol infusion or combined sevoflurane/propofol for laryngeal mask insertion: cardiovascular, movement and EEG Bispectral Index responses. Anaesth Intensive Care 26:360–365

Branson RD, Johannigman JA, Campbell RS, Davis K Jr (2002) Closed-loop mechanical ventilation. Respir Care 47:427–451

Bruhn J, Bouillon TW, Radulescu L, Hoeft A, Bertaccini E, Shafer SL (2003) Correlation of approximate entropy, Bispectral Index, and Spectral Edge Frequency 95 (SEF95) with clinical signs of "anesthetic depth" during coadministration of propofol and remifentanil. Anesthesiology 98:621–627

Brunner JX (2001) Principles and history of closed-loop controlled ventilation. Respir Care Clin N Am 7:341–362, vii

Camu F, Lauwers M, Vanlersberghe C (1998) Basic principles of pharmacokinetics and pharmacodynamics for the anesthesiologist. Acta Anaesthesiol Belg 49:55–64

Chee F, Fernando T, van Heerden PV (2002) Closed-loop control of blood glucose levels in critically ill patients. Anaesth Intensive Care 30:295–307

Chee F, Fernando T, van Heerden PV (2003) Closed-loop glucose control in critically ill patients using continuous glucose monitoring system (CGMS) in real time. IEEE Trans Inf Technol Biomed 7:43–53

Coetzee JF, Glen JB, Wium CA, Boshoff L (1995) Pharmacokinetic model selection for target controlled infusions of propofol. Assessment of three parameter sets. Anesthesiology 82:1328–1345

Cordato DJ, Mather LE, Gross AS, Herkes GK (1999) Pharmacokinetics of thiopental enantiomers during and following prolonged high-dose therapy. Anesthesiology 91:1693–1702

Cosgrove DM 3rd, Petre JH, Waller JL, Roth JV, Shepherd C, Cohn LH (1989) Automated control of postoperative hypertension: a prospective, randomized multicenter study. Ann Thorac Surg 47:678–682

Crankshaw DP, Morgan DJ, Beemer GH, Karasawa F (1993) Preprogrammed infusion of alfentanil to constant arterial plasma concentration. Anesth Analg 76:556–561

Dingemanse J, Haussler J, Hering W, Ihmsen H, Albrecht S, Zell M, Schwilden H, Schuttler J (1997) Pharmacokinetic-pharmacodynamic modelling of the EEG effects of Ro 48–6791, a new short-acting benzodiazepine, in young and elderly subjects. Br J Anaesth 79:567–574

Dojat M, Brochard L (2001) Knowledge-based systems for automatic ventilatory management. Respir Care Clin N Am 7:379–396, viii

Eger EI 2nd, Saidman LJ, Brandstater B (1965) Minimum alveolar anesthetic concentration: a standard of anesthetic potency. Anesthesiology 26:756–763

Fechner J, Albrecht S, Ihmsen H, Knoll R, Schwilden H, Schuttler J (1998) [Predictability and precision of "target-controlled infusion" (TCI) of propofol with the "Disoprifusor TCI" system]. Anaesthesist 47:663–668

Fechner J, Ihmsen H, Hatterscheid D, Jeleazcov C, Schiessl C, Vornov JJ, Schwilden H, Schuttler J (2004) Comparative pharmacokinetics and pharmacodynamics of the new propofol prodrug GPI 15715 and propofol emulsion. Anesthesiology 101:626–639

Fechner J, Ihmsen H, Schiessl C, Jeleazcov C, Vornov JJ, Schwilden H, Schuttler J (2005) Sedation with GPI 15715, a water-soluble prodrug of propofol, using target-controlled infusion in volunteers. Anesth Analg 100:701–706

Gentilini A, Schaniel C, Morari M, Bieniok C, Wymann R, Schnider T (2002) A new paradigm for the closed-loop intraoperative administration of analgesics in humans. IEEE Trans Biomed Eng 49:289–299

Gepts E, Shafer SL, Camu F, Stanski DR, Woestenborghs R, Van Peer A, Heykants JJ (1995) Linearity of pharmacokinetics and model estimation of sufentanil. Anesthesiology 83:1194–1204

Ghouri AF, Monk TG, White PF (1993) Electroencephalogram spectral edge frequency, lower esophageal contractility, and autonomic responsiveness during general anesthesia. J Clin Monit 9:176–185

Glass PS, Goodman DK, Ginsberg B, Reves JG, Jacobs JR (1989) Accuracy of pharmacokinetic model-driven infusion of propofol. Anesthesiology 71:A277

Glass PS, Glen JB, Kenny GN, Schuttler J, Shafer SL (1997) Nomenclature for computer-assisted infusion devices. Anesthesiology 86:1430–1431

Glen JB (1998) The development of 'Diprifusor': a TCI system for propofol. Anaesthesia 53 [Suppl 1]:13–21

Groetsch CW (1984) The theory of Tikhonov regularization for Fredholm equations of the first kind. Pitman, Boston

Hanaire H (2006) Continuous glucose monitoring and external insulin pump: towards a subcutaneous closed loop. Diabetes Metab 32:534–538

Hayes JK, Westenskow DR, East TD, Jordan WS (1984) Computer-controlled anesthesia delivery system. Med Instrum 18:224–231

Hengstmann JH, Stoeckel H, Schuttler J (1980) Infusion model for fentanyl based on pharmacokinetic analysis. Br J Anaesth 52:1021–1025

Hering WJ, Ihmsen H, Langer H, Uhrlau C, Dinkel M, Geisslinger G, Schuttler J (1996) Pharmacokinetic-pharmacodynamic modeling of the new steroid hypnotic eltanolone in healthy volunteers. Anesthesiology 85:1290–1299

Hoeksel SA, Schreuder JJ, Blom JA, Maessen JG, Penn OC (1996) Automated infusion of nitroglycerin to control arterial hypertension during cardiac surgery. Intensive Care Med 22:688–693

Hull CJ, Van Beem HB, McLeod K, Sibbald A, Watson MJ (1978) A pharmacodynamic model for pancuronium. Br J Anaesth 50:1113–1123

Ihmsen H, Geisslinger G, Schuttler J (2001) Stereoselective pharmacokinetics of ketamine: R(–)-ketamine inhibits the elimination of S(+)-ketamine. Clin Pharmacol Ther 70:431–438

Jaremko J, Rorstad O (1998) Advances toward the implantable artificial pancreas for treatment of diabetes. Diabetes Care 21:444–450

Jastremski M, Jastremski C, Shepherd M, Friedman V, Porembka D, Smith R, Gonzales E, Swedlow D, Belzberg H, Crass R, et al (1995) A model for technology assessment as applied to closed loop infusion systems. Technology Assessment Task Force of the Society of Critical Care Medicine. Crit Care Med 23:1745–1755

Kansanaho M, Olkkola KT (1995) Quantifying the effect of enflurane on atracurium infusion requirements. Can J Anaesth 42:103–108

Kansanaho M, Olkkola KT (1996a) Performance assessment of an adaptive model-based feedback controller: comparison between atracurium, mivacurium, rocuronium and vecuronium. Int J Clin Monit Comput 13:217–224

Kansanaho M, Olkkola KT (1996b) Quantifying the effect of isoflurane on mivacurium infusion requirements. Anaesthesia 51:133–136

Katoh T, Suzuki A, Ikeda K (1998) Electroencephalographic derivatives as a tool for predicting the depth of sedation and anesthesia induced by sevoflurane. Anesthesiology 88:642–650

Kenny GN, White M (1990) A portable computerised infusion system for propofol. Anaesthesia 45:692–693

Kissin I (1993) General anesthetic action: an obsolete notion? Anesth Analg 76:215–218

Kissin I, Gelman S (1988) Components of anaesthesia. Br J Anaesth 61:237–238

Kochs E, Bischoff P, Pichlmeier U, Schulte am Esch J (1994) Surgical stimulation induces changes in brain electrical activity during isoflurane/nitrous oxide anesthesia. A topographic electroencephalographic analysis. Anesthesiology 80:1026–1034

Kwok KE, Shah SL, Clanachan AS, Finegan BA (1995) Evaluation of a long-range adaptive predictive controller for computerized drug delivery systems. IEEE Trans Biomed Eng 42:79–86

Li YH, Xu JH, Yang JJ, Tian J, Xu JG (2005) Predictive performance of 'Diprifusor' TCI system in patients during upper abdominal surgery under propofol/fentanyl anesthesia. J Zhejiang Univ Sci B 6:43–48

Linkens DA, Rimmer SJ, Asbury AJ, Brown BH (1981) Identification of the model in the control of neuromuscular blockade using PRBS testing. Br J Anaesth 53:666P

Mandema JW, Veng-Pedersen P, Danhof M (1991) Estimation of amobarbital plasma-effect site equilibration kinetics. Relevance of polyexponential conductance functions. J Pharmacokinet Biopharm 19:617–634

Mapleson WW (1979) From clover to computer. Towards programmed anaesthesia? Anaesthesia 34:163–172

Marsh B, White M, Morton N, Kenny GN (1991) Pharmacokinetic model driven infusion of propofol in children. Br J Anaesth 67:41–48

Mayo CW, Bickford RG, Faulconer A Jr (1950) Electroencephalographically controlled anesthesia in abdominal surgery. J Am Med Assoc 144:1081–1083

Meijers RH, Schmartz D, Cantraine FR, Barvais L, d'Hollander AA, Blom JA (1997) Clinical evaluation of an automatic blood pressure controller during cardiac surgery. J Clin Monit 13:261–268

Mertens MJ, Engbers FH, Burm AG, Vuyk J (2003) Predictive performance of computer-controlled infusion of remifentanil during propofol/remifentanil anaesthesia. Br J Anaesth 90:132–141

Mortier E, Struys M (2003) Effect site modelling and its application in TCI. Adv Exp Med Biol 523:239–244

Mortier E, Struys M, De Smet T, Versichelen L, Rolly G (1998) Closed-loop controlled administration of propofol using Bispectral analysis. Anaesthesia 53:749–754

O'Hara DA, Derbyshire GJ, Overdyk FJ, Bogen DK, Marshall BE (1991) Closed-loop infusion of atracurium with four different anesthetic techniques. Anesthesiology 74:258–263

Olkkola KT, Kansanaho M (1995) Quantifying the interaction of vecuronium with enflurane using closed-loop feedback control of vecuronium infusion. Acta Anaesthesiol Scand 39:489–493

Olkkola KT, Tammisto T (1994a) Assessment of the interaction between atracurium and suxamethonium at 50% neuromuscular block using closed-loop feedback control of infusion of atracurium. Br J Anaesth 73:199–203

Olkkola KT, Tammisto T (1994b) Quantifying the interaction of rocuronium (Org 9426) with etomidate, fentanyl, midazolam, propofol, thiopental, and isoflurane using closed-loop feedback control of rocuronium infusion. Anesth Analg 78:691–696

Olkkola KT, Tammisto T (1994c) Quantitation of the interaction of rocuronium bromide with etomidate, fentanyl, midazolam, propofol, thiopentone, and isoflurane using closed-loop feedback control of infusion of rocuronium. Eur J Anaesthesiol Suppl 9:99–100

Pfeiffer EF, Thum C, Clemens AH (1974) The artificial beta cell—a continuous control of blood sugar by external regulation of insulin infusion (glucose controlled insulin infusion system). Horm Metab Res 6:339–342

Quasha AL, Eger EI 2nd, Tinker JH (1980) Determination and applications of MAC. Anesthesiology 53:315–334

Ruiz R, Borches D, Gonzalez A, Corral J (1993) A new sodium-nitroprusside-infusion controller for the regulation of arterial blood pressure. Biomed Instrum Technol 27:244–251

Salamonsen RF (1978) A vaporizing system for programmed anaesthesia. Br J Anaesth 50:425–433

Schiel R (2003) Continuous subcutaneous insulin infusion in patients with diabetes mellitus. Therap Apher Dial 7:232–237

Schüttler J, Schwilden H (1997) Closed-loop systems in clinical anaesthesia. Curr Opin Anaesthesiol 9:457–481

Schuttler J, Ihmsen H (2000) Population pharmacokinetics of propofol: a multicenter study. Anesthesiology 92:727–738

Schuttler J, Schwilden H (1999) Present state of closed-loop drug delivery in anesthesia and intensive care. Acta Anaesthesiol Belg 50:187–191

Schuttler J, Schwilden H, Stoekel H (1983) Pharmacokinetics as applied to total intravenous anaesthesia. Practical implications. Anaesthesia 38 [Suppl]:53–56

Schuttler J, Kloos S, Schwilden H, Stoeckel H (1988) Total intravenous anaesthesia with propofol and alfentanil by computer-assisted infusion. Anaesthesia 43 [Suppl]:2–7

Schwilden H (1981) A general method for calculating the dosage scheme in linear pharmacokinetics. Eur J Clin Pharmacol 20:379–386

Schwilden H, Olkkola KT (1991) Use of a pharmacokinetic-dynamic model for the automatic feedback control of atracurium. Eur J Clin Pharmacol 40:293–296

Schwilden H, Stoeckel H (1993) Closed-loop feedback controlled administration of alfentanil during alfentanil-nitrous oxide anaesthesia. Br J Anaesth 70:389–393

Schwilden H, Schuttler J, Stoekel H (1983) Pharmacokinetics as applied to total intravenous anaesthesia. Theoretical considerations. Anaesthesia 38 [Suppl]:51–52

Schwilden H, Schuttler J, Stoeckel H (1985) Quantitation of the EEG and pharmacodynamic modelling of hypnotic drugs: etomidate as an example. Eur J Anaesthesiol 2:121–131

Schwilden H, Schuttler J, Stoeckel H (1987) Closed-loop feedback control of methohexital anesthesia by quantitative EEG analysis in humans. Anesthesiology 67:341–347

Schwilden H, Honerkamp J, Elster C (1993) Pharmacokinetic model identification and parameter estimation as an ill-posed problem. Eur J Clin Pharmacol 45:545–550

Servin FS, Bougeois B, Gomeni R, Mentre F, Farinotti R, Desmonts JM (2003) Pharmacokinetics of propofol administered by target-controlled infusion to alcoholic patients. Anesthesiology 99:576–585

Shafer SL (1993) Constant versus optimal plasma concentration. Anesth Analg 76:467–469

Sheiner LB, Steimer JL (2000) Pharmacokinetic/pharmacodynamic modeling in drug development. Annu Rev Pharmacol Toxicol 40:67–95

Sheiner LB, Stanski DR, Vozeh S, Miller RD, Ham J (1979) Simultaneous modeling of pharmacokinetics and pharmacodynamics: application to d-tubocurarine. Clin Pharmacol Ther 25:358–371

Sheppard LC, Kouchoukos NT (1977) Automation of measurements and interventions in the systematic care of postoperative cardiac surgical patients. Med Instrum 11:296–301

Stanski DR, Hug CC Jr (1982) Alfentanil—a kinetically predictable narcotic analgesic. Anesthesiology 57:435–438

Stoeckel H, Hengstmann JH, Schuttler J (1979) Pharmacokinetics of fentanyl as a possible explanation for recurrence of respiratory depression. Br J Anaesth 51:741–745

Struys MM, De Smet T, Versichelen LF, Van De Velde S, Van den Broecke R, Mortier EP (2001) Comparison of closed-loop controlled administration of propofol using Bispectral Index as the controlled variable versus "standard practice" controlled administration. Anesthesiology 95:6–17

Struys MM, De Smet T, Greenwald S, Absalom AR, Binge S, Mortier EP (2004) Performance evaluation of two published closed-loop control systems using Bispectral Index monitoring: a simulation study. Anesthesiology 100:640–647

Tehrani F, Rogers M, Lo T, Malinowski T, Afuwape S, Lum M, Grundl B, Terry M (2004) A dual closed-loop control system for mechanical ventilation. J Clin Monit Comput 18:111–129

Van Poucke GE, Bravo LJ, Shafer SL (2004) Target controlled infusions: targeting the effect site while limiting peak plasma concentration. IEEE Trans Biomed Eng 51:1869–1875

Varvel JR, Donoho DL, Shafer SL (1992) Measuring the predictive performance of computer-controlled infusion pumps. J Pharmacokinet Biopharm 20:63–94

Visser K, Hassink EA, Bonsel GJ, Moen J, Kalkman CJ (2001) Randomized controlled trial of total intravenous anesthesia with propofol versus inhalation anesthesia with isoflurane-nitrous oxide: postoperative nausea with vomiting and economic analysis. Anesthesiology 95:616–626

Vozeh S, Steimer JL (1985) Feedback control methods for drug dosage optimisation. Concepts, classification and clinical application. Clin Pharmacokinet 10:457–476

Vuyk J, Engbers FH, Burm AG, Vletter AA, Bovill JG (1995) Performance of computer-controlled infusion of propofol: an evaluation of five pharmacokinetic parameter sets. Anesth Analg 81:1275–1282

Webster NR, Cohen AT (1987) Closed-loop administration of atracurium. Steady-state neuromuscular blockade during surgery using a computer controlled closed-loop atracurium infusion. Anaesthesia 42:1085–1091

Westenskow DR (1997) Fundamentals of feedback control: PID, fuzzy logic, and neural networks. J Clin Anesth 9:33S–35S

Advanced Technologies and Devices for Inhalational Anesthetic Drug Dosing

J.-U. Meyer(✉), G. Kullik, N. Wruck, K. Kück, and J. Manigel

Abstract Technological advances in micromechanics, optical sensing, and computing have led to innovative and reliable concepts of precise dosing and sensing of modern volatile anesthetics. Mixing of saturated desflurane flow with fresh gas flow (FGF) requires differential pressure sensing between the two circuits for precise delivery. The medical gas xenon is administered most economically in a closed circuit breathing system. Sensing of xenon in the breathing system is achieved with miniaturized and unique gas detector systems. Innovative sensing principles such as thermal conductivity and sound velocity are applied. The combination of direct injection of volatile anesthetics and low-flow in a closed circuit system requires simultaneous sensing of the inhaled and exhaled gas concentrations. When anesthetic conserving devices are used for sedation with volatile anesthetics, regular gas concentration monitoring is advised. High minimal alveolar concentration (MAC)

J.-U. Meyer
Drägerwerk AG, Moislinger Allee 53-55, 23542 Lübeck, Germany
joerg-uwe.meyer@draeger.com

J. Schüttler and H. Schwilden (eds.) *Modern Anesthetics.*
Handbook of Experimental Pharmacology 182.

values of some anesthetics and low-flow conditions bear the risk of hypoxic gas delivery. Oxygen sensing based on paramagnetic thermal transduction has become the choice when long lifetime and one-time calibration are required. Compact design of beam splitters, infrared filters, and detectors have led to multiple spectra detector systems that fit in thimble-sized housings. Response times of less than 500 ms allow systems to distinguish inhaled from exhaled gas concentrations. The compact gas detector systems are a prerequisite to provide "quantitative anesthesia" in closed circuit feedback-controlled breathing systems. Advanced anesthesia devices in closed circuit mode employ multiple feedback systems. Multiple feedbacks include controls of volume, concentrations of anesthetics, and concentration of oxygen with a corresponding safety system. In the ideal case, the feedback system delivers precisely what the patient is consuming.

In this chapter, we introduce advanced technologies and device concepts for delivering inhalational anesthetic drugs. First, modern vaporizers are described with special attention to the particularities of delivering desflurane. Delivery of xenon is presented, followed by a discussion of direct injection of volatile anesthetics and of a device designed to conserve anesthetic drugs. Next, innovative sensing technologies are presented for reliable control and precise metering of the delivered volatile anesthetics. Finally, we discuss the technical challenges of automatic control in low-flow and closed circuit breathing systems in anesthesia.

1 Introduction to Dosing of Anesthetics

Since the discovery of inhaled agents with anesthetic effect, dosing has been a major challenge because of potential adverse side effects and risks when delivered inappropriately. Accurate dosing relates to the delivery of the exact amount of drug in a specified volume over a defined time. Ambient conditions, such as pressure, gas flow rates, and temperatures, affect the delivery characteristics of the gas. Modern anesthesia devices compensate for the effects of fresh gas flow (FGF), carrier-gas composition, ambient temperatures, and pressure changes in the system. Commonly, inhaled anesthetics are physically present as volatile liquids or as gases. Nitrous oxide and xenon are delivered in their gas phase. The volatile agents halothane, enflurane, isoflurane, desflurane, and sevoflurane are administered as vapors after evaporation in devices known as vaporizers. Volatiles differ in regard to their physical, chemical, and physiological properties. Table 1 summarizes characteristic parameters of volatile gases, including their boiling point, vapor pressure, blood/gas partition coefficient, and their minimal alveolar concentration (MAC) (Stoelting and Hillier 2006).

The different physical properties of the gases require vaporizer designs that are particular for each of the volatile anesthetics. Dosing principles of vaporizers vary from passive evaporation to liquid injection. Control of delivered doses and consumption of gases is achieved with precise sensing and metering of delivered gas concentration. The monitoring of inhaled oxygen is mandatory for anesthesia

Table 1 Physical characteristics of inhalational anesthetics

	Nitrous Oxide	Halothane	Enflurane	Isoflurane	Desflurane	Sevoflurane	Xenon
Boiling point(C)@ 750 mmHg Ambient Pressure	-	50.2	56.5	48.5	22.8	58.6	-
Vapor pressure (mmHg) @ 20C	Gas	244	172	240	669	170	Gas
Blood / Gas Partition Coeffcient	0.46	2.54	1.90	1.46	0.42	0.69	0.115
MAC(%)	104	0.75	1.63	1.17	6.6	1.8	63-71

machines. Metering of single gases and gas compositions under low-flow conditions is most critical and therefore requires advanced sensing technologies. Volatile anesthetics are delivered in open, semi-open, or semi-closed circuit anesthesia systems. Fresh gas flows at higher levels (approx. 6 l/min) in non-rebreathing semi-open systems. Normal, low, and minimal FGFs are used in semi-closed anesthesia systems ranging from less than 1 l/min to 4 l/min. In an ideal closed system, the delivery of anesthetic agents corresponds precisely to the consumed gases. Patient individual consumption of anesthetic agents is approximated from the delivered drug concentration and from the end-tidal drug concentration in exhaled breath.

2 Dosing Technologies

2.1 Vaporizer

Typically, vaporizers are characterized by employing either high or low fresh gas control (FGC) in an out-of-circle mode. Vaporizers are categorized according to their physical and mechanical principle of drug delivery. Evaporation methods and direct liquid injection technologies constitute the main principles of volatile drug delivery (Scharmer 1995). Plenum vaporizers are devices that evaporate the volatile anesthetics without exerting external energy. Vaporization energy is replenished from the environment. They are commonly used for most agents and available from many manufacturers. The fresh gas stream is split into the dosage path and a bypass path. The flow through the dosage path is directly controlled by the control dial, the bypass flow by a temperature compensating cone. The gas flow is laminar over a wide flow range, and additional components compensate for back pressure fluctuations from the breathing circuit. Two additional valves inhibit intrusion of anesthetic agent into the dosage components during transport. During "off" mode, the fresh gas completely bypasses the dosage components. During "on" mode, part of the fresh gas flows through the vaporization chamber and is enriched with anesthetic vapor. The other part of the fresh gas bypasses the vaporization chamber through the vaporization chamber bypass. The two parts are combined downstream of the flow control slots and fed to the outlet. The desired concentration is achieved by the split of the gas and the saturation concentration of the anesthetic. The latter changes with temperature. A temperature compensation mechanism (thermal expansion of different materials) affects the split to compensate for this effect. When the temperature compensator heats up it opens the vaporizer chamber bypass. When the temperature compensator cools down it narrows the vaporizer chamber bypass. The pressure compensation effectively reduces the pumping effect that may otherwise cause the respiratory pressure variations to result in undesirable delivered gas concentrations (Fig. 1).

2.2 *Desflurane Vaporizer*

The concentration of desflurane and thus the thermal loss from vaporization needed to achieve comparable levels of anesthesia is four to six times higher than that of other volatile agents. Desflurane's high vapor pressure and its comparably steeper temperature vs vapor pressure curve create temperature compensation requirements that go well beyond what traditional plenum vaporizers can provide.

The Tec6 desflurane vaporizer electrically heats the anesthetic in a sealed chamber to 39°C, creating a pressure of approximately 1,550 mmHg. The pressure created from the agent flowing through a variable resistor (set by the user through the vaporizer control dial) is controlled to be the same pressure that is created from the FGF passing through a fixed resistor. The saturated agent flow and the FGF mix before their delivery into the breathing circuit. Desflurane vaporizers are calibrated for operation with an FGF of 100% O_2 concentration, resulting in differences between set and actual concentrations for other FGF mixtures. The desflurane vaporizer principle described here delivers a fixed volume percentage, making it different from conventional vaporizers, which deliver fixed partial pressures. A number of safety features are employed in desflurane vaporizers. Two instead of only one differential pressure sensor are typically used. If the difference between the two sensors is too high, if the liquid anesthetic agent level in the heated chamber reaches a minimum volume, if the vaporizer is tilted, or if there is a power failure, a valve completely switches off the desflurane flow into the breathing circuit (Andrews et al. 1993; Andrews and Johnston 1993; Fig. 2).

2.3 *Delivery of Xenon as an Anesthetic Agent*

Xenon is known for its advantageous properties in anesthesia: it is not metabolized, has no organ toxicity, and provides cardiovascular stability, neuroprotection, good

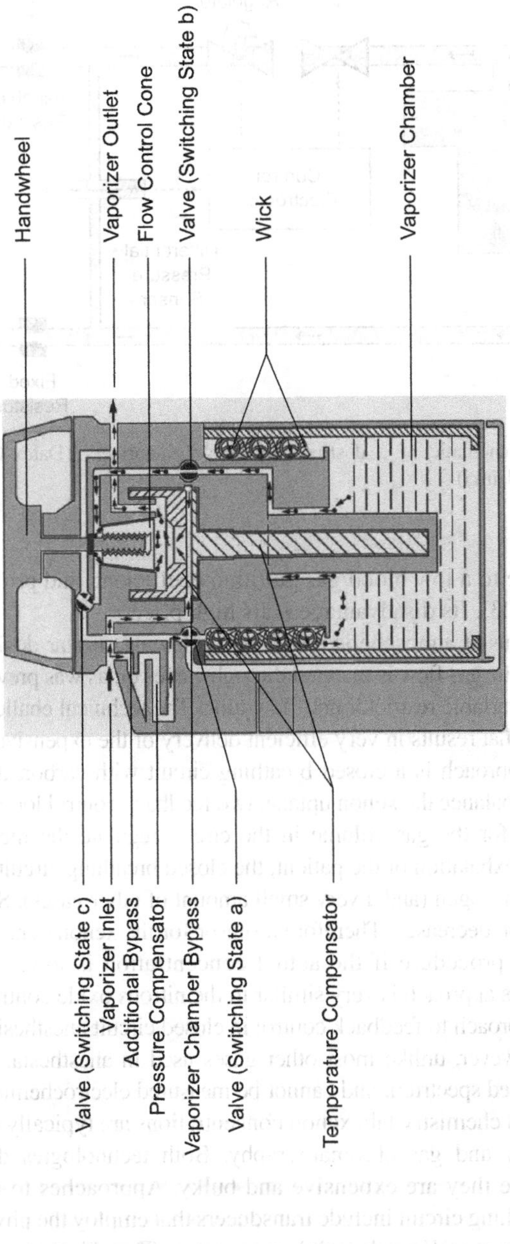

Fig.1 Dräger plenum vaporizer 2000

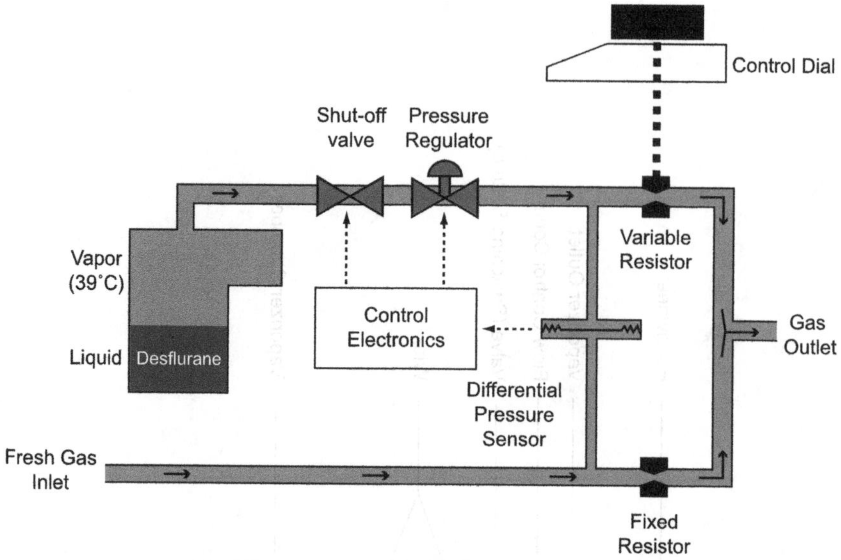

Fig. 2 Simplified schematic of a desflurane "Tec6"* vaporizer *(Datex-Ohmeda Division, Instrumentarium, Helsinki)

controllability due to a low blood/gas partition coefficient, and profound analgesia (Sanders et al. 2003). Its disadvantage is its high price.

Xenon is gaseous at atmospheric conditions, allowing similar dosing principles as for nitrous oxide. The gas flow is metered through valves or, as was previously common, is controlled by a variable restrictor and flow tube. The technical challenge is to design a delivery system that results in very efficient delivery of the expensive gas.

The obvious approach is a closed breathing circuit with carbon dioxide removal. In order to closely balance the xenon uptake, two feedback control loops for the oxygen concentration and for the gas volume in the circuit regulate the metering valve for xenon. Due to the exhalation of the patient, the closed breathing circuit is continuously accumulated with nitrogen (and a very small amount of other gases). Subsequently the xenon concentration decreases. Therefore a sensor for the xenon concentration is used to trigger a flush procedure if the actual concentration is lower than the target concentration. This approach is very similar to the nitrous oxide control system.

The general approach to feedback control in closed circuit anesthesia is well known (Baum 2005). However, unlike most other gases used in anesthesia, xenon does not absorb in the infrared spectrum, and cannot be measured electrochemically either.

In the analytical chemistry lab, xenon concentrations are typically measured using mass spectrometry and gas chromatography. Both technologies do not work in anesthesia because they are expensive and bulky. Approaches to measure xenon in the patient breathing circuit include transducers that employ the physical principles of thermal conductivity (Wiegleb 1998) or acoustics. The effect of xenon on thermal conductivity and sound velocity are distinct and different from other anesthetics.

The flushing of the breathing system before anesthesia induction and after recovery poses a challenge when xenon is meant to remain in the closed system. A release of xenon into the operating room or recovery room should be avoided. Attempts to collect any gas from the circuit and to recover the xenon include process-engineering technologies such as adsorption and liquefaction, either by instrumentation close to the anesthesia machine or in special process equipment (Georgieff et al. 1995). Employing xenon in conventional anesthesia systems also requires material and technical adaptations on patient gas flow measurements and radial blower volume delivery.

In the past, some conventional anesthesia machines have been modified to be used with xenon, but none of them has been made available commercially, since xenon has gained medical approval quite recently (in 2005). Dräger PhysioFlex and Dräger Cicero anesthesia machines (Dräger Medical, Lübeck, Germany) are prominent examples of anesthesia devices suited for the delivery of xenon. Both were equipped with thermal conductivity sensors and have been used in many scientific studies (Hecker et al. 2003). Efforts are underway to make commercially available a modern anesthesia device that is approved for the use of medical xenon as supplied by the company Air Liquide.

2.4 *Direct Injection of Volatile Anesthetics*

When uncoupling agent delivery and FGF, anesthetic agent can be titrated independently of the chosen FGF. The volatile anesthetics are injected directly into the breathing circuit. When combined with minimal FGF in a closed breathing system, this technique enables rapid control of agent concentrations as well as minimal consumption of anesthetics.

Direct injection of volatile agents has been implemented in the PhysioFlex anesthesia machine and the Zeus anesthesia machine (both from Dräger, Lübeck, Germany) as part of a closed loop volatile anesthetic drug delivery system.

The volatile agent dosing unit of the Zeus anesthesia machine comprises a reservoir unit, a dosing chamber, and a heating unit (Struys et al. 2005). The reservoir unit stores a quantity of anesthetic liquid in a tank and delivers it by means of an automatic injection system as schematically presented in Fig. 3. The volatile agent is injected from a pressurized chamber into a heated vaporizing chamber using a pulsed liquid injection valve. The anesthetic vapor is finally delivered to the breathing system via a heated pipe.

The Zeus anesthesia machine offers different agent dosing modes. In the conventional fresh gas mode, where the user sets a fresh gas agent concentration, the vapor is mixed with the fresh gas before being administered into the breathing system. In this dosing mode the agent dosage performance is equivalent to a conventional vaporizer.

An auto control mode provides the delivery of the anesthetics to the breathing system independent of the FGF settings. A closed loop feedback control is

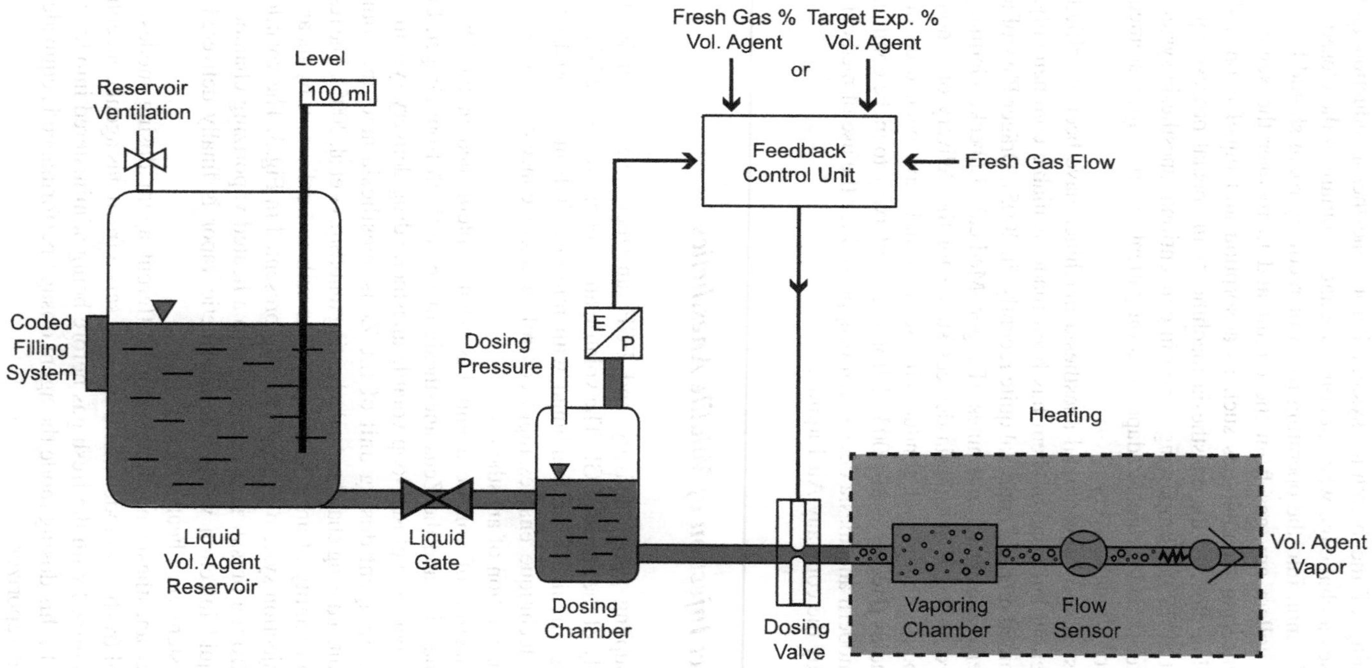

Fig. 3 Feedback-controlled volatile agent delivery system. The advanced vapor delivery unit of the Zeus anesthesia machine comprises a reservoir, a dosing chamber, and a heating unit. A closed loop feedback unit controls the direct injection of the liquid anesthetics into the vapor heating element

employed. The user can directly set the expiratory target concentration independent of the fresh gas concentration. Based on a simplified physiological model of the patient, a feedback controller calculates the amount of agent from the deviation between the expiratory target value and the expiratory concentration measured at the Y-piece. A second gas sensor in the inspiratory limb acts as a supervisor to ensure that the inspiratory concentration will not exceed a maximal value and to crosscheck the plausibility of the gas measurements. A circuit flow provided by a blower located in the inspiratory limb of the breathing system provides a homogeneous agent concentration within the breathing circuit (Fig. 4).

2.5 Anesthetic Conserving Device

An anesthetic conserving device (ACD) has been introduced recently (Tempia et al. 2003). The liquid anesthetic is administered via a syringe pump system to a porous rod for evaporation. The anesthetic is instantaneously vaporized inside the ACD by the inspiratory gas flow and is delivered to the lungs. During expiration, activated carbon fibers absorb a large fraction of the expired anesthetic vapor and desorb it during the next inspiration (Enlund et al. 2001). In combination with a standard critical care ventilator, the ACD functions as a vaporizer. The ACD can be used in an ICU environment, where it is connected to the patient's breathing circuit similar to a heat and moisture exchanger (HME). Instead of only water being reflected to the patient, as in the case of an HME, activated carbon fibers reflect common anesthetic gases, with the exception of nitrous oxide. Main applications include the sedation of patients with volatile anesthetic agents in the ICU. The ACD is especially suited for sedation of adults, because a large dead space volume of 100 ml is inherent to the system. Efforts are underway to achieve device approval for isoflurane and sevoflurane for indications of long-term sedation. Additional safety equipment is required when using the ACD for sedation in the ICU: (1) a gas monitor, (2) a syringe pump for the liquid anesthetic, and (3) an expiration gas conditioning system. The gas monitor detects the concentration administered to the patient. Ergonometric solutions of the monitor have to deal with the fluctuations of anesthetic concentrations that vary during the inspiration and expiration phase. Pump rates need careful control, since high pump rates are needed during filling of the ACD, but low rates are required later when simply compensating for the loss of anesthetic agent (the device features a reflection efficiency of about 90%). The administered concentration has to be checked regularly because a change in conditions (e.g., breathing pattern) can alter the reflection efficiency. Expiratory gases, which comprise anesthetic agents that are not taken up by the gas reflection material, are required to be fed into a gas suction system that is rarely available in common ICUs. The ACD is not designed for long-term use. The ACD has been well accepted in Europe, while safety issues are still under discussion (Berton et al. 2007).

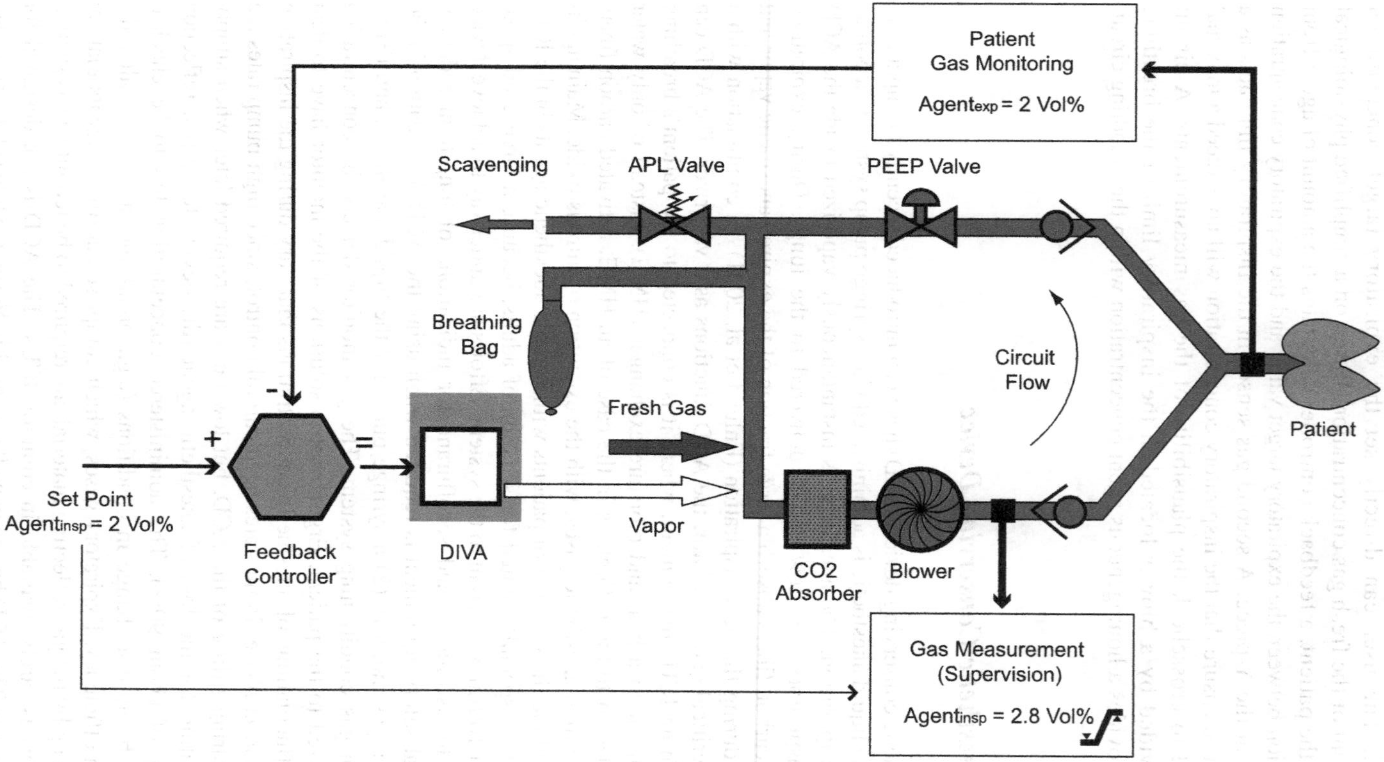

Fig. 4 Closed loop feedback control. Vapor is delivered separately from fresh gas to the breathing system as part of a closed loop feedback control system. The user can directly set the expiratory target concentration. Optical sensors measure the concentration of anesthetics in the exhalation branch of the Y-piece

3 Sensor Technologies and Modules to Meter Gas Dosing

3.1 Oxygen Gas Sensing

Oxygen concentration measurements are important to detect hypoxic mixtures when dosing anesthetic agents, particularly those with high MAC values. In the past, electrochemical cells were used, but their inherently limited lifetime led to the development of a physical sensor to measure oxygen extended lifetimes. The paramagnetic effect of oxygen has been well known for more than a century. The magnetic flux increases when oxygen is drawn in an air gap of a magnetic field. This principle has been employed in early paramagnetic oxygen sensors of anesthesia sensor modules, such as in the Datex OM101 and the Servomex PM1111E. The Dräger PATO (paramagnetic thermal oxygen analyzer) device (Dräger Medical, Lübeck, Germany) utilizes the effect of reduced thermal conductivity of oxygen in the presence of a magnetic field in a novel sensor approach. The operational principle of the PATO device is that a modulated magnetic field affects the thermodynamic characteristics of oxygen, which has an influence on the warming of the gas when in the immediate vicinity of a heating element (Seftleben and Pietzner 1933). This results in a temperature modulation whose magnitude is a function of the oxygen concentration. Figure 5 depicts the sensing principles and the alignment of oxygen molecules under the influence of a magnetic field.

Micromechanical techniques have been employed to integrate heating and sensing components on a chip with a dimension less than 4×3 mm^2. Thermal conductivity and the flow of oxygen is measured simultaneously in the same gas cell. The gas

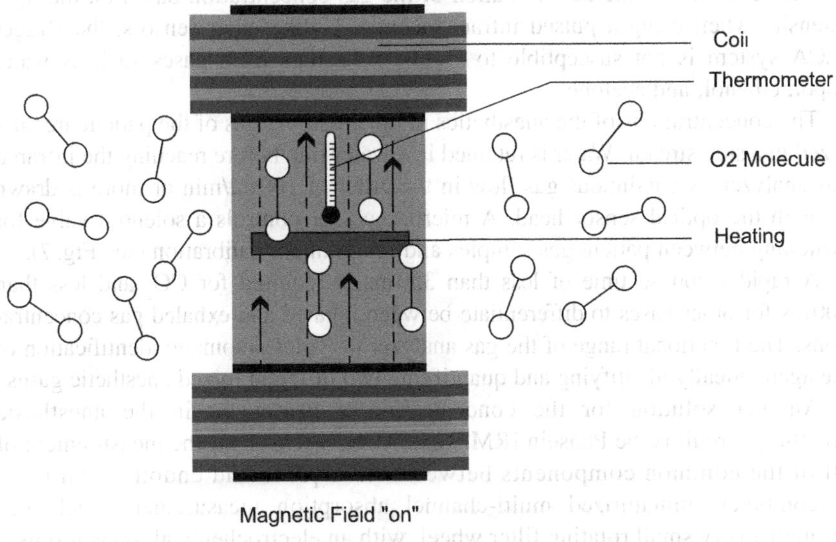

Fig. 5 Schematic of the working principle of the paramagnetic thermal oxygen analyzer (PATO)

cell and the magnets are packed in a rigid housing. Since there are no moving parts to wear out, the PATO module has a virtually unlimited lifespan and requires no recalibration. Another feature of the PATO is an exceptionally long zeroing time lag of 30 h or more. For this purpose, readjustment with ambient air suffices. The actual concentration measurement may be performed within the exhausted sample gas in combination with anesthetic agent detector, as described in the next section. The shock-resistant unit contributes to the highly stable signal of the sensor. The PATO is also suitable to be used as an independent oxygen sensor.

3.2 Integrated Gas Sensor Modules

In recent years, technology has advanced toward the compact integration of optical components in confined settings. The Dräger Medical ILCA (infrared low-cost analyzer, Dräger Medical, Lübeck, Germany) is a multi-gas sensor unit that incorporates integrated design techniques and solid-state technology for maximal compactness and reliability. The miniaturized sensor unit measures all five relevant anesthetic agents, as well as carbon dioxide and nitrous oxide. The highly shockproof system operates without moving parts, eliminating the risk of mechanical wear-out. The infrared technology comprises a pulsed infrared source and a multispectral detector that operates according to the principles of absorption and ray mixture. The infrared light is reflected in four directions after which it passes through infrared narrow-band filters onto a pyroelectric detector chip (Fig. 6).

The filters are laid out such that they are only permeable for the small wavelength bandwidth in which the analyzed gas shows a particular absorption characteristic. This allows the determination of the gas concentration based on the light intensity when using a pulsed infrared source. Unlike other sensors, the Dräger ILCA system is not susceptible to cross-sensitivities from gases such as water vapor, ethanol, and acetone.

The concentrations of the anesthetics in the breathing gas of the patient are analyzed in a side stream. Water is retained in a water trap before reaching the infrared gas analyzer. A continuous gas flow in the order of 100 ml/min or more is drawn through the optical sensor head. A microprocessor controls a solenoid valve for switching between patient gas samples and room air for calibration (see Fig. 7).

A rapid response time of less than 350 ms is required for CO_2 and less than 500 ms for other gases to differentiate between inhaled and exhaled gas concentrations. The functional range of the gas analyzer provides automatic identification of the agent, ideally identifying and quantifying two different mixed anesthetic gases.

Another solution for the concentration measurement in the anesthesia breathing circuit is the Phasein IRMA mainstream sensor for the measurement of all of the common components between the Y-piece and endotracheal tube. It combines miniaturized multi-channel absorption measurements, achieved through a very small rotating filter wheel, with an electrochemical oxygen sensor and a disposable airway adapter.

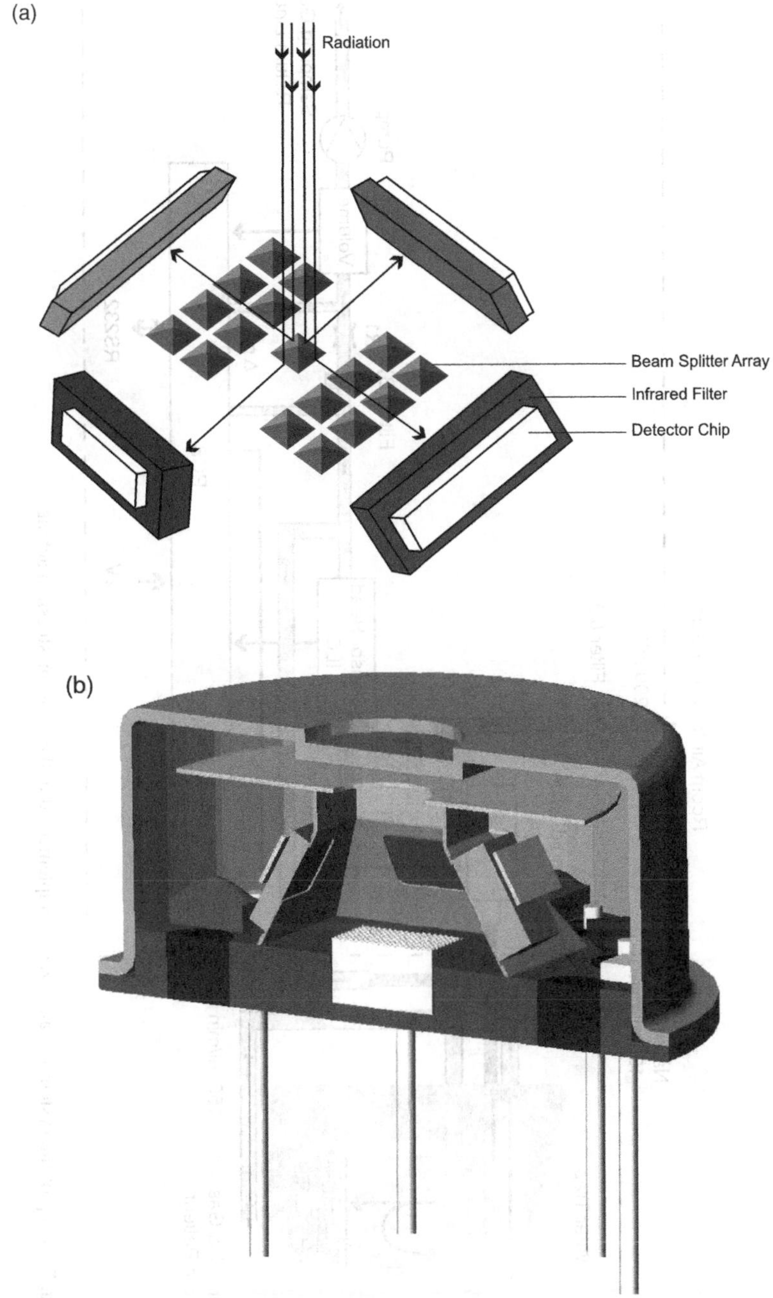

Fig. 6 Schematic of the multiple gas sensor system. **a** The filtered infrared light is reflected in four directions to measure gases at distinct narrow-banded wavelengths at their particular absorption characteristic. **b** Arrangement of filters and detector chips in a standard TO8 housing

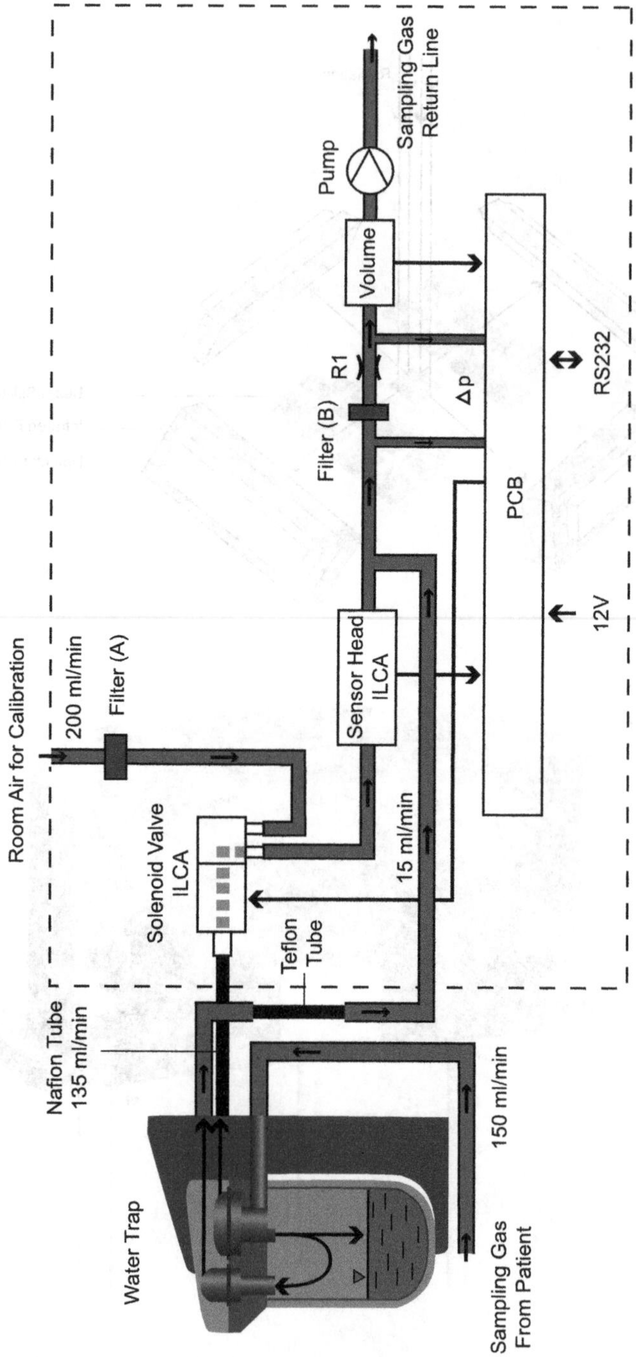

Fig. 7 Setup of the system gas analyzer, as implemented in the Zeus anesthesia machine

4 Ventilator Systems with Closed Breathing Circuits

A rebreathing system becomes a closed system if the amount of fresh gas and volatile anesthetics correspond exactly to the consumption of the patient. The gas volume inside of the rebreathing system stays constant with no surplus or deficit flow. If the fresh gas flow contains exactly the amount of oxygen, nitrous oxide, and agent the patient absorbs, the term "quantitative anesthesia" is more descriptive. Closed systems have been implemented in the PhysioFlex and in the Zeus anesthesia machines (both from Dräger, Lübeck, Germany) with a multi-parameter feedback system.

4.1 Zeus Anesthesia Machine Breathing System

The breathing system of the Zeus apparatus is a rebreathing system, as shown in Fig. 8. A central component of the breathing system is the high dynamic speed-controlled blower, which is designed for use in closed systems. Its function is to generate the pressure required for ventilation. The circuit flow is an advantage for patient ventilation as it supports spontaneous breathing. When interacting with the proportional positive end-expiratory pressure (PEEP) valve, the blower regulates the flow in the breathing circuit. Another role is to homogenize the anesthetic agent concentration in the breathing system. The blower is based on the radial principle and is regulated according to the requirements of an electronic activation circuit. The control variables used are the measured values from the pressure and flow sensors contained in the breathing system. The ventilation pressure and the circulatory flow during inhalation and exhalation are attained by means of defined activation of the blower and the flow valve in the breathing system (see Fig. 8). There are two separated inlets for fresh gas and saturated vapor (see the inlets indicated by A in Fig. 8). Mixed fresh gas is let in through a separate port (inlet B).

During the inspiratory breathing phase the blower delivers the tidal volume from the breathing bag, which is used as the breathing gas reservoir of the ventilator, via the CO_2 absorber, the non-return valve, and the flow sensor to the patient's lung. During this phase, the PEEP valve is more or less closed. However, depending on the ventilation mode, it allows spontaneous breathing in any ventilation phase. During the expiratory breathing phase the tidal volume is exhaled via the flow sensor, the non-return valve, and the PEEP valve back to the breathing bag. The PEEP valve controls the airway pressure while the blower ensures a circuit flow, which is superimposed to the expiratory patient flow. Surplus volume–if there is any–is evacuated through the surplus gas valve to the anesthetic gas scavenger system. A pressure preset of the opened surplus gas valve leads to an adequate filling level of the breathing bag. In the automatic controlled mode of the Zeus anesthesia machine, the surplus gas valve can be closed to prevent any loss of gas volume.

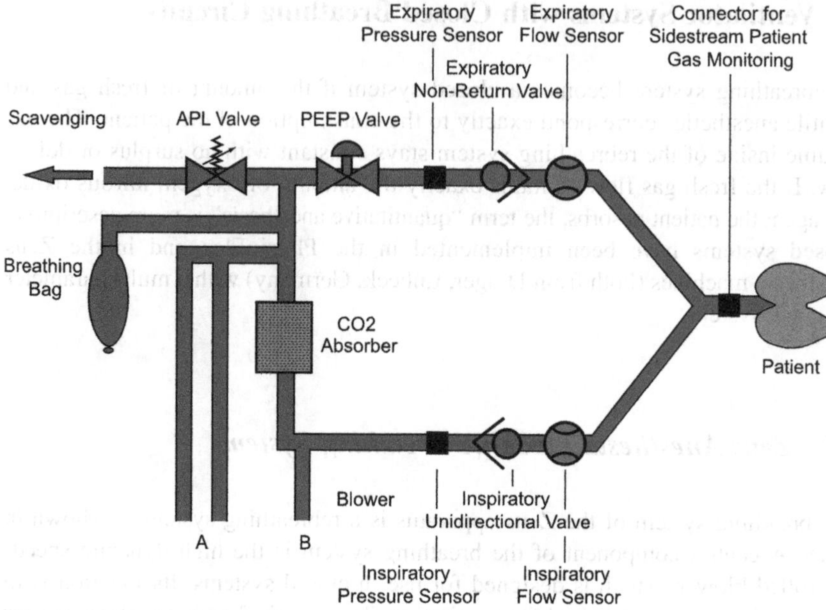

Fig. 8 The Zeus anesthesia machine breathing system in a simplified view

In automatic controlled mode FGF and saturated vapor will be inserted separately into the breathing system via inlets "A." Inlet "B" will be used only for the mixture of FGF and vapor in conventional fresh gas mode. The automatic controlled closed mode of the Zeus anesthesia machine is enabled by multiple, parallel, working feedback systems.

4.2 *Volume Feedback Control*

The task of the volume feedback controller is to keep the gas volume in the breathing system constant. The output control variable of the volume feedback controller is the amount of FGF, including agent flow (Fig. 9).

The gas volume of the breathing system is measured from the filling level of the breathing bag, which is calculated from the bag pressure at the end of the expiration phase. A bag pressure below the reference value of 1 mbar (which means lack of FGF) will lead to a higher amount of FGF. Similarly, a bag pressure above the reference value leads to a lower amount of FGF. Normally the surplus valve is closed during volume control. However, the volume feedback controller will open the surplus valve if the bag pressure steps up. The exact size of the breathing bag does not

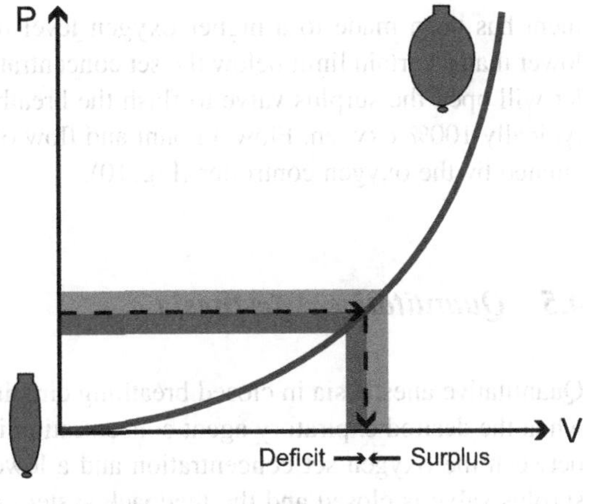

Fig. 9 Volume feedback control. The gas volume of the breathing system is measured from the filling level of the breathing bag

need to be known. However, different breathing bag sizes, classified during the system test, lead to different gains of the feedback controller.

4.3 Agent Feedback Control

The target of the agent feedback controller is to reach the desired expiratory agent concentration as fast as possible after an adjustment has been made and to then maintain a constant agent concentration.

If the agent level is lower than the set concentration, the output control variable of the feedback controller is the amount of agent liquid, which needs to be vaporized. In this case the surplus valve can stay closed. If the agent level is higher than a certain limit above the set concentration, the output control variable is the amount of FGF to flush the system. In this case the agent feedback controller will open the surplus valve. The anesthetic agent feedback control system is illustrated and described in Sect. 2.4.

4.4 Oxygen Feedback Control

The task of the oxygen feedback controller is to reach the desired inspiratory oxygen concentration and maintain a constant inspiratory oxygen concentration. The output control variable of this feedback controller is the oxygen concentration and the amount of FGF. If the oxygen level is higher than the set concentration, the amount of FGF will be limited to the flow calculated by the volume controller and the surplus valve will stay closed. This behavior leads to a slow decrease of oxygen concentration in the breathing system. A faster decrease can be achieved by setting a higher FGF manually–but it results in higher agent consumption. After an adjustment has been made to a higher oxygen level or in case the oxygen level drops lower than a certain limit below the set concentration, the oxygen feedback controller will open the surplus valve to flush the breathing system with a higher FGF of typically 100% oxygen. Flow amount and flow oxygen concentration are both calculated by the oxygen controller (Fig. 10).

4.5 Quantitative Anesthesia

Quantitative anesthesia in closed breathing circuit machines is practically achieved when the desired expiratory agent concentration is reached and the oxygen level is between the oxygen set concentration and a lower limit. Under this condition the surplus valve is closed and the feedback system nearly delivers what is consumed by the patient. In the ideal case, oxygen uptake closely corresponds to the oxygen flow delivered.

5 Conclusion and Outlook

The previous sections have described advanced technologies and devices for precise delivery and monitoring of inhalational anesthetic drugs. Novel actuator technologies, such as direct agent injection, have demonstrated sufficient maturity and reliability for the precise delivery of volatile anesthetics. New materials and alternative delivery principles, e.g., actuating components that are not exerted to mechanical wear, have the potential to further reduce the number of electromechanical components in vaporizers, and to provide higher reliability for less cost.

Advances in anesthesia delivery and control will emanate from a new breed of unobtrusive sensors. They are characterized by superior sensor performance through higher sensitivity and accuracy. Improved sensor operation will come from advances in the integration and miniaturization of optical and electromechanical components and from biochemical sensing. Precise and reliable measurements of delivered anesthetics will lead to improved studies of pharmacokinetics and enhance patient safety. Major breakthroughs are expected in the area of "pharmacodynamic sensing," which will offer unprecedented means to measure the effect of the drug on the body and the anesthetic state of the patient. Unobtrusive sensors will measure neural and muscular signals that are related to the state of anesthesia. In the future, anesthesiologists will be able to project activities at the cell and receptor level by continuously collecting acute individual genomic and proteomic profiles. Refined and standardized methods will emerge to measure molecular quantities of metabolic markers in samples taken from blood, saliva, through skin, or in breath.

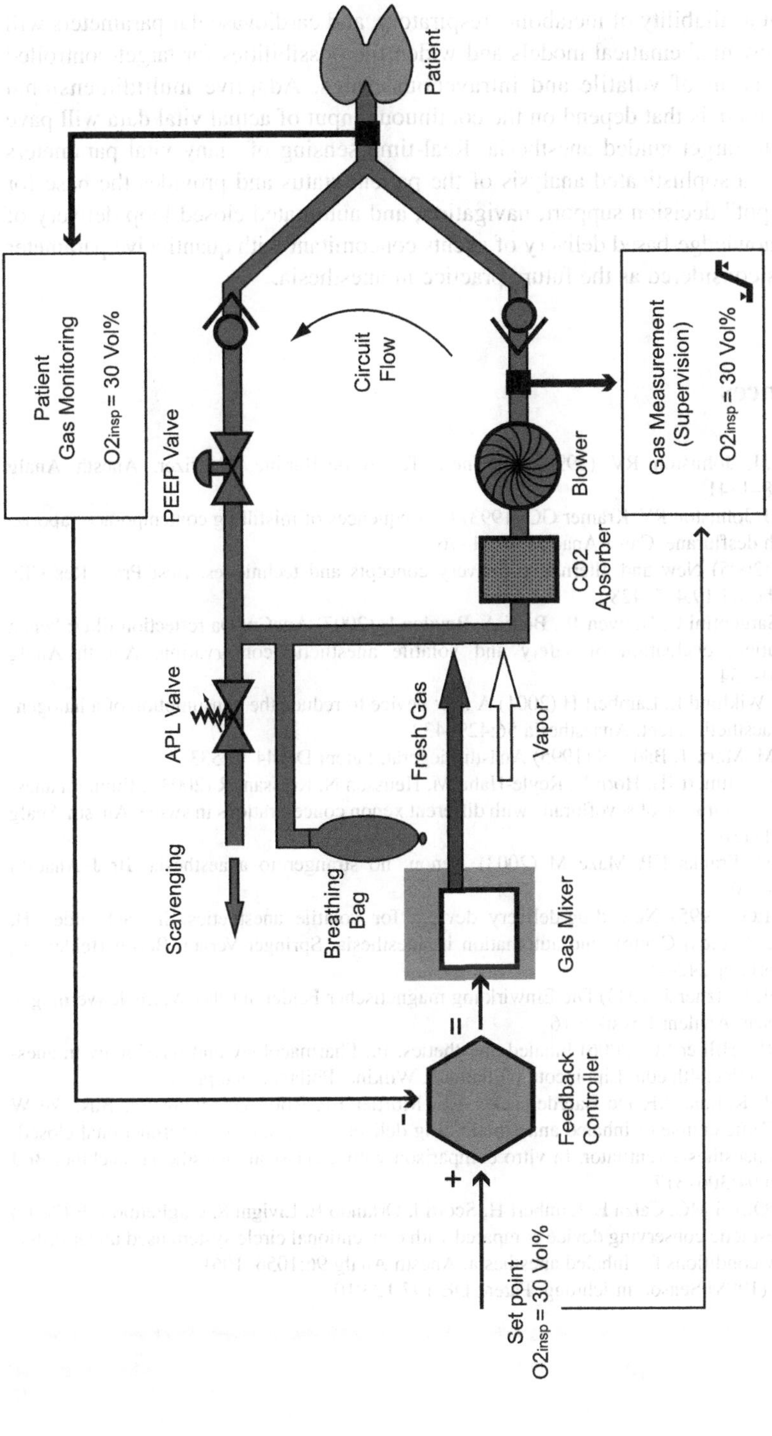

Fig. 10 Oxygen feedback control in a closed circuit breathing system

Instant availability of metabolic, respiratory, and cardiovascular parameters will lead to new mathematical models and widen the possibilities for target-controlled administration of volatile and intravenous drugs. Adaptive multidimensional run-time models that depend on the continuous input of actual vital data will pave the way to target-guided anesthesia. Real-time sensing of many vital parameters allows for a sophisticated analysis of the patient status and provides the base for "on the spot" decision support, navigation, and automated closed loop delivery of drugs. Knowledge-based delivery of agents concomitant with quantitative parameter control is considered as the future practice in anesthesia.

References

Andrews JJ, Johnston RV (1993) The new Tec 6 desflurane vaporizer. Anesth Analg 76:1338–1341

Andrews JJ, Johnston RV, Kramer GC (1993) Consequences of misfilling contemporary vaporizers with desflurane. Can J Anaesth 40:71–76

Baum JA (2005) New and alternative delivery concepts and techniques. Best Pract Res Clin Anaesthesiol 19:415–428

Berton J, Sargentini C, Nguyen JL, Belii A, Beydon L (2007) AnaConDa reflection filter: bench and patient evaluation of safety and volatile anesthetic conservation. Anesth Analg 104:130–134

Enlund M, Wiklund L, Lambert H (2001) A new device to reduce the consumption of a halogenated anaesthetic agent. Anaesthesia 56:429–432

Georgieff M, Marx T, Bäder S (1995) Anästhesiegerät. Patent DE 44 11 533

Hecker KE, Baumert JH, Horn N, Reyle-Hahn M, Heussen N, Roissant R (2003) Minimum anesthetic concentration of sevoflurane with different xenon concentrations in swine. Anesth Analg 97:1364–1369

Sanders RD, Franks NP, Maze M (2003) Xenon: no stranger to anaesthesia. Br J Anaesth 91:709–710

Scharmer EG (1995) New drug-delivery devices for volatile anesthetics. In: Schwilden H, Stoeckel H (eds) Control and automation in anesthesia. Springer-Verlag, Berlin Heidelberg New York, pp 242–251

Seftleben H, Pietzner J (1933) Die Einwirkung magnetischer Felder auf das Wärmeleitvermögen von Gasen. Analenr Physik 5:16

Stoelting RK, Hillier SC (2006) Inhaled anesthetics. In: Pharmacology and physiology in anesthetic practice, 4th edn. Lippincott Williams & Wilkins, Philadelphia, pp 42–86

Struys MM, Kalmar AF, De Baerdemaeker LE, Mortier EP, Rolly G, Manigel J, Buschke W (2005) Time course of inhaled anaesthetic drug delivery using a new multifunctional closed-circuit anaesthesia ventilator. In vitro comparison with a classical anaesthesia machine. Br J Anaesth 94:306–317

Tempia A, Olivei MC, Calza E, Lambert H, Scotti l, Orlando E, Livigni S, Guglielmotti E (2003) The anesthetic conserving device compared with conventional circle system used under different flow conditions for inhaled anesthesia. Anesth Analg 96:1056–1061

Wiegleb G (1998) Sensoreinrichtung. Patent DE 197 12 910

Hypnotic and Opioid Anesthetic Drug Interactions on the CNS, Focus on Response Surface Modeling

T.W. Bouillon

Abstract This chapter will present the conceptual and applied approaches to capture the interaction of anesthetic hypnotic drugs with opioid drugs, as used in the clinical anesthetic state. The graphic and mathematical approaches used to capture hypnotic/opiate anesthetic drug interactions will be presented. This chapter is not a review article about interaction modeling, but focuses on specific drug interactions within a quite narrow field, anesthesia.

1 Overview

Hypnotic and opioid drug interactions are the mainstay of both balanced and total intravenous anesthesia. Their exploitation results in reliable hypnosis/analgesia/autonomic stability, rapid recovery, and minimal residual effects. Before 1980, virtually no studies were available in the literature that had systematically investigated the interaction between opioids and hypnotics. Isobole-based approaches such as the minimal alveolar concentration (MAC) reduction paradigm previously used to quantify the interaction between nitrous oxide and volatile anesthetics were first applied to the problem in 1982. Initially, the MAC reduction/isobole-based approach was also used to quantify the interaction between propofol and opioids. The corresponding

T.W. Bouillon
Department of Anesthesia, Insepital Bern, 3010 Bern, Switzerland,
Current Address: Modeling & Simulation, Novartis AG, Novartis Campus 4002 Basel, Switzerland
thomas.bouillon@novartis.com

J. Schüttler and H. Schwilden (eds.) *Modern Anesthetics.*
Handbook of Experimental Pharmacology 182.

calculations yield the concentration of a volatile/hypnotic corresponding to the 50% probability of tolerating a certain stimulus (MAC or C_{50} hypnotic for the respective endpoint), the opioid concentration, which leads to a 50% decrease of MAC or C_{50} for the endpoint, and the value of an "interaction parameter," which denotes additivity, infraadditivity (antagonism), or supraadditivity (synergy). Intraoperative assessments of drug interactions based on the processed EEG have also been performed, in their most advanced and recent form using computer-controlled administration of the hypnotic to a certain endpoint while varying the opioid concentrations. Of course, the maintenance of a therapeutic "depth of anesthesia"/corresponding EEG endpoint forces the investigators to adhere to an isobole.

In 2000, a very important paradigm change away from the isobole toward response surface modeling took place, initially applied to characterize the interaction between propofol, alfentanil, and midazolam. Response surface methods yield the MAC of the volatile agent/C_{50} of the i.v. hypnotic, the C_{50} of the opioid, and the (not necessarily constant) slope of the entire surface, enabling investigators to describe the interaction at different effect levels, which is especially important when investigating the interactions of drugs on continuous endpoints but also yields meaningful results for quantal responses. Based on trial simulations, the so-called "criss-cross" design was identified as optimal for the identification of response surfaces in 2002. In 2004, a new paradigm mirroring specifically the interaction between stimulus, opioids, and hypnotics, the so-called sequential or hierarchical model, was introduced. Current research focuses on using isoboles and response surfaces for optimization of the ratio between opioid and hypnotic using criteria such as minimal wakeup time, alternative formulations of the interaction term, simulations to further optimize sampling/determine the study size for the assessment of quantal responses, and alternative formulations of the objective function, minimizing the sum of squared distances of the data points from the surface and not, as currently done, the sum of squared distances orthogonal to the plane representing the combined drug concentrations.

2 The MAC/C_{50} Reduction Paradigm for Investigation of Hypnotic Opioid Interactions

Soon after its introduction, MAC became the gold standard for quantification of the potency of volatile anesthetics. As defined by Eger et al., MAC is the minimum alveolar concentration of an anesthetic at 1 atm that produces immobility in 50% of those patients or animals exposed to a noxious stimulus (Eger et al. 1965). The noxious stimulus referred to is skin incision; however, other "calibrated stimuli," e.g., laryngoscopy, calling the volunteer's name/mild prodding ("MAC awake"), have been used. In complete analogy, the pseudo steady-state concentration of a hypnotic, which produces immobility in 50% of those patients or animals exposed to a noxious stimulus, can be termed the C_{50} with regard to this stimulus. The fact that opioids coadministered with volatiles/hypnotics reduce the amount of hypnotic needed to reach a certain clinical endpoint has been known qualitatively for as long as members of those substance groups have been combined in clinical anesthesia. Quantitation of the effect began in 1982, initially in dogs using "tail clamping" as the calibrated stimulus. While the measurement of exposure to volatile anesthetics had always used the end-tidal concentration, exposure to opioids was expressed both as a cumulative dose (Murphy and Hug 1982b) and, more precisely, as the plasma concentration of fentanyl (Murphy and Hug 1982a; Hall et al. 1987). The earlier study (Murphy and Hug 1982a) can be viewed as the prototype "MAC reduction by opioids study" investigating the influence of different plasma concentrations of fentanyl on the MAC of enflurane. Lacking target-controlled infusion (TCI) technology, but being aware of the pharmacokinetics of fentanyl in dogs, the authors achieved approximately constant plasma concentrations for the MAC determinations with a loading dose followed by a maintenance infusion. The covered concentration range was extensive (baseline and 6 steps, 0–100 ng/ml). For each concentration step, the MAC of enflurane was determined. Unfortunately, the authors did not estimate parameters describing the isobole. They did not test for the type of interaction, but applied confirmatory statistics only to assess the significance of the MAC reduction at different fentanyl concentrations. However, from their plot of enflurane concentration vs fentanyl concentration, a MAC isobole with the following qualitative properties was drawn: (1) small fentanyl concentrations (in the dog, <10 ng/ml) lead to a pronounced reduction of the MAC, (2) with increasing fentanyl concentrations (10 and 30 ng/ml), the MAC reduction becomes relatively less, and (3) a ceiling effect can be observed at very high opioid concentrations (30 ng/ml and 100 ng/ml). These three characteristics are generally valid and fundamental to the understanding and clinical use of MAC reduction by opioids. The raw data obtained and a MAC reduction isobole with an intuitively appealing parameterization are displayed in Fig. 1.

Ten years later, Sebel in collaboration with Murphy (Sebel et al. 1992) performed the prototype "MAC reduction by opioids study" in humans, investigating the influence of two bolus doses of fentanyl (3 and 6 μg/kg) on the MAC of desflurane (some patients received isoflurane, but no formal analysis of their data was performed). In this study, logistic regression was applied to estimate the parameters of the MAC isobole, a feature routinely applied thereafter. Although the investigators determined fentanyl concentrations, they were aware of their dubious value for pharmacodynamic assessments under non-steady-state conditions. Further refinements of the experimental procedure [using computer-controlled infusion pumps for target-controlled administration of the opioid and ascertaining near to equal concentrations of the opioid in plasma and at the effect site (pseudo steady-state) when the "calibration stimulus" was applied] led to the current "standard design" for MAC reduction studies (McEwan et al. 1993; Brunner et al. 1994; Westmoreland et al. 1994; Lang et al. 1996; Katoh and Ikeda 1998; Katoh et al. 1999).

The study paradigm has also been applied on the determination of MAC awake reduction by opioids (Katoh et al. 1994; Katoh and Ikeda 1998). Another common feature of MAC reduction studies is the low information content contributed by a single individual; a substantial number of patients are therefore needed (between 50 and 150).

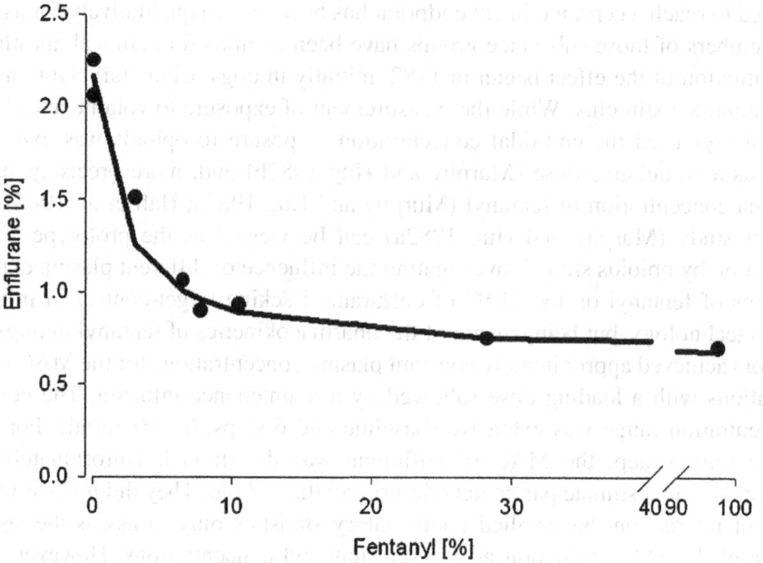

Fig. 1 Enflurane MAC reduction by fentanyl in dog. The data obtained by Murphy and Hug in dogs were plotted in the standard MAC reduction format and described by the author with an isobole. *Dots*, original data by Murphy; *line*, isobole expressed as $MAC_{enf}(fen) = MAC_{enf} * \left(1 - OSF * \frac{C_{fen}}{C_{50fen} + C_{fen}}\right)$ with $MAC_{enf(fen)}$, enflurane MAC in presence of Fentanyl, c_{fen}, fentanyl plasma concentration; MAC_{enf}, enflurane MAC (2.16%); *OSF*, opioid suppressible fraction of MAC (0.7); c_{50fen}, fentanyl concentration which leads to a 50% reduction of the opioid suppressible fraction (2 ng/ml), for OSF=0.7 this equals 0.35 MAC_{enf}

Similar to MAC reduction of volatile anesthetics, studies have been performed to elucidate the interaction of midazolam with fentanyl (Ben Shlomo et al. 1990) and propofol with fentanyl (Smith et al. 1994) and alfentanil (Vuyk et al. 1995; Vuyk et al. 1996) for tolerance of several clinically relevant stimuli. Ben-Shlomo investigated the interaction for loss of consciousness with an isobolographic method, testing the null hypothesis of additivity with confirmatory statistics instead of describing the entire isobole. He reported a supraadditive interaction of the drugs; however, a pseudo steady-state was not obtained, nor were drug concentrations measured. Vuyk et al. went beyond reporting the clinically not immediately useful parameters and performed simulations yielding specific dosing recommendations for maintenance of anesthesia while minimizing time to return of consciousness (ROC) (Vuyk et al. 1997). However, the isoboles chosen by them to describe tolerance of the surgical stimulus and ROC display the unfortunate properties of not providing an intersection with the propofol axis and yielding negative propofol concentrations at high opioid concentrations. As always, it is up to the individual clinician/scientist to decide whether he or she accepts the mathematics because it describes the measured data or rejects it because of anomalies occurring beyond the measured range.

The designs of all studies mentioned so far yield concentration pairs enveloping an isobole expressing a certain probability of response to the stimulus applied in the study; for MAC, by definition, the probability is 50%. The concentration of the opioid is usually treated as an independent variable, the concentration of the hypnotic as a dependent variable. These data undergo logistic regression, yielding both C_{50} values of the drugs and an interaction parameter denoting the type of interaction (additive, infraadditive, or supraadditive). Without exception, the interaction between hypnotics/volatiles and opioids with regard to suppression of response to noxious stimuli has been characterized as supraadditive. Regardless of the substance, relatively small concentrations of opioids yield a pronounced decrease of the MAC of volatiles/C_{50} of propofol. With increasing concentrations, there is limited return with regard to the hypnotic sparing effect, as already became evident from Murphy's pivotal study (Murphy and Hug 1982a) and has been pointed out in previous summaries (Glass et al. 1997; Glass 1998). However, questions have been raised concerning the validity of treating the opioid concentration as a true independent variable and minimizing the sum of the squared ordinate distances instead of the sum of the squared distances of the data points from the isobole (Schwilden et al. 2003). Inspecting the specific isobole plots, including raw data, for the interaction in question to decide whether the relevant part of the isobole is supported by measurements and to what extent the concerns of Schwilden et al. invalidate the conclusions by the authors is therefore recommended.

3 Intraoperative Assessments of Hypnotic Opioid Interaction Based on the Processed EEG

EEG-based interaction studies between opioids and hypnotics in presence of surgical stimulation are by definition isobolographic studies, since the investigators are "forced" to maintain a clinically adequate level of anesthesia, which corresponds to a certain numerical value of the EEG-derived parameter. The concentration pairs do not envelope an isobole, but are situated on the isobole, facilitating parameter estimation considerably. The study paradigm consists of choosing a suitable isobole, e.g., intraoperative Bispectral Index value (BIS; Aspect Medical Systems, Norwood, MA) of 45–55 (Röpcke et al. 2001) or a median value of the EEG power spectrum of 1.5–2.5 Hz (Fechner et al. 2003; Schwilden et al. 2003). Thereafter, the concentration of one interacting drug, usually the opioid, is maintained at several predetermined values, the concentration of the other drug, usually the hypnotic, is adjusted according to the continuously measured EEG-based signal. This adjustment is ideally done by closed-loop administration of the drug to be adjusted, yielding rapid and precise estimates of the concentration pair corresponding to the EEG endpoint. Schwilden's research group concluded that the closed-loop administration of drugs, besides yielding potential clinical benefit, is a highly suitable research tool for interaction studies. However, one caveat applies to the intraoperative approach: Since not only the concentration of both drugs, but also the intensity of the surgical stimulus influences the EEG-derived value, a constant level of stimulation must be maintained during intrasubject measurements (that is, a certain phase of the surgical procedure) as well as across subjects (identical procedures need to be chosen for the study). In any case, the isobole obtained for a BIS value of 50 during orthopedic surgery (Röpcke et al. 2001) will in all likelihood differ from the isobole for a BIS value of 50 during surgical procedures that have a different intensity of stimulation. Using this study paradigm, the type of interaction between propofol and opioids has been described both as supraadditive or additive, necessitating a closer look at the intricacies of the studies. Both Röpcke and Schwilden minimized the sum of the squared distances of the data points from the isobole. The most striking differences are the range of opioid concentrations and the minimal opioid concentration chosen. Röpcke investigated remifentanil concentrations from 2 to 15 ng/ml, Schwilden fixed three concentrations (5, 10, 15 ng/ml), which are clearly in the "flat," linear part of the isobole. It has already been shown for volatile opioid interactions that the most pronounced effect of opioids can be expected at rather low concentrations. Therefore it is not surprising that synergism has been identified from the data set covering a larger part of the isobole, admittedly including concentrations below and beyond the clinically useful range.

4 Response Surface Methods

A response surface is a $n+1$ dimensional structure connecting measures of drug exposure of n drugs with their corresponding combined effect. In its simplest and most recognizable form, it is a three-dimensional surface representing the concentrations of two drugs and their respective effects (for an overview see Greco et al. 1995; Jonker et al. 2005). As an example, Fig. 2 displays the interaction of propofol and remifentanil with regard to tolerance of laryngoscopy (TOL). Response surfaces should not be confused with the three-dimensional isoboles resulting from the interaction of three drugs to yield one specific effect size (e.g., Röpcke et al. 1999), since they express the concentration effect relationship for any magnitude of effect. Isoboles can be viewed as horizontal slices through the response surface, and concentration response curves as vertical slices. Therefore, information contained in a response surface encompasses information about any isobole and the concentration response curve of any combination of the drugs involved, making it by far the most powerful approach for the investigation of drug interactions and especially useful for dose finding including optimization of recovery times.

A seminal publication by Minto and colleagues (2000) introduced response surface modeling for the description of hypnotic opioid interactions in anesthesia (the Web enhancement of the publication contains additional valuable information on interaction modeling for the mathematically inclined reader).

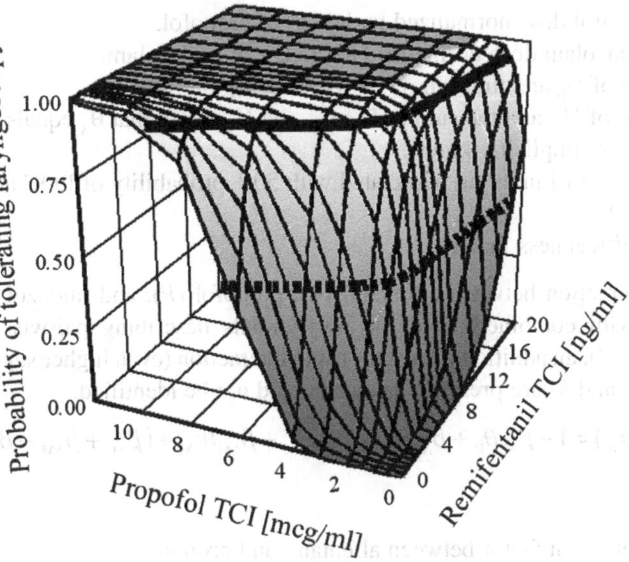

Fig. 2 Demonstration of the response surface concept, with the present example being the probability of tolerance of laryngoscopy for different propofol and remifentanil concentrations (Bouillon et al. 2004). The interacting drugs are plotted on the lower axes forming a plane or concentration grid, the response is plotted orthogonally to it. The *transparent mesh* denotes the probability of tolerating laryngoscopy depending on the respective combined concentrations of propofol and remifentanil. The *dotted line parallel to the concentration grid* is the 50% isobole (any drug combination on this line yields a 50% probability of tolerance of laryngoscopy), the *solid line parallel to the concentration grid* is the 95% isobole. Note the outward bulge representing synergy

They validated their model describing the interaction between midazolam, propofol, and alfentanil doses administered to 400 (!) patients with regard to loss of consciousness (proportion of patients failing to open the eyes on verbal command, LOC) (Short et al. 1992). The analysis was based on a logistic regression model expressing the proportion of patients experiencing LOC for all possible dose combinations. The drugs were treated as full agonists with regard to LOC (supported by the data not only for propofol and midazolam, but also for alfentanil) and the slope of the individual dose response curves set equal, yielding

$$P=\frac{\left(\dfrac{U_A+U_P+U_M}{U_{50}(\theta_P,\theta_M)}\right)^{\gamma}}{1+\left(\dfrac{U_A+U_P+U_M}{U_{50}(\theta_P,\theta_M)}\right)^{\gamma}}$$

with

- P: proportion of patients displaying LOC.
- U_A: alfentanil dose normalized to the D_{50} (dose, which causes LOC in 50% of the subjects).

- U_P: propofol dose normalized to the D_{50} of propofol.
- U_M: midazolam dose normalized to the D_{50} of midazolam.
- θ_P: ratio of U_P and the sum of U_A, U_P, and U_M.
- θ_M: ratio of U_M and the sum of U_A, U_P, and U_M. Note that θ_A equals $1-\theta_P-\theta_M$ and is therefore implicitly known.
- U_{50}: number of units (u) associated with 50% probability of LOC at the respective θ_P, θ_M.
- γ: slope/steepness factor.

The interaction between alfentanil (*A*), propofol (*P*), and midazolam (*M*) was modeled with combined quadratic polynomials describing pairwise interaction (*AP*, *AM*, *PM*), an additional term for triple interaction (even higher supraadditivity, when *A*, *P*, and *M* are present together), could not be identified.

$$\mathrm{U50}(\theta_P,\theta_M)=1-\beta_{AP}\theta_P+\beta_{AP}\theta^2{}_P-\beta_{AM}\theta_M+\beta_{AM}\theta^2{}_M+(\beta_{AP}+\beta_{AM}-\beta_{PM})^*\,\theta_P{}^*\theta_M$$

with

- β_{AP}: interaction factor between alfentanil and propofol.
- β_{AM}: interaction factor between alfentanil and midazolam.
- β_{PM}: interaction factor between propofol and midazolam.
- $\beta n=0$ would denote additive, $\beta n>0$ supraadditive interaction.

All three interaction parameters for the respective drug combinations showed synergy with regard to LOC, which is remarkable for two reasons. (1) Propofol and midazolam exert their action via the γ-aminobutyric acid $(\mathrm{GABA})_A$ receptor, and a common molecular target should always lead to additive interactions for full agonists. Perhaps they act on different parts of the receptor. (2) Opioids are notoriously poor hypnotics; however, the doses of alfentanil administered in this study were substantial. Another surprising aspect is the design of the study that the source data are derived from. Whenever a drug combination was given, the doses of both concomitantly administered substances were increased simultaneously, which is not the most efficient trial design for the definition of response surfaces (see below). However, the substantial amount of data from single administration of the three drugs very much facilitated the estimation of the respective D_{50} values. A most important aspect of this manuscript is its broader scope, including guidelines that an ideal pharmacodynamic interaction model should adhere to and a demonstration of the flexibility of the model (different maximal effects, different slopes of the concentration effect curves of the individual drugs, asymmetric isoboles, etc.). Although it is unlikely that this flexibility will ever be utilized analyzing "real world data," it is comforting to have this "Swiss knife" in the pocket. A modification of the Minto model using splines instead of polynomials to interpolate between the C_{50} values of two interacting drugs has been developed by Olofsen (Dahan et al. 2001; Nieuwenhuijs et al. 2003) and applied to the combined effect of sevoflurane and alfentanil as well as propofol and remifentanil on respiration. The most attractive feature of this parameterization is the ability to immediately identify the type of interaction and the symmetry of the isobole from two parameters, named I_{max} (a value of 1 denoting additive interaction) and Q_{max} (a value of 0.5

denoting symmetric interaction). The authors identified a supraadditive interaction between the respiratory effects of hypnotics and opioids. Although there were inconsistencies in parameter estimation, namely the C_{50} of propofol ranging from 0.7 μg/ml for depression of isohypercapnic ventilation to 34.3 μg/ml for causing hypercarbia (meaning it varied 40-fold for different respiratory endpoints), they are not a consequence of the applied interaction model, which is held in high esteem by this author.

Short et al. identified the most suitable design for robust parameter estimation of response surfaces (Short et al. 2002). Using computer-assisted trial design (CATD) techniques, the investigators compared different sampling paradigms ("radial, slices, criss-cross") and study sizes for a two-drug interaction on a continuous endpoint. The criss-cross design (keeping the concentration of drug 1 constant, escalating the concentration of drug 2 until the maximal effect has been observed and vice versa) was identified as most suitable for parameter estimation, with 20 patients sufficient to estimate the parameters of the response surface. However, this simulation study, as with any other CATD result, suffers from being sensitive to the underlying assumptions. Strictly spoken, the recommendation that "20 patients suffice," is only valid for a continuous response, a certain degree of supraadditivity (beta=1.6), the respective underlying interindividual variability of the parameters (cv=0.3), and taking 13 ideally spaced samples of both concentrations and the respective effect per observation unit. The situation becomes much more ambiguous if quantal responses, such as reaction to one or more stimuli at different pseudo steady-state concentrations, are used for parameter estimation. We concur with Jonker et al. (2005) and believe that CATD plays a predominant role in designing interaction studies complex enough to be evaluated with response surface methodology. It is unlikely that published "cookbooks" for all possible problem constellations will become available. However, since most software packages used for parameter estimation by nonlinear regression can be run in simulation mode, anybody able to apply response surface methodology and the population approach to analyze data can very easily perform simulations to determine study size, sampling schedules, and identifiability of parameters. Commercial packages specifically geared toward CATD are also available. Very recently, software packages based on the evaluation of the Fisher information matrix became available, which can be used to formalize study design even further. However, none of them are (yet) geared towards isolated pharmacodynamic, not to mention interaction, problems.

The interaction between propofol and remifentanil on tolerance of noxious stimuli and loss/return of consciousness (ROC) has been investigated extensively using response surface methodology (Mertens et al. 2003; Kern et al. 2004; Bouillon et al. 2004). Since the investigators used different populations, different pharmacodynamic endpoints, different sampling strategies, and different modeling approaches, a close comparison of these studies and the respective findings might prove interesting.

Mertens et al. investigated 30 patients with regard to tolerance of intubation (TOI), laryngoscopy (TOL), adequate anesthesia during abdominal surgery, and ROC. With the exception of the intraoperative data (isobolographic analysis), he used the response surface model by Bol et al. (2000), which is based on the model by Greco et al. (1995).

This model is a straightforward extrapolation from the 50% effect isobole expressed according to Loewe.

$$P = \frac{\left(\frac{CP}{C50P} + \frac{CR}{C50R} + \varepsilon * \frac{CP}{C50P} * \frac{CR}{C50R}\right)^{\gamma}}{1 + \left(\frac{CP}{C50P} + \frac{CR}{C50R} + \varepsilon * \frac{CP}{C50P} * \frac{CR}{C50R}\right)^{\gamma}}$$

with

- P: proportion of patients displaying either TOL, TOI or ROC
- c_P, c_R: propofol and remifentanil concentrations
- c_{50P}, c_{50R}: concentrations of propofol and remifantanil leading to tolerance of the respective stimulus in 50% of the patients in absence of the other drug
- ε: Interaction parameter (ε=0: additive interaction, ε<0: infraadditive interaction, ε<0: supraadditive interaction)
- γ: slope/steepness factor

The authors introduced two different equations useful for identification of a response surface in case supraadditivity was observed and one or both of the drugs were unable to cause the investigated effect in absence of the other or the study design was not suited to estimate the respective C_{50} values. Especially for endpoints requiring loss of consciousness it is questionable whether such endpoints can be reliably achieved with opioids alone, at least in the clinically relevant concentration range.

If the C_{50} of the opioid cannot be identified, the equation can be rewritten as:

$$P = \frac{\left(\frac{CP}{C50P} + \varepsilon' * \frac{CP}{C50P} * CR\right)^{\gamma}}{1 + \left(\frac{CP}{C50P} + \varepsilon' * \frac{CP}{C50P} * CR\right)^{\gamma}}$$

$$\varepsilon' = \frac{\varepsilon}{C50R}$$

If both C_{50} values are unobtainable from the data and supraadditivity exists, the equation becomes

$$P = \frac{\left(\varepsilon'' * CP * CR\right)^{\gamma}}{1 + \left(\varepsilon'' * CP * CR\right)^{\gamma}}$$

$$\varepsilon'' = \frac{\varepsilon}{C50P * C50R}$$

Compared to the model of Minto et al., the Greco/Bol model is inherently less flexible. In particular, it assumes identical slope factors and identical maximal effects for the single concentration effect courses of the interacting drugs.

Mertens et al. identified a supraadditive interaction between propofol and remifentanil for all endpoints investigated, the C_{50} of remifentanil was not identifiable for TOL, TOI, and ROC, the C_{50} of propofol was not identifiable for TOI.

Kern et al. investigated the interaction between remifentanil and propofol in 24 volunteers using the same model as Mertens. Endpoints were OAA/S (observer assessment of alertness/sedation scale) grades, algometry (tibial pressure and electrical titanic stimulus applied to the posterior tibial nerve), and laryngoscopy. The drugs were administered according to the criss-cross design, additionally obtaining a single drug concentration response curve for either propofol or remifentanil in each volunteer. Therefore, individual concentration response curves were available and C_{50} values for both drugs could be independently estimated. For analysis of the response surfaces, these C_{50} values were fixed to the predetermined values and a single slope of the surface determined. Although clearly different slopes of the individual concentration response curves were found, the use of the Bol/Greco model precluded expressing these in the response surface equation.

Similar to Mertens, Kern identified profound synergy between propofol and remifentanil for all endpoints.

Finally, Bouillon et al. investigated the interaction of propofol and remifentanil in 20 volunteers using a criss-cross design (Bouillon et al. 2004). Endpoints were changes of the Bispectral Index and approximate entropy, tolerance of shaking the volunteer and shouting his or her name (TOSS), and TOL. The EEG-derived data were evaluated with a Minto response surface model. For the quantal response data, a mechanistic model was used. It is based on the notion that an incoming (noxious) stimulus can be attenuated by an opioid prior to affecting the concentration effect curve of the hypnotic. Since the originally published form of the model was overparameterized for the description of the experimental data (in this author's view), this discussion will confine itself to the most parsimonious form of the model; Fig. 2 illustrates the underlying logic.

The following equation describes the attenuation of an incoming stimulus by an opioid, e.g., remifentanil:

$$A_{out} = A_{in} * \left(1 - \frac{\left(\frac{CR}{C50R} \right)}{1 + \left(\frac{CR}{C50R} \right)} \right)$$

with

- A_{in}: Strength of applied stimulus in the absence of opioid
- c_R: remifentanil concentration
- c_{50R}: concentrations of remifentanil leading to a 50% decrease of A_{in}
- A_{out}: resulting stimulus strength after opioid effect, equal to A_{in} in absence of opioid

Tolerance to a certain stimulus can be expressed as

$$P = \frac{\left(\frac{CP}{C50P * Aout}\right)^{\gamma}}{1+\left(\frac{CP}{C50P * Aout}\right)^{\gamma}}$$

with

- *P*: Proportion of patients displaying either TOSS or TOL
- c_P: propofol concentration
- c_{50P}: concentration of propofol leading to tolerance of the respective stimulus in 50% of the patients in absence of opioid/remifentanil
- γ: slope/steepness factor

The model displays several peculiarities:

- It implies that A_{in} always equals 1 if only one stimulus is tested, however, it can be used to evaluate the relative strength of several stimuli by comparison of the respective values for A_{in}.
- It does not contain a specific interaction parameter, but always displays strongly supraadditive behavior.
- In the absence of a hypnotic, tolerance to the stimulus can never be achieved, in accordance to the notion that opioids are not able to provide hypnosis/amnesia in clinically useful concentrations (Hug 1990).
- It implies that the identical concentration of opioid always suppresses A_{in} to the same relative extent (c_R=$c50_R$ yields A_{out}=0.5 A_{in}, regardless of the absolute value of A_{in}, which appears to be highly speculative.
- It can be transformed into a reduced Greco (G_{red}) model, which will be shown below.

As long as the interaction only occurs on potency and not on slope of the surface as well, all interaction models discussed so far can be reduced to

$$P = \frac{N^{\gamma}}{1+N^{\gamma}}$$

For equal steepness of the surface, the reduced Greco and the sequential models are identical if:

$$N_{Gred} = N_S \; or \; \frac{Cp}{C50p} + \varepsilon' * \frac{Cp}{C50p} * Copi = \frac{Cp}{C50p * Aout}$$

Division by $\frac{Cp}{c50_p}$ yields

$$1+\varepsilon' * Copi = \frac{1}{Aout}$$

Solving for A_{out} and resubstitution yields:

$$1-\frac{Copi}{C50opi+Copi}=\frac{1}{1+\varepsilon'*Copi}$$

Multiplication with both denominators and simplification yields:

$$C50opi+Copi-Copi=\frac{C50opi+Copi}{1+\varepsilon'*Copi}$$

$$C50opi+C50opi*\varepsilon'*Copi=C50opi+Copi$$

$$C50_{opi}*\varepsilon'=1$$

and therefore:

$$C50opi=\frac{1}{\varepsilon'}$$

The fact that Bouillon et al. described their quantal response data adequately with this model points towards supraadditivity for TOSS and TOL in their study population.

Comparison between recalculated C_{50} values from Mertens for ROC and TOL (1.39 ng/ml, 1.45 ng/ml of remifentanil) are in adequate agreement with our C_{50} value recalculated from the simplified model (common C_{50} of 1.16 ng/ml) and support the notion that one C_{50} of an opioid can be used to describe suppression of stimuli of a different intensity.

Since this C_{50} value is *not* the concentration of opioid to exert 50% of the maximal effect in question, but the concentration to decrease the C_{50} of the hypnotic to 50% of its initial value, it is not surprising that the remifentanil concentration for reduction of the MAC of isoflurane is matched (Lang et al. 1996).

It is likely that the sequential response model (Fig. 3) can be used to construct response surfaces for all permutations of hypnotics and opioids, as long as the concentration response curve of the hypnotic and the hypnotic-independent "C_{50} for stimulus reduction" are known.

With regard to interaction on the EEG in absence of stimulation, Bouillon et al. identified an additive interaction with a remifentanil C_{50} of 19.3 ng/ml, clearly beyond the clinically relevant range. In conclusion, considering an unnpublished investigation (isoflurane and alfentanil) (P.M. Schumacher, T.W. Bouillon, R. Wymann, M. Luginbühl, T.W. Schnider; data on file, University of Bern) and the findings by Olofsen for sevoflurane and remifentanil (Olofsen et al. 2002), it can be said that, in the absence of stimulation, opioids contribute negligibly to the pronounced effects of hypnotics on the EEG (inert interaction). This is the reason why at the same EEG parameter setpoint the opioid concentrations determine the likelihood of response to noxious stimulation.

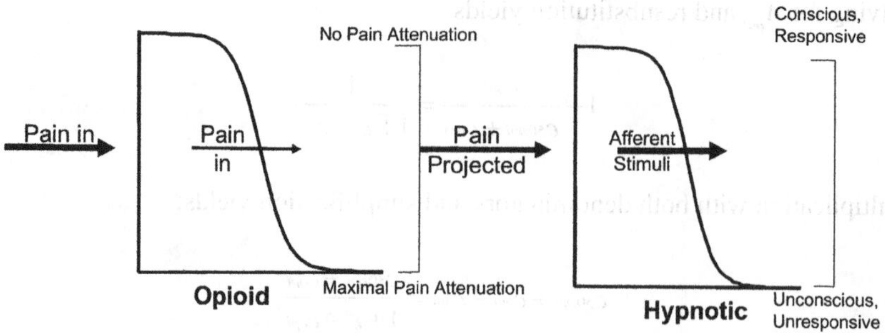

Fig. 3 Underlying logic of the sequential response model. The opioid attenuates the incoming arousal stimulus (*Pain in*) in a concentration-dependent manner (*left*). The output of the model, the residual arousal stimulus (*Pain Projected*) is then fed into a model describing the effect of the hypnotic on the probability of response to the arousal stimulus (*right*). Probability of response depends on the intensity of the incoming arousal stimulus, the concentration of opioid, and the concentration of hypnotic. In the absence of opioid, "Pain in" equals "Pain Projected." In the absence of hypnotic, the probability of response to "Pain Projected" is always 1, regardless of opioid concentration

5 Future Directions of Response Surface Research

Similar to the problems described when discussing isoboles, the current approaches minimize the squared distances of the data points from the plane formed by the drug concentrations, instead of the sum of squared distances from the isobole. It remains to be seen whether this problem can be adequately solved, especially to describe the interaction of more than two drugs. CATD approaches have already been mentioned. Since interaction studies require more raw data than single drug studies and this comes at a price, it is almost negligent not to simulate at least the expected result for the most preferred design, if only to confirm the expectations. We are currently investigating a formal optimization method for interaction studies based on design methodology such as D- and product design optimality.

Despite the fact that most experimental data sets can adequately be described with relatively inflexible response surfaces, e.g., assuming identical steepness of the entire response surface, a complex interaction model has recently been presented (Fidler and Kern 2006). Since this model did not outperform the Minto model on all data sets tested, it appears to be unlikely that one "great unifying interaction model" will make its predecessors obsolete. Real world interaction modeling will in all likelihood "suffer from real world data" with limitations on the number of observations within an individual as well as interindividual variability. Theoretical advantages of models might therefore disappear when applied on actual data sets.

Finally, we will in all likelihood see simultaneous assessments of several response surfaces, as already presented (Fig. 4; Bouillon et al. 2004. Combined desired/undesired effect interaction studies/analyses, where the response surfaces for desired and undesired effects will be combined to yield the so-called "well being surface," promise to be especially helpful for dose finding. Similar to utility curves for single drugs, this approach will yield an optimal concentration range of

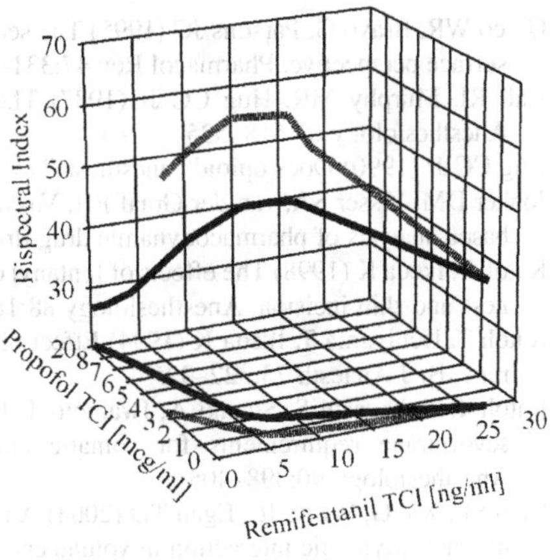

Fig. 4 Combination of response surfaces: BIS values for the 95% probability of tolerating a profound arousal stimulus (*broken lines*) and laryngoscopy (*solid lines*) vary according to the relative contribution of hypnotic and opioid. The isoboles for the 95% probability of tolerating a profound arousal stimulus and laryngoscopy are plotted as combination of propofol and remifentanil in the concentration plane and as combination of the drug concentrations and the respective BIS values (ascending curves). From this combined analysis of response surfaces for BIS suppression and tolerance of quantal stimuli it becomes obvious that a certain BIS value does not refer to a certain "depth of anesthesia," expressed as probability of response to a certain "calibration stimulus" (the MAC paradigm)

a drug combination by searching for a balance between desired and undesired effects, depending on their relative weights. A detailed description of the methods and its potential usefulness has been recently published (Zanderigo et al. 2006).

References

Ben Shlomo I, abd-el-Khalim H, Ezry J, Zohar S, Tverskoy M (1990) Midazolam acts synergistically with fentanyl for induction of anaesthesia. Br J Anaesth 64:45–47

Bol CJ, Vogelaar JP, Tang JP, Mandema JW (2000) Quantification of pharmacodynamic interactions between dexmedetomidine and midazolam in the rat. J Pharmacol Exp Ther 294:347–355

Bouillon TW, Bruhn J, Radulescu L, Andresen C, Shafer TJ, Cohane C, Shafer SL (2004) Pharmacodynamic interaction between propofol and remifentanil regarding hypnosis, tolerance of laryngoscopy, bispectral index, and electroencephalographic approximate entropy. Anesthesiology 100:1353–1372

Brunner MD, Braithwaite P, Jhaveri R, McEwan AI, Goodman DK, Smith LR, Glass PS (1994) MAC reduction of isoflurane by sufentanil. Br J Anaesth 72:42–46

Dahan A, Nieuwenhuijs D, Olofsen E, Sarton E, Romberg R, Teppema L (2001) Response surface modeling of alfentanil-sevoflurane interaction on cardiorespiratory control and bispectral index. Anesthesiology 94:982–991

Eger EI, Saidman LJ, Brandstater B (1965) Minimum alveolar anesthetic concentration: a standard of anesthetic potency. Anesthesiology 26:756–763

Fechner J, Hering W, Ihmsen H, Palmaers T, Schuttler J, Albrecht S (2003) Modelling the pharmacodynamic interaction between remifentanil and propofol by EEG-controlled dosing. Eur J Anaesthesiol 20:373–379

Fidler M, Kern SE (2006) Flexible interaction model for complex interactions of multiple anesthetics. Anesthesiology 105:286–296

Glass PS (1998) Anesthetic drug interactions: an insight into general anesthesia—its mechanism and dosing strategies. Anesthesiology 88:5–6

Glass PS, Gan TJ, Howell S, Ginsberg B (1997) Drug interactions: volatile anesthetics and opioids. J Clin Anesth 9:18S–22S

Greco WR, Bravo G, Parsons JC (1995) The search for synergy: a critical review from a response surface perspective. Pharmacol Rev 47:331–385
Hall RI, Murphy MR, Hug CC Jr (1987) The enflurane sparing effect of sufentanil in dogs. Anesthesiology 67:518–525
Hug CC Jr (1990) Does opioid "anesthesia" exist? Anesthesiology 73:1–4
Jonker DM, Visser SA, van der Graaf PH, Voskuyl RA, Danhof M (2005) Towards a mechanism-based analysis of pharmacodynamic drug-drug interactions in vivo. Pharmacol Ther 106:1–18
Katoh T, Ikeda K (1998) The effects of fentanyl on sevoflurane requirements for loss of consciousness and skin incision. Anesthesiology 88:18–24
Katoh T, Uchiyama T, Ikeda K (1994) Effect of fentanyl on awakening concentration of sevoflurane. Br J Anaesth 73:322–325
Katoh T, Kobayashi S, Suzuki A, Iwamoto T, Bito H, Ikeda K (1999) The effect of fentanyl on sevoflurane requirements for somatic and sympathetic responses to surgical incision. Anesthesiology 90:398–405
Kern SE, Xie G, White JL, Egan TD (2004) A response surface analysis of propofol-remifentanil pharmacodynamic interaction in volunteers. Anesthesiology 100:1373–1381
Lang E, Kapila A, Shlugman D, Hoke JF, Sebel PS, Glass PS (1996) Reduction of isoflurane minimal alveolar concentration by remifentanil. Anesthesiology 85:721–728
McEwan AI, Smith C, Dyar O, Goodman D, Smith LR, Glass PS (1993) Isoflurane minimum alveolar concentration reduction by fentanyl. Anesthesiology 78:864–869
Mertens MJ, Olofsen E, Engbers FH, Burm AG, Bovill JG, Vuyk J (2003) Propofol reduces perioperative remifentanil requirements in a synergistic manner: response surface modeling of perioperative remifentanil-propofol interactions. Anesthesiology 99:347–359
Minto CF, Schnider TW, Short TG, Gregg KM, Gentilini A, Shafer SL (2000) Response surface model for anesthetic drug interactions. Anesthesiology 92:1603–1616
Murphy MR, Hug CC Jr (1982a) The anesthetic potency of fentanyl in terms of its reduction of enflurane MAC. Anesthesiology 57:485–488
Murphy MR, Hug CC Jr (1982b) The enflurane sparing effect of morphine, butorphanol, and nalbuphine. Anesthesiology 57:489–492
Nieuwenhuijs DJ, Olofsen E, Romberg RR, Sarton E, Ward D, Engbers F, Vuyk J, Mooren R, Teppema LJ, Dahan A (2003) Response surface modeling of remifentanil-propofol interaction on cardiorespiratory control and bispectral index. Anesthesiology 98:312–322
Olofsen E, Sleigh JW, Dahan A (2002) The influence of remifentanil on the dynamic relationship between sevoflurane and surrogate anesthetic effect measures derived from the EEG. Anesthesiology 96:555–564
Röpcke H, Lier H, Hoeft A, Schwilden H (1999) Isoflurane, nitrous oxide, and fentanyl pharmacodynamic interactions in surgical patients as measured by effects on median power frequency. J Clin Anesth 11:555–562
Röpcke H, Konen-Bergmann M, Cuhls M, Bouillon T, Hoeft A (2001) Propofol and remifentanil pharmacodynamic interaction during orthopedic surgical procedures as measured by effects on bispectral index. J Clin Anesth 13:198–207
Schwilden H, Fechner J, Albrecht S, Hering W, Ihmsen H, Schuttler J (2003) Testing and modelling the interaction of alfentanil and propofol on the EEG. Eur J Anaesthesiol 20:363–372
Sebel PS, Glass PS, Fletcher JE, Murphy MR, Gallagher C, Quill T (1992) Reduction of the MAC of desflurane with fentanyl. Anesthesiology 76:52–59
Short TG, Plummer JL, Chui PT (1992) Hypnotic and anaesthetic interactions between midazolam, propofol and alfentanil. Br J Anaesth 69:162–167
Short TG, Ho TY, Minto CF, Schnider TW, Shafer SL (2002) Efficient trial design for eliciting a pharmacokinetic-pharmacodynamic model-based response surface describing the interaction between two intravenous anesthetic drugs. Anesthesiology 96:400–408
Smith C, McEwan AI, Jhaveri R, Wilkinson M, Goodman D, Smith LR, Canada AT, Glass PS (1994) The interaction of fentanyl on the Cp50 of propofol for loss of consciousness and skin incision. Anesthesiology 81:820–828

Vuyk J, Lim T, Engbers FH, Burm AG, Vletter AA, Bovill JG (1995) The pharmacodynamic interaction of propofol and alfentanil during lower abdominal surgery in women. Anesthesiology 83:8–22

Vuyk J, Engbers FH, Burm AG, Vletter AA, Griever GE, Olofsen E, Bovill JG (1996) Pharmacodynamic interaction between propofol and alfentanil when given for induction of anesthesia. Anesthesiology 84:288–299

Vuyk J, Mertens MJ, Olofsen E, Burm AG, Bovill JG (1997) Propofol anesthesia and rational opioid selection: determination of optimal EC50-EC95 propofol-opioid concentrations that assure adequate anesthesia and a rapid return of consciousness. Anesthesiology 87:1549–1562

Westmoreland CL, Sebel PS, Gropper A (1994) Fentanyl or alfentanil decreases the minimum alveolar anesthetic concentration of isoflurane in surgical patients. Anesth Analg 78:23–28

Zanderigo E, Sartori V, Sveticic G, Bouillon T, Schumacher P, Morari M, Curatolo M (2006) The well-being model: a new drug interaction model for positive and negative effects. Anesthesiology 104:742–753

Index

M

N

9783540728139